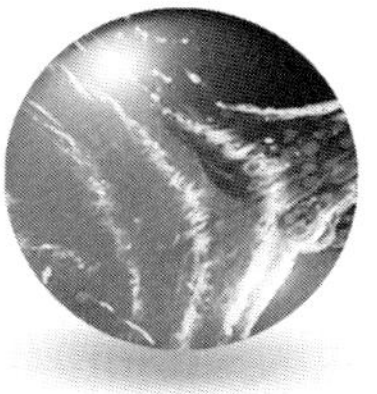

Biologically-responsive Hybrid Biomaterials

A Reference for Material Scientists and Bioengineers

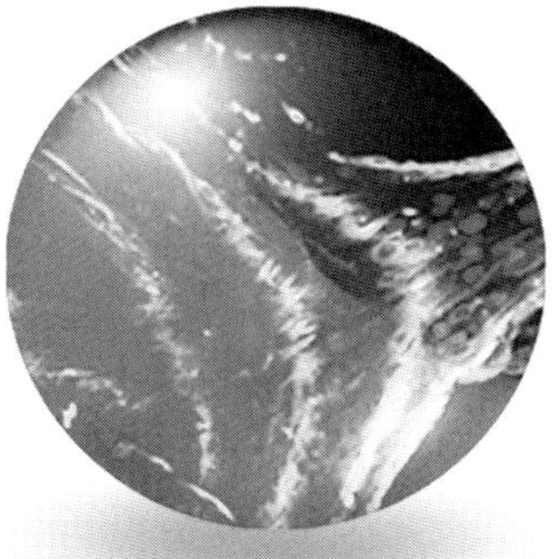

Biologically-responsive Hybrid Biomaterials

A Reference for Material Scientists and Bioengineers

Editors

E. Jabbari
University of South Carolina, USA

A. Khademhosseini
Harvard-MIT, USA

World Scientific

NEW JERSEY · LONDON · SINGAPORE · BEIJING · SHANGHAI · HONG KONG · TAIPEI · CHENNAI

Published by

World Scientific Publishing Co. Pte. Ltd.
5 Toh Tuck Link, Singapore 596224
USA office: 27 Warren Street, Suite 401-402, Hackensack, NJ 07601
UK office: 57 Shelton Street, Covent Garden, London WC2H 9HE

British Library Cataloguing-in-Publication Data
A catalogue record for this book is available from the British Library.

BIOLOGICALLY-RESPONSIVE HYBRID BIOMATERIALS
A Reference for Material Scientists and Bioengineers

ISBN-13 978-981-4295-67-3
ISBN-10 981-4295-67-1

Printed by FuIsland Offset Printing (S) Pte Ltd. Singapore

CONTENTS

INTRODUCTION

ENGINEERING THE TISSUE EXTRACELLULAR MATRIX WITH HYBRID BIOMATERIALS

Esmaiel Jabbari*

Biomimetic Materials and Tissue Engineering Laboratory, Department of Chemical Engineering, University of South Carolina, Columbia, SC 29208, USA
E-mail: jabbari@engr.sc.edu

1. Introduction

Synthetic materials are finding widespread applications as a replacement for tissue extracellular matrix in medicine.[1] These include, among others, biomaterials for total hip and knee replacement, bone grafts, intraocular lenses, vascular grafts, breast implants, sutures, artificial heart, vascular stents, dental implants, as a scaffold in cranial and maxillofacial reconstruction, and as a carrier in drug delivery. Autologous grafts, the gold standard for tissue replacement, have limited supply and suffer from donor site morbidity. Allografts are limited by reduced rates of graft incorporation. The flexibility in the design of synthetic materials allows the synthesis of a wide range of tissue replacement grafts with varying physical, mechanical, biologic and degradation properties to suit various medical applications. However, there are also limitations, especially in regenerative medicine, in the use of synthetic materials. For example, titanium cages coated with collagen and loaded with osteoinductive factors are being used in spine fusion but the metallic cage shield stress from the regenerating region during the remodeling phase resulting in lower than expected bone density.[2] Bioactive ceramics augmented with bioactive factors promote mineralization and bone formation but their drawbacks are fatigue fracture and low tensile strength.[3] Synthetic hydrolytically degradable polymers like poly(L-lactide), poly(glycolide), and their lactide-co-glycolide copolymers can provide some structural support to the regenerating region and their surface can be treated to support cell adhesion, but these hydrophobic matrices have limited ability to support solubilization and diffusion of proteins and their interaction with the cellular environment. Hydrogels like poly(ethylene glycols) (PEG), due to their hydrophilicity and high water content, exhibit excellent biocompatibility, and immobilized biomolecules retain higher biological activity within hydrogels[4] but their low strength and soft tissue compression limits their application in regenerative medicine.

It is now well-established that synthetic materials alone or in combination with soluble growth factors can not provide the microenvironment and the signaling factors required to initiate the cascade of cell migration, homing, adhesion, differentiation, matrix formation and remodeling in tissue regeneration. Furthermore, synthetic macromolecules do not possess in their structure the pattern of weak non-polar, polar, hydrogen bonding, and electrostatic interactions to produce functional specificity for drug targeting, imaging, or biological sensing. On the other hand, scaffolds produced from bioactive sequences alone are potentially immunogenic and have low metabolic stability in-vivo.[5] An attractive alternative is to use synthetic materials grafted/conjugated/hybridized with bioactive motifs, originating from the amino acid and carbohydrate sequences on proteoglycans and glycoproteins in the ECM. These biomimetic materials and structures possess biological recognition motifs as well as desired engineering properties. In addition, synthetic materials hybridized with bioactive motifs represent a multivalent form of the ligand for interaction with cluster of biological receptors, resulting in stronger interaction or stimulating particular subsets of receptors.[6] In the following sections, an overview of the synthesis, characterization, structure, and applications of hybrid biomaterials is presented, followed by the book structure.

2. Synthesis

Poly(lactide-co-glycolide) (PLGA) is the most widely used biodegradable polymer in the biomedical field. It is used in fabrication of pre-formed tissue engineering scaffolds in regenerative medicine and nano-/micro- particles in drug delivery because its degradation products, lactic and glycolic acids, are resorbed through the metabolic pathways. Furthermore, the flexibility in its design allows the synthesis of a wide range of polymers with varying mechanical, biologic and degradation properties to suit various applications. To further expand the application of PLGA in minimally-invasive procedures, a star lactide-co-glycolide (SLGA) macromer consisting of a hydrophilic multi-arm (2, 3, 4, 6, or 8) polyethylene glycol (PEG) core with very short lactide-glycolide (LG) chains terminated with an acrylate group attached to each arm is designed, as shown in Figure 1. The ethylene oxide core provides hydrophilicity and controlled water uptake to improve biomolecule and cell viability. The short LG chains provide

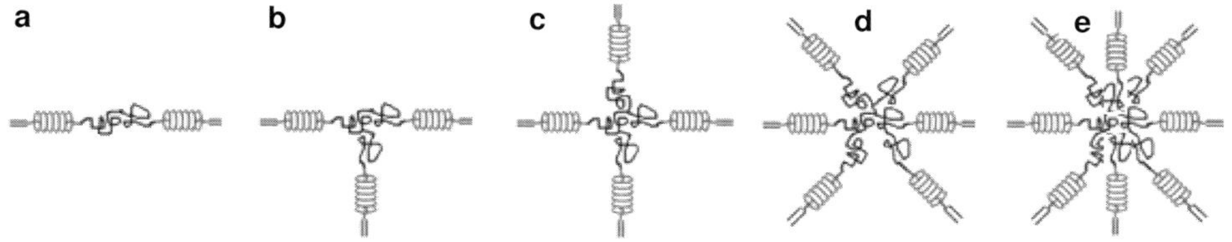

Fig. 1. The molecular structure of the star lactide-co-glycolide acrylate (SLGA) macromer with a polyethylene glycol (PEG) core. The macromer consists of a multi-arm PEG core (blue) with a lactide-co-glycolide (LG) segment (green) terminated with an acrylate group (red) at one end attached to each arm of the PEG core. The distinguishing feature of this macromer is the very short LG segments allowing the macromer to crosslink, via the unsaturated acrylate groups, to form a solid 3D network. The rate of network formation and crosslink density depend on the number of arms and the macromer molecular weight, respectively. The modulus depends on the number of arms and PEG:LG ratio. The water uptake of the crosslinked network depends on the ratio of hydrophilic PEG core to hydrophobic LG segments and the extent of crosslinking. The rate of degradation of the crosslinked network depends on the ratio of lactide to glycolide in LG segments. (a), (b), (c), (d), and (e) show the structure of the SLGA macromer with 2-arm (linear), 3, 4, 6, and 8 arms, respectively.

degradability and hydrophobicity to control water uptake while the unsaturated acrylate groups provide functionality for crosslinking. The rate of network formation is controlled by the number of arms on each macromer. The crosslink density can be controlled by the number of arms and the macromer molecular weight. The water uptake is controlled by PEG:LG ratio and crosslink density. The modulus of the crosslinked SLGA depends on PEG:LG ratio, number of arms, and macromer molecular weight. The degradation characteristic depends on lactide to glycolide ratio in the LG units and the PEG:LG ratio. Some SLGA compositions spontaneously self-assemble to form hydrolytically degradable nanoparticles for drug delivery. The unsaturated acrylate groups or the hydroxyl end groups of SLGA can be utilized for hybridization with bioactive motifs.

Different reaction schemes for conjugation of synthetic macromers to bioactive motifs are shown in Figure 2. Macromers with hydroxyl end-groups can be succinimide-functionalized by treating with N,N'-Disuccinimidyl carbonate (DSC) and conjugated with lysine-terminated peptides by the reaction of succinimide end-group of the macromer with amine group of the lysine, as shown in reaction scheme (a) in Figure 2.[7] Carboxylic-acid terminated macromers can be conjugated by the reaction between amine group of the peptide with carboxylic acid end-group of the macromer in the presence of N,N′-diisopropylcarbodiimide (DIC) coupling agent and N,N-dimethylaminopyridine (DMAP) catalyst, as shown in Figure 2(b). Michael's addition reaction can be

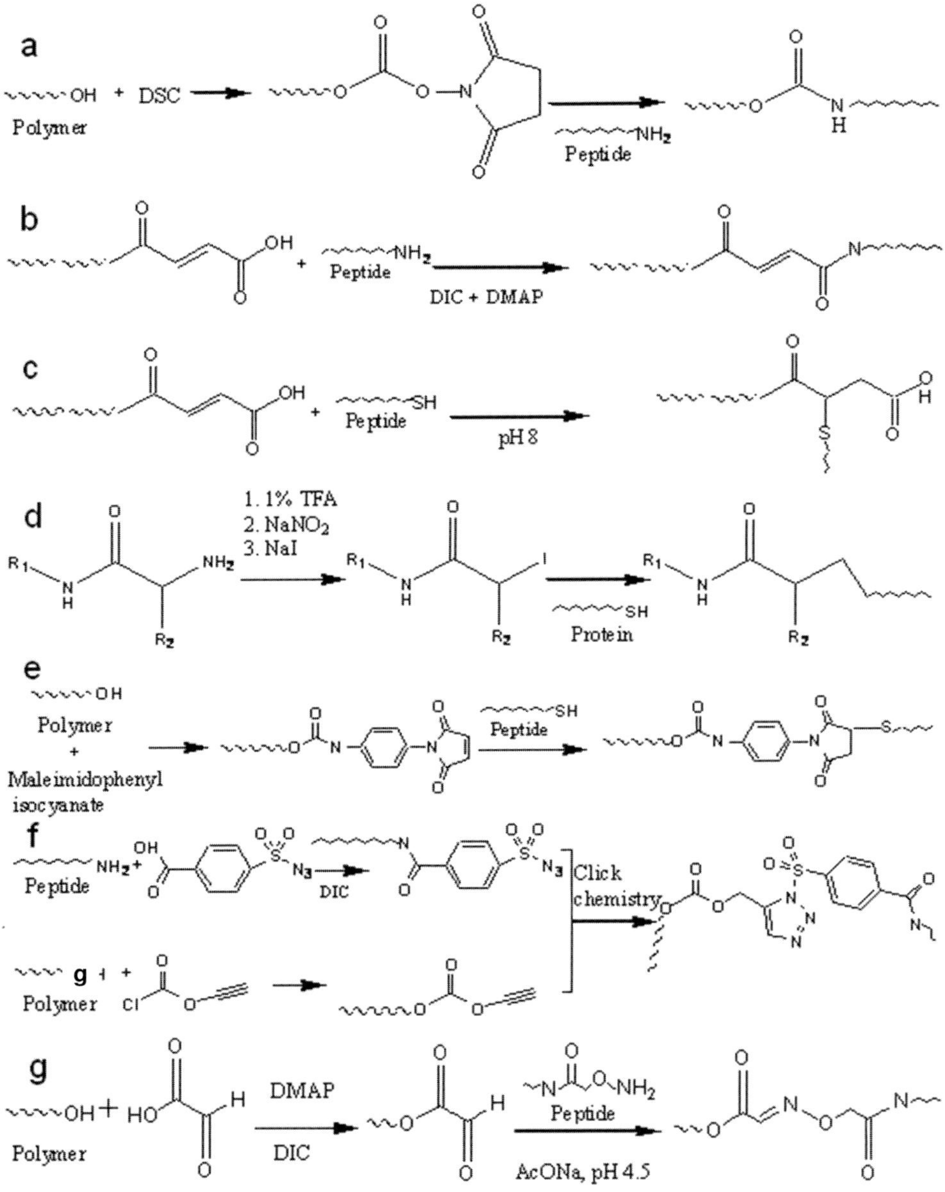

Fig. 2. Reaction schemes for conjugation: (a) succinimide-terminated macromer with lysine-terminated peptide; (b) carboxylic acid-terminated macromer with amine group of peptide; (c) unsaturated group-terminated macromer with sulfhydryl group of cysteine-functionalized peptide; (d) iodine-functionalized macromer with thiol-containing peptide; (e) maleimide-functionalized macromer with thiol-containing peptide; and (f) propargyl-functionalized macromer with azide-functionalized peptide; (g) aldehyde-functionalized macromer with amine group of peptide.

used to conjugate cysteine-functionalized peptides to acrylate-terminated macromers, as shown in Figure 2(c).[8] Another method is selective iodination of the peptide at the N-terminal using nitrite catalysts, followed by the reaction of iodinated peptide with thiol-containing compounds such as N-acetylcysteine and glutathione to form peptide conjugates, as shown in Figure 2(d).[9] Bioactive motifs with free thiol functionality can be conjugated to macromers by the thiol-maleimide conjugation. In this approach, p-maleimidophenyl isocyanate is used for functionalization of hydroxyl-terminated macromer, as shown in reaction (e) of Figure 2.[10] The "click reaction" between the azide group on the peptide and propargyl group on the macromer can also be used for conjugation, as shown in reaction (f) of Figure 2.[11] In "click reaction" the peptide is functionalized with an azide group by reacting with 4-carboxybenzenesulfonazide while the macromer is functionalized with a propargyl group by reacting with propargyl ester chloride. The "Oxime" reaction between an aldehyde-functionalized macromer with the amine group of the peptide can be used for conjugation, as shown in Figure 2(g).[12]

3. Characterization

The chemical structure of the macromer can be characterized by nuclear magnetic resonance (NMR) while the molecular weight distribution can be characterized by gel permeation chromatography (GPC) and mass spectrometry (MS). NMR is particularly useful for determining the ratio of different monomers in the macromer. The sequence distribution of the hybrid macromer can be determined by matrix-assisted laser desorption-ionization time-of-flight (MALDI-TOF) mass spectrometry. Size exclusion chromatography combined with MALDI mass spectrometry (SEC/MALDI) or pulsed gradient spin-echo (PGSE) NMR combined with MALDI can be used to accurately determine molecular weight distribution of the macromers.[13] The secondary structure of the hybrids can be characterized by circular dichroism (CD; 200-300 nm range) and Fourier Transform Infrared Spectrometry (FTIR; 1500-1800 nm range). The interaction of the macromer with conjugated peptide can be studied by x-ray reflectivity as well as CD and FTIR. Site-specific iodine labeling can be used to determine topology of the peptide within the conjugate. The effect of amino acid sequence on morphology of the peptide conjugate can be imaged with scanning electron microscopy (SEM), transmission electron microscopy (TEM), and atomic force microscopy (AFM) at micro-, nano-, and angstrom-scale resolution, respectively. In-vitro bioactivity of the hybrids can be directly measured by two-photon excitation fluorescence cross-correlation spectroscopy (TPE-FCCS) coupled with fluorescence correlation spectroscopy (FCS).[14] The Kaiser test can be used to quantify the density of the peptides conjugated to a substrate.[15] In-vitro toxicity of the hybrids can be determined by cell count after exposure, and their macrophage cell uptake can be quantified by live cell confocal microscopy and flow cytometry. Radioisotope labeling can be used for quantitative measurement of in-vivo biodistribution with a gamma scintillation counter.

4. Structure

Bioactive motifs conjugated to synthetic macromers can alter the nano-scale structure of these biomaterials. The side groups of the amino acids in the peptide can dictate secondary structures and preference for a specific shape in the aggregates. For example, the synthetic macromer poly(lactide fumarate) (PLAF), due to its hydrophobic nature forms solid nanopsheres with a relatively wide size distribution range (50-800 nm) in combination with the amphiphilic poly(lactide-ethylene oxide fumarate) (PLEOF) macromer, as shown in Figure 3.[16] The amino acid sequence Val-Val-Val-Val-Val-Val-Lys-Lys (V6K2) is known to self-assemble into vesicles (hollow spheres) with very narrow size distribution (see Figure 3).[17] Interestingly, when the V6K2 is conjugated to PLAF macromer via Michael's addition reaction, the hybrid macromer self-assembles into hollow spheres with a very narrow size distribution, even in the absence of the amphiphilic PLEOF macromer, as shown in Figure 3.[18] Cryogenic scanning electron microscopy images of the V6K2-PLAF hybrids demonstrate that the vesicles have a structure similar to that of V6K2 peptide. These results clearly

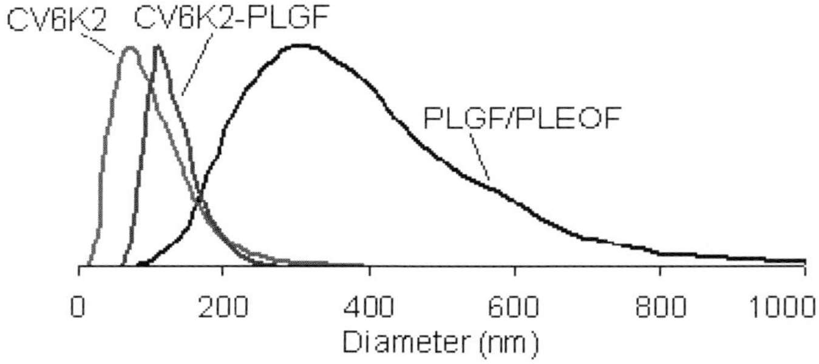

Fig. 3. Particle size distribution of V6K2-PLGF nanoparticles (red) compared to V6K2 vesicles (green) and PLGF stabilized with the amphiphilic poly(lactide-co-ethylene oxide fumarate) (PLEOF) macromer.

demonstrate that short peptide chains can dominate the nanostructure of the hybrids, producing novel biomaterials possessing unique nanostructures as well as biological recognition motifs.

5. Applications

Synthetic biomaterials conjugated with bioactive motifs have exciting applications in molecularly targeted diagnosis and imaging, targeted delivery of chemotherapeutic agents to tumor microenvironment, targeted antigen delivery to the most efficient dendritic cells to initiate an antigen-specific immune response in vaccination, receptor-mediated intracellular delivery using cell

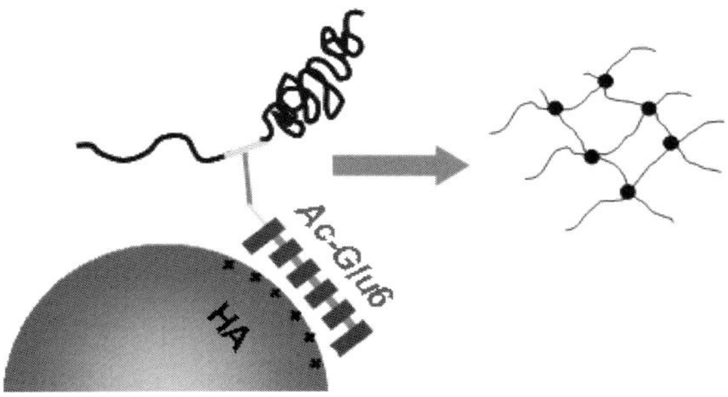

Fig. 4. Schematic diagram showing ionic and covalent interaction of an acrylate-functionalized glutamic acid sequence (red), a sequence in the terminal region of the osteonectin glycoprotein, with apatite (HA) crystals (gray) and the polymer matrix (blue), respectively, to produce a peptide-reinforced biocomposite. The reinforcement effect of the Glu6 peptide is modulated by the size of the HA crystals and it is specific to the glutamic acid sequence.

penetrating peptides in gene and siRNA delivery, controlling cellular expression in regenerative medicine, and in the design of mechanically robust biocomposites. Bioactive motifs based on amino acid sequences of the ECM proteins can be utilized to design peptide-reinforced composites in skeletal tissue engineering. For example, a glutamic acid sequence from the osteonectin glycoprotein is believed to be involved in linking the collagen network to the apatite (HA) crystal phase in the bone matrix.[19] When a glutamic acid sequence with ionic affinity to HA crystals, as shown in Figure 4, is functionalized with an acrylate group (Ac-Glu6) to covalently link the peptide to a poly(lactide-ethylene oxide-fumarate) (PLEOF) polymer matrix, it strongly affected the modulus of the composite matrix.[20] Addition of Ac-Glu6 peptide to nano-HA crystals increased modulus by ten-fold and the reinforcement effect was specific to the glutamic acid sequence (a glycine or lysine sequence did not have a similar effect). These findings demonstrate that hybrid biomaterials are potentially attractive for developing robust biomimetic composites for skeletal tissue regeneration.

In regenerative medicine, the synthetic scaffold is required to initiate and guide the cascade of cell differentiation and matrix formation. For example, reconstruction of large skeletal defects is limited by the lack of vascularization in the interior parts of the implanted biomaterial. Although the addition of soluble growth factors like bone morphogenetic proteins (BMPs) can substantially improve the extent of mineralization, their loss by diffusion away from the

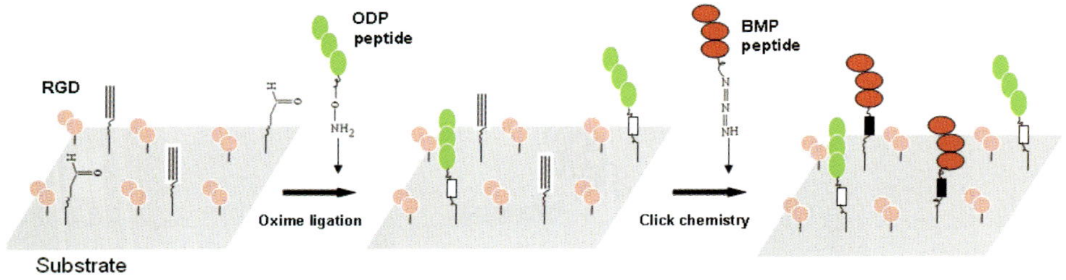

Fig. 5. Schematic diagram showing ligation of a substrate with multiple bioactive peptides by acrylation (RGD peptide), oxime reaction (osteopontin-derived peptide; ODP), and click reaction (peptide based on bone morphogenetic protein; BMP peptide).

intended site of regeneration, degradation, and soft tissue compression requires high doses to induce bone formation. Such high doses cause side effects such as bone overgrowth, abnormal vascular growth, and immunological reactions. An attractive alternative is to graft peptides, based on the active domains of osteogenic and vasculogenic growth factors, to a synthetic biomaterial substrate to initiate the process of vascularized osteogenesis. As an example, when the integrin binding focal-adhesion RGD peptide and a bioactive peptide from the recombinant human bone morphogenetic protein-2 (BMP peptide) were grafted to a synthetic biodegradable substrate, the extent of mineralization (measured by calcium content) of seeded mesenchymal stem cells increased by 12-fold compared to the inert substrate, as shown in Figure 5.[15] Furthermore, when a vasculogenic peptide derived from osteopontin protein was grafted to the substrate, parallel sheets of cells positive for PECAM was observed. These results demonstrate that synthetic hybrid biomaterials can mimic the cell-matrix interactions required for differentiation and maturation of stem cells into multiple lineages.

Another exciting application of hybrid biomaterials is in targeted tumor delivery. Intravenous administration of antitumor drugs allows targeted delivery to tumor vasculature but these less invasive systemic methods are limited by non-selectivity of antitumor drugs to normal cells. It is well established that chemotherapeutic drugs loaded into nanoparticles with narrow size distribution and diameter <200 nm, and conjugated with ligands that bind with high specificity to tumor vasculature can significantly reduce the undesired side effects of chemotherapy. In this regard, hybridization with bioactive motifs can confer biological recognition motifs as well as engineering properties to self-assembled synthetic nanoparticles for targeting to tumor microenvironment. For example, NPs self-assembled from a blend of poly(lactide fumarate) and poly(lactide-co-ethylene oxide fumarate) (PLAF/PLEOF) possess a wide 50-800 nm particle size distribution and have relatively low efficiency of crossing the leaky tumor vasculature. But hybridization of the PLAF macromer with V6K2 peptide produces NPs with very narrow size distribution (50-150 nm), as shown in Figure 3, that can potentially cross the tumor vasculature with high efficiency while delivering the chemotherapeutic agent at a sustained rate during the course of chemotherapy.[18] Interestingly, the hybridized V6K2-PLAF NPs, due to specific electrostatic interactions, show >90% uptake after 2 h by tumor cells.

These and many other examples in this book show that synthetic macromers hybridized with bioactive motifs are very promising as the next generation of biomaterials for biological recognition, imaging, sensing, targeting, and guiding the process of tissue regeneration.

6. Book Structure

This book is divided into three sections. In the first section, synthesis and characterization, conformation, self-assembly, micro-/nano- structure, and host response of hybrid biomaterials are covered. The second section is devoted to the applications of hybrid biomaterials in drug and intracellular delivery and vaccination. The third section is devoted to tissue engineering applications of hybrid biomaterials including cell adhesion, control of the stem cell niche, cartilage regeneration, neural and vascular tissue engineering, and dynamic cell culture systems for functionalized biomaterials. Undoubtedly, biologically-responsive hybrid biomaterials play a vital role in the design of biologics and medical devices. The salient feature of this book that sets it apart from other published books on Biomaterials is that synthesis, characterization, structure-activity, 3D assembly/fabrication, and applications of hybrid biomaterials are covered in one volume.

References

1. Peppas NA, Langer R, New challenges in biomaterials. Science 263(5154):1715-1720 (1994).
2. Ohyama T, Kubo Y, Iwata H, Taki W, Beta-tricalcium phosphate combined with recombinant human bone morphogenetic protein-2: A substitute for autograft, used for packing interbody fusion cages in canine lumbar spine. *Neurol. Med. Chir.* 44:234-241 (2004).
3. Akamaru T, Suh D, Boden SD, Kim HS, Minamide A, Louis-Ugbo J, Simple carrier matrix modifications can enhance delivery of recombinant human bone morphogenetic protein-2 for posterolateral spine fusion. *Spine* 28(5):429-34 (2003).
4. Slaughter BV, Khurshid SS, Fisher OZ, Ali Khademhosseini A, Peppas NA, Hydrogels in regenerative medicine. *Adv. Mater.* 21:1-23 (2009).
5. Latham PW, Therapeutic peptides revisited. *Nat. Biotechnol.* 17(8):755-757 (1999).
6. Rossi EA, Sharkey RM, McBride W, Karacay H, Zeng L, Hansen HJ, Goldenberg DM, Chang CH, Development of new multivalent-bispecific agents for pretargeting tumor localization and therapy. *Clin. Cancer Res.* 9(10):3886S-3896S (2003).
7. Fernandez-Megia, E, Novoa-Carballal R, Quinoa E, Riguera R, Conjugation of bioactive ligands to PEG-grafted chitosan at the distal end of PEG. *Biomacromolecules* 8(3):833-842 (2007).
8. Lutolf MP, Tirelli N, Cerritelli S, Cavalli L, Hubbell JA, Systematic modulation of michael-type reactivity of thiols through the Use of charged amino acids. *Bioconj. Chem.* 12(6):1051-1056 (2001).
9. Deng HT, Nitrite-assisted peptide iodination and conjugation. *J. Pept. Sci.* 13(2):107-112 (2007).
10. Ananda K, Nacharaju P, Smith PK, Acharya SA, Manjula BN, Analysis of functionalization of methoxy-PEG as maleimide-PEG. *Anal. Biochem.* 374(2):231-242 (2008).
11. Ossipov DA, Hilborn J, Poly(vinyl alcohol)-based hydrogels formed by "Click Chemistry". *Macromolecules* 39(5):1709-1718 (2006).
12. Dirksen A, Dawson PE, Rapid oxime and hydrazone ligations with aromatic aldehydes for biomolecular labeling. *Bioconj. Chem.* 19(12):2543-2548 (2008).
13. Mazarin M, Viel S, Allard-Breton B, Thevand A, Charles L, Use of pulsed gradient spin-echo NMR as a tool in MALDI method development for polymer molecular weight determination. *Anal. Chem.* 78(8):2758-2764 (2006).
14. Swift JL, Burger MC, Massotte D, Dahms TES, Cramb DT, Two-photon excitation fluorescence cross-correlation assay for ligand-receptor binding: Cell membrane nanopatches containing the human mu-opioid receptor. *Anal. Chem.* 79(17):6783-6791 (2007).
15. He X, Ma J, Jabbari E, The effect of grafting RGD and BMP peptides to a model hydrogel substrate on osteogenic differentiation of bone marrow stromal cells, *Langmuir* 24(21):12508-12516 (2008).
16. Mercado AE, He X, Xu W, Jabbari E, Release characteristics of a model protein from self-assembled succinimide-terminated poly(lactide-co-glycolide ethylene oxide fumarate) nanoparticles, *Nanotechnology* 19(32):325609 (2008).
17. Zhao X, Design of self-assembling surfactant-like peptides and their applications. *Curr. Opin. Colloid Inter. Sci.* 14950 340-348 (2009).
18. Mercado AE, Jabbari E, Peptide-induced self-assembly of synthetic poly(lactide fumarate) macromer, *Trans. Soc. Biomaterials* p. 118 (2009).

19. Hoang QQ, Sicheri F, Howard AJ, Yang DSC, Bone recognition mechanism of porcine osteocalcin from crystal structure. *Nature* 425:977-980 (2003).
20. Sarvestani AS, He X, Jabbari E, The Effect of osteonectin-derived peptide on the viscoelasticity of hydrogel/apatite nanocomposite scaffolds. *Biopolymers* 85(4):370-378 (2007).

Section 1

Synthesis, Characterization and Self-Assembly

CHAPTER 1

BULK AND SOLUTION PROPERTIES OF PEPTIDE-POLYMER CONJUGATES

Autumn Carlsen[1], Harm-Anton Klok[2] and Sébastien Lecommandoux[1*]

[1]*Université de Bordeaux, ENSCPB, 16 avenue Pey Berland, 33607 Pessac Cedex, France*

CNRS, Laboratoire de Chimie des Polymères Organiques, UMR5629, Pessac, France

[2]*École Polytechnique Fédérale de Lausanne (EPFL), Institut des Matériaux, Laboratoire des Polymères, Bâtiment MXD, Station 12, 1015 Lausanne, Switzerland*

[*]*E-mail: lecommandoux@enscbp.fr*

1. Introduction

Considerable effort has been devoted to elucidating the process by which block copolymers self-assemble into structures [1–5]. It is widely recognized that block copolymer morphologies result from the interplay of competing forces – one that minimizes the interfacial area of the chemically incompatible copolymer blocks and another that minimizes the entropically unfavorable chain stretching resulting from the segregation of those blocks [6,7]. Through variation of the volume fraction [2] and block properties [8,9] (more rigid or more liquid), a range of morphologies can be produced.

A large portion of the research up to this point has been carried out on materials composed of a synthetic block and a peptide block. These peptide-polymer conjugates combine the advantages of synthetic polymers (such as solubility, processability, and rubber elasticity) with those of polypeptides or protein-like polymers (such as secondary structure, functionality, and biocompatibility). While synthetic polymers generally present a coil structure, peptide sequences can adopt ordered conformations such as α-helices or β-strands (Figure 1). The former case produces block copolymers with a rod-coil character; such rod-coil block copolymers have generated unconventional nanoscale structures not observed for purely amorphous block copolymers. Copolymers containing peptide sequences with a β-strand conformation offer an additional means to direct nanoscale structure formation through intermolecular hydrogen-bonding.

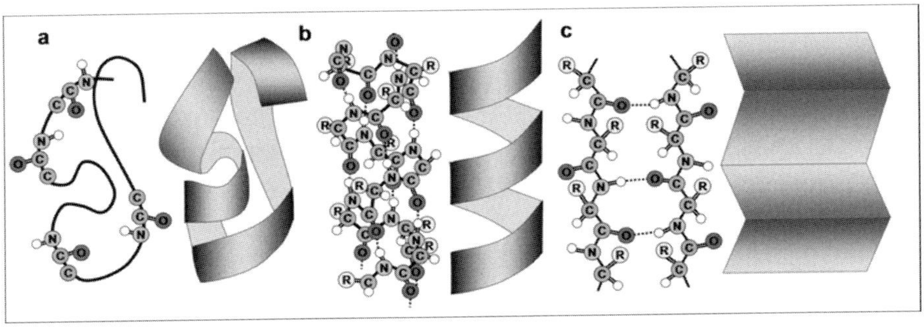

Fig. 1. Schematic diagram of secondary structures commonly adopted by polypeptides: (a) random coil, (b) α-helix, and (c) antiparallel β-sheet.

Combining peptide sequences and synthetic polymers is useful not only for enhanced control over nanoscale structure formation, but also for production of biologically interactive materials. Biomimetic hybrid polymers may also produce sophisticated superstructures with new material properties. "Smart" materials based on polypeptides may reversibly change conformation and associated properties in response to an environmental stimulus, such as a shift in pH or temperature [10]. Polypeptide block copolymers may also be used as model systems to study generic self-assembly processes in natural proteins. Obviously, such materials could be of significant interest for a variety of biomedical and bioanalytical applications.

This chapter will focus on linear polymer structures composed of synthetic polypeptide or polypeptide-polymer systems formed under bulk or solution conditions. The first section presents an overview of bulk self-assembled structures from polypeptide-based conjugates, specifically diblock and triblock architectures. The second section follows with a description of solution self-assembled structures obtained from peptide-polymer hybrid systems. The first part of this section is devoted to those copolymer micelles in which the polypeptide block exhibits high aqueous solubility (corona-forming peptidic copolymers), the second to those in which the polypeptide block exhibits low aqueous solubility (core-forming peptidic copolymers), and the third to those in which experimental conditions shift the micellar role of the polypeptide block (schizophrenic peptidic copolymers). The final part of the section reviews advances in the investigation of vesicle formation, including those based on peptide-polymer systems (polypeptide hybrid copolymer vesicles) and on purely peptidic systems (copolypeptide vesicles). A brief portion of the chapter then relates developments in polypeptide-based hydrogels, Finally, we summarize and offer a perspective on the future of research in the field of peptide-based copolymers.

2. Bulk Self-assembled Structures from Polypeptide-based Conjugates

2.1. *Diblock copolymer architectures*

Polydiene-based diblock copolymers

One of the first reports on the nanoscale solid-state structure of peptide–synthetic hybrid block copolymers was published by Gallot *et al.* [11] in 1976. In this publication, the solid-state structure of a series of polybutadiene-*block*-poly(γ-benzyl L-glutamate) (PB-*b*-PBLG) and polybutadiene-*block*-poly(N^5-hydroxyethyl L-glutamine) (PB-*b*-PHLGln) diblock copolymers was investigated using a combination of techniques, including infrared and circular dichroism (CD) spectroscopy, x-ray scattering (SAXS), and transmission electron microscopy (TEM). The block copolymers covered a broad composition range with peptide contents ranging from 19 to 75%. Interestingly, SAXS and TEM revealed a well-ordered lamellar superstructure characterized by up to four higher-order Bragg spacings for all of the investigated samples. Wide-angle x-ray scattering (WAXS) experiments indicated that the α-helical peptide blocks were assembled in a hexagonal array. For a number of block copolymer samples it was found that the calculated length of the peptide helix was larger than the thickness of the polypeptide layer. To accommodate this difference, it was proposed that the peptide helices were folded in the peptide layer. The lamellar structure consists of planar, parallel equidistant sheets. Each sheet is obtained by superposition of two layers; (i) the PB chains in a more or less random coil conformation and (ii) the α-helical polypeptide blocks in a hexagonal array of folded chains. The hexagonal-in-lamellar structure was also found for polybutadiene-*block*-poly(ε-benzyloxycarbonyl L-lysine) (PB-*b*-PZLLys) and polybutadiene-*block*-poly(L-lysine) (PB-*b*-PLLys) block copolymers by the same authors [12–15].

More recently, the solid-state nanoscale structure of polyisoprene-*block*-poly(ε-benzyloxycarbonyl L-lysine) (PI-*b*-PZLLys) diblock copolymers was reported [16]. Diblock copolymers composed of a PI block with a number-average degree of polymerization of 49 and a PZLLys block containing 61-178 amino acid residues were investigated with dynamic mechanical analysis (DMA) and x-ray scattering (SAXS and WAXS). For the PI_{49}-*b*-$PZLLys_{35}$, PI_{49}-*b*-

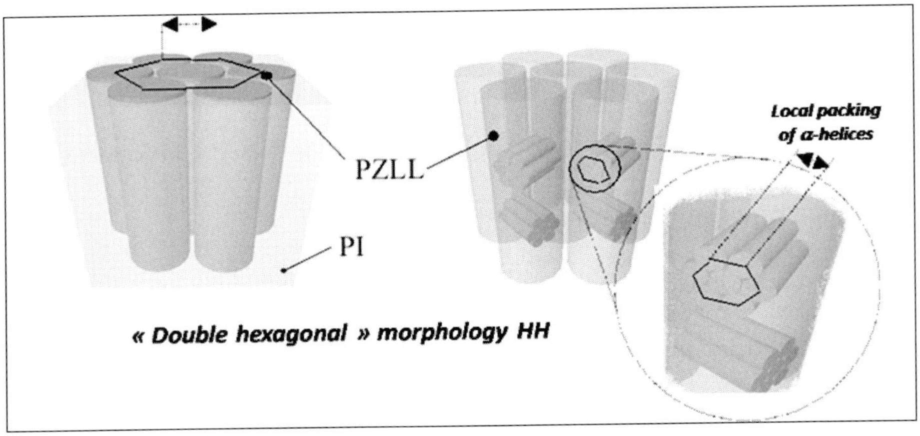

Fig. 2. Schematic model representation of the hexagonal in hexagonal (HH) morphology obtained for PI_{49}-*b*-$PZLLys_{178}$ copolymer cast from dioxane solution. Adapted from [16].

$PZLLys_{61}$ and PI_{49}-*b*-$PZLLys_{92}$, the x-ray scattering data were in agreement with a hexagonal-in-lamellar morphology. Interestingly, for PI_{49}-*b*-$PZLLys_{123}$ and PI_{49}-*b*-$PZLLys_{178}$ a hexagonal-in-hexagonal structure was found. This morphology is illustrated in Figure 2. This structure is unprecedented for polydiene-based peptide hybrid block copolymers, but has also been found for low molecular weight polystyrene-*block*-poly(γ-benzyl L-glutamate) (PS-*b*-PBLG) copolymers [17].

Polystyrene-based diblock copolymers

In an early study, Gallot *et al.* [13] reported on the bulk nanoscale structure of PS-*b*-PZLLys diblock copolymers, which were based on a PS block with a number-average molecular weight of M_n = 37 kg/mol and had peptide contents ranging from 18-80 mol %. X-ray scattering patterns of dry samples following evaporation from dioxane showed two sets of signals, characteristic again of a hexagonal-in-lamellar superstructure. For several samples, the calculated length of the peptide helix was larger than the peptide layer thickness as determined from the x-ray data. In these cases, it was proposed that the helical PZLLys chains were folded in the peptide layer. Thus, the bulk nanoscale structure of the PS-*b*-PZLLys copolymers can be described in terms of the same hexagonal-in-lamellar model as it was also proposed for the PB-based block copolymer described earlier (Figure 3).

Along the same lines, Douy and Gallot [15] also studied the bulk nanoscale organization of PS-*b*-PBLG. For block copolymers composed of a PS block with

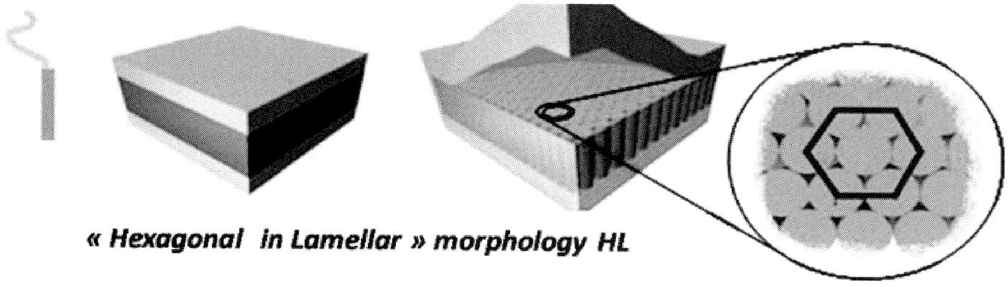

Fig. 3. Schematic model representation of the hexagonal-in-lamellar (HL) morphology obtained for polypeptide-based rod-coil diblock copolymers cast from solutions.

M_n = 25 kg/mol and containing 31-94 mol % peptide, the same hexagonal-in-lamellar morphology as described above for the PS-*b*-PZLLys was found. The biocompatibility of PS-*b*-PBLG copolymers has been discussed by Mori *et al.* [18] They studied the thrombus formation by exposing films of the diblock copolymers and the corresponding homopolypeptides to fresh canine blood. It was found that thrombus formation on the diblock copolymer films was reduced compared to the corresponding homopolymers. For the block copolymers, thrombus formation decreased with decreasing PBLG block length. Also, adsorption of plasma proteins such as bovine serum albumine, bovine γ-globulin, and bovine plasma fibrinogen was reduced on the block copolymers compared to PS homopolymer.

The characterization of the solid-state nanoscale organization of PS-polypeptide hybrid block copolymers has more recently been refined in a series of publications by Schlaad *et al.* [19–21] In a first report, three PS-*b*-PZLLys diblock copolymers were investigated [19] by SAXS from dimethylformamide (DMF) cast films, confirming the hexagonal-in-lamellar morphology published earlier by Gallot *et al.* [13] In their paper, Schlaad and coworkers went a step further and analyzed their SAXS data using the interface-distribution concept and the curvature-interface formalism. These evaluation techniques suggested that the bulk nanoscale structure of the PS-*b*-PZLLys diblock copolymers does not consist of plain but undulated lamellae. The concept of the interface distribution function and the curvature-interface formalism were also applied to compare the solid-state structure of two virtually identical PS-based diblock copolymers; PS_{52}-*b*-$PZLLys_{111}$ ($\phi_{peptide}$ = 0.82) and PS_{52}-*b*-$PBLG_{104}$ ($\phi_{peptide}$ = 0.79) [20]. Analysis of the SAXS data obtained on DMF cast films indicated a hexagonal-in-undulated (or zigzag) lamellar morphology for both block copolymers.

In addition, the influence of the polydispersity of the polypeptide block on the solid-state morphology of PS-*b*-PZLLys diblock copolymers has been studied

[21]. To this end, a series of five diblock copolymers was prepared from an identical ω-amino-polystyrene macroinitiator ($P_n = 52$; polydispersity index, PDI = 1.03). The peptide content in these diblock copolymers varied between 0.43 and 0.68 and the PDI ranged from 1.03 to 1.64. Evaluation of the SAXS data with the interface distribution function and the curvature–interface formalism confirmed, as expected, the hexagonal-in-undulated (or zigzag) lamellar solid-state morphology. Fractionation of the peptide helices according to their length leads (locally) to the formation of a nearly planar, parallel lamellar interface, which is disrupted by kinks (undulations).

Reiter and Schlaad *et al.* [22] used atomic force microscopy (AFM) to investigate the formation of hierarchical structures of PS_{52}-*b*-$PBLG_{104}$ in thin films. Thin films with a thickness of ~4 and 40 nm were prepared by spin-coating of dilute polymer solutions on silicon substrates and were subsequently annealed in saturated tetrahydrofuran (THF) vapor to achieve a controlled crystallization of the α-helical PBLG. On the smallest length-scale, the structure was found to be built of short ribbons or lamellae of interdigitated polymer chains. PBLG helices were fully stretched in thin films, in contrast to what has been observed in the 3D organized bulk mesophase (see above). Depending on the time of solvent annealing, different ordered structures on the micrometer length-scale could be observed (Figure 4).

The examples discussed so far all involved relatively high molecular weight diblock copolymers. In this case, the molecular weight of the polypeptide block is usually sufficiently high so that it forms a stable α-helix and the common hexagonal-in-lamellar morphology is found. The situation changes, however, when the molecular weight of the block copolymers is significantly decreased. The influence of molecular weight on the solid-state organization of polystyrene-

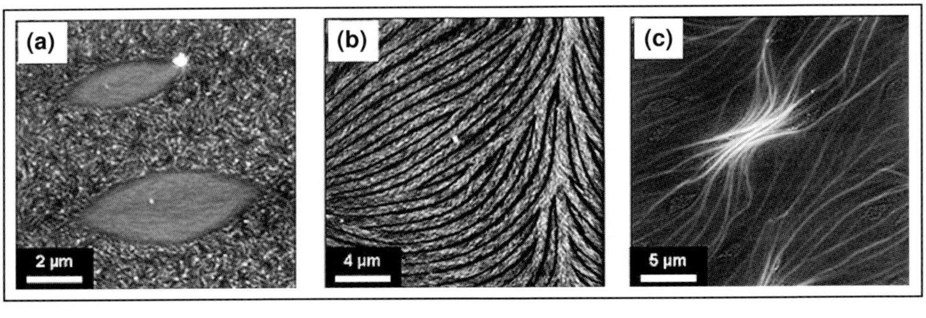

Fig. 4. AFM height images of a film of PS_{52}-*b*-$PBLG_{104}$ obtained by spin-coating from a 5 mg/mL THF solution and subsequent exposure to saturated THF vapor for 3.5 (a), 22.5 (b), and 42 hours (c). Adapted from [22].

based peptide–synthetic hybrid block copolymers has been studied for a series of low-molecular weight PS-*b*-PBLG and PS-*b*-PZLLys [23,24]. These diblock copolymers, consisting of a short PS block with P_n ~ 10 and a polypeptide block containing ~10 to 80 amino acid repeat units were characterized by means of variable temperature Fourier transform infrared (FTIR) spectroscopy and x-ray scattering. These experiments allowed the construction of "phase diagrams", which are shown in Figure 5. The phase diagrams reveal a number of interesting features. At temperatures below 200 °C and for sufficiently long polypeptide blocks, a hexagonal arrangement of the diblock copolymers was found, analogous to the hexagonal-in-lamellar morphology of the high-molecular weight analogues. Upon decreasing the length of the peptide block, however, several novel solid-state structures were discovered. For very short peptide block lengths (PS_{10}-*b*-$PBLG_{10}$, PS_{10}-*b*-$PZLLys_{20}$, PS_{10}-*b*-$PZLLys_{40}$ and PS_{10}-*b*-$PZLLys_{60}$) a lamellar supramolecular structure was found. This is due to the fact that, for such short peptide block lengths, a substantial fraction of the peptide blocks adopts a β-strand secondary structure.

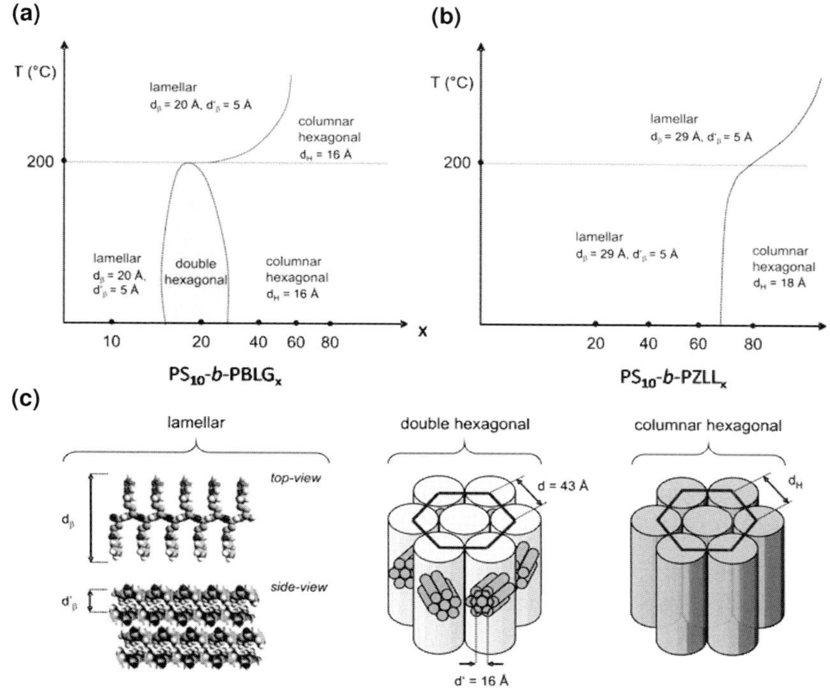

Fig. 5. Phase diagrams describing the solid-state nanoscale structure of (a) PS-*b*-PBLG and (b) PS-*b*-PZLLys diblock copolymers; (c) Illustration of the lamellar, double hexagonal and hexagonal morphologies found for the low molecular-weight hybrid block copolymers. Adapted from [23,24].

Self-assembly of these diblock copolymers in a β-sheet type fashion results in the lamellar structures observed by SAXS. For PS_{10}-*b*-$PBLG_{20}$ a peculiar and previously unprecedented structure was found. This structure, which consisted of hexagonally packed diblock copolymer molecules that are organized in a hexagonal superlattice, has been referred to as the double hexagonal or hexagonal-in-hexagonal morphology.

Apart from several unconventional solid-state nanoscale structures, another factor that distinguishes the phase diagrams in Figure 5 from those of the majority of conventional, conformationally isotropic block copolymers is the influence of temperature. For a number of diblock copolymers, increasing the temperature above 200 °C results in a change from a hexagonal-in-hexagonal (PS_{10}-*b*-$PBLG_{20}$) or hexagonal (PS_{10}-*b*-$PBLG_{40}$, PS_{10}-*b*-$PZLLys_{80}$) to a lamellar morphology. FTIR spectroscopy experiments suggested that these morphological transitions are induced by an increase in the fraction of peptide blocks that have a β-strand conformation. Interestingly, the self-assembly of the amphiphilic form of these diblock copolymers, namely polystyrene-*block*-poly(glutamic acid) (PS-*b*-PGA) revealed that the high immiscibility between PS and PGA blocks (conformational asymmetry) drove all of these rod-coil block copolymers to self-assemble in a hexagonal in lamellar (HL) morphology in the nanometer size range, regardless of their composition and architecture [25].

Polyether-based diblock copolymers

Poly(ethylene glycol)–polypeptide block copolymers are of particular interest, from both a structural and a functional point of view. In addition to microphase separation and the tendency of the peptide blocks towards aggregation, crystallization of poly(ethylene glycol) (PEG) introduces an additional factor that can influence the structure formation of these hybrid block copolymers. Ma *et al.* [26] have investigated the solid-state structure and properties of three poly(ethylene glycol)-*block*-poly(L-Alanine) (PEG-*b*-PLAla) copolymers that were prepared from a PEG macroinitiator with M_n = 2 kg/mol. The diblock copolymers contained 39.8, 49.6 and 65.5 mol % alanine. From FTIR spectra and differential scanning calorimetry (DSC) measurements, the authors proposed a microphase-separated bulk structure.

AB diblock and ABA triblock copolymers composed of PEG as the A block and random coil segments of poly(D,L-valine-*co*-D,L-leucine) as the B block(s) were investigated by Cho, Kim and Jung [27]. DSC experiments revealed PEG crystallization and showed that the PEG melting temperature was decreased compared to that of PEG homopolymer. TEM micrographs suggested a lamellar microphase-separated structure for one of the triblock copolymer samples.

Polyester-based diblock copolymers

One of the first studies focusing on the solid-state properties of polypeptide–polyester synthetic hybrid block copolymers was reported by Jérôme *et al.* [28] Differential scanning calorimetry (DSC) experiments on a poly(ε-caprolactone)$_{50}$-*block*-poly(γ-benzyl L-glutamate)$_{40}$ (PCL_{50}-*b*-$PBLG_{40}$) diblock copolymer revealed two endotherms. The first endotherm was found at 60 °C and is due to the melting of the PCL. The second endotherm which was located at 110 °C, was, mistakenly, interpreted as the melting transition of PBLG. This transition, however, is not a melting transition, but instead reflects the conformational transition of the PBLG helix from a 7/2 to an 18/5 helical structure. Although no further structural investigations were carried out, the observation of two separate endotherms occurring at temperatures identical to the transitions found for the respective homopolymers is a first indication for the existence of a microphase-separated structure. Similar results were reported by Chen *et al.* [29] who investigated the thermal properties of a series of PCL-*b*-PBLG copolymers composed of PCL blocks containing 13-51 repeat units peptide segments with and 22-52 amino acid repeat units.

Caillol *et al.* [30] have studied the solid-state structure and properties of a series of poly(L-lactide)-*block*-poly(γ-benzyl L-glutamate) (PLLac-*b*-PBLG) copolymers. The PLLac block in these copolymers contained 10-40 repeat units and the peptide segments were composed of 20-100 repeat units. DSC thermograms of the block copolymers revealed three transitions corresponding to the glass transition temperature (T_g) of PLLac (~50 °C), the 7/2 to 18/5 helix transition of PBLG (~100 °C) and the melting temperature of PLLac (~160 °C), respectively. This observation already provided a first hint towards a microphase-separated bulk morphology. WAXS experiments, which were performed at 100 °C, indicated the existence of hexagonally ordered assemblies of α-helical PBLG chains. With decreasing glutamate content, the peaks corresponding to this hexagonal organization decreased in intensity and another scattering peak appeared, which was ascribed to a lamellar assembly of PBLG chains with a β-strand secondary structure. Increasing the temperature to 200 °C resulted in the melting of PLLac, but also led to a decrease in intensity of the diffraction peaks corresponding to the hexagonally ordered α-helical PBLG segments and an increase in the fraction of PBLG segments that are ordered in a lamellar β-strand fashion.

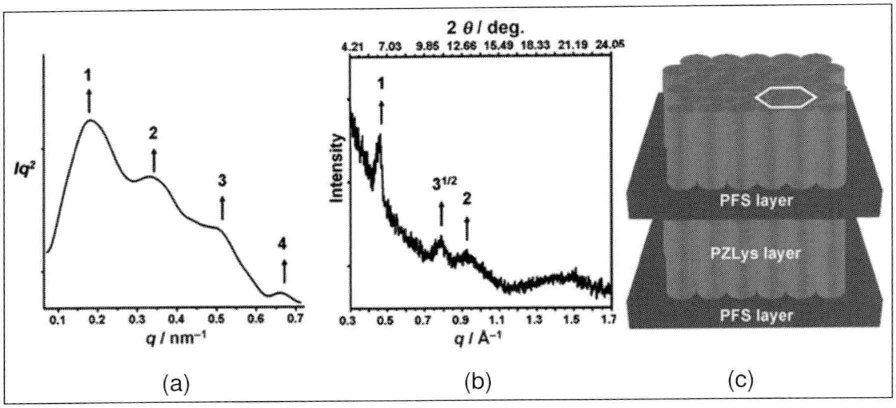

Fig. 6. (a) SAXS and (b) WAXS Patterns for a PFS-*b*-PZLys film. (c) schematic representation of HL morphology for PFS-b-PZLys (not to scale). Helices are presented as rods. Adapted from [32].

Diblock copolypeptides

A step forward in the design of hierarchically ordered structures with bio-functionality has been the recent reports on the synthesis of block copolymers based on polypeptides. Despite important synthetic efforts, the solid-state morphology of purely peptidic block copolymers remains largely unexplored. Hadjichristidis *et al.* [31] investigated recently the self-assembly of a series of narrow polydispersity poly(γ-benzyl L-glutamate)-*block*-poly(L-glycine) (PBLG-*b*-PLGly) diblock copolymer within the composition range $0.67 < f_{PBLG} < 0.97$ and the temperature range $303 < T < 433$ K. SAXS, WAXS, ^{13}C NMR and DSC were used for the structure investigation coupled with dielectric spectroscopy for both the peptide secondary structure and the associated dynamics. Not only did these techniques provide insight into the nanophase morphology, but they also gave information about the type and persistence of peptide secondary structures. Hexagonal-in-lamellar and cylinder-on-hexagonal nanostructures have been especially evidenced. In addition, nanoscale confinement proves to be important in controlling the persistence length of secondary peptide motifs.

Miscellaneous

Recently, the enhanced control of bulk and surface ordering of polypeptides has been employed to drive the processing and self-assembly of conductive rigid segments. Mainly triblock copolymer structures have been studied (see the following section). Manners and Winnik [32] synthesized a new type of metallopolymer-polypeptide block copolymer poly(ferrocenyldimethylsilane)-*b*-

poly(ε -benzyloxycarbonyl- L-lysine) (PFS-*b*-PZLLys) and studied their self-organization behavior in both the bulk state and in solution. In the bulk state, a cylindrical in-lamellar structure was observed in a compositionally asymmetric sample. Rod-like micelles with a polyferrocenylsilane core formed in a polypeptide-selective solvent alone or in the presence of a common solvent.

2.2. *Triblock copolymer architectures*

Polydiene-based diblock copolymers

Whereas Gallot *et al.* have mainly studied the solid-state organization of PB-based diblock copolymers, Nakajima *et al.* concentrated on ABA-type hybrid block copolymers containing PB as the B component ("once-broken rods"). In a first series of publications, the structure and properties of PBLG-*b*-PB-*b*-PBLG triblock copolymers containing 7.5-32.5 mol % (= 3.0-14.3 vol %) PB were investigated [33–35]. Infrared spectroscopy and WAXS experiments on films of the triblock copolymers indicated that the PBLG blocks were predominantly α-helical. From the WAXS experiments, it was concluded that the PBLG blocks assembled into different structures, depending on the type of solvent that was used to cast the films. In benzene cast films, the peptide helices were relatively poorly ordered, similar to the so-called form A morphology of PBLG [36]. In contrast, the PBLG segments in films cast from chloroform ($CHCl_3$) were well-ordered and contained paracrystalline and mesomorphic regions. Based on TEM analysis, a cylindrical microstructure was proposed for a triblock copolymer containing 8 vol % PB. Interestingly, copolymers having the same composition but polypeptide segments made of either enantiomerically pure or racemic γ-benzyl glutamate exhibited not only different secondary structures (α-helix or random coil, respectively; FTIR and WAXS), but also different supersturctures (TEM). A cylindrical or lamellar morphology was proposed in the first case and a more spherical superstructure in the second case [37].

The bulk and surface structure of solvent cast films from a series of PBLG-*b*-PB-*b*-PBLG triblock copolymers with much higher PB contents (50-80 mol %) than the samples discussed above have been discussed by Gallot *et al.* [38] The organization of these copolymers was compared with that of three other triblock copolymers with approximately the same PB content (~50 mol %) but which were composed of poly(N^{ε}-trifluoroacetyl L-lysine) (PTLLys), poly(N^5-hydroxyethyl L-glutamine) (PHLGln) or polysarcosine (PSar) as the peptide block. For any sample investigated, x-ray scattering experiments indicated a hexagonal-in-lamellar bulk morphology. X-ray photoelectron spectroscopy

(XPS) measurements revealed that for the triblock copolymers with hydrophobic peptide blocks, i.e. PBLG or PTLLys, the surface composition was identical to that in the bulk of the sample. In contrast, the surfaces of films prepared from the triblock copolymers with the more hydrophilic peptide segments, i.e. PHLGln or PSar, were PB-enriched. Furthermore, the XPS data suggested that the lamellar superstructures formed by the triblock copolymers were perpendicular to the air-polymer interface.

In addition, the solid-state organization and properties of PZLLys-*b*-PB-*b*-PZLLys triblock copolymers have been investigated. Nakajima *et al.* [39,40] have studied copolymers composed of a central PB block with M_n = 3.6 kg/mol and PB contents ranging from 12-52 mol %. WAXS patterns obtained from solution cast triblock copolymer films were in agreement with the α-helical secondary structure of the peptide blocks. The bulk microphase-separated structure of the five different block copolymer samples could be successfully characterized by means of TEM. For the samples with the largest PB volume fraction (56 and 65 vol %), a lamellar superstructure was found. For triblock copolymers with smaller PB volume fractions, the electron micrographs suggested cylindrical and spherical microphase-separated structures.

Other polybutadiene-based ABA type triblock copolymers that have been investigated include poly(γ-methyl L-glutamate)-*block*-polybutadiene-*block*-poly(γ-methyl L-glutamate) (PMLG-*b*-PB-*b*-PMLG) and poly(γ-methyl D,L-glutamate)-*block*-polybutadiene-*block*-poly(γ-methyl D,L-glutamate) (PMGlu-*b*-PB-*b*-PMGlu) [37,41]. Infrared spectroscopy experiments on solvent cast films indicated that the incorporation of 50% of the D-isomer disrupts the α-helical secondary structure and induces a random coil conformation in significant portions of the peptide blocks. Interestingly, different morphologies were observed when comparing the TEM images of PMLG-*b*-PB-*b*-PMLG and PMGlu-*b*-PB-*b*-PMGlu samples with the same PB content (≈ 30 mol %). For the first, a cylindrical morphology and for the second a spherical structure was proposed [37]. The attenuated total reflection infrared (ATR-IR) spectra further showed that adsorption of bovine serum albumine (BSA) and bovine fibrinogen (BF) did not lead to denaturation. From these observations, the authors concluded that the surfaces of the PMGlu-*b*-PB-*b*-PMGlu membranes only weakly or reversibly interact with these plasma proteins and it was predicted that this may also lead to a good overall biocompatibility.

The solid-state structure and properties of PELGlu-*b*-PB-*b*-PELGlu (PELGlu = poly(γ-ethyl L-glutamate)) triblock copolymers containing 31.5-94.5 mol % (= 17-88 vol %) PELGlu have been studied using the same techniques as described above for the other triblock copolymers [42,43]. Based on the electron micrographs, a spherical microphase-separated structure was proposed for the copolymer containing 17 vol % PB, while cylindrical and lamellar morphologies were suggested for triblock copolymers containing 28 and 44 vol % PB or 68 and 88 vol % PB, respectively. The biocompatibility of the PELGlu-*b*-PB-*b*-PELGlu triblock copolymers was assessed by coating the samples onto a polyester mesh fiber cloth, which was subsequently subcutaneously implanted in mongrel dogs for four weeks. It was found that the foreign body reaction and degradation of the PELGlu-*b*-PB-*b*-PELGlu samples were less pronounced as compared to PMLG-*b*-PB-*b*-PMLG, PBLG-*b*-PB-*b*-PBLG and PZLLys-*b*-PB-*b*-PZLLys triblock copolymers.

The bulk nanoscale structure of a series of PBLG-*b*-PI-*b*-PBLG copolymers containing 37.4-81.1 mol % PBLG was studied by means of infrared spectroscopy, WAXS, dynamic mechanical analysis and electron microscopy [44–47]. Based on the electron micrographs, a cylindrical morphology was proposed for triblock copolymers containing 74.6 and 81.1 mol % PBLG. Water permeability measurements also supported the microphase-separated bulk morphology [45].

Treatment of a PBLG-*b*-PI-*b*-PBLG film with a mixture of 3-amino-1-propanol and 1,8-octamethylenediamine led to the formation of hydrophilic, crosslinked PHLGln-*b*-PI-*b*-PHLGln membranes [48]. The swelling ratio of these membranes in pseudoextracellular fluid (PECF) was found to decrease with increasing PI content and increasing crosslink density. Enzymatic degradation experiments using papain showed that the triblock copolymer films were more resistant towards degradation than the corresponding homopolypeptide membranes. The half-times for sample degradation increased with decreasing peptide content, which was in agreement with the swelling behaviour of the membranes.

Polystyrene-based triblock copolymers

Tanaka *et al.* [49] studied ABA type triblock copolymers composed of a central PS block flanked by two polypeptide segments (PBLG, PZLLys or PSar). TEM of a $CHCl_3$-cast film of $PBLG_{25}$-*b*-PS_{165}-*b*-$PBLG_{25}$ revealed a lamellar phase separated structure. In contrast, no microphase separation was observed in a film of $PSar_{73}$-*b*-PS_{421}-*b*-$PSar_{73}$. The authors proposed that the different block copolymer morphologies could be related to the different secondary structure of the peptide block; while the PBLG segments are predominantly helical, the PSar may not form any regular secondary structure. Fibrinogen adsorption on the block copolymer films was studied with ATR-IR spectroscopy and compared with that on the corresponding homopolymer films [50]. It was found that fibrinogen adsorption on PS and PSar homopolymer films and on PSar-*b*-PS-*b*-PSar triblock copolymer films led to denaturation of the protein. In contrast, protein adsorption on the microphase-separated PBLG-*b*-PS-*b*-PBLG surfaces was reported to stabilize the protein's secondary structure. Blood clotting tests suggested that thrombus formation was retarded compared to the respective homopolymers.

Samyn *et al.* [51] extended the investigations of ABA triblock copolymers and studied the solid-state organization of three different PBLG-*b*-PS-*b*-PBLG copolymers containing 34, 55 and 92 wt % PBLG. TEM micrographs of ultramicrotomed and RuO_4-stained specimens and SAXS experiments indicated a lamellar morphology for the copolymers with 34 and 55 wt % PBLG. The sample containing 92 wt % PBLG did not form a lamellar structure. WAXS patterns yielded d-spacings reflecting the intermolecular distance between neighboring peptide α-helices.

Polysiloxane-based triblock copolymers

Imanishi *et al.* [52] have studied the structure, antithrombogenicity and oxygen permeability of ABA triblock copolymers composed of polydimethylsiloxane (PDMS) as the B block and PBLG, PBGlu (poly(γ-benzyl D,L-glutamate)), PZLLys or PSar as the A block. TEM images of DMF-cast films provided evidence for a microphase-separated morphology for $PZLLys_{49}$-*b*-$PDMS_{400}$-*b*-$PZLLys_{49}$ and $PZLLys_{91,160}$-$PDMS_{256}$-$PZLLys_{91,160}$. The images revealed a spherical morphology composed of PDMS islands in a PZLLys matrix. The formation of these spherical domains was attributed to the solvent that was used for sample preparation. While DMF is a good solvent for PZLLys, it is a poor solvent for PDMS. In a separate publication, the same authors also described non-spherical microphase-separated structures [53]. In CH_2Cl_2-cast films of a triblock copolymer with a very high PDMS content ($PBLG_{48}$-*b*-$PDMS_{508}$-*b*-$PBLG_{48}$, 83 mol % PDMS) more extended, rod-like PBLG aggregates in a matrix of PDMS were observed. The TEM experiments also provided insight into the effects of peptide secondary structure and the nature of the casting solvent on the thin film morphology [52]. $PBLG_x$-*b*-$PDMS_{30}$-*b*-$PBLG_x$ (x=8, 20, 43) triblock copolymers have also been studied by Papon *et al.* [54] Their self-assembly into a double-hexagonal structure was addressed using x-ray scattering and AFM imaging. The thermal behavior of these structures was investigated using dynamic mechanical analysis and differential scanning calorimetry.

Studies on adsorption/denaturation of proteins and oxygen permeation measurements from these triblock copolymers also describe the relationship between the film morphology and these properties. A detailed study of the gas permeation properties of PBLG-*b*-PDMS-*b*-PBLG films (PDMS = polydimethylsiloxane) cast from dichloromethane (CH_2Cl_2) and DMF solution with PDMS contents ranging from 46 to 83 mol % was reported [55] and revealed that the oxygen permeability of the triblock copolymer films in water exponentially increased with increasing PDMS content, in agreement with a microphase-separated morphology of the membranes. Similar results were reported by Kugo, Nishioka, and Nishino, who studied oxygen and nitrogen transport across PBLG-*b*-PDMS-*b*-PBLG triblock copolymers containing 63-81 mol % PBLG [56].

Polyether-based triblock copolymers

Kugo *et al.* [50] studied the solid-state conformation of the peptide segment of a series of PBLG-*b*-PEG-*b*-PBLG copolymers containing a PEG segment with a molecular weight of 4 kg/mol and 36-86 mol % PBLG. FTIR spectroscopy experiments on $CHCl_3$-cast films revealed that the PBLG blocks, which had degrees of polymerization of 25 to 276, had an α-helical secondary structure. The helix content of the triblock copolymer containing $PBLG_{276}$ blocks was found to be similar to that of the PBLG homopolymer. Swelling the triblock copolymer films with water resulted in a decrease in helix content, as indicated by the CD spectra. This decrease in helicity was attributed to competition of water clusters to form hydrogen bonds with the peptide backbone. The effect was even more pronounced when pseudo-extracellular fluid was used instead of water.

A first detailed study of the solid-state nanoscale structure of peptide–PEG hybrid block copolymers was published by Cho *et al.* [57] These authors investigated thin, $CHCl_3$-cast films of PBLG-*b*-PEG-*b*-PBLG copolymers, which were composed of a PEG block of 2 kg/mol and contained 25-76 mol % PBLG. TEM micrographs of RuO_4-stained specimens revealed a lamellar morphology for triblock copolymers containing 25-64 mol % PBLG. The microphase-separated structure was proposed to consist of chain folded, crystalline PEG domains and helical PBLG domains (IR). WAXS patterns were consistent with the ordered, crystalline-like solid-state modification of PBLG. In contrast, in films cast from benzene, the peptide blocks only formed poorly ordered arrays. The sensitivity of the organization of the PBLG blocks towards the nature of the casting solvent is identical to the behavior of the PBLG homopolymer.

While the data reported by Cho *et al.* described the structure and organization of thin solvent cast films of PBLG-*b*-PEG-*b*-PBLG, Floudas and coworkers have extensively studied the bulk nanoscale organization of these materials [58]. To this end, a series of triblock copolymers with PBLG volume fractions (f_{PBLG}) ranging from 0.07-0.89 was investigated using SAXS/WAXS, polarizing optical microscopy (POM), DSC and FT-IR spectroscopy. For triblock copolymers with $f_{PBLG} \leq 0.25$, PEG crystallization was observed, but with significant undercooling. Triblock copolymers with $f_{PBLG} \geq 0.43$ did not show PEG crystallization. SAXS experiments, which were carried out at 373 K, i.e. above the melting point of PEG, also revealed a different behaviour for triblock copolymers with small and large PBLG volume fractions. For triblock copolymers with $f_{PBLG} \geq 0.43$ only a weakly phase separated structure was found, whereas for samples with $f_{PBLG} \leq 0.25$ the SAXS data clearly indicated a microphase-separated structure. WAXS patterns showed that in the microphase-separated state the PEG phase was semi-crystalline and the peptide phase consisted of hexagonally ordered assemblies of PBLG α-helices that coexisted with β-sheet structures. For triblock copolymers with $f_{PBLG} \geq 0.43$, PEG is amorphous and interspersed with aggregates of α-helical PBLG segments and unordered peptide chains (Figure 7).

Additional insight into the solid-state nanoscale organization of the triblock copolymers just discussed could be obtained by combining SAXS/WAXS with different microscopic techniques (TEM and AFM) [59]. A "broken lamellar" morphology was observed in the TEM micrographs of $PBLG_{58}$-*b*-PEG_{90}-*b*-$PBLG_{58}$ ($f_{PBLG} = 0.58$). Annealing converted this metastable structure into a non-uniform microphase-separated pattern, which was proposed to consist of "puck-like" PEG domains in a PBLG matrix. For $PBLG_{105}$-*b*-PEG_{90}-*b*-$PBLG_{105}$ ($f_{PBLG} =$ 0.67), a lamellar morphology was found in the as-cast film, which was transformed into a "broken lamellar" structure upon annealing. Based on the results, a morphology map was constructed.

Cho *et al.* [60] reported on the solid-state structure of a series of PZLLys-*b*-PEG-*b*-PZLLys composed of a PEG block with M_n = 2 kg/mol and PZLLys contents of 25.2, 49.9 and 83.0 mol % (= 68, 86 and 98 vol %). Infrared spectra of $CHCl_3$-cast films were in agreement with a helical secondary structure of the peptide blocks. DSC experiments provided a first hint for the existence of a microphase-separated structure and revealed two T_g's for all samples. The higher T_g was very close to that of the PZLLys homopolymer and the lower T_g approximately 20 °C higher than that of PEG homopolymer. A PEG melting transition was not observed. These results were interpreted in terms of a microphase-separated structure with hard, crystalline PZLLys domains and soft,

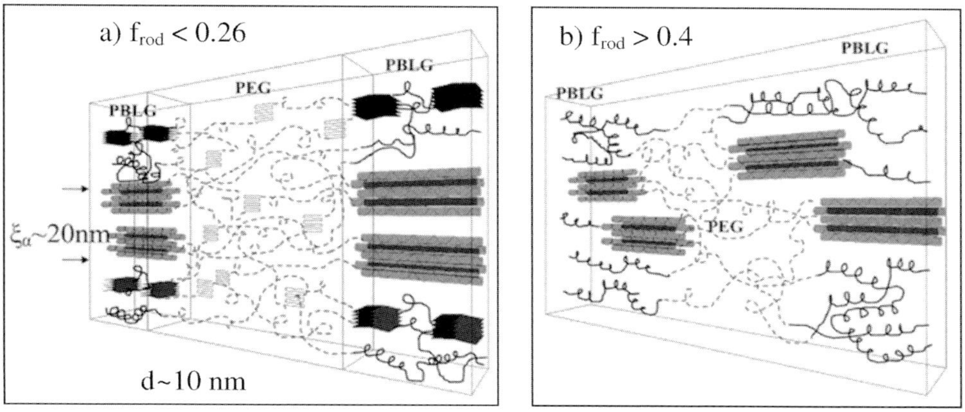

Fig. 7. Highly schematic model of the phase state in the PBLG-*b*-PEG-*b*-PBLG triblock copolymers. (a) Phase state corresponding to low peptide volume fractions depicting a microphase-separated copolymer consisting of all the peptide and PEG secondary structures. (b) Phase state corresponding to f_{rod} > 0.4 depicting phase mixing resulting in the appearance of only one (α-helical) secondary structure. Adapted from [58].

amorphous PEG segments. The presence of a microphase-separated structure was confirmed by TEM micrographs of RuO_4-stained thin films.

Akashi *et al.* [61] reported on the solid-state nanoscale structure of ABA type triblock copolymers composed of a central PEG block flanked by two poly(β-benzyl L-aspartate) (PBLAsp) blocks. The molecular weight of the central PEG block was 11 or 20 kg/mol and the degrees of polymerization of the peptide blocks ranged from 12 to 32. WAXS and POM studies on CH_2Cl_2-cast films showed PEG crystallization in all samples. DSC experiments showed that the melting temperature of the crystalline PEG domains decreased linearly with increasing PBLAsp content, reflecting the strong influence of the peptide segments on PEG crystallization. More interestingly, the authors found that heating the as-cast films above 333 K and cooling down to 303 K converted a certain fraction of the α-helical PBLAsp chains into β-strands and was accompanied by a decrease in PEG crystallinity. On a macroscopic level, this led to increased strength and elasticity of the films.

Cho *et al.* [62] have studied triblock copolymers composed of a middle block of poly(propylene glycol) (PPG) with a molecular weight of 2,000 flanked by two PBLG segments. Three triblock copolymer samples were investigated with PPG contents of 17.0, 26.0 and 60.0 mol %, respectively. According to infrared spectra and WAXS that were recorded from $CHCl_3$-cast films, the PBLG blocks possessed an α-helical secondary structure. No further details on the solid-state nanoscale structure and the possibility of microphase separation were reported.

Platelet adhesion on glass beads coated with block copolymers containing 33 or 47 mol% PPG was reduced compared to beads modified with PMLGlu homopolymer or block copolymers with 70.0 mol% PPG. These differences were attributed to differences in surface composition and morphology, which, unfortunately, were not further discussed.

Finally, Hayashi, Kugo and Nakajima [63] have reported on PMLG-*b*-PTHF-*b*-PMLG (PTHF = polytetrahydrofuran) triblock copolymers that were prepared from an amino-functionalized PTHF macroinitiator with a molecular weight of 9.6 kg/mol. Three different triblock copolymers were studied with PMLGlu contents and degrees of polymerization of 86.8 mol %/460, 89.7 mol %/605 and 91.3 mol %/730, respectively. With respect to the solid-state structure and organization, only infrared spectra and WAXS data were discussed.

Miscellaneous

The structure and properties of an ABA triblock copolymer composed of a polyetherurethaneurea (PEUU) B block with M_n = 15.8 kg/mol and two $PBLG_{29}$ B blocks were described by Ito and coworkers [64]. DSC thermograms showed a single endotherm located between the T_g of the PEUU and the 7/2 to 18/5 helix transition of PBLG, suggesting that there was no phase separation. Platelet adhesion on DMF-cast films of the triblock copolymer was significantly reduced compared to the respective homopolymers and a PEUU/PBLG blend. Thrombus formation on block copolymer films was found to be ~50% less compared to a glass surface. However, no significant difference in antithrombogenicity between PEUU, PBLG, their blend and the block copolymer was observed.

Another, very early study focused on two PBLG-*b*-PBAN-*b*-PBLG (PBAN = poly(butadiene-*co*-acrylonitrile)) triblock copolymers [65]. These block copolymers were composed of a PBAN block with M_n = 3.4 kg/mol and

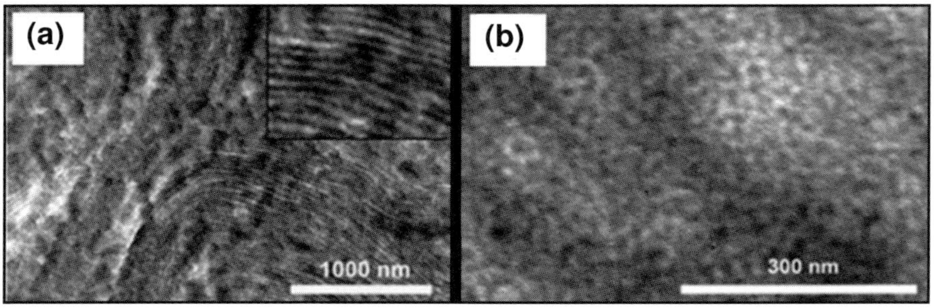

Fig. 8. TEM micrographs of triblock PBLG-*b*-PHF-*b*-PBLG copolymers in (a) coil-rod-coil conformation and (b) rod-rod-rod conformation. Adapted from [67].

two PBLG segments containing either 80 or 160 repeat units. TEM micrographs of OsO_4-stained films cast from dioxane, which is a selective solvent for PBLG, revealed a lamellar morphology. When the non-selective solvent $CHCl_3$ was used for the preparation of the TEM specimens, the images were more homogeneous and phase separation was less distinct. This suggests that, depending on the solvent conditions, the PBAN block can affect PBLG secondary structure.

Electro- and photoactive peptide–synthetic hybrid triblock copolymers have been prepared using bis(benzyl amine)-terminated poly(9,9-dihexylfluorene-2,7-diyl) (PHF) as a macroinitiator for the ring-opening polymerization of BLGlu-NCA [66]. The electroactive and photoactive properties of the triblock copolymers were similar to those of the PHF homopolymer, indicating that the introduction of the PBLG segments did not interfere with charge injection and transport and other materials properties. The thin film morphologies of the triblock copolymers were investigated with SFM using different casting solvents. Depending on solvent preparation, spherical and fibrillar nanostructures have been obtained. Later, triblock copolymer structures PBLG-*b*-PHF-*b*-PBLG with different PBLG ratio have been studied by Mezzenga *et al.* [67] Depending on the solvent casting history, the copolymers exhibit two different conformations: a rod-rod-rod or coil-rod-coil configuration. The observed photoluminescence spectra and dominant excited lifetimes of the poly(9,9-dihexylfluorene-2,7-diyl) block were found to differ markedly in rod-rod-rod and coil-rod-coil configurations and were correlated to the morphology of the self-assembled triblock copolymers.

Pseudo-phase diagram

Based on all the experimental work on hybrid polypeptide block copolymers, one can attempt to draw a pseudo-phase diagram presenting the different morphologies obtained as a function of the polypeptide volume fraction. Because we do not have a sufficiently large series of diblock copolymers with the same chemical blocks, we cannot define a real phase diagram and calculate the Flory-Huggins χ parameter. We decided to combine the data obtained from different systems based on polypeptides (PBLG or PZLLys) and polyvinyl segments (polystyrene, polyisoprene and polybutadiene) with a diblock architecture. All these diblock copolymers behave as rod-coils. We have thus been able to represent this pseudo-phase diagram plotting the total number of monomer unit N_{total} as a function of the polypeptide (or rod) volume fraction (Figure 9). The first observation is that most of the phase diagram consists of the previously described hexagonal in Lamellar (HL) morphology, consisting of a local order of

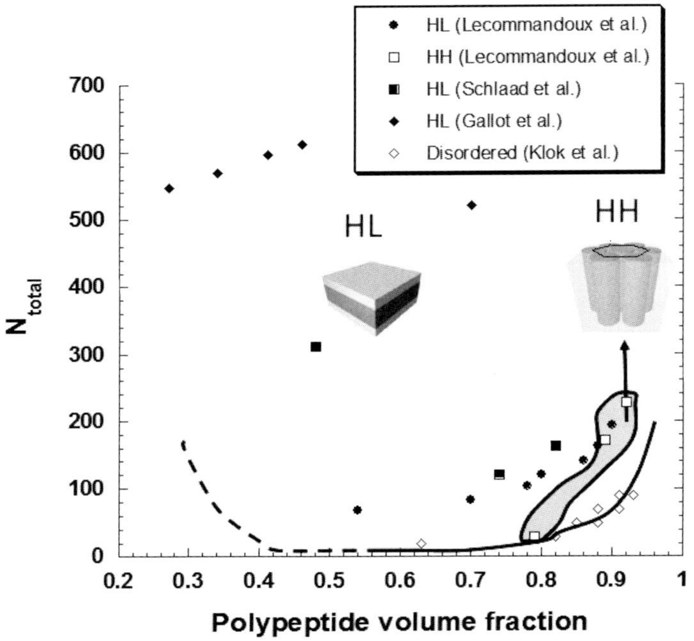

Fig. 9. Pseudo phase diagram for polypeptide-based diblock copolymers. HL: Hexagonal in Lamellar morphology. HH: double hexagonal morphology.

the polypeptide chains and a lamellar phase separation between both blocks. In a very small part of the phase diagram, a double hexagonal (HH) structure can be observed, mainly for short and highly asymmetric block copolymers. Considering the polypeptide in α-helical conformation as rigid rods, one can see an excellent agreement of this experimental pseudo-phase diagram with the theoretical one calculated for rod-coil block copolymers [68].

3. Solution Self-assembled Micellar Structures from Polypeptide-based Conjugates

3.1. *Polypeptide-based micelles*

Peptide core-forming micelles

In aqueous solution, micellization can occur due to the complexation of water-soluble chains containing equal lengths of oppositely charged copolymers. For example, Harada and Kataoka [69–71] observed the formation of monodisperse micelles (R_H = 15 nm, as determined by DLS) from a mixture of equal parts polyanionic PEG_{113}-*b*-$PAsp_{18,\ 78}$ and polycationic PEG_{113}-*b*-$PLLys_{18,\ 78}$. Charge neutralization drove the self-assembly of the polyion complex (PIC) core, while phase separation necessitated the formation of the PEG corona. These forces together produced the "chain length recognition" phenomenon, in which micelles preferentially formed from chains with equivalent anionic and cationic segments [71].

CD spectra obtained from aqueous solutions of PEG_{113}-*b*-$PMLG_{20,50}$ and lactose-modified PEG_{75}-*b*-$PMLG_{32}$ revealed an associative tendency for the α-helical PMLG portion [72]. This tendency could provide the impetus for the observed aggregation through an initial formation of planar bilayers followed by closure of the bilayers into vesicles [73]. Although attributed to spherical micelles, the 250 nm hydrodynamic radius determined by DLS could more reasonably be assigned to vesicles or micellar aggregates.

Investigation of similarly sized aggregates by Cho *et al.* [74,75] revealed aggregation numbers less than 100, a value inconsistent with typical vesicle-produced aggregation numbers measuring in the thousands [76]. Despite the known LCST behavior of the PNIPAM block, no size evolution was reported for the PNIPAM-containing aggregates at that temperature. Zhang and collaborators [77] reported micelle formation from poly(N-isopropylacrylamide)-*b*-poly(lysine-*co*-glutamic acid). Since the copolypeptide portion was insoluble in water between pH 6.0 and 10, it formed the core of micelles with hydrodynamic radius measuring 1800 nm according to light scattering data.

TEM was performed on spherical aggregates measuring from 200 to 700 nm obtained from aqueous dissolution of a triblock copolymer composed of two poly(L-alanine) or PBLG blocks flanking a central poly(2-acryloyloxyethyllactoside) (PAELA) portion [78,79]. A decrease in aggregate size corresponding to an increase in copolymer concentration suggested a micellar structure, despite the TEM-observed compact structures similar to those of multilamellar vesicles. Variation in initial polymer concentration was reported to produce micelle morphologies ranging from spherical to wormlike [80].

Large aggregates (R_H = 425 nm, as determined by DLS) were obtained from poly(acetyliminoethylene)-*b*-poly(L-phenylalanine) (PAI-*b*-PLPhe) at neutral pH in 0.05 M phosphate buffer [81]. Infrared spectroscopy supplied a possible explanation for the high aggregation rate, which was unexpected due to the notably weak presence of hydrophobic L-phenylalanine: hydrogen bridging between amino acids. Hydrophobic interactions may also have contributed to the observed micellar clusters and coacervates.

Poly(acrylic acid)-*b*-poly(L-valine) (PAA-*b*-PLVal) block copolymers (i.e., PAA_{40}-*b*-$PLVal_{100}$, PAA_{80}- *b*-$PLVal_{100}$, PAA_{80}-*b*-$PLVal_{80}$, and PAA_{80}-*b*-$PLVal_{60}$) were reported to form core-shell spherical micelles [82]. In the presence of a urea solution (0.2 M), micelles composed of PAA_{40}-*b*-$PLVal_{100}$ exhibited greater uniformity and smaller diameters (90 nm compared to 245 nm) as observed by TEM. Further, hydrodynamic radius of micelles composed of PAA_{80}-*b*-$PLVal_{80}$ increased from nearly 70 nm at pH 0.15 to nearly 90 nm at pH 0.2, due to the rearrangement of the PAA chains to accommodate increasing charge density (Figure 10).

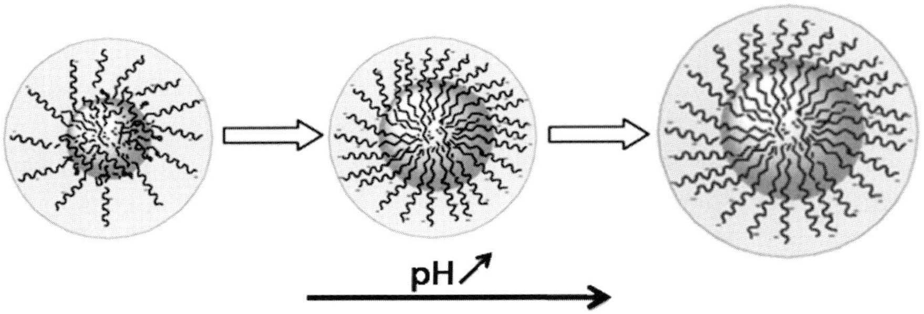

Fig. 10. Schematic diagram showing effects of pH increase on micelles formed from PAA-*b*-PLVal. The blue circle represents the radius of gyration, while the green circle represents the hydrodynamic radius. Adapted from [82].

Micellization was reported with a system employing poly(γ-benzyl-L-glutamate)-*g*-poly(ethylene glycol) graft copolymer (PBLG-*g*-PEG) in distilled water with various degrees of grafting and mixtures composed of PBLG-*g*-PEG and poly(γ-benzyl-L-glutamate)-*b*-poly(ethylene glycol) block copolymer (PBLG-*b*-PEG). Analysis of TEM data revealed a shape change of micelles from irregular to spindle with variation in grafting from 20% to 36% [83]. Another group observed by TEM the formation of compound spherical aggregates upon addition of trifluoroacetic acid to PBLG-*g*-PEG micelles in an ethanol solution due to a conformational transition of the PBLG from alpha helix to random coil and reordering of the PEG chains [84].

Peptide shell-forming micelles

When a component of a block copolymer exhibits greater affinity for the solvent, that block tends to form a protective corona surrounding a core composed of the less solvo-philic material. This section focuses on micellar aggregates in which the polypeptide portion of the material forms a corona or shell around a core of polymer.

Three decades ago, Nakajima *et al.* [85] first reported the formation of micelles in organic solvents from a polypeptide copolymer material consisting of a coiled poly(*trans*-1,4-butadiene) block flanked by two rod-like blocks of poly(γ-benzyl L-glutamate) to form $PBLG_{53\text{-}188}$-*block*-PB_{64}-*block*-$PBLG_{53\text{-}188}$ (subscripts indicate average number of repeat units). Contact-angle-based estimation of the surface tension of the component copolymer blocks, in addition to consideration of their interfacial free energy, enabled thermodynamic calculation of micellar structures likely to result from various copolymer compositions. The presence of these predicted morphologies – spherical, cylindrical, and lamellar structures with calculated micelle dimensions of 25 to 45 nm – was confirmed by transmission electron microscope (TEM). A later study [86] revealed similar behavior for a different rod-coil block copolymer with rod-like poly(γ-methyl L-glutamate) (PMLG) dissolved in the continuous phase, suggesting that the aggregation of such samples may be handled similarly to those of conformationally isotropic samples [87].

The past decade has seen micellar structures obtained in water using hydrophilic poly(amino-acids) that exhibit secondary structure transitions similar to those of proteins. For example, the hydrodynamic radius of polyisoprene-*b*-poly(L-lysine) (PI_{49}-*b*-$PLLys_{123}$) micelles nearly doubled following a decrease of pH from 11 to 6 in saline solution [88]. At pH 11, the poly(L-lysine) presented α-helical structure corresponding to a hydrodynamic radius of 23 nm (determined by dynamic light scattering or DLS). At pH 6, micelle radius swelled to 44 nm due to a shift from helical to coil PLLys structure. For polybutadiene-*b*-poly(L-glutamate) (PB-*b*-PLGA) with similarly sized segments (PB_{48}-*b*-$PLGA_{114}$ compared to PI_{49}-*b*-$PLLys_{123}$) the effect was significantly smaller at about 8% [89]. The minimal pH-induced size response in the PB-*b*-PLGA system may be a consequence of folding or disruption [90] of the PLGA helices, whereas the PLLys helices may be in a more extended state. Moreover, addition of 2,2'-(ethylenedioxy)bisethylamine to PB_{48}-*b*-$PLGA_{114}$ and of glutaric dialdehyde to PI_{49}-*b*-$PLLys_{178}$ promoted crosslinking in either system [91], without affecting aggregate size or morphology.

Micelle formation was observed from the material poly(L-cysteine)-*b*-poly(L-lactide) or PLCys-*b*-PLLac [92]. In this case, addition of dithiothreitol (DTT) reversibly removed cross-linking of the hydrophilic poly(L-cysteine) corona or shell through the cleaving of disulfide bonds into two separate thiol groups. Extension of the polycysteine segments resulted in a slight, but measurable, increase in hydrodynamic radius (determined by DLS) from 47.1 nm for the crosslinked micelle to 55.1 nm for the DTT-reduced micelles.

In contrast to the PB-*b*-PLGA system in which morphological changes (from micelles to vesicles) were induced by variation of the hydrophobic content or pH, no such morphological changes were observed with the poly(L-lactide)-*b*-poly(aspartic acid) system despite similar variation [93]. Throughout the considered range of hydrophobic content (21 to 74 mol % aspartic acid) and pH (4.4 to 8.6), scanning force microscopy and light scattering data continued to reveal the presence of solely spherical aggregates with hydrodynamic radius varying from 10 to 80 nm. Two possible explanations for this behavior have been postulated. On one hand, a metastable state adopted by the semi-crystalline PLLac core material could be locking each vesicle into a spherical conformation [94]. On the other hand, the system may have attained a state of equilibrium, in which an interplay of core/corona forces – hydrogen bonding of the PAsp corona, hydrophobic forces in the PLLac core, and electrostatic repulsion between the two – could produce similar aggregation behaviour [93].

Another block copolymer, polystyrene-*b*-poly(L-lysine) ($PS_{8,\,10}$-*b*-$PLLys_{9\text{-}72}$), described by Klok *et al.* [95] exhibited original behavior at neutral pH and in aqueous dilute solution. Despite variation of the PLLys block length, solely cylindrical micelles were observed by dynamic/static light scattering (DLS/SLS), small angle neutron scattering (SANS), and analytical ultracentrifugation (AUC).

Micelles were formed by the block copolymer $polystyrene_{388}$-*b*-poly(L-$lysine)_{138}$. Circular dichroism (CD) spectroscopy reveals a conformational change of the poly(L-lysine) portion from random coil to β-sheet as pH increases beyond 11. Data obtained by atomic force microscopy (AFM) corroborates this pH-dependent conformational transition: material deposited by solvent evaporation on graphite at pH 8 shows less wetting ability than the same material deposited at pH 11 [96].

$Poly(butadiene)_m$-*b*-poly(L-$lysine)_n$ (m–n = 107–200, 107–100, and 60–50) was reported by Savin *et al.* [97] to form spherical or rod-like micelles depending on the block composition at high pH. Specifically, TEM and DLS data supported the appearance of more elongated rod-like shape in addition to spherical micelles at pH 9 than at pH 2 in the PB_{107}-$PLLys_{100}$ and PB_{60}-$PLLys_{50}$ systems. Further, micelles shrank with decreasing pH from 82 ± 2 nm at pH 2 to 62 ± 2 nm at pH 9.2, as determined by DLS.

Recently, formation of micellar aggregates was reported for a material with polytetrahydrofuran (PTHF) as a central hydrophobic block flanked by two segments of poly(L-lysine) as outer hydrophilic blocks to form the ABA triblock copolymer [poly(L-lysine)-*b*-polytetrahydrofuran-*b*-poly(L-lysine) or ($PLLys_{30}$-*b*-

PTHF-*b*-PLLys$_{30}$)]. This material was further modified with sugar moieties – either D-gluconolactone or lactobionolactone – and employed as a nano-carrier for doxorubicin as a model anticancer drug [98].

The diameter of the micelles formed with the ABC triblock copolymer poly(ethylene glycol)-*b*-poly(L-lactide)-*b*-poly(L-glutamic acid) (PEG-*b*-PLLac-*b*-PLGA) was found to depend on the PLGA block length and on the ratio of water to dimethylformamide (DMF) in solution. The system exhibits a reversible transition at or below pH 3.2 with spherical micelles shifting to a connected-rod morphology [99].

Using AFM and light scattering, micelles were observed from a triblock copolymer containing a central oligopeptide segment sandwiched between hydrophilic poly(ethylene oxide) (PEO) and hydrophobic poly(butyl acrylate) (PBA) blocks [PEO-*b*-Arg$_{10}$-*b*-PBA] [100]. The biofunctional arginine segment, mimicking cell penetrating peptides, is interestingly confined at the hydrophilic and hydrophobic interface, between micelle core and corona. A recent approach employed the co-micellization of poly(L-glutamic acid)-*b*-poly(propylene oxide)-*b*-poly(L-glutamic acid) (PLGA-*b*-PPO-*b*-PLGA) and poly(ethylene glycol)-*b*-poly(propylene oxide) (PEG-*b*-PPO) in water to produce PPO core blocks surrounded by poly(L-glutamic acid) and poly(ethylene glycol) mixed corona chains [101]. DLS showed that micelle radii increased at lowered temperatures (approaching 20 °C) due to expansion of the PPO core and decreased at acidic

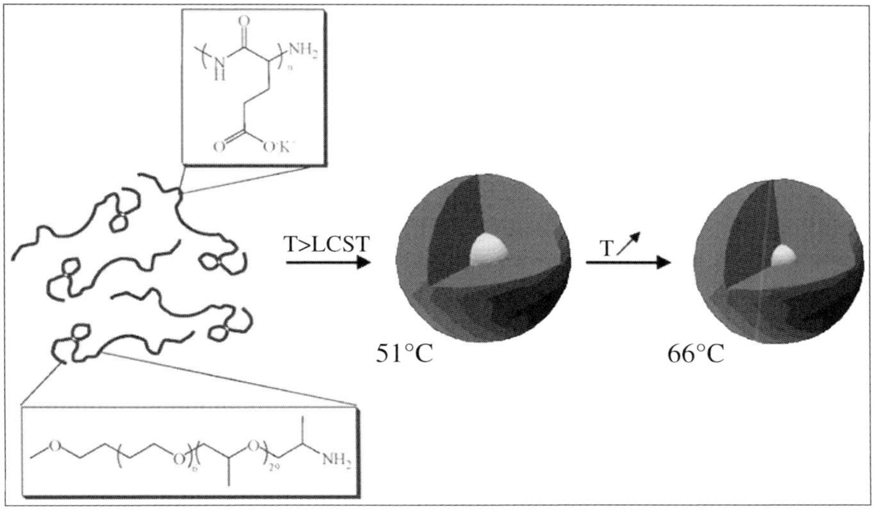

Fig. 11. Schematic diagram showing effect of temperature increase from 51°C to 66°C on micelles formed from Jeffamine-*b*-PLGA$_{30}$. Adapted from [102].

pH (less than 7) due to the conformational shift from extended coil to alpha helix of the PLGA segment, as confirmed by CD spectroscopy.

Similar micelles composed of poly(L-glutamic acid) in a protective corona enveloping a core of Jeffamine were previously described by Agut *et al.* [102] DLS revealed the micellar hydrodynamic radius of the doubly hydrophilic block copolymer Jeffamine-*b*-$PLGA_{30}$ (Jeffamine being $P(EO_6$-*r*-$PO_{29}))$ to increase from 11.2 nm at 36 °C to 13.5 nm at 66 °C. Micelle formation and core dehydration upon heating (as seen in Figure 11) was quantitatively evaluated by SANS.

Schizophrenic micelles

In some material sets, experimental conditions (such as pH and temperature) dramatically affect the structure of the micelle. This section focuses on micellar systems in which experimental conditions determine the role – core or corona – of the polypeptide block.

Rao *et al.* [103] observed pH and thermo-responsive micelles from the copolymer poly(N-isopropylacrylamide)-*b*-poly(L-glutamic acid) (PNIPAM-*b*-PLGA). Under basic heated conditions, the PLGA block formed a corona around the PNIPAM, as revealed by proton nuclear magnetic resonance (^{1}H NMR) spectra. However, the PLGA migrated to the core of the micelle under acidic conditions at room temperature. This behavior was attributed to a decrease in water solubility of the PLGA with decreasing pH, corresponding to a secondary structure transition from random coil to α-helical rod (CD spectroscopy). Based on light-scattering data obtained at 25 °C, the hydrodynamic radius of $PNIPAM_{65}$-*b*-$PLGA_{110}$ shifted from 10 nm at pH 10 to 53 nm at pH 2, offering further evidence of the material's pH responsiveness.

The PLGA portion of micelles formed from $PNIPAM_{55}$-*b*-$PLGA_{35}$ was also observed to shift from core to corona with changing experimental conditions [104]. As confirmed by CD spectroscopy, a pH-induced transition of the PLGA chain from random coil (pH 11) to alpha helix (pH 3.0) causes formation of micelles in aqueous solution at 25 °C. At a constant pH of 10, micellization occurred with an increase in temperature from 25 to 45 °C, due to the temperature-dependent coil to globule transition of PNIPAM in water. SANS and TEM data showed spherical, PLGA-core micelles at pH 3 and 25 °C. At pH 10 and 45 °C, cylindrical, PLGA-corona micelles were observed.

3.2. *Polypeptide-based vesicles*

Peptide-polymer conjugate vesicles

The formation of fluid-filled sacs, or vesicles, has been observed for a range of block copolymer systems. This section describes developments in the formation of vesicles from copolymer systems containing both a synthetic polymer and a polypeptide block.

With variation of the hydrophobic to hydrophilic ratio of the block copolymer polybutadiene-*b*-poly(L-glutamate) or PB-*b*-PLGA in aqueous saline solution, Schlaad [105], Lecommandoux [89], and their collaborators observed a shift from micellar aggregates to unilamellar vesicles. Despite earlier findings [106,107] of vesicle formation by PB_{40}-*b*-$PLGA_{100}$ (71% glutamate content), sub-40 nm spherical micelles were produced by the same block copolymer at a glutamate composition of 70 to 75% and examined using light scattering, TEM, and SANS. The same techniques were applied to unilamellar vesicles with hydrodynamic radii in the range of 50 to 90 nm obtained at a glutamate composition of 17 to 54%. A decrease in pH might be expected to shrink PB-*b*-PLGA micelles, since the poly(L-glutamate) chain length is more than halved in the transition from coil to α-helical secondary structure that occurs in the range of pH 6 to 5. Despite confirmation of the secondary structure change by CD spectroscopy, no corresponding decrease in hydrodynamic radius was observed in the case of $PB_{27\text{-}119}$-*b*-$PLGA_{24\text{-}64}$ [105]. A minor radial decrease of 20% or less did occur in the case of PB_{48}-*b*-$PLGA_{56\text{-}145}$ [89]. Although the aggregates equilibrated with a dynamic exchange of polymer chains [105], data obtained by SANS suggested no change in aggregation number [89].

Various combinations of hydrophobic to hydrophilic content of the triblock copolymer poly(L-glutamic acid)-*b*-poly(propylene oxide)-*b*-poly(L-glutamic acid) (PLGA-*b*-PPO-*b*-PLGA) can form spherical micelles under alkaline conditions (pH 11) or a combination of vesicles and micelles under acidic conditions (pH 4.1), as seen by TEM. The hydrodynamic radius of the micelles is also observed by DLS to decrease from 167 nm at 20 °C to 110 nm at 40 °C. The same technique revealed a radius shift from 147 nm at pH 4.1 to 130 nm at pH 6.7 [108]. These values are notably more consistent with polymer vesicles.

By varying the polymer composition and the helicogenic common solvents of poly(N-isopropylacrylamide)-*b*-poly(ε-benzyloxycarbonyl L-lysine) (PNIPAM-*b*-PZLLys), Huang *et al.* also recently obtained spherical micelles, wormlike micelles, and vesicles [109]. The block copolymer poly(butadiene)$_{107}$-*b*-poly(L-lysine)$_{27}$ (PB_{107}-*b*-$PLLys_{27}$) formed vesicles that increased in size with high temperature and pH due to conformational changes from coil to β-sheet motifs, with supporting data obtained by CD spectroscopy, TEM, and light scattering. The vesicles increased in hydrodynamic radius from 72 ± 2 nm under more alkaline conditions (pH between 5.5 and 10) to 92 ± 2 nm under acidic conditions (pH between 2 and 5.5). Varying the temperature at pH 10.9 produced a wider range of vesicle sizes, with a hydrodynamic radius of around 70 nm at 25 °C increasing to about 140 nm at 65 °C [110].

The material poly(γ-benzyloxycarbonyl L-lysine)-*b*-poly(diethylene glycol bis(3-amino propyl)ether)-*b*-poly(γ-benzyloxycarbonyl L-lysine) (PZLLys-*b*-DGBE-*b*-PZLLys) formed both vesicles and large compound micelles in aqueous solution [111]. Distinction of vesicles versus large compound micelles was achieved with the use of a shorter PZLLys segment. DLS revealed the hydrodynamic radius of the vesicles to range from 10 to 160 nm depending on the DGBE to PZLLys ratio.

In addition, Kataoka *et al.* [112] reported formation of the first semi-permeable vesicles using a charge-driven approach with a poly(ethylene glycol)-*b*-poly(β,α-aspartic acid)/ poly(ethylene glycol)-*b*-poly([5-aminopentyl]-β,α-aspartamide) or PEG-P(Asp)/PEG-P(Asp-AP) system in water. As described in the core-forming polypeptide-based copolymer micelle section of this review, "chain length recognition" of oppositely charged block copolymers (polyion complexes or PICs) produces a membrane of matched polymer chains. Figure 12 illustrates the formation of vesicles known as PICsomes with a layer of PEG shielding the PIC membrane in aqueous solution.

Finally, dextran-*b*-poly(γ-benzyl L-glutamate) vesicles were very recently synthesized and investigated by Schatz and Lecommandoux *et al.* [113] This material represents a new category of polypeptide-polymer structure utilizing a natural sequence – the polysaccharide block – and accesses an interesting

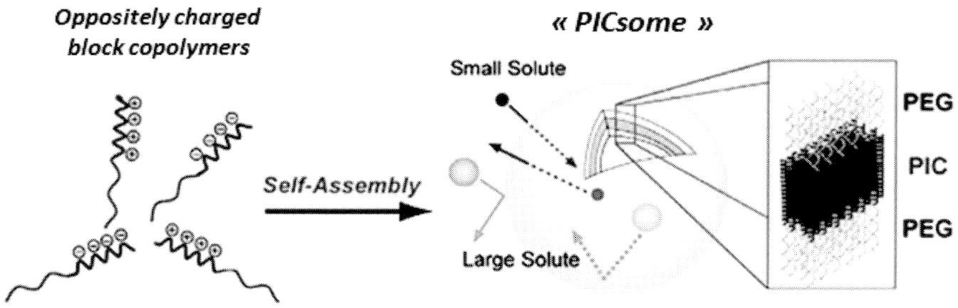

Fig. 12. Schematic diagram showing formation of PICsome from oppositely charged block copolymers. Adapted from [112].

potential route for mimicking glycoprotein structure and function. DLS showed a homogeneous population of 45 nm hydrodynamic radius. SANS and TEM supported a hollow vesicular structure with a wall thickness of around 20 nm.

Copolypeptide vesicles

Inclusion of a polypeptide segment in the vesicle membrane offers advantages such as stimuli-responsive secondary structure and biocompatibility. Besides pairing a polypeptide segment with a synthetic polypeptide, researchers have reported the formation of vesicles from copolymers consisting solely of polypeptides, without the presence of a synthetic polymer block. This section of the review summarizes efforts in the formation of vesicles from such copolypeptide systems.

Evolution of the aggregate morphology of phosphate-head-group-bearing $PMLG_{10}$ occurred in water, as observed by Doi *et al.* [114,115] Within an hour of initial preparation, inter-chain hydrogen bonding drove a shift from globular structures (measuring 50 to 100 nm in diameter, as determined by TEM) to fibrous aggregates. After twenty-four hours, hydrophobic interactions promoted the formation of 4-nm-thick twisted ribbons through anti-parallel stacking of the β-sheet conformation adopted by $PMLG_{10}$-P (as determined by CD and Fourier transform infrared (FTIR) spectroscopy.)

Unilamellar vesicles were formed in water from the zwitterionic material $PLGA_{15}$-*b*-$PLLys_{15}$ [116]. According to DLS data, the initial hydrodynamic radius near 110 nm increased to 175 nm with an increase in pH from 3 to 12. At intermediate pH, free chains in solution were observed. Based on NMR analysis and zeta-potential measurements, the size change was attributed to a structural inversion of the membrane. Authors thus evidenced for the first time the formation of "schizophrenic vesicles" that could be reversibly produced as a function of pH in pure water. Formation of hollow spheres rather than micelles may be attributed to the low interfacial curvature induced by the presence of a rod-like polypeptide in the hydrophobic portion of the block copolymer membrane.

This was also evidenced by the range of structures produced by $PLLeu_{10\text{-}75}$-*b*-$PELLys_{60\text{-}200}$ [117]. The α-helical tendencies of either non-ionic residue – the L-leucine and the ethylene glycol-modified L-lysine – produced sheets, irregular structures, and vesicles measuring less than 1 μm in diameter.

The poly(L-glutamate) brush portion of $PLLeu_{180}$-*b*-$PLGA_{180}$ provided electrosteric stability to selectively precipitated particles suspended in water or in 0.15 M phosphate saline buffer (pH 7.4) [118]. Particle shape varied according to chain composition (as determined by NMR): a strong glutamate presence in the chain produced cylindrical or spherical micelles, while large hexagonal platelets resulted from a strong leucine presence. TEM revealed the width of the platelets to be 200 nm, while data from a combination of CD spectroscopy and x-ray diffraction suggested the platelet core material was constructed from a three-dimensional array of leucine zippers.

Deming *et al.* [119] employed extrusion to produce vesicles from poly(L-lysine)-*b*-poly(L-leucine) or $PLLys_{20\text{-}80}$-$PLLeu_{10\text{-}30}$. The positively charged poly(L-lysine) portion was included to promote solubility and lend a greater degree of flexibility to the vesicle membrane. However, the length of this positively charged portion was shortened (20 to 80 monomers) relative to the length considered in an earlier study [120] (80 to 380 monomers) so as to discourage the formation of twisted fibrils due to repulsive interchain reactions. The copolymer was dissolved in a THF/water solution prior to dialysis against distilled water. In the considered range of hydrophobic to hydrophilic content, $PLLys_{60}$-*b*-$PLLeu_{20}$ was selected as the best candidate for further investigation, due to its formation of giant, unilamellar vesicles (LSCM/TEM). Vesicles formed from its anionic counterpart – poly(L-glutamic acid)-*b*-poly(L-leucine) or $PLGA_{60}$-$PLLeu_{20}$ – were also produced for the sake of comparison. The 0.8 μm to 5 μm vesicles (size determined by DLS) were extruded through filters with pore sizes ranging from 0.1 to 1 μm, and post-extrusion measurement of the vesicle size showed good agreement with the pore size. Extrusion was also found to be an effective way of encapsulating solute (specifically Texas Red-tagged dextran) within the vesicles. Subsequent osmotic stress tests revealed that the vesicles were permeable to water, but impermeable to larger molecules such as sucrose.

The same technique was reported to produce vesicles from poly(L-arganine)$_{60}$-*b*-poly(L-leucine)$_{20}$, $PLArg_{60}$-*b*-$PLLys_{20}$ [121]. A substitution of arganine for lysine was made in order to equip the vesicle membrane with protein-transduction domains for therapeutic application, specifically intracellular delivery of vesicle contents (Figure 13). Laser confocal scanning microscopy (LCSM) revealed rapid cellular uptake for dextran-filled $PLArg_{60}$-*b*-$PLLys_{20}$ with no apparent disruption to the vesicle or its contents.

The triblock copolymer PLLys-*b*-PBLG-d7-*b*-PLLys (where PLLys and PBLG-d7 are poly(L-lysine hydrochloride) and poly(γ-benzyl-d7- L-glutamate) respectively) was found to form vesicles in water at neutral pH by Hadjichristidis and collaborators [122]. Vesicle formation occurred within a broad range of hydrophobic block content – from 19 to 74% of the total molecular weight. According to the authors, the triblock nature of PBLG-d7-*b*-PLLys is particularly

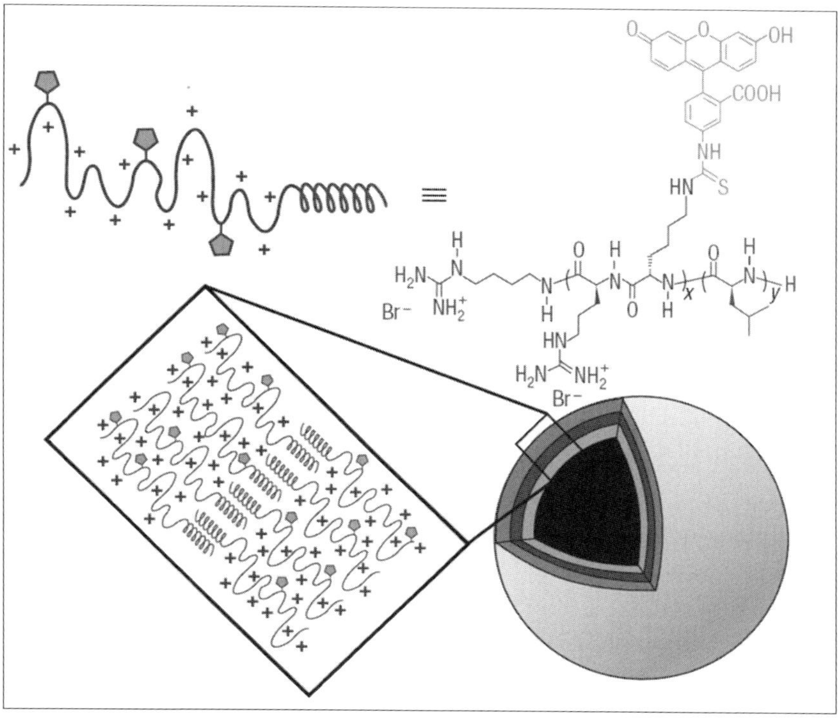

Fig. 13. Schematic diagram of vesicles formed from PLArg$_{60}$-*b*-PLLys$_{20}$. Adapted from [121].

well-suited for vesicle formation, since the middle block promotes membrane assembly due to its insolubility but discourages micelle assembly due to its rigidity. Vesicle size increased considerably with temperature increase due to a shift in the PLLys from a compact α-helix to an elongated β-sheet secondary structure (CD spectroscopy). Light scattering data showed that the hydrodynamic radius of PLLys$_{134}$-(PBLG-d7)$_{64}$-PLLys$_{134}$ vesicles increased from 92.5 nm at 25 °C to 148 nm at 37 °C at pH 11.5. The formation of vesicles from a solution containing plasmid DNA and copolypeptides was also investigated with a number of techniques, including AFM, cryo-TEM, and scanning electron microscopy (SEM). Plasmid DNA was found to be partially encapsulated by the vesicle and partially condensed on the PLLys phase of the vesicle membrane.

Jing and collaborators [123] reported vesicle formation from simple aqueous dissolution of a copolypeptide material – poly(L-lysine)-*b*-poly(L-phenylalanine) (PLLys-*b*-PLPhe) (specifically PLLys$_{53}$-*b*-PLPhe$_{12}$). Water selectively dissolved hydrophilic PLLys, while intra-chain hydrogen bonding and hydrophobic interactions of the PLPhe phase drove subsequent vesicle assembly. Increasing the number of repeat PLLys monomers (from 53 to 65) while maintaining a constant number of PLPhe monomers (12) roughly tripled vesicle diameter (from 2.2 ± 0.4 μm to 6.2 ± 2.0 μm), as visualized by AFM. The opposite operation, in which the number of PLLys monomer was held constant (53) while the number of PLPhe monomers was increased (from 6 to 12) also increased vesicle diameter, in this case by a factor of roughly 2 (from to 1.1 ± 0.2 μm to 2.2 ± 0.4 μm.) AFM data also revealed a significant increase in vesicle size corresponding to a decrease in solution pH. The diameter of vesicles swelled from 1.5 μm at pH 9 to 2.6 μm at pH 2.5 due to the increase in repulsive forces in the PLLys chain and its gradual transition from α-helical toward random coil conformation. UV absorbance, fluorescence, and SEM provided supporting evidence for the complexation of calf thymus DNA upon mixing of the copolymer with a DNA solution.

3.3. *Polypeptide-based hydrogels*

Applications for protein-based hydrogels range from food and cosmetic thickeners to support matrices for drug delivery and tissue replacement. These materials are usually prepared using proteins extracted from natural resources, which can give rise to inconsistent properties unsuitable for medical applications.

Recently, Deming *et al.* [124–127] designed and synthesized diblock copolypeptide amphiphiles containing charged and hydrophobic segments. It was demonstrated that gelation depends not only on the amphiphilic nature of the polypeptides, but also on chain conformation, meaning α-helix, β-strand or random coil. Specific rheological measurements were performed to evidence the self-assembly process responsible for gelation: the rod-like helical secondary structure of enantiomerically pure PLLeu blocks is instrumental for gelation at polypeptide concentrations as low as 0.25 wt % [126]. The hydrophilic polyelectrolyte segments have stretched coil configurations and stabilize the twisted fibrillar assemblies by forming a corona around the hydrophobic cores (Figure 14).

Interestingly, these hydrogels can retain their mechanical strength up to temperatures of about 90 °C and recover rapidly after stress. This new mode of assembly was found to give rise to polypeptide hydrogels with a unique combination of properties, such as heat stability and injectability. Such properties are attractive for applications in food engineering, personal care, and medicine. More specifically, investigation has been made into biological application of the polypeptide hydrogels as tissue engineering scaffolds [128].

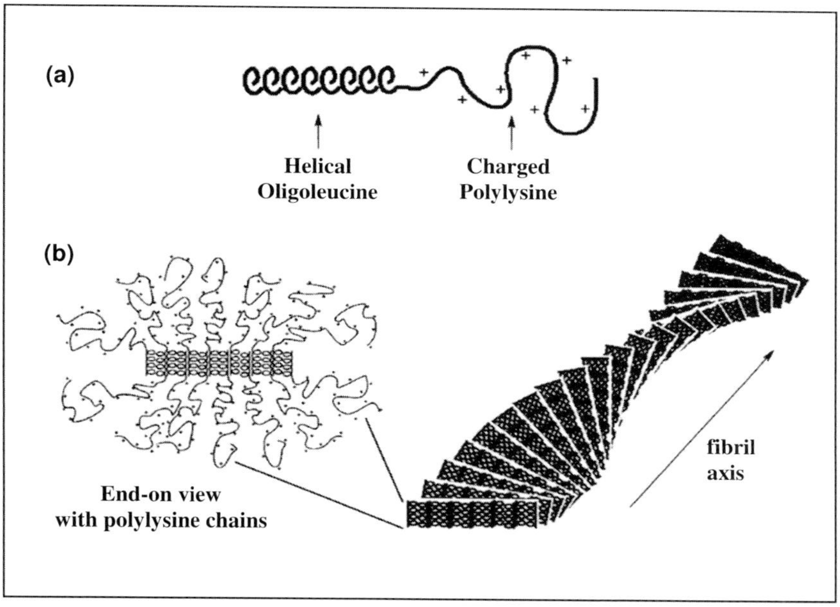

Fig. 14. Drawings showing (a) representation of a block copolypeptide chain and (b) proposed packing of block copolypeptide amphiphiles into twisted fibrillar tapes, with helices packed perpendicular to the fibril axes. Polylysine chains were omitted from the fibril drawing for clarity. Adapted from [126].

4. Conclusion and Outlook

Polypeptide-based block copolymers are an attractive and promising class of block copolymer structures with a proven ability to mimic some of the basic properties of proteins. The most notable difference between peptide-based block copolymers and their fully synthetic and amorphous analogues is their hierarchical solid-state organization. In contrast to most synthetic amorphous block copolymers (which typically exhibit structural order only over a single length scale) peptide-based block copolymers can form hierarchically organized nanoscale structures that cover several different length scales. At the smallest length scale, peptide sequences fold into regular secondary structures, such as α-helices or β-strands. At the next level, peptide α-helices and β-strands can assemble into hexagonal superstructures and β-sheets, respectively. Finally, phase separation between the peptide and synthetic blocks leads to the formation of ordered domains with the largest characteristic length scales. This behavior is very similar to that of proteins for which the primary structure controls the secondary, tertiary and quaternary structures.

Lamellar phase-separated morphologies have been observed for a large number of peptide-based block copolymers. In comparison to conventional, fully amorphous diblock copolymers, these lamellar structures are typically observed over a much broader range of compositions. This behavior in bulk, as in solution, can be easily explained with a consideration of the flat interface generated by the rod-rod packing. In addition to these more conventional morphologies, structural investigation of peptide-based block copolymers has also revealed novel phase-separated structures, previously unknown for fully amorphous diblock copolymers. These observations underscore the fact that the solid-state structure formation of peptide-based block copolymers is not solely dictated by phase separation (as is the case for amorphous diblock copolymers), but is also influenced by other factors such as intra- and intermolecular hydrogen bonding and chain conformation. While much of the early interest in peptide-polymer conjugates was driven by their potential application as membrane materials or for the development of antithrombogenic surfaces, more recent studies reveal that these materials can also possess interesting mechanical properties [61] and can also be used as templates for nanofabrication and devices [94].

Mainly over the last 10 years, different structures have been obtained from solution-based assembly, including spherical aggregates, wormlike micelles, and vesicles. Depending on its hydrophilicity, the polypeptide chain can be found in the core or shell of the structure. In both situations, the ability of the peptide chains to stabilize a well-defined conformation (generally α-helix or β-sheet)—and to reversibly shift this secondary structure in response to stimuli—allows increased control over morphologies and so-called "smart" properties. For instance, the use of charged hydrophilic polypeptide chains (such as PLGA and PLLys) in shell-forming micelles or vesicles allows the formation of stimuli-responsive systems with a higher amplitude and tolerance to the presence of salts as compared to classical polyelectrolytes. Recent work from the groups of Deming [117], Lecommandoux [118], and Hadjichristidis [122] also evidenced that the use of a hydrophobic polypeptide chain in α-helical (or rod-like) conformation drives the self-assembly process into vesicle formation, independent of the copolymer composition and structure (diblock or triblock).

The block copolymer structures currently under development are progressively more complex. They may include stimuli-responsiveness to temperature, pH, or both, possibly in addition to biological function. For instance, Lin *et al.* [101] reported micelles with a poly(propylene oxide) core encased in a mixed shell of poly(L-glutamic acid) and polyethylene glycol. Micellar radii increased at lowered temperatures and decreased with decreased pH. Morphological changes due to pH variation were shown to be directly related to the release rate of encapsulated drugs. Another interesting strategy was reported by Kataoka *et al.* [112] regarding the first semi-permeable vesicles, called PICsomes, that were formed using a charge-driven approach with a PEG-P(Asp)/PEGP(Asp-AP) system in water. In addition, a recent development in this research area consists of employing building blocks with a specific functionality. Deming *et al.* [121] reported highly relevant work on the formation of poly(L-leucine)-*b*-poly(arginine) block copolymers. In this system, the poly(arginine) segment was used both to direct structure for vesicle formation and to provide biofunctionality for efficient intracellular delivery of the vesicles, mimicking the arginine-rich sequences identified as significant in protein-transduction domains.

Though outside the peptide-polymer focus of this chapter, the field of protein-like polymers merits mention as a promising area for future research. Recombinant DNA techniques allow fine-tuning of amino acids within the polymer chain, thereby determining specific biological functions (including properties such as degradation), in addition to imparting intrinsic biocompatibility. The most studied polypeptide sequences thus far exhibit elastin-like structures. For example, Dreher *et al.* [129] and Chaikof *et al.* [130] reported on the temperature-triggered formation of spherical micelles with elastin-like polypeptide (ELP) motifs.

We have no doubt that the published literature in this domain, which has matured dramatically in the last 2–3 years, will continue to exhibit tremendous growth in the next few years. A range of scientific communities, from materials sciences to colloidal sciences, stand to benefit in the near future. The potential impact is profound for biological applications, particularly in the area of drug delivery, but also in biomaterials and tissue engineering.

Materials

AP, 5-aminopentyl; BF, bovine fibrinogen; BSA, bovine serum albumine; DGBE, poly(diethylene glycol bis(3-amino propyl) ether); DMF, dimethylformamide; DTT, dithiothreitol; ELP, elastin-like polypeptide; PAA, poly(acrylic acid); PAELA, poly(2-acryloyloxyethyllactoside); PAI, poly(acetyliminoethylene); PAP, poly(5-aminopentyl); PAsp, poly(β,α-aspartic acid); PB, polybutadiene; PBA, poly(butylacrylate); PBAN, poly(butadiene-*co*-acrylonitrile; PBGlu (poly(γ-benzyl D,L-glutamate); PBLAsp, poly(β-benzyl L-aspartate); PBS, phosphate buffer solution; PBLG, poly(γ-benzyl L-glutamate); PCL, poly(ε-caprolactone); PDMS, polydimethylsiloxane; PECF, pseudoextracellular fluid; PEG, poly(ethylene glycol); PELGlu, poly(γ-ethyl L-glutamate); PELLys, ethylene glycol-modified poly(L-lysine); PEO, poly(ethylene oxide); PEUU, polyetherurethaneurea; PFS, poly(ferrocenyldimethylsilane); PGA, polyglutamic acid; PHF, (benzyl amine)-terminated poly(9,9-dihexylfluorene-2,7-diyl); PHLGln, poly(N^5-hydroxyethyl L-glutamine); PI, polyisoprene; PIC, polyion complex; PLAla, poly(L-alanine); PLArg, poly(L-arginine); PLCys, poly(L-cysteine); PLGA, poly(Lglutamate) or poly(glutamic acid); PLGly, poly(L-glycine); PLLac, poly(L-lactide); PLLeu, poly(L-leucine); PLLys, poly(L-lysine); PLPhe, poly(L-phenylalanine); PLVal, poly(L-valine); PMGlu, poly(γ-methyl D,L-glutamate); PMLG, poly(γ-methyl L-glutamate); PNIPAM, poly(N-isopropylacrylamide); PPG, poly(propylene glycol); PPO, poly(propylene oxide); PS, polystyrene; PSar, polysarcosine; PTHF, polytetrahydrofuran; PTLLys, poly(N^{ε}-trifluoroacetyl L-lysine); PZLLys, poly(ε-benzyloxycarbonyl L-lysine); THF, tetrahydrofuran.

Technical analysis

AFM, atomic force microscopy; ATR-IR, attenuated total reflection infrared; AUC, analytical ultracentrifugation; CD, circular dichroism; DLS, dynamic light scattering; DMA, dynamic mechanical analysis; DSC, differential scanning calorimetry; FTIR, Fourier transform infrared; LCSM, laser confocal scanning microscopy; 1H NMR, proton nuclear magnetic resonance; POM, polarizing optical microscopy; SANS, small angle neutron scattering; SAXS, x-ray scattering; SEM, scanning electron microscopy; SLS, static light scattering; TEM, transmission electron microscope; WAXS, wide-angle x-ray scattering; XPS, x-ray photoelectron spectroscopy.

References

[1] Förster, S., and M. Antonietti, "Amphiphilic Block Copolymers in Structure-Controlled Nanomaterial Hybrids," *Advanced Materials*, Vol. 10, 1998, pp. 195–217.

[2] Bates, F. S., and G. H. Fredrickson, "Block copolymers – Designer soft materials," *Physics Today*, Vol. 52, 1999, pp. 32–39.

[3] Cölfen, H., "Double-hydrophilic block copolymers: Synthesis and application as novel surfactants and crystal growth modifiers," *Macromolecular Rapid Communications*, Vol. 22, 2001, pp. 219–252.

[4] Förster, S., and M. Konrad, "From self-organizing polymers to nano-and biomaterials," *Journal of Materials Chemistry*, Vol. 13, 2003, pp. 2671–2688.

[5] Antonietti, M., and S. Förster, "Vesicles and liposomes: A self-assembly principle beyond lipids," *Advanced Materials*, Vol. 15, 2003, pp. 1323–1333.

[6] Bates, F. S., and G. H. Fredrickson, "Block copolymer thermodynamics: theory and experiment," *Annual Review of Physical Chemistry*, Vol. 41, 1990, pp. 525–557.

[7] Hamley, I. W. *The physics of block copolymers*, Oxford New York Tokyo: Oxford University Press, 1998.

[8] Walther, M., and H. Finkelmann, "Structure Formation of Liquid Crystalline Block Copolymers," *Progress in Polymer Science*, Vol. 21, 1996, pp. 951–980.

[9] Mao, G., and C. K. Ober, "Block copolymers containing liquid crystalline segments," Acta Polymerica, Vol. 48, 1997, 405–422.

[10] Rodriguez-Hernandez, J., F. Checot, Y. Gnanou, and S. Lecommandoux, "Toward 'smart' nano-objects by self-assembly of block copolymers in solution," *Progress in Polymer Science*, Vol. 30, 2005, pp. 691–724.

[11] Perly, B., A. Douy, and B. Gallot, "Block copolymers polybutadiene/poly(benzyl-L-glutamate) and polybutadiene/poly(N^5-hydroxypropylglutamine) preparation and structural study by X-ray and electron microscopy," *Die Makromolekulare Chemie,* Vol. 177, 1976, pp. 2569–2589.

[12] Billot, J.-P., A. Douy, and B. Gallot, "Synthesis and structural study of block copolymers with a hydrophobic polyvinyl block and a hydrophilic polypeptide block: Copolymers polystyrene/poly(L-lysine) and polybutadiene/poly(L-lysine)," *Die Makromolekulare Chemie*, Vol. 177, 1976, pp. 1889–1893.

[13] Billot, J.-P., A. Douy, and B. Gallot, "Preparation, fractionation, and structure of block copolymers polystyrene-poly(carbobenzoxy-L-lysine) and polybutadiene-poly(carbobenzoxy-L-lysine)," *Die Makromolekulare Chemie*, Vol. 178, 1977, pp. 1641–1650.

[14] Douy, A., and B. Gallot, "Structure of AB block copolymers with a polypeptide block: Effect of the chain conformation," *Polymer Engineering and Science*, Vol. 17, 1977, pp. 523–526.

[15] Douy, A., and B. Gallot, "Block copolymers with a polyvinyl and a polypeptide block: factors governing the folding of the polypeptide chains," *Polymer*, Vol. 23, 1982, pp. 1039–1044.

[16] Babin, J., J. Rodríguez-Hernández, S. Lecommandoux, H.-A. Klok, and M.-F. Achard, "Self-assembled nanostructures from peptide–synthetic hybrid block copolymers: Complex, stimuli-responsive rod–coil architectures," *Faraday Discussions*, Vol. 128, 2005, pp. 179–192.

[17] Klok, H.-A., and S. Lecommandoux, "Supramolecular Materials via Block Copolymer Self-Assembly," *Advanced Materials*, Vol. 13, 2001, pp. 1217–1229.

[18] Mori, A., Y. Ito, M. Sisido, and Y. Imanishi, "Interaction of polystyrene/poly(gamma-benzyl L-glutamate) and poly(methyl methacrylate)/poly(gamma-benzyl L-glutamate) block copolymers with plasma proteins and platelets," *Biomaterials*, Vol. 7, 1986, pp. 386–392.

[19] Schlaad, H., H. Kukula, B. Smarsly, M. Antonietti, and T. Pakula, "Solid-state morphologies of linear and bottlebrush-shaped polystyrene–poly(Z-l-lysine) block copolymers," *Polymer*, Vol. 43, 2002, pp. 5321–5328.

[20] Losik, M., S. Kubowicz, B. Smarsly, and H. Schlaad, "Solid-state structure of polypeptide-based rod-coil block copolymers: Folding of helices," *The European Physical Journal E*, Vol. 15, 2004, pp. 407–411.

[21] Schlaad, H., B. Smarsly, and M. Losik, "The Role of Chain-Length Distribution in the Formation of Solid-State Structures of Polypeptide-Based Rod- Coil Block Copolymers," *Macromolecules*, Vol. 37, 2004, pp. 2210–2214.

[22] Ludwigs, S., G. Krausch, G. Reiter, M. Losik, M. Antonietti, and H. Schlaad, "Structure Formation of Polystyrene-block-poly ([gamma]-benzyl l-glutamate) in Thin Films," *Macromolecules*, Vol. 38, 2005, pp. 7532–7535.

[23] Klok, H.-A., J. F. Langenwalter, and S. Lecommandoux, "Self-assembly of peptide-based diblock oligomers" *Macromolecules*, Vol. 33, 2000, pp. 7819–7826.

[24] Lecommandoux, S., M. F. Achard, J. F. Langenwalter, and H.-A. Klok, "Self-Assembly of Rod- Coil Diblock Oligomers Based on [alpha]-Helical Peptides"*Macromolecules*, Vol. 34, 2001, pp. 9100–9111.

[25] Babin, J.; Taton, D.; Brinkmann, M.; Lecommandoux, S. "Synthesis and self-assembly in bulk of linear and mikto-arm star block copolymers based on polystyrene and poly(glutamic acid)", *Macromolecules*, Vol. 41, 2008, pp 1384-1392.

[26] Zhang, G., J. Ma, Y. Li, and Y. Wang, "Synthesis and characterization of poly (L-alanine)-block-poly (ethylene glycol) monomethyl ether as amphiphilic biodegradable co-polymers," *Journal of Biomaterials Science, Polymer Edition*, Vol. 14, 2003, pp. 1389–1400.

[27] Cho, I., J.-B. Kim, H.-J. Jung, "Synthesis and characterization of di-and triblock copolymers of poly (ethylene oxide) and poly (DL-valine-co-DL-leucine)," *Polymer*, Vol. 44, 2003, pp. 5497–5500.

[28] Degée, P., P. Dubois, R. Jérôme, and P. Theyssié, "Synthesis and characterization of biocompatible and biodegradable poly(ε-caprolactone-b- γ -benzylglutamate) diblock copolymers," *Journal of Polymer Science Part A: Polymer Chemistry*, Vol. 31, 1993, pp. 275–278.

[29] Rong, G., M . Deng, C. Deng, Z. Tang, L. Piao, X. Chen, and X. Jing, "Synthesis of Poly(ε-caprolactone)-*b*-Poly(γ-benzyl-l-glutamic acid) Block Copolymer Using Amino Organic Calcium Catalyst,"*Biomacromolecules*, Vol. 4, 2003, pp. 1800–1804.

[30] Caillol, S., S. Lecommandoux, A.-F. Mingotaud, M. Schappacher, A. Soum, N. Bryson, and R. Meyrueix. "Synthesis and Self-Assembly Properties of Peptide- Polylactide Block Copolymers," *Macromolecules*, Vol. 36, 2003, p. 1118–1124.

[31] Papadopoulos, P., G. Floudas, I. Schnell, T. Aliferis, H. Iatrou, and N. Hadjichristidis, "Nanodomain-Induced Chain Folding in Poly(γ-benzyl-l-glutamate)-*b*-polyglycine Diblock Copolymers," *Biomacromolecules*, Vol. 6, 2005, 2352–2361.

[32] Wang, Y., S. Zou, K. T. Kim, I. Manners, and M. A. Winnik, "Organometallic–Polypeptide Block Copolymers: Synthesis and Self-Assembly of Poly(ferrocenyldimethylsilane)-b-Poly(e-benzyloxycarbonyl-l-Lysine)," *Chemistry - A European Journal*, Vol. 14, 2008, pp. 8624–8631

[33] Nakajima, A., T. Hayashi, K. Kugo, and K. Shinoda, "Synthesis and Structural Study of the A-B-A Type Block Copolymer Consisting of Poly(γ-benzyl L-glutamate) as the A Component and Polybutadiene as the B Component," *Macromolecules*, Vol. 12, 1979, pp. 840–843.

[34] Nakajima, A., K. Kugo, and T. Hayashi, "Microheterophase Structure of the A-B-A Type Block Copolymer Consisting of α-Helical Poly(γ-benzyl L-glutamate) as the A Component and Polybutadiene as the B Component," *Macromolecules*, Vol. 12, 1979, pp. 844–848.

[35] Nakajima, A., K. Kugo, and T. Hayashi, "Mechanical Properties and Water Permeability of A–B–A Tri-Block Copolymer Membranes Consisting of Poly(γ-benzyl L-glutamate) as the

A-Component and Polybutadiene as the B-Component," *Polymer Journal*, Vol. 11, 1979, pp. 995–1001.

[36] McKinnon, A. J., and A. V. Tobolsky, "Structure and properties of poly(.gamma.-benzyl-L-glutamate) cast from dimethylformamide," *Journal of Physical Chemistry*, Vol. 72, 1968, pp. 1157–1161.

[37] Hayashi, T., G.-W. Chen, and A. Nakajima, "Synthesis and Structural Study of the A–B–A Tri-Block Copolymer Consisting of Poly(γ-benzyl D,L-glutamate) or Poly(γ-methyl D,L-glutamate) as the A Component and Polybutadiene as the B Component," *Polymer Journal*, Vol. 16, 1984, 739–749.

[38] Gervais, M., A. Douy, B. Gallot, and R. Erre, "X-ray photoelectron spectroscopy of ABA polypeptide-polybutadiene-polypeptide triblock copolymers," *Polymer*, Vol. 29, 1988, pp. 1779–1783.

[39] Kugo, K., T. Hayashi, and A. Nakajima, "Synthesis, Structure, and Mechanical Properties of A-B-A Tri-Block Copolymers Consisting of Poly(ε-N-benzyloxy-carbonyl-L-lysine) as the A Component and Polybutadiene as the B Component," *Polymer Journal*, Vol. 14, 1982, pp. 391–399.

[40] Kugo, K., T. Hayashi, and A. Nakajima, "Studies on Membrane Surfaces of A-B-A Tri-Block Copolymers Consisting of Poly(ε-N-benzyloxycarbonyl-L-lysine) as the A Component and Polybutadiene as the B Component," *Polymer Journal*, Vol. 14, 1982, pp. 401–410.

[41] Kugo, K., M. Murashima, T. Hayashi, and A. Nakajima, "Structure and Properties of Membrane Surfaces of A-B-A Tri-Block Copolymers Consisting of Poly(γ-methyl D,L-glutamate) as the A Component and Polybutadiene as the B Component," *Polymer Journal*, Vol. 15, 1983, pp. 267–277.

[42] Chen, G.-W., T. Hayashi, and A. Nakajima, "Synthesis and Molecular Characterization of A–B–A Tri-Block Copolymers Composed of Poly(γ-ethyl L-glutamate) as the A Component and Polybutadiene as the B Component," *Polymer Journal*, Vol. 13, 1981, pp. 433 – 442.

[43] Sato, H., A. Nakajima, T. Hayashi, G.-W. Chen, and Y. Noishiki, "Microheterophase structure, permeability, and biocompatibility of A-B-A triblock copolymer membranes composed of poly(γ-ethyl L-glutamate) as the A component and polybutadiene as the B component," *Journal of Biomedical Materials Research*, Vol. 19, 1985, pp. 1135–1155.

[44] Yoda, R., S. Komatsuzaki, E. Nakanishi, and T. Hayashi, "Microheterophase structure of A-B-A type block copolymer consisting of poly(γ-benzyl -glutamate) as the a component and polyisoprene as the B component," *European Polymer Journal*, Vol. 31, 1995, pp. 335–339.

[45] Yoda, R., S. Komatsuzaki, and T. Hayashi, "Membrane properties of A-B-A type block copolymer consisting of poly(γ-benzyl- L -glutamate) as the a component and polyisoprene as the B component," *European Polymer Journal*, Vol. 32, 1996, pp. 233–237.

[46] Yoda, R., M. Shimoda, S. Komatsuzaki, T. Hayashi, and T. Nishi, "Morphology study of poly(γ-benzyl L-glutamate) and polyisoprene copolymer by pulsed proton NMR," *European Polymer Journal*, Vol. 33, 1997, pp. 815–821.

[47] Yoda, R., S. Komatsuzaki, and T. Hayashi, "Surface properties and biocompatibility of A-B-A type block copolymer membranes consisting of poly(γ-benzyl-L -glutamate) as the A

component and polyisoprene as the B component," *Biomaterials*, Vol. 16, 1995, pp. 1203–1209.

[48] Yoda, R., S. Komatsuzaki, E. Nakanishi, H. Kawaguchi, and T. Hayashi, "Preparation and properties of A-B-A type block copolymer membranes consisting of poly(N-hydroxypropyl-L-glutamine) as the A component and polyisoprene as the B component," *Biomaterials*, Vol. 15, 1994, pp. 944–949.

[49] Imanishi, Y., M. Tanaka, and C. H. Bamford, "Block copolymerization of vinyl compounds by the terminal - group activation of poly(γ - amino acids) and the characterization of the block copolymers," *International Journal of Biological Macromolecules*, Vol. 7, 1985, pp. 89–99.

[50] Kugo, K., A. Ohji, T. Uno, and J. Nishino, "Synthesis and Conformations of A-B-A Tri-Block Copolymers with Hydrophobic Poly(γ-benzyl l-glutamate) and Hydrophilic Poly(ethylene oxide)," *Polymer Journal*, Vol. 19, 1987, pp. 375 – 381.

[51] Janssen, K., M. Van Beylen, C. Samyn, R. Scherrenberg,and H. Reynaers, "Morphology of ABA triblock copolymers consisting of poly(γ -benzyl L-glutamate) as the A component and polystyrene as the B component," *Die Makromolekulare Chemie*, Vol. 191, 1990, pp. 2777–2785.

[52] Kumaki, T., M. Sisido, and Y. Imanishi, "Antithrombogenicity and oxygen permeability of block and graft copolymers of polydimethylsiloxane and poly(-amino acid)," *Journal of Biomedical Materials Research*, Vol. 19, 1985, pp. 785–811.

[53] Kang, I.-K., Y. Ito, M. Sisido, and Y. Imanishi, "Adsorption of plasma proteins and platelet adhesion on to polydimethylsiloxane/poly(gamma-benzyl L-glutamate) block copolymer films," *iomaterials*, Vol. 9, 1988, pp. 138–144.

[54] Ibarboure, E., E. Papon, and J. Rodriguez-Hernandez, "Nanostructured thermotropic PBLG-PDMS-PBLG block copolymers," *Polymer*, Vol. 48, 2007, pp. 3717–3725.

[55] Kang, I.-K., Y. Ito, M. Sisido, and Y. Imanishi, "Gas permeability of the film of block and graft copolymers of polydimethylsiloxane and poly(gamma-benzyl L-glutamate)," *Biomaterials*, Vol. 9, 1988, pp. 349–355.

[56] Kugo, K., H. Nishioka, and J. Nishino, *Chemistry Express*, Vol. 2, 1987, pp. 21

[57] Cho, C.-S., S.-W. Kim, and T. Komoto, "Synthesis and structural study of an ABA block copolymer consisting of poly(γ-benzyl L-glutamate) as the a block and poly(ethylene oxide) as the B block," *Die Makromolekulare Chemie*, 191, 1990, pp. 981–991.

[58] Floudas, G., P. Papadopoulos, H.-A. Klok, G. W. M. Vandermeulen, and J. Rodríguez-Hernandez, "Hierarchical Self-Assembly of Poly(γ-benzyl-l-glutamate)–Poly(ethylene glycol)–Poly(γ-benzyl-l-glutamate) Rod–Coil–Rod Triblock Copolymers," *Macromolecules*, Vol. 36, 2003, pp. 3673–3683.

[59] Parras, P., V. Castelletto, I. W. Hamley, H.-A. Klok, "Nanostructure formation in poly(γ-benzyl-L-glutamate)–poly(ethylene glycol)–poly(γ-benzyl-L-glutamate) triblock copolymers in the solid state," *Soft Matter*, Vol. 1, 2005, pp. 284–291.

[60] Cho, C. S., B.-W. Jo, J. K. Kwon, and T. Komoto, "Synthesis and structural study of an ABA block copolymer consisting of poly(ε-benzyloxycarbonyl-L-lysine) as the a block and poly(ethylene oxide) as the B block ," *Macromolecular Chemistry and Physics*, Vol. 195, 1994, pp. 2195–2206.

[61] Tanaka, S., A. Ogura, T. Kaneko, Y. Murata, and M. Akashi, "Precise Synthesis of ABA Triblock Copolymers Comprised of Poly(ethylene oxide) and Poly(β-benzyl-L-aspartate):

A Hierarchical Structure Inducing Excellent Elasticity," *Macromolecules*, Vol. 37, 2004, 1370–1377.
[62] Cho, C.-S., S.-W. Kim, Y.-K. Sung, and K.-Y.Kim, "Synthesis and structural study of an ABA block copolymer consisting of poly(γ-benzyl L-glutamate) as the A component and poly(propylene glycol) as the B component," *Die Makromolekulare Chemie*, Vol. 189, 1988, pp. 1505–1510.
[63] Hayashi, T., K. Kugo, and A. Nakajima, *Cont Topics Polym Sci*, Vol. 4, 1984, pp. 685–688.
[64] Ito Y., K. Miyashita, T. Kashiwagi, and Y. Imanishi, "Synthesis and Interactions with Blood of Polyetherure-Thaneurea/Polypeptide Block Copolymers," *Biomaterials, Artificial Cells, & Immobization Biotechnology*, Vol. 21, 1993, pp. 571–580
[65] Barenberg, S., J. M. Anderson, and P. H. Geil, "Structure and Properties of two plastic peptide triblock, ABA, copolymers of poly (-benzyl-l-glutamate), A, and poly (butadiene/acrylonitrile), B," *International Journal of Biological Macromolecules*, Vol. 3, 1981, p. 82–90.
[66] Kong, X., and S. A. Jenekhe, "Block Copolymers Containing Conjugated Polymer and Polypeptide Sequences: Synthesis and Self-Assembly of Electroactive and Photoactive Nanostructures," *Macromolecules*, Vol. 37, 2004, pp. 8180 - 8183.
[67] Rubatat, L., X. Kong, S. A. Jenekhe, J. Ruokolainen, M. Hojeij, and R. Mezzenga, "Self-assembly of polypeptide/π-conjugated polymer/polypeptide triblock copolymers in rod–rod–rod and coil –rod–coil conformations," *Macromolecules*, Vol. 41, 2008, pp. 1846–1852.
[68] Reenders, M., and G. T. Brinke, "Compositional and Orientational Ordering in Rod- Coil Diblock Copolymer Melts," *Macromolecules*, Vol. 35, 2002, pp. 3266–3280.
[69] Harada, A., and K. Kataoka, "Formation of polyion complex micelles in an aqueous milieu from a pair of oppositely-charged block copolymers with poly(ethylene glycol) segments," *Macromolecules*, Vol. 28, 1995, pp. 5294-5299.
[70] Harada, A., and K. Kataoka, "Formation of stable and monodispersive polyion complex micelles in aqueous medium from poly(L-lysine) and poly(ethylene glycol)-poly(aspartic acid) block copolymer," *Journal of Macromolecular Science Pure and Applied Chemistry*, Vol. A34, 1997, pp. 2119-2133.
[71] Harada, A., and K. Kataoka, "Chain length recognition: core-shell supramolecular assembly from oppositely charged block copolymers," *Science*, Vol. 283, 1999, pp. 65–67.
[72] Toyotama, A., Kugimiya, S.-I., Yamanaka, J., and M. Yonese, "Preparation of a novel aggregate like sugar-ball micelle composed of poly(methylglutamate) and poly(ethyleneglycol) modified by lactose and its molecular recognition by lectin," *Chemical and Pharmaceutical Bulletin*, Vol. 49, 2001, pp. 169–172.
[73] Antonietti, M., and S. Förster, "Vesicles and liposomes: A self-assembly principle beyond lipids," *Advanced Materials*, Vol. 15, 2003, pp. 1323–1333.
[74] Cheon, J.-B., Y.-I. Jeong, and C.-S. Cho, "Self-assembly of rigid polypeptides," *Korea Polymer Journal*, Vol. 6, 1998, pp. 34–40.
[75] Cheon, J.-B., Y.-I. Jeong, and C.-S. Cho, "Effects of temperature on diblock copolymer micelle composed of poly (γ-benzyl L-glutamate) and poly(N-isopropylacrylamide)," *Polymer*, Vol. 40, 1999, pp. 2041– 2050.
[76] Discher, D.E., and A. Eisenberg, "Polymer Vesicles," *Science*, Vol. 297, 2002, pp. 967-973.

[77] Li, J., T. Wang, D. Wu, X. Zhang, J. Yan, S. Du, Y. Guo, J. Wang, and A. Zhang, "Stimuli-responsive zwitterionic block copolypeptides: Poly(N-isopropylacrylamide-*block*-poly(lysine-*co*-glutamic acid)," *Biomacrolecules*, Vol. 9, 2008, pp. 2670–2676.

[78] Dong, C.-M., X.-L Sun, K. M. Faucher, R. P. Apkarian, and E. L. Chaikof, E.L., "Synthesis and characterization of glycopolymer-polypeptide triblock copolymers," *Biomacromolecules*, Vol. 5, 2004, pp. 224-231.

[79] Dong, C.-M., K. M. Faucher, and E.L. Chaikof, "Synthesis and properties of biomimetic poly(L-glutamate)-*b*-poly (2-acryloyloxyethyllactoside)-*b*-poly(L-glutamate) triblock copolymers," *Journal of Polymer Science Part A: Polymer Chemistry*, Vol. 42, 2004, pp. 5754-5765.

[80] Dong, C.-M., and E.L. Chaikof, "Self-assembled nanostructures of a biomimetic glycopolymer-polypeptide triblock copolymer," *Colloid and Polymer Science*, Vol. 283, 2005, pp. 1366-1370.

[81] Naka, K., R. Yamashita, T. Nakamura, A. Ohki, and S. Maeda, "Aggregates of peptide-containing block copolymers and their interactions with a lipase in aqueous solution," *Macromolecular Chemistry and Physics*, Vol. 198, 1997, pp. 89-100.

[82] Sinaga, A., T. A. Hatton, and K. C. Tam, "Hydrogen bonded assembly of poly(acrylic acid)-*block*-poly(L-valine) in dilute solutions," *Macromolecules*, Vol. 40, 2007, pp. 9064 – 9073.

[83] Li, T., J. Lin, T. Chen, S. and Zhang, "Polymeric micelles formed by polypeptide graft copolymer and its mixtures with polypeptide block copolymer," *Polymer*, Vol. 47, 2006, pp. 4485-4489.

[84] Lin, J., G. Zhu, X. Zhu, S. Lin, T. Nose, and W. Ding, "Aggregate structure change induced by intramolecular helix–coil transition," *Polymer*, Vol. 49, 2008, pp. 1132-1136.

[85] Nakajima, A., K. Kugo, and T. Hayashi, "Synthesis and structural study of the ABA type block copolymer consisting of poly(γ-benzyl L-glutamate) as the A component and polybutadiene as the B component," *Macromolecules*, Vol. 12, 1979, pp. 840-843.

[86] Hayashi, T. In *Developments in Block Copolymers*, pp. 109, I. Goodman (ed.), London: Elsevier Applied Science Publishers, 1985.

[87] Förster, S., M. Zisenis, E. Wenz, and M. Antonietti, "Micellization of strongly segregated block copolymers," *Journal of Chemical Physics*, Vol. 104, 1996, pp. 9956–9970.

[88] Babin, J., J. Rodríguez-Hernández, S. Lecommandoux, H.-A. Klok, M.-F. Achard, "Self-assembled nanostructures from peptide–synthetic hybrid block copolymers: Complex, stimuli-responsive rod–coil architectures," *Faraday Discussions*, Vol. 128, 2005, pp. 179-192.

[89] Chécot, F., A. Brûlet, J. Oberdisse, Y. Gnanou, O. Mondain-Monval, and S. Lecommandoux, "Structure of polypeptide-based diblock copolymers in solution: Stimuli-responsive vesicles and micelles," Langmuir, 21, 2005, pp. 4308-4315.

[90] Hayashi, T. In *Developments in Block Copolymers*, pp. 109, I. Goodman (ed.) London: Elsevier Applied Science Publishers, 1985.

[91] Rodríguez-Hernández, J., J. Babin, B. Zappone, and S. Lecommandoux, "Preparation of shell cross-linked nano-objects from hybrid-peptide block copolymers," *Biomacromolecules*, Vol. 6, 2005, pp. 2213-2220.

[92] Sun, J., X. Chen, T. Lu, S. Liu, H. Tian, Z. Guo, and X. Jing. "Formation of reversible shell cross-linked micelles from the biodegradable amphiphilic diblock copolymer poly(L-cysteine)-*block*-poly(L-lactide)," *Langmuir*, Vol. 24, 2008, pp. 10099-10106.

[93] Arimura, H., Y. Ohya, and T. Ouchi, "Formation of core-shell type biodegradable polymeric micelles from amphiphilic poly (aspartic acid)-*block*-polylactide diblock copolymer," Biomacromolecules, Vol. 6, 2005, pp. 720-725.

[94] Lecommandoux, S., H.-A. Klok, and H. Schlaad, "Self assembly of linear polypeptide-based diblock copolymers," In Block Copolymers in Nanoscience. Lazzari, M., Liu G, Lecommandoux S. (eds.) Wiley-VCH Verlag; 2006:4.

[95] Lübbert, A., V. Castelletto, I. W. Hamley, H. Nuhn, M. Scholl, L. Bourdillon, C. Wandrey, and H.-A. Klok, "Nonspherical assemblies generated from polystyrene-*b*-poly(L-lysine) polyelectrolyte block copolymers," *Langmuir*, Vol. 21, 2005, pp. 6582-6589.

[96] Gil, G.O., M. Łosik, H. Schlaad, M. Drechsler, and T. Hellweg, "Properties of pH-responsive mixed aggregates of polystyrene-*block*-poly(L-lysine) and nonionic surfactant in solution and adsorbed at a solid surface," *Langmuir*, Vol. 24, 2008, pp. 12823-12828.

[97] Gebhardt, K.E., S. Ahn, G. Venkatachalam, and D. A. Savin, "Rod-sphere transition in polybutadiene–poly(L-lysine) block copolymer assemblies," *Langmuir*, Vol.23, 2007, pp. 2851-2856.

[98] Tian, Z., M. Wang, A. Zhang, and Z. Feng, "Preparation and evaluation of novel amphiphilic glycopeptide block copolymers as carriers for controlled drug release," Polymer, Vol. 49, 2008, pp. 446-454.

[99] Sun, J., C. Deng, X. Chen, H. Yu, H. Tian, J. Sun, and X. Jing, "Self-assembly of polypeptide-containing ABC-type triblock copolymers in aqueous solution and its pH dependence," *Biomacromolecules*, Vol. 8, 2007, pp. 1013-1017.

[100] ten Cate, M.G.J., and H. G. Börner, "Synthesis of ABC-triblock peptide-Polymer Conjugates for the Positioning of Peptide Segments within Block Copolymer Aggregates," *Macromolecular Chemistry Physics*, Vol. 208, 2007, pp. 1437–1446.

[101] Lin, J., J. Zhu, T. Chen, S. Lin, C. Cai, L. Zhang, Y. Zhuang, and X.-S. Wang, "Drug releasing behavior of hybrid micelles containing polypeptide triblock copolymer," *Biomaterials*, Vol. 30, 2009, pp. 108-117.

[102] Agut, W., A. Brûlet, D. Taton, and S. Lecommandoux, "Thermoresponsive micelles from Jeffamine-*b*-poly(L-glutamic acid) double hydrophilic block copolymers," *Langmuir*, Vol. 23, 2007, pp. 11526-11533.

[103] Rao, J., Z. Luo, Z. Ge, H. Liu, and S. Liu, "'Schizophrenic' micellization associated with coil-to-helix transitions based on polypeptide hybrid double hydrophilic rod–coil diblock copolymer," *Biomacromolecules*, Vol. 8, 2007, pp. 3871-3878.

[104] Deng, L., K. Shi, Y. Zhang, H. Wang, J. Zeng, X. Guo, Z. Du, and B. Zhang, "Synthesis of well-defined poly(N-isopropylacrylamide)-*b*-poly(L-glutamic acid) by a versatile approach and micellization," *Journal of Colloid and Interface Science*, Vol. 323, 2008, pp. 169-175.

[105] Kukula, H., H. Schlaad, M. Antonietti, and S. Förster, "The formation of polymer vesicles or 'peptosomes' by polybutadiene-*block*-poly(L-glutamate) s in dilute aqueous solution," *Journal of American Chemical Society*, Vol. 124, 2002, pp. 1658-1663.

[106] Chécot, F., S. Lecommandoux, Y. Gnanou, and H.-A. Klok, "Water-soluble stimuli-responsive vesicles from peptide-based diblock copolymers," *Angewandte Chemie International Edition English*, Vol. 41, 2002, pp. 1340-1343.

[107] Chécot, F., S. Lecommandoux, H.-A Klok, and Y. Gnanou, "From supramolecular polymersomes to stimuli-responsive nano-capsules based on poly(diene-*b*-peptide) diblock copolymers," *The European Physical Journal E*, Vol. 10, 2003, pp. 25-35.

[108] Cai, C., L. Zhang, J. Lin, and L. Wang, "Self-assembly behavior of pH-and thermosensitive amphiphilic triblock copolymers in solution: Experimental studies and self-consistent field theory simulations," *Journal of Physical Chemistry B*, Vol. 112, 2008, pp. 12666-12673.

[109] Huang, C.-J., and F.-C. Chang, "Polypeptide diblock copolymers: Syntheses and properties of poly(N-isopropylacrylamide)-*b*-polylysine," *Macromolecules*, Vol. 41, 2008, pp. 7041-7052.

[110] Gebhardt, K.E., S. Ahn, G. Venkatachalam, and D. Savin, "Role of secondary structure changes on the morphology of polypeptide-based block copolymer vesicles," *Journal of Colloid and Interface Science*, Vol. 317, 2008, pp. 70-76.

[111] Sun, J., Q. Shi, X. Chen, J. Guo, and X. Jing, "Self-assembly of a hydrophobic polypeptide containing a short hydrophilic middle segment: Vesicles to large compound micelles," *Macromolecular Chemistry and Physics*, Vol. 209, 2008, pp. 1129-1136.

[112] Koide, A., A. Kishimura, K. Osada, W.-D. Jang, Y. Yamasaki, and K. Kataoka, "Semipermeable polymer vesicle (PICsome) self-assembled in aqueous medium from a pair of oppositely charged block copolymers: Physiologically stable micro-/nanocontainers of water-soluble macromolecules," *Journal of American Chemical Society*, Vol. 128, 2006, pp. 5988-5989.

[113] Schatz, C., S. Louguet, J.-F. Le Meins, and S. Lecommandoux. "Polysaccharide-*block*-polypeptide copolymer vesicles: towards synthetic viral capsids," *Angewandte Chemie International Edition*, Vol. 48, 2009, pp. 2572-2575.

[114] Doi, T., T. Kinoshita, H. Kamiya, Y. Tsujita, and H. Yoshimizu, "A spontaneous aggregate formed by polypeptide-based amphiphile in water," *Chemistry Letters*, Vol. 29, 2000, pp. 262-263.

[115] Doi, T., T. Kinoshita, H. Kamiya, S. Washizu, Y. Tsujita, and H. Yoshimizu, "Aggregation of Polypeptide-Based Amphiphiles in Water," *Polymer Journal*, Vol. 33, 2001, pp. 160-164.

[116] Rodríguez-Hernández, J., and S. Lecommandoux, "Reversible inside-out micellization of pH-responsive and water-soluble vesicles based on polypeptide diblock copolymers," *Journal of American Chemical Society*, Vol. 127, 2005, pp. 2026-2027.

[117] Bellomo, E.G., M.D. Wyrsta, L. Pakstis, D. J. Pochan, and T. J. Deming, "Stimuli Responsive Polypeptide Vesicles via Conformation Specific Assembly," *Nature Materials*, Vol. 3, 2004, pp. 244-248.

[118] Constancis, A., R. Meyrueix, N. Bryson, S. Huille, J.-M. Grosselin, T. Gulik-Krzywicki, and G. Soula, "Macromolecular colloids of diblock poly(amino acids) that bind insulin," *Journal of Colloid and Interface Science*, Vol. 217, 1999, pp. 357-368.

[119] Holowka, E.P., D. J. Pochan, and T. J. Deming, "Charged Polypeptide Vesicles with Controllable Diameter," *Journal of the American Chemical Society*, Vol. 127, 2005, pp. 12423-12428.

[120] Breedveld, V., A. P. Nowak, J. Sato, T. J. Deming, and D. J. Pine, "Rheology of Block Copolypeptide Solutions: Hydrogels with Tunable Properties," *Macromolecules*, Vol. 37, 2004, pp. 3943-3953.

[121] Holowka, E. P., V. Z. Sun, D. T. Kamei, and T. J. Deming, "Polyarginine segments in block copolypeptides drive both vesicular assembly and intracellular delivery," *Nature Materials*, Vol. 6, 2007, pp. 52-57.

[122] Iatrou, H., H. Frielinghaus, S. Hanski, N. Ferderigos, J. Ruokolainen, O. Ikkala, D. Richter, J. Mays, and N. Hadjichristidis, "Architecturally induced multiresponsive vesicles from well-defined polypeptides. Formation of gene vehicles," *Biomacromolecules*, Vol. 8, 2007, pp. 2173-2181.

[123] Sun, J., X. Chen, C. Deng, H. Yu, Z. Xie, and X. Jing. "Direct Formation of Giant Vesicles from Synthetic Polypeptides," *Langmuir*, Vol. 23, 2007, pp. 8308-8315.

[124] Deming, T. J. "Polypeptide Hydrogels via a Unique Assembly Mechanism," *Soft Matter*, Vol. 1, 2005, p. 28–35.

[125] Nowak A.P., V. Breedveld, L. Pakstis, B. Ozbas, D. J. Pine, D. Pochan, and T. J. Deming, "Rapidly recovering hydrogel scaffolds from self-assembling diblock copolypeptide amphiphiles," *Nature*, Vol. 417, 2002, pp. 424–428.

[126] Breedveld, V., A. P. Nowak, J. Sato, T. J. Deming, and D. J. Pine, "Rheology of Block Copolypeptide Solutions: Hydrogels with Tunable Properties," *Macromolecules*, Vol. 37, 2004, pp. 3943-3953.

[127] Pochan D. J., L. Pakstis, B. Ozbas, A. P. Nowak and T. J. Deming, "SANS and Cryo-TEM Study of Self-Assembled Diblock Copolypeptide Hydrogels with Rich Nano- through Microscale Morphology," *Macromolecules*, Vol. 35, 2002, pp. 5358–5360.

[128] Pakstis L. M., B. Ozbas, K. D. Hales, A. P. Nowak, T. J. Deming, and D. Pochan, "Effect of chemistry and morphology on the biofunctionality of self-assembling diblock copolypeptide hydrogels," *Biomacromolecules*, Vol. 5, 2004, pp. 312–318.

[129] Dreher, M. R., A. J. Simnick, K. Fischer, R. J. Smith, A. Patel A, M. Schmidt, et al. "Temperature triggered self-assembly of polypeptides into multivalent spherical micelles," *Journal of American Chemical Society*, Vol. 130, 2008, pp. 687–94.

[130] Sallach, R. E., M. Wei, N. Biswas N, V. P. Conticello, S. Lecommandoux, R. A. Dluhy, et al. "Micelle density regulated by a reversible switch of protein secondary structure," *Journal of American Chemical Society*, Vol. 128, 2006, pp. 12014–12019.

CHAPTER 2

POLYMER-PEPTIDE CONJUGATE NETWORKS: FORMATION, SWELLING AND DEGRADATION

Donald L. Elbert

Department of Biomedical Engineering and Center for Materials Innovation, Washington University in St. Louis, Campus Box 1097, One Brookings Dr., St. Louis, MO 63130
E-mail: Elbert@biomed.wustl.edu

1. Introduction

The use of synthetic polymers for the fabrication of bioactive hybrid hydrogels has enabled the development of highly advanced scaffolds for tissue engineering. Synthetic water-soluble polymers such as poly(ethylene glycol) (PEG), poly(vinyl alcohol) (PVA), poly(N-(2-hydroxypropylmethacrylamide) (PHMPA), poly(acrylic acid), poly(hydroxyethylmethacrylate) and poly(vinyl pyrrolidone) (PVP) are easily modified with a variety of functional groups, allowing crosslinking and/or modification with biologically active molecules. The history of the synthesis of hydrogels and their use in medicine is extensive and pre-dates the field of tissue engineering [1, 2]. In this chapter, hydrogels based on PEG will be used to illustrate principles governing the formation, swelling and degradation of bioactive hybrid materials. The principles described here may be readily applied to hydrogels synthesized using other hydrophilic polymers.

PEG-based hydrogels may be produced via three major crosslinking strategies: 1) 'vulcanization', 2) physical crosslinking, and 3) chemical crosslinking via end-groups [3]. Many of the reactions that lead to the formation of pure PEG hydrogels are easily adapted to form hybrid hydrogels. Thus, the most commonly used crosslinking chemistries will be described, followed by their application to produce hybrid materials.

2. Vulcanization

Vulcanization of PEG chains is possible by ionizing radiation (e.g. gamma-radiation or electron beam irradiation). Merrill and colleagues described the properties of both PEG and PVA hydrogels crosslinked in this manner

[4-6]. Similar to classic vulcanization used to crosslink natural rubber, the crosslinks may occur at any site along the backbone of the original polymer chains. Although ionizing radiation is not ideal for the production of protein/peptide hydrogels, radiation crosslinked PEG hydrogels have been post-functionalized with monosaccharides to promote cell adhesion [6].

2.1. *Physical crosslinking*

Physical crosslinking may be via multiple non-covalent interactions, for example between heparin and a heparin-binding peptide end-attached to multiarm-PEG [7, 8]. Crosslinks may also be formed between coiled coil-forming proteins and PHMPA copolymers via histidine tags [9]. Further examples of hydrogels formed by interactions of peptides have been recently reviewed [10]. Other biological molecules may be used to physically crosslink PEG. Hybridization between complementary DNA strands may also be used to form hydrogels [11]. The threading interaction between the PEG backbone and the cyclic oligosaccharide cyclodextrin produces hydrogels simply by mixing unmodified star PEG with cyclodextrins [12]. In cases where stoichiometric physical interactions occur, multi-arm PEG may be needed for gel formation, while less specific interactions may allow aggregation between multiple chains such that linear PEG is sufficient for gel formation. Most hybrid self-assembled hydrogels will be of the former type. While physical gelation has many attractive properties such as rapid yet readily reversible *in situ* gelation, stable chemical crosslinks are much more commonly utilized to produce hybrid materials.

2.2. *Chemical crosslinking of PEG — commonly used reactions*

Chemical crosslinking by free-radical polymerization of PEG modified with unsaturated groups may be initiated by thermal or photolytic degradation of an initiator [13]. Chemical groups subject to free-radical polymerization are typically reacted with the hydroxyl groups present at both termini of the linear PEG chain. Each group that is subject to free-radical polymerization has a functionality of two, meaning that each unsaturated group may propagate polymerization of a linear polymer. Linear PEG chains have two hydroxyl termini such that each modified PEG has a total functionality of four. Any molecule with a functionality greater than two may serve as a crosslink site. Thus, PEG molecules with more than one unsaturated group may be used to form crosslinked materials. The most commonly utilized unsaturated groups are acrylates, methacrylates and fumarates [3]. Hydrogels formed with macromonomers such as PEG-diacrylate (PEG-DA) are structurally similar to polyacrylamide gels used in electrophoresis, with PEG-DA serving the same role as N,N'-methylenebisacrylamide. Although free-radical crosslinking is generally used to produce macroscopic hydrogels, micron-scale hydrogels may also be produced and further crosslinked into modular scaffolds [14, 15].

Chemical crosslinking also occurs by reaction of two groups that each have a functionality of one ('step growth'), a characteristic that is distinct from the chain growth mechanism of free-radical crosslinking. Linear PEG modified with groups that participate in step growth reactions may only form high molecular weight linear polymers. For example, Kohn and colleagues formed such high molecular weight PEG polymers by reacting PEG-di(N-hydroxysuccinimide) with both amines on a carboxyl-protected lysine. After deprotection and activation of the multiple lysine carboxyl groups along the backbone of the PEG/lysine polymer, the high functionality chains were crosslinked using a diamine to form a hydrogel [16]. A similar strategy was employed with a linear, thiol-containing PEG-co-2-mercaptosuccinic acid that was then crosslinked with PEG-divinylsulfone [17]. These examples demonstrate that linear PEG must be reacted with molecules of higher functionality to produce hydrogels in a one-step process. The higher functionality molecules in non-hybrid materials may be multifunctional monomers, dendrimers, or star/multiarm polymers [5, 18-20]. Hydrogels produced by reaction of linear unmodified PEG and a small, multifunctional isocyanate were described over twenty years ago by Rempp and colleagues [18]. Lysine-based dendrons may also be reacted with PEG-dialdehyde to produce hydrogels for use as a tissue sealant [20]. The availability of high quality multiarm PEG from the NOF Corporation in the late 1990's enabled a number of new reaction schemes, many of which were first described by Milton Harris and colleagues [21]. Subsequently, other groups demonstrated that nucleophilic substitution between four-arm PEG-active esters and four-arm PEG-thiols or four-arm PEG-amines produced stable hydrogels in a one-step reaction [22, 23]. Multiarm PEG-nucleophiles and PEG-electrophiles also may react via Michael-type additions to form hydrogels. Reaction of multiarm PEG-acrylate and PEG-dithiol produced hydrolytically degradable hydrogels [24], while reaction of multiarm PEG-vinylsulfone and PEG-diamine produced stable materials [25]. Multiarm PEG-thiol may also be oxidized to produce disulfide-bonded hydrogels [26]. Click chemistry has recently been applied to the synthesis of PEG hydrogels. PEG-diacetylene was reacted with tetraazide-modified tetraethylene glycol in the presence of copper sulfate and sodium ascorbate to produce hydrogels that were much less brittle than their photopolymerized counterparts [27]. Bowman, Anseth and colleagues introduced mixed-mode PEG-DA polymerization based on the transfer of free radicals to thiol groups from a photoinitiator [28]. The radical is transferred from the thiol group to acrylate groups. A polyacrylate chain may grow by reaction with another acrylate, with the chain growth terminated by capture of the radical by another thiol. At low thiol:acrylate ratios, chain growth is predominantly observed, and thus is similar to standard free radical polymerization. At high ratios of thiol:acrylate a step growth mechanism is favored, as termination may occur after the formation of a single acrylate dimer. In another type of mixed-mode strategy, Messermith and colleagues produced PEG hydrogels end-modified with L-3,4-dihydroxyphenylalanine (DOPA). DOPA undergoes oxidation to a quinone or semi-quinone that may undergo either free radical polymerization or Michael-type addition [29].

2.3. *Chemical crosslinking to produce hybrid PEG materials*

Similar reactions may be used to couple biologically active molecules into a PEG network, before or after crosslinking [30-33]. The reactions may also be modified such that proteins or peptides are part of the network. By incorporating proteins or peptides in the backbone of the network, hydrogels may become sensitive to the actions of proteases. Enzymatic degradability is most commonly imparted by incorporating peptides between the main PEG chain and the polymerizable end groups [34-36]. Three routes to produce enzymatically degradable PEG hydrogels are shown in Figure 1. One method relies on liquid phase peptide synthesis, with linear PEG serving the same role as a peptide synthesis resin (Figure 1A) [37]. Amino acids of the desired sequence are added one at a time, with precipitation of PEG in diethyl ether at the end of each coupling reaction and deprotection step. Although laborious, the reaction efficiency is quite high. The free amine group present on the final amino acid is acrylated, producing a photopolymerizable, enzymatically degradable precursor. Similar degradable precursors may be synthesized by reacting a bifunctional acrylate-PEG-NHS ester with peptides (Figure 1B). Reacting a bifunctional PEG with amines on both ends of the peptide produces a photopolymerizable, enzymatically degradable precursor [36]. Similarly, reaction of denatured, reduced fibrinogen with an excess of PEG-DA by Michael-type addition leads to a product that may be photopolymerized [38].

Enzymatically degradable peptides may be reacted with PEG via Michael addition in a one step process to produce hydrogels (Figure 1C). Linear PEG-vinylsulfone that is reacted with an enzymatically degradable peptide containing

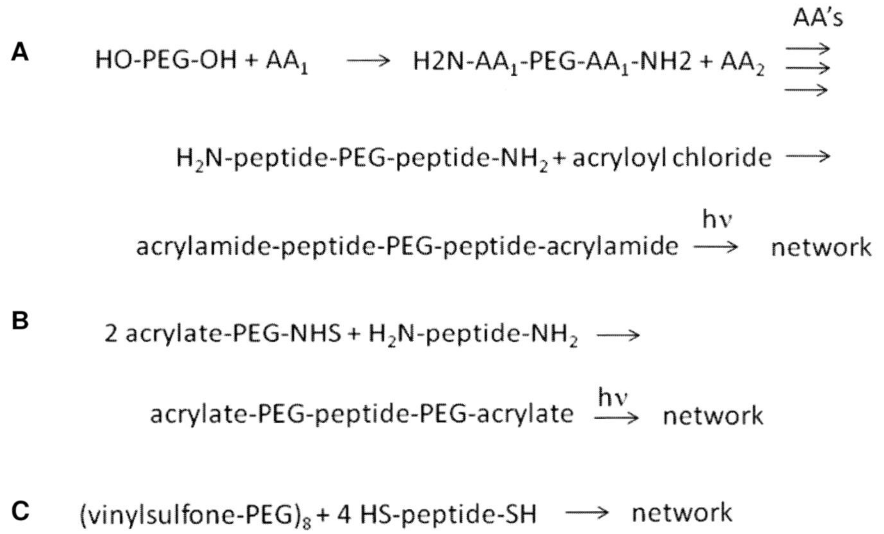

Fig. 1. Three routes to synthesize enzymatically degradable hydrogels. A. An enzymatically degradable peptide is synthesized one amino acid at a time on both ends of a linear PEG. This product is then reacted with acryloyl chloride. The diacrylamide derivative may be photopolymerized to form a network. B. A bifunctional PEG may be reacted with an enzymatically degradable peptide, and the product may be photopolymerized. C. An eight arm PEG-vinylsulfone is reacted with an enzymatically degradable peptide to directly form a network.

three or more cysteine residues forms a degradable hydrogel [39]. Alternatively, multiarm PEG-vinylsulfone may be reacted with an enzymatically degradable peptide containing two cysteines to produce a hydrogel [35]. Reaction of multiarm PEGs may also be performed enzymatically in a two step process. Initially, the hydroxyl groups on multiarm PEG are activated with a good leaving group. This leaving group is reacted with a nucleophilic amine group on a peptide containing either lysines or glutamines. Complementary peptides on different multiarm PEGs are then crosslinked via enzymatic catalysis with transglutaminases [40]. By including sequences in the peptide that are susceptible to specific proteases, enzymatically degradable hydrogels are produced [41]. Instead of using enzymatically degradable peptides, entire proteins can crosslink PEG. Proteins generally have multiple lysine groups that may be used to crosslink activated linear PEG, as first described by Fortier and colleagues [19, 21]. Reaction of multiarm PEG-vinylsulfone with bovine serum albumin or fibrinogen produces biohybrid materials [25]. Proteins may be specifically engineered to contain enzymatically degradable sites, adhesion sites and free cysteines to react with PEG by a Michael-type addition [42]. The enzyme adenylate kinase was engineered to have two free cysteines that were used to crosslink four arm PEG-maleimide. Incubation of the hydrogels with ATP resulted in a 20% contraction of the hydrogels [43].

Mixed mode thiol-acrylate hybrid hydrogels have been formed by reaction of PEG-DA with peptides containing two cysteines. The chain growth nature of the mixed mode reaction may be exploited to eliminate the need for multi-arm PEG [44]. Because the free radicals are generated photochemically, this allows patterning that is not possible with the typical step growth reactions. Click chemistry may also used to produce hydrogels from PEG-tetraazide and an acetylene-modified peptide [45]. Biologically active polysaccharides such as hyaluronan may be modified with thiols and used to crosslink PEG-diacrylate [46]. Alternatively, acrylated hyaluronan may be reacted with enzymatically degradable peptides by Michael-type addition and subsequently photo-polymerized [47]. Other strategies to produce hybrid hydrogels have been recently reviewed [48].

3. Swelling Properties of PEG Hydrogels

Regardless of the physical/chemical route to hydrogel formation, the use of reaction conditions that are well-tolerated by living cells is highly desirable. While this requirement initially limited progress in the field, the list of cell-compatible reactions continues to increase, as illustrated by the numerous crosslinking schemes listed above. However, one principle that does not change with the introduction of new crosslinking schemes is that the swelling and degradation of hydrogels are determined by the balance between the number of crosslinks in the hydrogel and the affinity of water for the constituent polymers. Mechanical and degradation properties of hydrogel scaffolds ultimately determine their clinical relevance and are thus of paramount importance in the design of hybrid biomaterials.

A starting point for understanding the mechanical properties of biohybrid hydrogels is the classic gel swelling model of Flory and Rehner. Building on earlier work in the field of statistical mechanics, Flory and Rehner calculated the probabilities for a polymer chain to adopt a particular end-to-end distance in the presence of solvent and crosslinks [49, 50]. They imagined the assembly of the swollen network from 'network chains' of uniform length. The network chains were postulated to result from the cleavage of much larger original polymer chains. The network chains would first assemble into four-arm molecules that were then reacted to form infinite networks. The postulated four-arm molecule arose from considering two long polymer chains coming together in a vulcanization reaction through a single small crosslinker. The resulting primary network unit would consist of four smaller polymer chains emanating from the point crosslink. Further reaction between the same two long polymer chains would result in the formation of a loop between two polymer segments. Loops do not contribute to the network and are difficult to detect experimentally. Loops were assumed to only occur when crosslinking occurred at low concentrations of polymer and were neglected in the analysis. If two crosslinked chains reacted with a third polymer chain, the resulting structure would be identical to that obtained by an end-linking reaction between two four-armed polymer chains. The length of each arm depends on the locations of the crosslinks, but a uniform molecular weight of the arms (i.e. molecular weight between crosslinks, M_c) may be assumed when averaging over a large number of chains and crosslinks. This greatly simplifies development of the statistical mechanical model.

In the Flory-Rehner model, polymer chains were assumed to crosslink as multiarm polymers to form perfect, infinite polymer networks (i.e. no loops or surface effects). Upon exposure to solvent, the network swelled as the polymer chains interacted with the solvent enthalpically, characterized by the Flory-Huggins interaction parameter χ. The favorability of dispersing the polymer chains into the solvent is balanced by the resistance of the crosslinks introduced mechanical stress in the polymer chains, which Flory and Rehner modeled in a companion publication [51]. The equilibrium amount of solvent incorporated in the network led to an observed volumetric swelling ratio (Q, the ratio of the final volume in excess solvent to the initial volume).

Flory & Rehner assumed that crosslinking occurred within pure polymer without solvent, typical for vulcanization of rubber. The network chains were considered to be near their most favorable conformations in the solid/melt. The crosslinks locked in this favorable structure, such that this was a state of zero stress. Addition of solvent and subsequent swelling deformed the chains from this state. The probability that the chains would spontaneously adopt the deformed state versus the original state dictated the stress on the polymer chains. Flory alluded to the possibility that the polymer chains may be crosslinked in solvent but did not propose a solution until 1950 [49]. If crosslinked in solution, the polymer chains would be in a state of zero stress at the polymer concentration during crosslinking. Thus, removal of solvent may introduce supercoils in the network as the crosslink sites collapse to a greater extent than the polymer chains

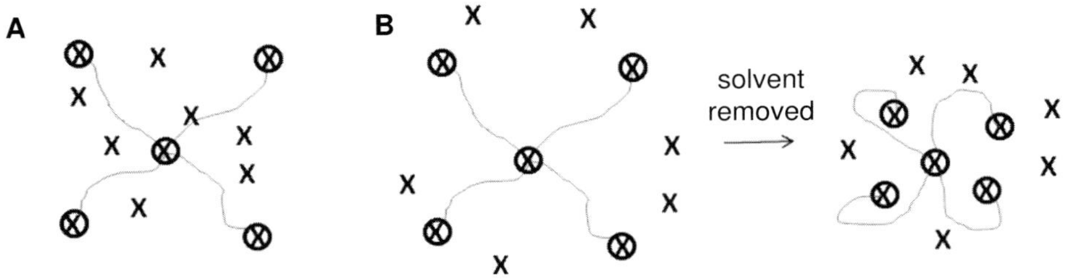

Fig. 2. Location of crosslinks for the reaction of four arm polymers. A single four arm polymer chain is shown (gray lines), with crosslinks represented as X's. The circled X's are the crosslinks associated with this polymer chain. A. With crosslinking in the absence of solvent or at high concentrations of polymer, the polymer chain ends extend past the nearest neighbors. The entanglements contribute to the network mechanical properties. B. With crosslinking in dilute solution, reaction with nearest neighbors is more likely, as well as the formation of non-productive loops (not shown). Upon removal of solvent, the crosslinks sites collapse more than the polymer chains, leading to the formation of supercoils and a highly extensible network. Flory postulated that the concentration of polymer at the crosslinking condition was a state of zero stress and should be used to reference swelling calculations. Adapted from reference 53 (Mark & Erman, 1988).

(Figure 2) [52, 53]. A modified Flory-Rehner equation has been applied to hydrogels by Bray, Peppas and Merrill [4, 54, 55]. The modified form of the Flory-Rehner equation is typically used to describe the swelling of networks of water-soluble polymers crosslinked in aqueous solutions. The equation for hydrogels formed in solution as derived by Flory in 1950 is:

$$-\left[\ln(1-v_{2,s})+v_{2,s}+\chi_{12}(v_{2,s})^2\right]=\frac{1}{Z}\left((v_{2,0})^{\frac{2}{3}}(v_{2,s})^{\frac{1}{3}}-\frac{2v_{2,s}}{f}\right) \quad [1]$$

where $v_{2,s}$ is the volume fraction of polymer in the swollen hydrogel, $v_{2,0}$ is the volume fraction of polymer at the crosslinking state, f is the functionality of the crosslink site (i.e. number of arms emanating from the crosslink site; $f = 4$ for vulcanization), χ_{12} is the Flory-Huggins interaction parameter and Z is the volume ratio of solvent to elastically active chains [49]. Z is related to the volume fraction of polymer by:

$$v_2 = \frac{Z\nu}{n+Z\nu} \quad [2]$$

where ν is the number of elastically active chains in the network and n is the number of solvent molecules. In a perfect network, each arm emanating from a crosslink is an elastically active chain. The volume ratio *Z* is related to more useful parameters by:

$$Z = \frac{M_c}{\rho V_1} = \frac{\bar{v} M_c}{V_1} = \frac{V_0}{\nu V_1} \qquad [3]$$

where M_c is the molecular weight between crosslinks, ρ is the density of polymer, V_1 is the molar volume of solvent (18 mL/mol for water), $\bar{v}$ is the specific volume of the polymer and V_0 is the volume of polymer in the hydrogel. For the case of PEG, these parameters are available from a number of sources [18, 56].

Vulcanization of long polymer chains along the backbone leads to two dangling polymer ends per original chain that do not contribute to the structure of the network. The number of dangling polymer ends can be subtracted from the total number of chains:

$$\nu_e = \nu_0 - 2\nu' \qquad [4]$$

where ν_e is the number of elastically active chains in the network, ν_0 is the total number of chains attached to crosslink sites and ν' is the number of original long polymer chains present prior to crosslinking. For each original long polymer chain, neither end of the chain will be elastically active because the crosslinks do not occur at the terminal groups on the chains except by chance. The number of elastically active chains ν_e may be substituted for ν in equation 3. Furthermore, the ratio ν'/ν_0 is equal to M_c/M_0, where M_0 is the average molecular weight of the original long chains from which the network was formed. Equation 1 corrected for dangling ends is:

$$-\left[\ln(1-v_{2,s}) + v_{2,s} + \chi_{12}(v_{2,s})^2\right] = \frac{V_1}{\bar{v} M_c}\left(1 - \frac{2M_c}{M_0}\right)\left((v_{2,0})^{\frac{2}{3}}(v_{2,s})^{\frac{1}{3}} - \frac{2v_{3,s}}{f}\right) \qquad [5]$$

This form of the equation is only valid for hydrogels formed by vulcanization or an equivalent process. Hydrogels formed by radiation crosslinking of PEG may be readily analyzed using this equation [5]. Radiation crosslinking of star or multiarm PEG leads to a dangling end on each reacted arm and requires a modified version of equation 5 [57].

Free radical crosslinking of multifunctional monomers such as PEG-diacrylate produces network structures that generally resemble crosslinking by vulcanization but with important differences. Polyacrylamide gels used for electrophoresis are a familiar example of this type of network structure. Gels for electrophoresis have low ratios of N,N'-methylenebisacrylamide crosslinker (functionality = 4) compared to acrylamide monomer (functionality = 2). The polyacrylamide backbones that form during crosslinking serve the same role as the backbone chains of vulcanized networks. An N,N'-methylenebisacrylamide crosslinker may join two backbone polyacrylamide chains consisting primarily of acrylamide monomers. The dangling ends of the polyacrylamide chains may be accounted for by using equation 5, with the average molecular weight of the polyacrylamide chains as M_0 and the ratio of acrylamide to N,N'-methylenebisacrylamide used to calculate M_c. Thus, the polyacrylamide gels can be analyzed as vulcanized networks, although crystallization of the crosslinker complicates analysis of these familiar gels [58]. The structure of PEG-DA hydrogels is more difficult to analyze. PEG-DA is frequently mixed with N-vinylpyrrolidone (NVP) in an aqueous solution and photopolymerized [59]. Within these hydrogels, the crosslinker is PEG-DA, which has a high molecular weight and is present in high molar amounts compared to NVP. Similar to polyacrylamide hydrogels, the relevant backbone chain is not the PEG but rather the poly(acrylate-VP) copolymer that forms during crosslinking. The M_c may be calculated using the molar ratio of PEG-DA to VP assuming equal reactivity of the acrylate and vinyl groups, but the molecular weight of the PEG chain is generally so large that treating the PEG-DA as a point crosslink is not appropriate. A simplifying strategy has emerged to analyze PEG-DA hydrogels by the Flory-Rehner equation, in which swelling data are used to calculate an M_c assuming a hypothetical, all-PEG network [59, 60]. This approach assumes that the structure of the hydrogel is identical to that expected for vulcanization of PEG [5]. The calculated 'mesh size' may be compared with the rate of diffusion of proteins of different molecular weights through the hydrogel, with the mesh size calculated from M_c [61]. Hydrogel swelling and thus the calculated mesh sizes are well correlated with the rate of release of proteins of different molecular weights [60].

PEG-DA is often synthesized with degradable polyester linkages between the PEG and the acrylate group, producing hydrolytically degradable hydrogels [13]. The poly(α-hydroxy acid) subunits have a profound effect on the solubility of the PEG, leading to the formation of micelles in aqueous solution [62, 63]. This may lead to high molecular weight poly(acrylate) formed within a single micelle, with crosslinking due to bridging of two micelles by a single PEG. Such a model of crosslinking is supported by small angle neutron scattering studies with PEG-dimethacrylate [64]. Crosslinking without vinyl pyrrolidone is possible and thus the hydrogels are formed with 100% crosslinker [62]. The crosslinked network might be best described by a model that treats each polyacrylate backbone as a high functionality point crosslink. Perhaps an even better model might incorporate the bimodal nature of M_c, using the number average of the smaller M_c along the polyacrylate backbone and a larger M_c equal to the molecular weight of PEG. Polysiloxane gels with bimodal distributions of M_c are tougher than gels with a unimodal distribution [65], which may have some impact on the mechanical properties of PEG-DA hydrogels.

Considering that the Flory-Rehner model was developed with four-arm polymers in mind, application of the model to gels formed by end-linking multiarm PEG may be more straightforward, but some limitations still remain. Flory imagined that each four arm polymer filled its own tetrahedron and the crosslinks occurred with the nearest neighbor. However, most crosslinking reactions occur at relatively high concentrations of PEG. The concentration at which overlap of chains becomes significant is called c* [66]. The c* concentration depends on the molecular weight of the PEG and may be determined by viscometry, e.g. c* for four arm PEG 10,000 in water is about 6%(w/v) [23]. Typical PEG concentrations used for end-crosslinking are 10-20%(w/v) PEG [25, 35]. Thus, multiarm polymer chains may form crosslinks well beyond their nearest neighbors, producing an interdigitated, entangled structure (Figure 2).

The presence of entanglements is intimately linked with the relative success of the Flory-Rehner equation. The equation assumes an affine network, in which the crosslink sites expand relative to one other to the same degree as the expansion of the macroscopic network. An alternative possibility is a phantom network, in which the crosslink sites may fluctuate within the network. The position of the crosslink sites in a phantom network deforms affinely, but the fluctuations about the mean are invariant [67]. The phantom model is more relevant than the former for highly swollen networks, while real networks typically lie somewhere in between the two models [53]. Entanglements increase the stress in a swollen network by restricting fluctuations in the crosslink sites, enhancing agreement with the affine model [67]. Flory later proposed a model of the following form:

$$-\left[\ln(1-v_{2,s})+v_{2,s}+\chi_{12}(v_{2,s})^2\right]=\frac{1+K}{2Z}\left((v_{2,0})^{\frac{2}{3}}(v_{2,s})^{\frac{1}{3}}\right) \qquad [6]$$

where K depends on the average number of crosslink sites within the volume of a single four-arm crosslink site. The 'constrained junction model' was derived from the phantom model accounting for constriction of fluctuations due to entanglements [65, 68, 69].

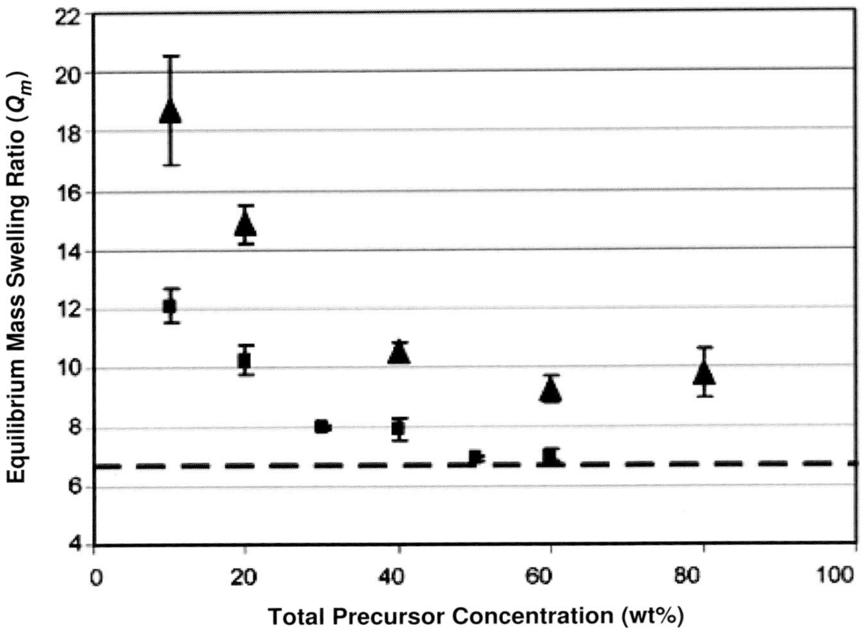

Fig. 3. The concentration of polymer during crosslinking affects subsequent swelling. The swelling ratio predicted by the Flory-Rehner equation for a perfectly crosslinked gel is shown (---). Eight arm PEG crosslinked with linear PEG (squares) approaches an asymptote in swelling at high precursor concentration that is in good agreement with the Flory-Rehner equation. Four arm PEG crosslinked with linear PEG (triangles) also reaches an asymptote in swelling, but this is not predicted by the Flory-Rehner equation. Reprinted from Metters A. & Hubbell J. (2005). Network formation and degradation behavior of hydrogels formed by Michael-type addition reactions. Biomacromolecules 6(1): 290–301. Copyright 2005 American Chemical Society.

The formation of gels in solution also introduces complications. Flory corrected for the effects of solvent present during crosslinking (equation 1), but dilution in solvent also encourages loop formation, i.e. non-productive crosslinks [50]. Accounting for loops is a challenge. For this reason, the model may accurately predict the swelling of a gel as it approaches perfection, but may be inaccurate under many crosslinking conditions, or as the gel degrades by hydrolysis or enzymatic activity. Figure 3 illustrates that gel swelling is strongly affected by the concentration of PEG in the crosslinking reaction [70]. Swelling of the hydrogels was predicted using the Flory-Rehner equation with $v_{2,0} = 1$ (shown as dotted line). As the concentration of polymer in the crosslinking solution increased, swelling reached an asymptotic value. The asymptotic value was accurate for the eight-arm PEG but not for four-arm PEG. End-linked PEG hydrogels thus represent a class of model network that may be used to test the accuracy of various swelling models. However, an extensive literature on model networks already exists, typically using end-linked PDMS [52, 53].

Another limitation of the Flory-Rehner model was the assumption of Gaussian chains, which is not an accurate model for chains less than 100 mers long or for polymers in a better than theta solvent [2]. Although simulations of 1000 Da PEG chains show that the end-to-end distances are reasonably well approximated by a Gaussian function [71], the limitations of the Gaussian chain assumption may be overcome by introducing more accurate probability distribution functions, as demonstrated by Huang, Szleifer and Peppas [72]. Such improved models may lead to more accurate models of swelling, particularly of complex and imperfect gels. However, the success of the Flory-Rehner model results from the cancelation of two large errors of opposite sign such that improvement upon one assumption alone may actually lead to worse results [66].

The stiffness of a hydrogel is related to the swelling in a simple manner. The equation for the elastic modulus of a swollen gel by the affine model for small deformations is:

$$E_{affine} = \frac{3RT}{\bar{v}M_c} v_2^{\frac{1}{3}} \qquad [7]$$

where R is the gas constant and T is the temperature [50, 51]. Thus, the molecular weight between crosslinks may be calculated from measurements of the elastic modulus or equilibrium swelling, with qualitative agreement [35, 73]. Typically, rheometry is used to measure the shear modulus of hydrogels, due to the difficulty in gripping the ends of hydrogel for linear extension. The relationship between the elastic modulus, E_{affine}, and the shear modulus, G_{affine}, is $E_{affine} = 3G_{affine}$. Rheometry is also useful to study gelation, wherein the crossover between the storage modulus G' and the loss modulus G'' may be used to define the gel point. Rheometric characterization is particularly useful for physically crosslinked hydrogels, as changes in temperature, salt concentration, pH and other factors may affect the crosslink density [7].

4. Predicting Degradation of PEG Hydrogels

Predictions of the swelling and degradation of hybrid gels may be important in the design of scaffolds for tissue engineering. The scaffold will presumably be replaced by tissue due to degradation by host cells or proliferation of transplanted cells. During the dissolution process, the scaffold will become weaker as bonds are broken, either by hydrolysis or by cell-derived enzymatic activity. In either case, the timing of degradation is crucial as the scaffold may dissolve before the strength of the new tissue has developed. Mechanical conditioning strengthens a variety of engineered tissues [74, 75], while stem cell differentiation is influenced by mechanical properties [76, 77]. Changes in the scaffold stiffness during degradation may thus complicate production of new tissues.

In a hydrolytically degradable gel, the kinetics of bond breakage may be assumed to be pseudo-first order due to buffering of the aqueous solution. In highly swollen gels, the hydrolysis rate constants may be further assumed to be similar to the solution values or at least constant throughout the degradation process [24, 78]. For enzymatic degradation, Michaelis-Menten kinetics apply [35]. With these assumptions, predicting when a PEG chain is released from the gel is a simple matter of combinatorics. In Figure 4A, four-arm PEG-acrylate is assumed to react with an enzymatically degradable peptide to form a network [70]. The probability that exactly three of the arms are still attached to the network as illustrated on the figure is $\binom{4}{3}p^3(1-p)$ where p is the fraction of peptides that are intact and $\binom{4}{3}$ is a binomial coefficient. Similarly, the amount of PEG released by the hydrogel is given as $(1\text{-}p)^4$. Degradation of more complex hydrogels, such as those formed from the free-radical polymerization of acrylate-oligolactide-PEG-oligolactide-acrylate, may also be predicted in a similar manner (Figure 4B) [78-80]. Calculation of mass loss from the hydrogel as bonds are hydrolyzed relies primarily on accurate values for the bond hydrolysis rate constant, the length of the formed polyacrylate chain and the number of lactide units connecting the PEG to the polyacrylate chain. If bonds are broken on both sides of a PEG, the PEG is released from the gel. An entire polyacrylate chain may similarly be released at high conversions [79]. The fraction of intact bonds decays exponentially over time due to the pseudo-first order nature of the process. Predicted release of PEG or polyacrylate over time may be compared to the experimentally measured mass loss, with excellent agreement [79]. Final dissolution of the hydrogel may be predicted by considering the degradation to be a reverse gelation process. The critical extent of reaction for gelation, p_c, may also be used to predict the time to dissolution for photopolymerized or end-linked hydrogels that are dissolved by hydrolysis or proteases [35, 79].

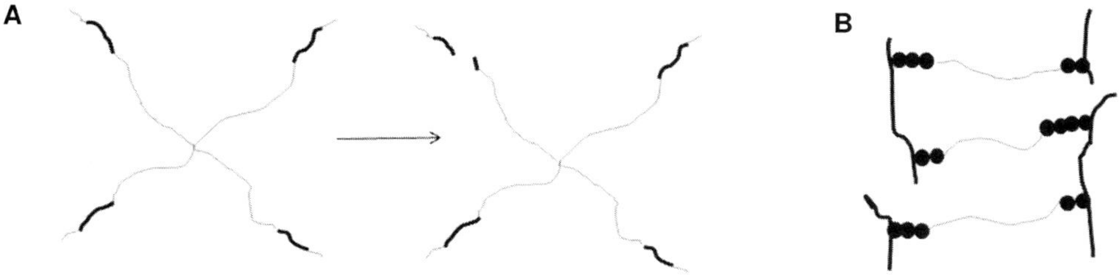

Fig. 4. Degradation of PEG hydrogels. A. Hydrogel formed from reaction of four-arm PEG-vinylsulfone (thin grey lines) with an enzymatically degradable peptide (thick black lines). Even after degradation of one of the four peptide that attach the four-arm PEG to the network, the four-arm PEG is still connected to the network but now has a functionality of three. B. Hydrogel formed by free radical polymerization acrylate-lactide-PEG-actide-acrylate in the presence of PVP. The PEG chains (thin grey lines) are connected through poly(acrylate-co-VP) segments (thick black line). Degradable lactide groups are represented as filled black circles.

Much more challenging is the prediction of swelling during degradation of the hydrogels. Inaccuracies in the Flory-Rehner model may result in poor predictions of the initial swelling of the hydrogels [70]. Network imperfections are also likely present that are not well described and not included in the model. In these cases, a scaling law may be applied to describe swelling from the initial state during the degradation process:

$$Q \propto Z^{\frac{3}{5}} \propto M_c^{\frac{3}{5}} \propto \left(\frac{\nu}{V_0} \right)^{-\frac{3}{5}} \qquad [8]$$

Thus, as the gel degrades, the average molecular weight between crosslinks increases and the density of crosslinks decreases [49]. The scaling law approach is successful in fitting the swelling of degrading acrylate-oligolactide-PEG-oligolactide-acrylate hydrogels to the predicted crosslink density [80]. For end-linked hydrogels, the Flory-Rehner equation may be used directly if it is assumed that the gels only reach a fraction of complete end group reaction, which may vary with gel formation conditions and becomes an adjustable parameter [70]. As hydrogels formed from end-linked multiarm polymers degrade, the number of elastically inactive dangling ends may become quite large, while the presence of multiarm polymer with only two chains linked to the network leads to an increase in M_c (Figure 5). Despite these complexities, analysis using relatively simple combinatorics leads to excellent predictions.

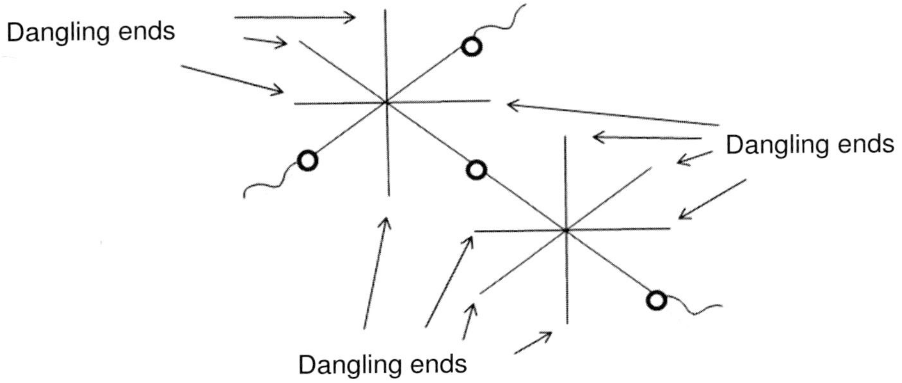

Fig. 5. Degradation of a network made from end-linked eight-arm PEG leads to the formation of dangling ends and an increase in the average molecular weight between crosslinks. Circles represent bonds, wavy lines represent the rest of the network. Dangling ends become numerous just prior to dissolution of the gel. The eight-arm polymer in the lower right only has two arms joined to the network, thus increasing the molecular weight between crosslinks.

Another scaling law is useful to relate the shear modulus to the swelling of network:

$$E_s \propto Q^{-\frac{3v}{3v-1}} \qquad [9]$$

Where E_s is the modulus of the gel in the swollen state and v here is not the number of crosslinks but the universal exponent relating the Flory radius to the size of the polymer chain [81]. In a good solvent, v is 3/5, leading to $E_s \propto Q^{-2.25}$. In a theta solvent or concentrated solution, v is 1/2, leading to $E_s \propto Q^{-3}$. A power law plot of E_s versus Q yielded a slope of -2.8 for photopolymerized PEG hydrogels [82]. A slope close to -3 was found for end-linked hybrid PEG hydrogels [32].

5. Conclusions

Characterization of hybrid hydrogels may be aided by the application of classic statistical mechanical models of rubberlike elasticity and swelling. Although the

Flory-Rehner model is an excellent starting point, more recent theoretical advancements must be considered. The limitations of the mathematical models are numerous, but an extensive literature on model networks may aid in the design of experiments and analysis of the results. In particular, the use of scaling laws may allow predictions of swelling and mechanical properties based on prior results. The introduction of peptides into the backbone of the polymers has to date not presented obstacles to the analysis of the thermodynamics of swelling as polymer networks. Given the compact nature of proteins and the small size of peptides, this approach may prove to be reasonable. The measurements required for the calculation of network properties, i.e. swelling and/or stiffness, are typically already performed in characterizing hybrid hydrogels. Thus, a more detailed analysis of hybrid hydrogels may allow true engineering of the properties of these promising materials.

References

[1] Andrade JD, ed. Hydrogels for Medical and Related Applications. Washington, DC: American Chemical Society 1976.

[2] Peppas NA. Hydrogels in Medicine & Pharmacy. Boca Raton: CRC Press 1986.

[3] Tessmar JK, Göpferich AM. Customized PEG-Derived Copolymers for Tissue-Engineering Applications. Macromolecular Bioscience. 2007;7:23-39.

[4] Bray JC, Merrill EW. Poly(vinyl Alcohol) Hydrogels. Formation by Electron Beam Irradiation of Aqueous Solutions and Subsequent Crystallization. J Appl Polym Sci. 1973;17:3779-94.

[5] Merrill EW, Dennison KA, Sung C. Partitioning and Diffusion of Solutes in Hydrogels of Poly(Ethylene Oxide). Biomaterials. 1993;14:1117-26.

[6] Lopina ST, Wu G, Merrill EW, GriffithCima L. Hepatocyte culture on carbohydrate-modified star polyethylene oxide hydrogels. Biomaterials. 1996;17:559-69.

[7] Seal BL, Panitch A. Physical Polymer Matrices Based on Affinity Interactions between Peptides and Polysaccharides. Biomacromolecules. 2003;4:1572-82.

[8] Yamaguchi N, Kiick KL. Polysaccharide-poly(ethylene glycol) star copolymer as a scaffold for the production of bioactive hydrogels. Biomacromolecules. 2005;6:1921-30.

[9] Wang C, Stewart RJ, KopeCek J. Hybrid hydrogels assembled from synthetic polymers and coiled-coil protein domains. Nature. 1999;397:417-20.

[10] Kopecek J, Yang JY. Peptide-directed self-assembly of hydrogels. Acta Biomater. 2009;5:805-16.

[11] Nagahara S, Matsuda T. Hydrogel formation via hybridization of oligonucleotides derivatized in water-soluble vinyl polymers. Polym Gels Netw. 1996;4:111-27.

[12] Sabadini E, Cosgrove T. Inclusion Complex Formed between Star-Poly(ethylene glycol) and Cyclodextrins. Langmuir. 2003;19:9680-3.

[13] Sawhney AS, Pathak CP, Hubbell JA. Bioerodible Hydrogels Based on Photopolymerized Poly(Ethylene Glycol)-Co-Poly(Alpha-Hydroxy Acid) Diacrylate Macromers. Macromolecules. 1993;26:581-7.

[14] Yeh J, Ling Y, Karp JM, Gantz J, Chandawarkar A, Eng G, et al. Micromolding of shape-controlled, harvestable cell-laden hydrogels. Biomaterials. 2006;27:5391-8.

[15] Du Y, Lo E, Ali S, Khademhosseini A. Directed assembly of cell-laden microgels for fabrication of 3D tissue constructs. Proceedings of the National Academy of Sciences. 2008;105:9522-7.

[16] Nathan A, Zalipsky S, Ertel SI, Agathos SN, Yarmush ML, Kohn J. Copolymers of lysine and polyethylene glycol: a new family of functionalized drug carriers. Bioconjugate chemistry. 1993;4:54-62.

[17] Qiu B, Stefanos S, Ma J, Lalloo A, Perry BA, Leibowitz MJ, et al. A hydrogel prepared by in situ cross-linking of a thiol-containing poly(ethylene glycol)-based copolymer: a new biomaterial for protein drug delivery. Biomaterials. 2003;24:11-8.

[18] Gnanou Y, Hild G, Rempp P. Molecular Structure and Elastic Behavior of Poly(ethylene oxide) Networks Swollen to Equilibrium. Macromolecules. 1987;20:1662-71.

[19] Gayet JC, Fortier G. Drug-Release from New Bioartificial Hydrogel. Artificial Cells Blood Substitutes and Immobilization Biotechnology. 1995;23:605-11.

[20] Wathier M, Jung PJ, Camahan MA, Kim T, Grinstaff MW. Dendritic macromers as in situ polymerizing biomaterials for securing cataract incisions. J Am Chem Soc. 2004;126:12744-5.

[21] Zhao X, Harris JM. Novel degradable poly(ethylene glycol) hydrogels for controlled release of protein. Journal of Pharmaceutical Sciences. 1998;87:1450-8.

[22] Wallace DG, Cruise GM, Rhee WM, Schroeder JA, Prior JJ, Ju J, et al. A tissue sealant based on reactive multifunctional polyethylene glycol. J Biomed Mater Res. 2001;58:545-55.

[23] Sakai T, Matsunaga T, Yamamoto Y, Ito C, Yoshida R, Suzuki S, et al. Design and fabrication of a high-strength hydrogel with ideally homogeneous network structure from tetrahedron-like macromonomers. Macromolecules. 2008;41:5379-84.

[24] Elbert DL, Pratt AB, Lutolf MP, Halstenberg S, Hubbell JA. Protein delivery from materials formed by self-selective conjugate addition reactions. J Control Release. 2001;76:11-25.

[25] Wacker BK, Scott EA, Kaneda MM, Alford SK, Elbert DL. Delivery of sphingosine 1-phosphate from poly(ethylene glycol) hydrogels. Biomacromolecules. 2006;7:1335-43.

[26] Goessl A, Tirelli N, Hubbell JA. A hydrogel system for stimulus-responsive, oxygen-sensitive in situ gelation. Journal of biomaterials science. 2004;15:895-904.

[27] Malkoch M, Vestberg R, Gupta N, Mespouille L, Dubois P, Mason AF, et al. Synthesis of well-defined hydrogel networks using Click chemistry. Chemical Communications. 2006:2774-6.

[28] Cramer NB, Bowman CN. Kinetics of thiol-ene and thiol-acrylate photopolymerizations with real-time Fourier transform infrared. J Polym Sci Pol Chem. 2001;39:3311-9.

[29] Lee BP, Dalsin JL, Messersmith PB. Synthesis and gelation of DOPA-Modified poly(ethylene glycol) hydrogels. Biomacromolecules. 2002;3:1038-47.

[30] Hern DL, Hubbell JA. Incorporation of adhesion peptides into nonadhesive hydrogels useful for tissue resurfacing. J Biomed Mater Res. 1998;39:266-76.

[31] Elbert DL, Hubbell JA. Conjugate Addition Reactions Combined with Free-radical Cross-linking for the Design of Materials for Tissue Engineering. Biomacromolecules. 2001;2:430-41.
[32] Lutolf MP, Hubbell JA. Synthesis and Physicochemical Characterization of End-Linked Poly(ethylene glycol)-co-peptide Hydrogels Formed by Michael-Type Addition. Biomacromolecules. 2003;4:713-22.
[33] Singh N, Bridges AW, Garcia AJ, Lyon LA. Covalent tethering of functional microgel films onto poly(ethylene terephthalate) surfaces. Biomacromolecules. 2007;8:3271-5.
[34] West JL, Hubbell JA. Polymeric biomaterials with degradation sites for proteases involved in cell migration. Macromolecules. 1999;32:241-4.
[35] Lutolf MP, Lauer-Fields JL, Schmoekel HG, Metters AT, Weber FE, Fields GB, et al. Synthetic matrix metalloproteinase-sensitive hydrogels for the conduction of tissue regeneration: engineering cell-invasion characteristics. Proc Natl Acad Sci U S A. 2003;100:5413-8.
[36] Mann BK, Gobin AS, Tsai AT, Schmedlen RH, West JL. Smooth muscle cell growth in photopolymerized hydrogels with cell adhesive and proteolytically degradable domains: synthetic ECM analogs for tissue engineering. Biomaterials. 2001;22:3045-51.
[37] West J, Hubbell J. Polymeric biomaterials with degradation sites for proteases involved in cell migration. Macromolecules. 1999;32:241-4.
[38] Almany L, Seliktar D. Biosynthetic hydrogel scaffolds made from fibrinogen and polyethylene glycol for 3D cell cultures. Biomaterials. 2005;26:2467-77.
[39] Pratt AB, Weber FE, Schmoekel HG, Muller R, Hubbell JA. Synthetic extracellular matrices for in situ tissue engineering. Biotechnology and bioengineering. 2004;86:27-36.
[40] Sperinde JJ, Griffith LG. Control and prediction of gelation kinetics in enzymatically cross-linked poly(ethylene glycol) hydrogels. Macromolecules. 2000;33:5476-80.
[41] Ehrbar M, Rizzi SC, Schoenmakers RG, San Miguel B, Hubbell JA, Weber FE, et al. Biomolecular Hydrogels Formed and Degraded via Site-Specific Enzymatic Reactions. Biomacromolecules. 2007;8:3000-7.
[42] Halstenberg S, Panitch A, Rizzi S, Hall H, Hubbell JA. Biologically engineered protein-graft-poly(ethylene glycol) hydrogels: A cell adhesive and plasm in-degradable biosynthetic material for tissue repair. Biomacromolecules. 2002;3:710-23.
[43] Yuan W, Yang J, Kopecková P, Kopecek J. Smart Hydrogels Containing Adenylate Kinase: Translating Substrate Recognition into Macroscopic Motion. Journal of the American Chemical Society. 2008;130:15760-1.
[44] Salinas CN, Anseth KS. Mixed Mode Thiol-Acrylate Photopolymerizations for the Synthesis of PEG-Peptide Hydrogels. Macromolecules. 2008;41:6019-26.
[45] Polizzotti BD, Fairbanks BD, Anseth KS. Three-dimensional biochemical patterning of click-based composite hydrogels via thiolene photopolymerization. Biomacromolecules. 2008;9:1084-7.
[46] Shu XZ, Liu YC, Palumbo FS, Lu Y, Prestwich GD. In situ crosslinkable hyaluronan hydrogels for tissue engineering. Biomaterials. 2004;25:1339-48.
[47] Khetan S, Katz JS, Burdick JA. Sequential crosslinking to control cellular spreading in 3-dimensional hydrogels. Soft Matter. 2009;5:1601-6.
[48] Jia XQ, Kiick KL. Hybrid Multicomponent Hydrogels for Tissue Engineering. Macromol Biosci. 2009;9:140-56.

[49] Flory PJ. Statistical mechanics of swelling of network structures. J Chem Phys. 1950;18:108-11.

[50] Flory PJ, Rehner J. Statistical Mechanics of Cross-Linked Polymer Networks II. Swelling. J Chem Phys. 1943;11:521-6.

[51] Flory PJ, Rehner J. Statistical Mechanics of Cross-Linked Polymer Networks I. Rubberlike Elasticity. J Chem Phys. 1943;11:512-20.

[52] Urayama K, Kohjiya S. Extensive stretch of polysiloxane network chains with random- and super-coiled conformations. Eur Phys J B. 1998;2:75-8.

[53] Mark JE, Erman B. Rubberlike elasticity: A molecular primer. New York: John Wiley & Sons 1988.

[54] Peppas NA, Merrill EW. Poly(vinyl Alcohol) Hydrogels: Reinforcement of Radiation-Crosslinked Networks by Crystallization. J Polym Sci. 1976;14:441-57.

[55] Peppas NA, Merrill EW. Determination of Interaction Parameter Chi, for Poly(vinyl Alcohol) and Water in Gels Crosslinked from Solutions. J Polym Sci. 1976;14:459-64.

[56] Eliassi A, Modarress H, Mansoori GA. Densities of Poly(ethylene glycol) + Water Mixtures in the 298.15–328.15 K Temperature Range. Journal of Chemical & Engineering Data. 1998;43:719-21.

[57] Cima LG, Lopina ST. Network Structures of Radiation-Cross-Linked Star Polymer Gels. Macromolecules. 1995;28:6787-94.

[58] Hino T, Prausnitz JM. Swelling equilibria for heterogeneous polyacrylamide gels. Journal of Applied Polymer Science. 1996;62:1635-40.

[59] Cruise GM, Scharp DS, Hubbell JA. Characterization of permeability and network structure of interfacially photopolymerized poly(ethylene glycol) diacrylate hydrogels. Biomaterials. 1998;19:1287-94.

[60] Lu S, Anseth KS. Release Behavior of High Molecular Weight Solutes from Poly(ethylene glycol)-Based Degradable Networks. Macromolecules. 2000;33:2509-15.

[61] Peppas NA, Barr-Howell BD. Characterization of the cross-linked structure of hydrogels. In: Peppas NA, ed. *Hydrogels in Medicine and Pharmacy, Vol 1.* Boca Raton: CRC Press 1987:27-56.

[62] Jarrett P, Lalor CB, Chan L, Redmon MP, Hickey AJ. Micelle formation and reaction kinetics of a bioabsorbable polyethylene glycol-oligolactide ABA block copolymer hydrogel. Colloids and Surfaces B-Biointerfaces. 2000;17:11-21.

[63] Vilenchik LZ, Barman S, Pathak CP. Method for studying micelle formation using size exclusion chromatography, light scattering, and UV spectroscopy. Strategies in Size Exclusion Chromatography. 1996;635:328-46.

[64] Lin-Gibson S, Jones RL, Washburn NR, Horkay F. Structure-Property Relationships of Photopolymerizable Poly(ethylene glycol) Dimethacrylate Hydrogels. Macromolecules. 2005;38:2897-902.

[65] Andrady AL, Llorente MA, Mark JE. Model networks of end-linked polydimethylsiloxane chains. VII. Networks designed to demonstrate non-Gaussian effects related to limited chain extensibility. The Journal of Chemical Physics. 1980;72:2282-90.

[66] DeGennes PG. Scaling Concepts in Polymer Physics. Ithaca, NY: Cornell University Press 1979.

[67] Flory PJ. Theory of elasticity of polymer networks. The effect of local constraints on junctions. The Journal of Chemical Physics. 1977;66:5720-9.

[68] Flory PJ. The Elastic Free Energy of Dilation of a Network. Macromolecules. 1979;12:119-22.
[69] Erman B, Flory PJ. Relationships between stress, strain, and molecular constitution of polymer networks. Comparison of theory with experiments. Macromolecules. 1982;15:806-11.
[70] Metters A, Hubbell J. Network formation and degradation behavior of hydrogels formed by Michael-type addition reactions. Biomacromolecules. 2005;6:290-301.
[71] Lee KJ, Eichinger BE. Computer-Simulation of End-Linked Networks - Telechelic Poly(Oxyethylene) Cross-Linked with Plurifunctional Isocyanates. Macromolecules. 1989;22:1441-8.
[72] Huang YB, Szleifer I, Peppas NA. A molecular theory of polymer gels. Macromolecules. 2002;35:1373-80.
[73] Gnanou Y, Hild G, Rempp P. Molecular structure and elastic behavior of poly(ethylene oxide) networks swollen to equilibrium. Macromolecules. 1987;20:1662-71.
[74] Mann BK, West JL. Tissue engineering in the cardiovascular system: Progress toward a tissue engineered heart. The Anatomical Record. 2001;263:367-71.
[75] Wendt D, Jakob M, Martin I. Bioreactor-based engineering of osteochondral grafts: from model systems to tissue manufacturing. Journal of Bioscience and Bioengineering. 2005;100:489-94.
[76] Kraehenbuehl TP, Zammaretti P, Van der Vlies AJ, Schoenmakers RG, Lutolf MP, Jaconi ME, et al. Three-dimensional extracellular matrix-directed cardioprogenitor differentiation: Systematic modulation of a synthetic cell-responsive PEG-hydrogel. Biomaterials. 2008;29:2757-66.
[77] Engler AJ, Griffin MA, Sen S, Bonnemann CG, Sweeney HL, Discher DE. Myotubes differentiate optimally on substrates with tissue-like stiffness: pathological implications for soft or stiff microenvironments. J Cell Biol. 2004;166:877-87.
[78] Metters AT, Anseth KS, Bowman CN. A statistical kinetic model for the bulk degradation of PLA-b- PEG-b-PLA hydrogel networks: Incorporating network non- idealities. J Phys Chem B. 2001;105:8069-76.
[79] Metters AT, Bowman CN, Anseth KS. A statistical kinetic model for the bulk degradation of PLA-b- PEG-b-PLA hydrogel networks. J Phys Chem B. 2000;104:7043-9.
[80] Martens P, Metters AT, Anseth KS, Bowman CN. A generalized bulk-degradation model for hydrogel networks formed from multivinyl cross-linking molecules. J Phys Chem B. 2001;105:5131-8.
[81] Urayama K, Kawamura T, Kohjiya S. Elastic modulus and equilibrium swelling of networks crosslinked by end-linking oligodimethylsiloxane at solution state. The Journal of Chemical Physics. 1996;105:4833-40.
[82] Metters AT, Bowman CN, Anseth KS. Verification of scaling laws for degrading PLA-b-PEG-b-PLA hydrogels. Aiche J. 2001;47:1432-7.

CHAPTER 3

PEPTIDE SELF-ASSEMBLY BIOMATERIALS DESIGN AND APPLICATION

Xiaojun Zhao[1,3*], Songtao Wang[1], Yangrong Lu[2] and Jingqiu Cheng[2]

[1]*Institute for Nanobiomedical Technology and Membrane Biology, West China Hospital, Sichuan University, Chengdu, 610041, P. R. China*

[2]*Key Lab of Transplant Engineering and Immunology, Ministry of Health, West China Hospital, Sichuan University, Chengdu, 610041, Chengdu, P. R. China*

[3]*Center for Biomedical Engineering, NE47-379, Massachusetts Institute of Technology, Cambridge, MA 02139-4307, USA*

[*]*E-mail: xiaojunz@mit.edu*

1. Introduction

Nature has selected and evolved numerous and diverse chemical and molecular structural motifs through billions of years of molecular selection and evolution, these motifs are the basic building blocks of a wide range of sophisticated nanomachines that work at astonishing speed and efficiency with the finest controls, such as directly and efficiently harvesting solar power by converting it into chemical energy that we depend on today, using the same building blocks to faithfully copy and evolve all life forms on Earth, and balancing the complex ecosystem.

Only now we begin to learn from Nature—in its finest molecular details and intricate interactions of numerous fine parts—to go one step further and reap Nature's power to benefit humankind while maintaining its delicate balance. We are learning the basic molecular engineering principles for nano- and micro-fabrication at the exquisitely fine scale through the understanding of molecular self-assembly phenomena.

Molecular self-assembly phenomena are ubiquitous in nature: lattice packing in crystals and minerals, shell and tooth growth, oil droplets forming in water, triple helical collagen structures, and the formation of numerous complex molecular machines (such as ribosomes and light-harvesting photo systems). Molecular self-assembly is not only well-studied chemistry as we know it, but essential in all chemical and life sciences. The key elements in molecular self-assembly are chemical complementarity and structural compatibility through numerous noncovalent weak interactions.

Molecular self-assembly is a rather broad and fast-moving field; it is impossible to fully cover the entire spectrum, so here we will only focus on the self-assembling peptide systems from our own laboratories.

Several self-assembling peptide systems have been developed, ranging from models for studying protein folding and protein conformational diseases, to molecular materials that produce peptide nanofibers, peptide scaffolds, peptide surfactants and peptide ink. These self-assembling peptide systems are rather simple, versatile, economically affordable and easy to produce on a large-scale to spur new industries. These self-assembling peptide systems represent a significant advance in molecular design and engineering for diverse technological innovations. Those who are interested in a broad view are encouraged to consult earlier reviews.

Molecular self-assembly is facilitated through numerous weak, noncovalent bonds—especially hydrogen bonds, ionic bonds (also called electrostatic interactions, or salt bridges as commonly referred to in biology), hydrophobic interactions, van der Waals interactions, and water-mediated hydrogen bonds. Although these weak bonds are rather insignificant in isolation, when combined they not only govern the 3-D structural conformations of all proteins, nucleic acids and other molecules, but also dictate their interaction with other molecules. The water-mediated hydrogen bond is particularly important for living systems since all biological molecules interact with water.

These weak interactions promote the assembly of molecules into units of well-defined and stable hierarchical macroscopic structures. Although each of the bonds or interactions is rather weak, the collective interactions can result in very stable structures and materials. Like hands and gloves, both the size/shape and the correct orientation, i.e. chirality, are important in order to have a complementary and compatible fit.

Molecular self-assembly is ubiquitous in Nature and has recently emerged as a new approach in chemical synthesis, nanotechnology, polymer science, materials and engineering. Molecular self-assembly systems lie at the interface between molecular biology, protein science, biochemistry, polymer science, materials science and engineering. Many self-assembling systems have been developed, and they represent a significant advance in the molecular engineering of simple molecular building blocks useful for a wide range of applications (Figure 1). This field is growing at an accelerating pace, riding on the tide of biotechnology and nanotechnology.

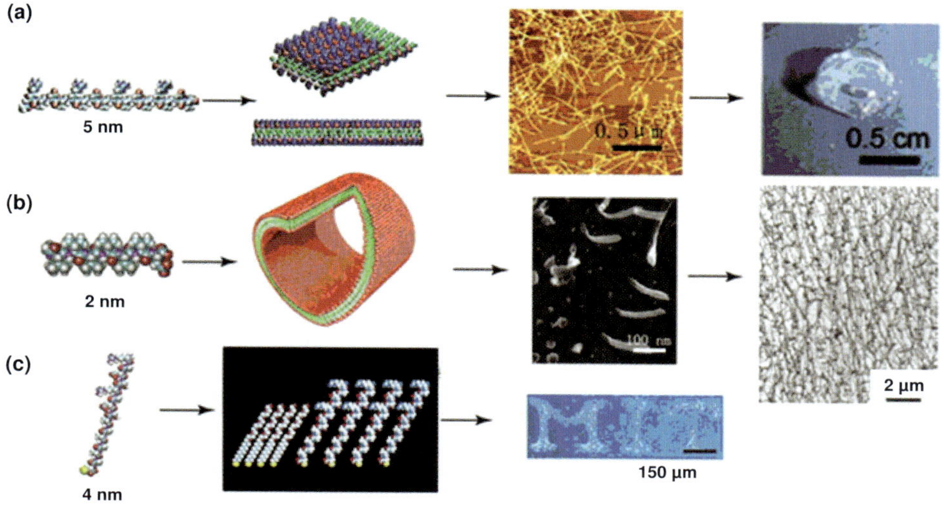

Fig. 1. Fabrication of various peptide materials. (a) Peptide Lego, also called ionic self-complementary peptide has 16 amino acids, ≈5 nm in size, with an alternating polar and nonpolar pattern. They form stable β-strand and β-sheet structures, thus the side chains partition into two sides, one polar and the other nonpolar. They undergo self-assembly to form nanofibers with the nonpolar residues inside (green) and positive (blue) and negative (red) charged residues forming complementary ionic interactions, like a checkerboard. These nanofibers form interwoven matrices that produce a scaffold hydrogel with very high water content, ≈99.5% water. (b) Peptide surfactant/detergent, ≈2 nm in size, has a distinct head group, either positively charged or negatively charged, and a hydrophobic tail consisting of six hydrophobic amino acids. They can self-assemble into nanotubes and nanovesicles with a diameter of ≈30–50 nm. These nanotubes go on to form an inter-connected network, which has been observed in other nanotubes. (c) Peptide ink. This type of peptide has three distinct segments: a functional segment where it interacts with other proteins and cells; a linker segment that is either flexible or stiff and sets the distance from the surface, and an anchor for covalent attachment to the surface. These peptides can be used as ink for an inkjet printer to directly print on a surface, instantly creating any arbitrary pattern, as shown here. Neural cells from rat hippocampal tissue form defined patterns. (Images courtesy of Sawyer Fuller, Neville Sanjana and Shuguang Zhang).

2. Self-assembling Peptides as Structural Building Motifs

In the construction of a building, the doors, windows, and other components can be prefabricated, programmed, and assembled according to the architectural plans. If we shrink the construction units millions or billions of times into nanoscale, we can apply similar principles to construct molecular materials and nanodevices through molecular self-assembly and programmed molecular assembly. Due to space constraints, only four self-assembling construction units are summarized here. They are: peptide Lego that forms well-ordered nanofiber scaffolds for 3D cell culture and for regenerative medicine; peptide surfactants or detergents for drug, protein and gene deliveries as well as for solubilizing and stabilizing membrane proteins; and "peptide ink" for surface biological engineering. These designed construction peptide motifs are structurally simple and versatile for a wide spectrum of applications.

Peptide lego

Molecular-designed peptide Lego, at the nanometer scale, resembles the Lego bricks that have both pegs and holes in a precisely determined organization that can be programmed to assemble in well-formed structures. This class of peptide Lego can spontaneously assemble into well-formed nanostructures at the molecular level. The first member of the peptide Lego was serendipitously discovered from a segment in a left-handed Z-DNA binding protein in yeast and named Zuotin (Zuo means left in Chinese, tin means protein in biology) [1, 2].

This class of designer self-assembling peptides forms β-sheet structures in water and in aqueous solution, thus forming two distinct surfaces: one hydrophilic and the other hydrophobic, like the pegs and holes in Lego bricks. In aqueous solution, the hydrophobic sides shield themselves from water, thus facilitating the peptide to undergo intermolecular self-assembly, similar to what is seen in the case of intramolecular protein folding. The unique structural feature of these ''peptide Lego'' systems is that they form complementary ionic bonds with regular repeats on the hydrophilic surface (Figure 2). The complementary ionic sides have been classified into several modules, i.e. modules I, II, III, IV,

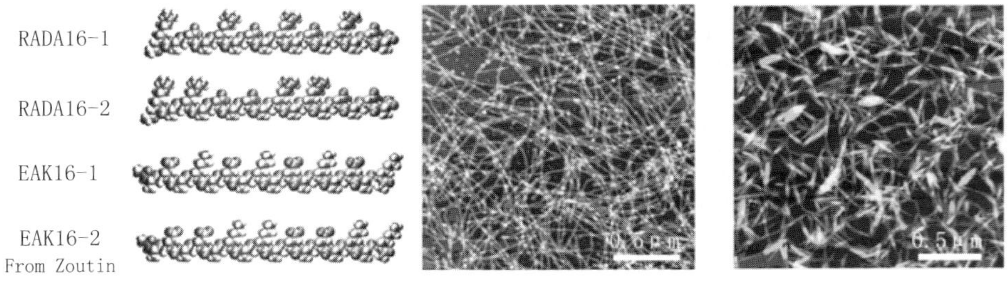

Fig. 2. Molecular models of several self-assembling peptides, RAD16-I, RAD16-II, EAK16-I and EAK16-II. Each molecule is ≈5 nm in length with 8 alanines on one side and 4 negative and 4 positive charged amino acids in an alternating arrangement on the other side. AFM image of RADA16-I nanofiber scaffold (PuraMatrix). Note the nanofiber scale fiber with pores ranging from 5–200 nm, the correct pore size for biomolecular diffusion. This is in contrast to the microfibers of traditional polymer scaffolds, in which the fiber diameter is ≈10-50 micron and the pores range from 10~200 microns.

etc., and mixed modules. This classification is based on the hydrophilic surface of the molecules that have alternating + and – charged amino acid residues, either alternating by 1, 2, 3, 4 and so on. For example, charge arrangements for the different modules are as follows: module I, – + – + – + – +; module II, – – + + – – + +; module III, – – – + + +; and module IV, – – – – + + + +. The charge orientation can also be designed in reverse orientations that yield entirely different molecules with distinct molecular behaviors. These well-defined sequences allow them to undergo ordered self-assembly, resembling some situations found in well-studied polymer assemblies [3, 4].

3. Dynamic Behavior of the Peptide Re-assemblies

The self-assembly process is reversible and dynamic since these peptides are short and simple [5], thus numerous individual peptides can be readily self-organized through weak interactions that include hydrogen bonds, ionic bonds, hydrophobic and *van der Waals* interactions, as well as water-mediated hydrogen-bond formation. These nanofibers can be broken mechanically with sonication. However, they can undergo dynamic re-assembly repeatedly, which

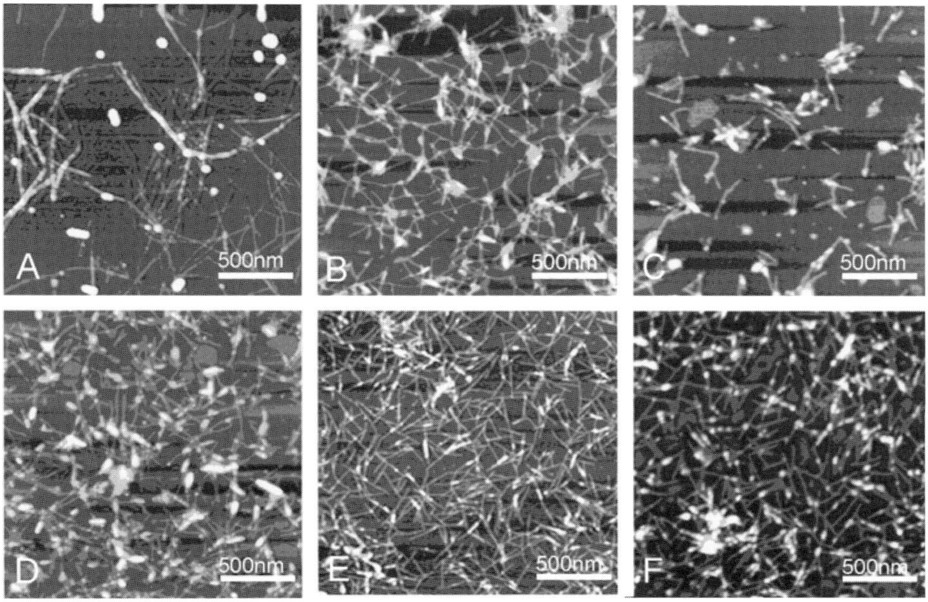

Fig. 3. AFM images of RADA16-I nanofiber at various time points before sonication (*A*) and after sonication (*B-F*). Sample time points, 2 min (*B*), 30 min (*C*), 2h (*D*), 4h (*E*) and 24h (*F*), were taken after sonication. Note the elongation and reassembly of the peptide nanofibers over time.

is similar to a material self-healing process (Figure 3). The driving energy of the assembly in water is not only hydrophobic, but also the arrays of ionic interactions as well as the peptide backbone hydrogen bonds. This phenomenon can be further exploited for the production and fabrication of many such materials.

Unlike processed polymer microfibers in which the fragments of polymers cannot readily undergo reassembly without addition of catalysts or through material processing, the super-marcomolecular self-assembly and re-assembly event uncovered here is likely to be widely spread in many unrelated fibrous biological materials where there are numerous weak interactions involved. Self-assembly and re-assembly are very important properties for the fabrication of novel materials, and it is necessary to fully understand the detailed process in order to design better biological materials.

Table 1. A diversity of cells and tissues cultured on PuraMatrix. These cells include stable cell lines, primarily isolated cells from animals, progenitor, and stem cells.

Animal	**Human**
Mouse fibroblas	Human cervical carcinoma
Chicken embryo fibroblast	Human hepato-cellular carcinoma
Chinese hamster ovary	Human embryonic Kidney
Rat pheochromocytoma	Human epidermal keratinocytes
Rat neural stem cells	Human hepatocytes
Mouse embryonic stem cells	Human osteosarcoma
Mouse cerebellum granule cells	Human neuroblastoma
Bovine osteoblasts	Human foreskin fibroblast
Bovine calf & adult chondrocytes	Human neural stem cells
Bovine endothelial cells	Human embryonic stem (ES) cells
Rat adult liver progenitor cells	
Rat cardiac myocytes	
Rat hippocampal neural tissue slice	
Mouse neural colony stem cells	
Mouse & rat hippocampal cells	
Hamster pancreas cells	

4. Peptide Scaffolds for Three-dimensional (3D) Cell Cultures

In aqueous solutions, the Lego peptides spontaneously assemble to form well-ordered nanofibers of ≈10 nm in diameter and these nanofibers further self-assemble into scaffolds. These nanofiber scaffolds contain an extremely high water content >99.5–99.9% or 1~5 mg/mL (w/v) due to their massive nano-scale pores (~5~200 nm) [6], and have been used as 3D cell-culture scaffolds. These scaffolds closely mimic the porosity and structure of extra-cellular matrices, which allow tissue cells to reside and migrate in a 3D environment. Moreover, molecules, such as growth factors and nutrients diffuse in and out of the scaffold very slowly. These peptide scaffolds have been used for 3D cell culture, controlled cell differentiation, tissue engineering, cancer research, and regenerative medicine applications (Figure 4, Table 1). For example, Zhao's lab has investigated the influence of nanofiber matrix of self-assembling peptide RADA16 in comparison with collagen I and Matrigel on the malignant phenotype of human breast cancer cell MDA-MB-231 in 3D cultures, including the morphology, survival, proliferation rate, migration potential and the effect of these matrices on the malignancy of cancer cells in vivo. Cellular phenomena indicated cells presented different phenotype in 3D matrices in vitro and distinct tumorigenicity in vivo. RADA16 as an extracellular matrix could effectively reduce the malignant phenotype of cells in vitro and in vivo.

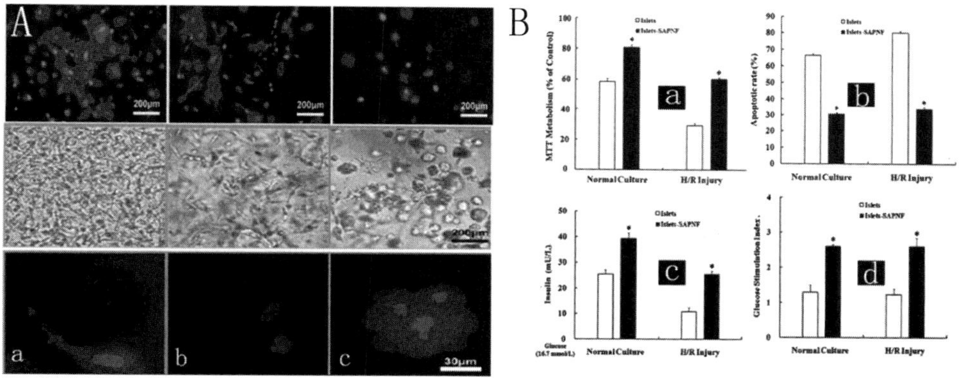

Fig. 4. **(A)** Encapsulation of MDA-MB-231 cells in different matrices. In upper and middle panels: Encapsulation of breast cancer MDA-MB-231 cells in different matrices of collagen I (left row), RADA16 (middle row) and Matrigel (right row) hydrogels using calcein-AM staining for the living cells for three days. These results reveal that cells in collagen I and RADA16 have an elongated form in cell shape while in Matrigel changed to spheroid form. In bottom panel: Light microscope images of cells encapsulated in collagen I, RADA16 and Matrigel matrices for 5 days. F-actin (red) and nuclear (blue) fluorescence images of morphology in collagen I (a), RADA16 (b) and Matrigel (c). 3D cultures were stained for F-actin and nuclei were counterstained with DAPI. In collagen I and RADA16 3D cultures, cells with elongated cell body and projections indicate a spindle-shaped morphology. In Matrigel, cells form colonies with disorganized nuclei which are in sharp contrast with cells in the other two matrices. **(B)** Protective effects of self-assembling peptide nanofiber (SAPNF) on islet viability and apoptosis. The viability of islets was detected by MTT assay *(a)*. The apoptotic rate was determined by flow cytometry *(b)*. And Function improving effects of self-assembling peptide nanofiber (SAPNF) on islets. The actual quantity of insulin released under high-glucose stimulation was detected by radioimmunoassay *(c)*. The glucose stimulation index was calculated as described previously *(d)*. Results are presented as means ± standard deviations ($n = 3$). $^*P < .05$ versus islets alone. (Images courtesy of Yangrong Lu)

One of the Lego peptides, RADA16-I, now called PuraMatrix for its single component purity, is commercially available for research (BD Bioscience). PuraMatrix has been used to culture diverse types of tissue cells including stem and progenitor cells, as well as differentiated cell types and tissues. The examples of cell types cultured in PuraMatrix are listed in Table 1 and the list is rapidly expanding as more and more people use such scaffolds for their research and clinical tissue repair studies[7~10].

5. Peptide Surfactants or Detergents

Inspired from building blocks of cell membranes using Nature's lipids as a guide, a class of peptide surfactants containing hydrophobic tails and hydrophilic heads has been designed by taking advantage of their self-assembly properties in water. These peptides have a hydrophobic tail with various degrees of hydrophobicity and a hydrophilic head, either negatively charged aspartic and glutamic acids or positively charged lysine or histidine. These peptide monomers contain 7~16 amino acid residues and have a hydrophilic head composed of aspartic acid and a tail of hydrophobic amino acids, such as alanine, valine or leucine. The length of each peptide is ≈2 nm, similar to that of biological phospholipids. The length can also be varied by adding more amino acids, one at a time to a desired length as shown in Figure 5.

Although individually these peptide surfactants have completely different composition and sequences, they share a common feature: the hydrophilic heads have 1~2 charged amino acids and the hydrophobic tails have four or more consecutive hydrophobic amino acids. For example, A6K (AAAAAAK), $A6K^{\pm}$ ($AAAAAAK^{\pm}$) peptide has six hydrophobic alanine residues from the N-terminus followed by a positive charged lysines acid residue, thus having two negative charges, one from the side chain and the other from the C-terminus [11, 12]. Likewise, G8DD (GGGGGGGGDD) has eight glycines following by two asparatic acids with three negative charges. By contrast, K2V6 (KKVVVVVV) has two positively charged lysines as the hydrophilic head, followed by six valines as the hydrophobic tail [11~15].

These peptides undergo self-assembly in water to form nanotubes and nanovesicles with an average diameter of 30–50 nm. The tails consisting of alanines and valines produce more homogeneous and stable structures than those of glycines, isoleucine and leucine. This property might be due to their hydrophobic and hydrophilic ratios. Besides, the surfactant peptides were used for molecular modeling and data suggest that they form tubular and vesicle structures. It is interesting that these simple surfactant peptides can produce remarkable complex and dynamic structures by the bottom-up method.

Figure 5 explains how these simple surfactant peptides can form such well-ordered nanotubes and nanovesicles. Although the lipids and these peptides share some similarities, both containing hydrophilic head and a hydrophobic tail, the packing between lipids and peptides is likely to be quite different. In lipids, the hydrophobic tails pack tightly against each other to completely displace water, precluding the formation of hydrogen bonds. In addition to hydrophobic tail packing between the amino acid side chains, surfactant peptides also interact through intermolecular hydrogen bonds along the backbone.

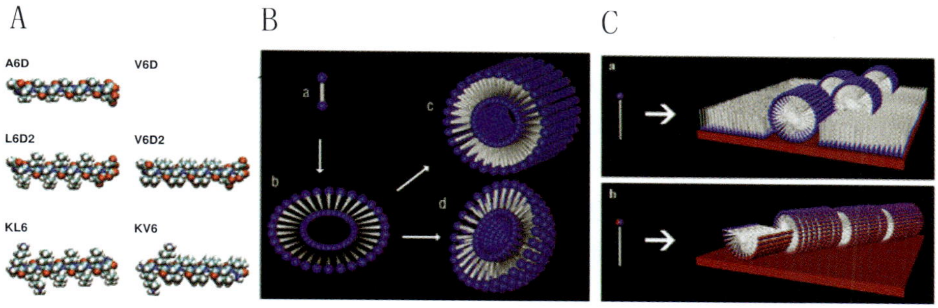

Fig. 5. (A) Molecular models of peptide surfactants/detergents. In left panel: A6D, V6D, V6D2 and L6D2. KL6, KV6. D (Aspartic acid) bears negative charges but A (alanine); V (valine) and L (leucine) constitute the hydrophobic tails with increasing hydrophobicity. Each peptide is ~2–3 nm in length, similar to biological phospholipids. K (lysine) bears positive charges. (B) Proposed molecular model for the self-assembly of the bolaamphiphilic peptide. Single peptide molecules (a) aggregate together in the form of a micelle (b) and self-assemble into cylindrical (c) or spherical (d) nanostructures with a hydrophilic core and surface. (C) Proposed self-assembling mechanism of A6K and A6K± on mica surface. (a) A6K forms cylindrical micelles and monolayer membrane. (b) A6K± only forms cylindrical micelles. White, hydrophobic tail; blue, positive charge; red, negative charge.

6. Peptide Surfactants Stabilize Membrane Proteins

These lipid-like peptide surfactants have been found to be excellent materials not only for solubilizing and stabilizing several diverse membrane proteins and membrane protein complexes but also for crystallizing membrane protein. Although membrane proteins make up approximately one-third of total cellular proteins and carry out some of the most important functions in cells, only several dozen membrane protein structures have been elucidated. This is in striking contrast to ≈25, 000 non-membrane protein structures that have been solved. The main reason for this delay is the difficulty in purifying and crystallizing membrane proteins because removal of lipids from membrane proteins affects protein solubility and conformational stability. Despite a variety of detergents and lipids behaved as surfactants has been used to solubilize, stabilize, purify and crystallize membrane proteins over decades, the way surfactants interact with membrane proteins to influence structure and function and therefore criteria for choosing good surfactants remain largely unknown. This is partly due to the complexity of membrane protein–detergent–lipid interactions and lack of a "magic material" surfactant. Hence the need to develop new membrane compatible material is acute [16, 17].

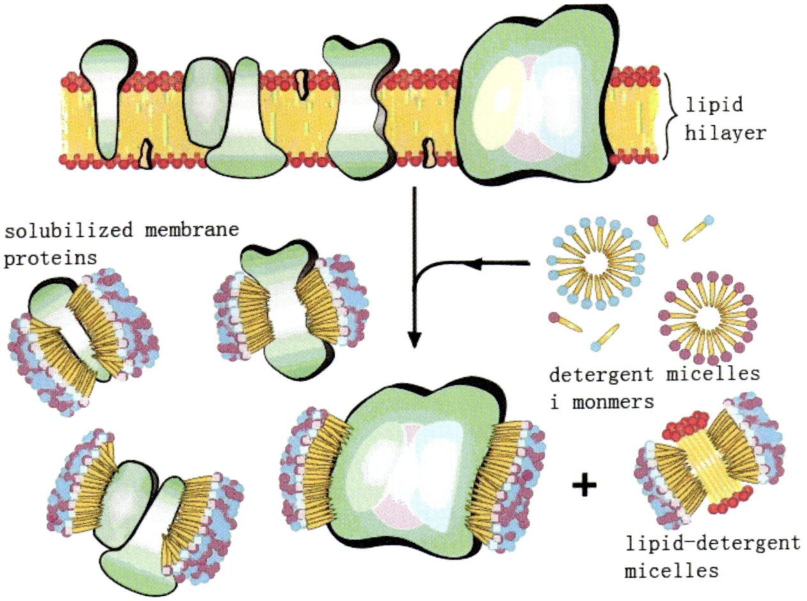

Fig. 6. A proposed model for the lipid-like peptides to stabilize membrane proteins. These simple self-assembling lipid-like peptides have been used to solubilize, stabilize, and crystallize membrane proteins. These peptides have a hydrophilic head and a hydrophobic tail, much like other biological lipids. They use their tail to sequester the hydrophobic part of the membrane proteins, and the hydrophilic heads are exposed to water. Thus, they make membrane proteins soluble and stable outside of their native cellular lipid milieu. These lipid-like peptides are very important for accelerating determination of the high resolutions of molecular structure for challenging membrane proteins.

These simple designer peptide surfactants may now open a new avenue to overcome one of the biggest challenges in biology: not only to obtain large numbers of high-resolution structures of membrane proteins and but also to understand their important biological functions.

Photosynthetic system I (PS-I) is one of the first examples that clearly demonstrate how designer lipid like peptides stabilize membrane protein complexes. It is plausible that peptide surfactants, similar to other surfactants, may directly interact with the hydrophobic domains of membrane proteins (Figure 6). It is likely that numerous peptide surfactant molecules, approximately 2.4 nm in size, like lipids, can effectively surround the hydrophobic trans-membrane domains of membrane proteins, thus sequestering them from directly interacting with water molecules and preventing them from undergoing self-aggregation. Some other membrane proteins, including a membrane protein enzyme glycerol-3- phosphate dehydrogenase and a G-protein coupled receptor bovine rhodopsin, have also been stabilized with various peptide surfactants [14, 18].

Applications of peptide surfactants

This new type of molecularly engineered peptide surfactant may have a broad range of applications, not only as surfactants, but also in growing biotechnologies and emerging nanobiotechnologies. Since the individual molecules can be designed and modified, they can be easily tailored for a variety of uses. These include encapsulation of water-insoluble molecules and delivery of drugs and other biological molecules. Because these surfactants are made of amino acids that can be bio-absorbed and reused, they may also be useful for cosmetic industries where other surfactants are used. Furthermore, for the positively charged peptide surfactants, they can compact and encase negatively charged DNA and RNA for gene delivery. Currently, gene therapy endeavors still lack optimal DNA delivery systems that are highly efficient, non-toxic, non-immunogenic, widely available through commercial synthesis vendors, and simple to produce in large scales. Preliminary experiments using the cationic surfactant peptides presented here showed promise to compact DNA and to deliver DNA into several types of cells in a cell culture. We should not be surprised if many unexpected findings and applications emerge in the coming years.

Peptide ink

Whitesides and coworkers developed a microcontact printing technology that combines semi-conducting industry fabrication, chemistry, and polymer science to produce defined features on a surface down to the micrometer or nanometer scale. Following microcontact printing, a surface can be functionalized with different molecules using a variety of methods, such as covalent coupling, surface adhesion and coordination chemistry [19~21]. Surfaces have now been modified with a variety of chemical compounds. Furthermore peptides and proteins as inks have also been printed onto surfaces. This development has spurred new research into the control of molecular and cellular patterning, cell morphology, and cellular interactions, and fueled new technology development.

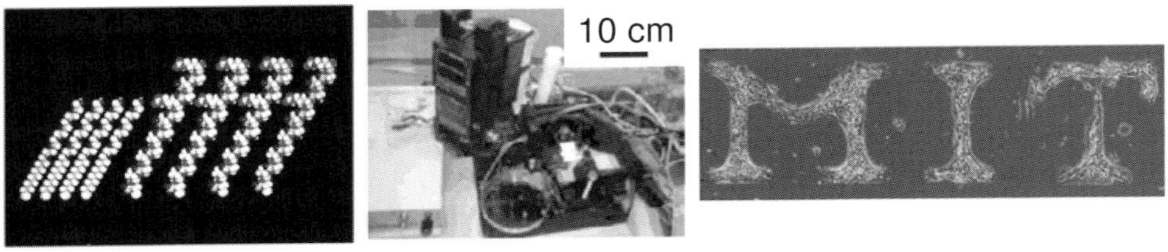

Fig. 7. Molecular structure of peptide ink. This class of peptide ink has three general regions along their lengths: a ligand for specific cell recognition and attachment, a linker for physical separation from the surface, and an anchor for covalent attachment to the surface. Color code: carbon, green; hydrogen, white; oxygen, red; nitrogen, blue; thiol group, yellow. Cells adhere to printed patterns. The protein was printed onto a uniform PEG inhibitory background. Cells adhered to patterns after 8–10 days in culture spelling MIT. (Images courtesy of Shuguang Zhang).

Molecular surface assembly can be targeted to alter the chemical and physical properties of a material's surface. Surface coatings instantly alter a material's texture, color and compatibility with and responsiveness to the environment.

Peptide or protein inks have been directly printed on surfaces to allow adhesion molecules to interact with cells and adhere to the surface (Figure 6). These peptides have three general regions along their lengths: *(i)* a ligand for specific cell recognition and attachment; *(ii)* a linker for physical separation from the surface; and *(iii)* an anchor for covalent attachment to the surface. The ligands might be of the RGD (arginine–glycine–aspartic acid) motif that is known to promote cell adhesion, or other sequences for specific molecular recognition, or specific cell interactions. The linker is usually a string of hydrophobic amino acids such as alanine or valine. The anchor can be a cysteine residue for gold surfaces, asparatic acid linking on amine surfaces, or lysine linking on carboxylic surfaces. This approach could facilitate research into cell–cell communication. Recently, they have moved one step further: using proteins or peptides as ink we have directly microprinted specific features onto the non-adhesive surface of polyethylene glycol to write any arbitrary patterns rapidly without preparing the mask or stamps (Figure 7). The process is similar to using an ink pen for writing here, the printing device is the pen and the biological substances are the inks.

This simple and rapid printing technology allowed us to design arbitrary patterns to address questions in neurobiology that would not have been possible before. Because understanding of correct complex neuronal connections is absolutely central to comprehension of our own consciousness, human beings are always interested in finding ways to further investigate this. However, the neuronal connections are exceedingly complex; we must dissect the complex neuronal connections into smaller and more-manageable units to study them in a well-controlled manner through systematic biomedical engineering approaches. Therefore, nerve fiber guidance and connections can now be studied on special engineered pattern surfaces that are printed with protein and peptide materials. The surface substrate can either be from purified native proteins or from self-assembling peptides containing cell adhesion motifs, prepared through systematic molecular engineering of amino acids. Previous studies have shown that nerve fibers attach and outgrow extensively on the self-assembling peptide matrices [22].

We are interested in studying the nerve fiber navigation on designed pattern surfaces in detail. Studies of nerve fiber navigation and nerve cell connections undoubtedly enhance our general understanding of the fundamental aspects of neuronal activities in the human brain and brain–body connections. It probably also has applications in screening neuropeptides and drugs that stimulate or inhibit nerve fiber navigation and nerve cell connections.

7. Other Peptide Construction Motifs as Material Building Blocks

Zhao and colleagues reported formation nanowebs by using a peptide (AC-PSFCFKFEP-$CONH_2$) that contains only half-sequence ionic self-complementarity together with turn-making residues of Pro at its termini to generate turns or bended structures, creating self-complementary cohesive or staggering ends for knitting and tethering peptide components (Figure 8) [23].

Building blocks beyond natural peptide construction motifs can be used to create peptide materials. Stupp and colleagues have designed a "peptide-amphiphile" derivitized with non-polar hydrocarbon tails, demonstrating that a composite of hydrophobic polymer tails and hydrophilic peptide heads can be used to form nanocyclinders. These molecules have a long alkyl chain at the N-terminus of a peptide that acts as the hydrophobic tail. By incorporating a phosphorylated serine within the peptide ends, calcium or other ions can be attracted, organized, and regulated to facilitate the mineralization of hydroxyapatite. The C-terminus of the peptide can be further functionalized with the RGD motif, thereby promoting cell attachment onto the nanofibers [24, 25].

Reches and Gazit have demonstrated using the shortest peptide, a Phe–Phe dipeptide can form stable nanotubes [26]. By diffusing silver ions into the well-formed tubes, then removing the peptide either enzymatically, chemically, or through heat burning, the silver wire was revealed.

Amyloid protein nanofibers have also been used as scaffold to align gold nanocrystals. Scheibel, Lindquist and colleagues reported that a bioengineered prion-determining (NM) domain of yeast prion protein Sup35 provided a scaffold for fabricating nanowires. They also tested the conducting capability of the resulting wires [27].

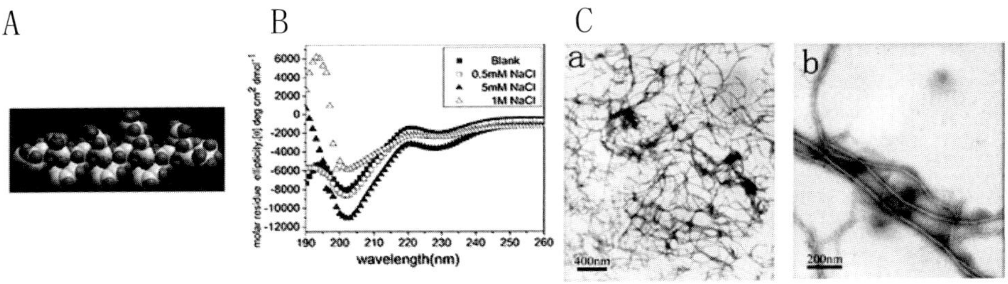

Fig. 8. **(A)** Schematic three-dimensional molecular model of P9: (AC- PSFCFKFEP -NH2). In this conformation, all of the hydrophobic phenylalanine side chains face in one direction, and the residues of serine, asparagine, lysine and glutamic acid side chains face in the other direction to create two distinct faces. The dimensions are about 3.1 nm long, 1.2 nm in height and 0.4 nm thick. **(B)** The far-UV CD spectra of the peptide (200 μM) at different sodium chloride concentrations from 190 to 260 nm were shown: pure water (■); 0.5 mM sodium chloride (□); 5 mM sodium chloride (▲); and 1 M sodium chloride (△). (C) TEM images of the peptide at 0.2 mg/mL. (a) Low magnification (25,000-fold), showing high-density fiber networks. (b) Higher magnification (60,000-fold) for a single fiber, and the fibrils were twisted together to form fibers. The scales are marked in each panel.

Belcher and colleagues take a very different approach, not only to discover but also to fabricate electronic and magnetic materials, departing sharply from the traditional materials process technology [27-30]. Their strategy is to genetically engineer self-assembling bacteriophage so that they can be used to select conducting, semi-conducting and magnetic materials. They have also evolved the phages (and other microbial organisms) for additional material fabrications. This strategy might lead to the discovery of new electronic and magnetic materials.

8. Future Trends in Nanobiotechnology

One of the trends in nanobiotechnology is the development of new biological materials and nanobiotechnologies that in turn often broaden the questions we can address therefore deepening our understanding of seemingly intractable biological phenomena. Self-assembling peptide systems will create a new class of materials at the molecular scale and will have a high impact in many fields. One of the benefits of studying self-assembling peptide systems unexpectedly emerged recently.

We found that the simple peptide surfactant/detergents can be excellent materials for solubilizing and stabilizing membrane proteins that have been extremely difficult to work with a lag far behind in solving their high-resolution structures. In one case, a membrane protein was crystallized in a very short time. This surprising finding encouraged the attention to work on membrane proteins that we would not have considered before.

We believe that application of these simple and versatile molecular self-assembly systems will provide us with new opportunities for studying complex and previously intractable biological phenomena. Molecular engineering through molecular design of self-assembling peptides is an enabling technology that will likely play an increasingly important role in the future of nanobiotechnology and will change our lives in the coming decades. We have encountered many surprises since we started our serendipitous journey of working on various self assembling peptide systems: from developing a class of pure peptide nanofiber scaffolds for 3D tissue culture and for tissue engineering, studying of the model system of protein conformational diseases, and designing peptide or protein inks for surface printing to finding peptide surfactant/detergents that solubilize and stabilize membrane proteins.

Acknowledgements

We would like to thank the members of our laboratories, past and present, for making discoveries and carrying out exciting research. We gratefully acknowledge the support of grants to Xiaojun Zhao from Chinese National '985 Project' of Education Ministry to Sichuan University, Chengdu, China. We would like to thank Prof. Shuguang Zhang for his suggestive discussion and encouragement in this project.

References

[1] Zhang S., Holmes T., Lockshin C., Rich A. Spontaneous assembly of a self-complementary oligopeptide to form a stable macroscopic membrane. *Proc. Natl. Acad. Sci. USA* **1993**, 8, 3334-3338.

[2] Zhang S., Lockshin C., Herbert A., Winter E., Rich A. Zuotin, a putative Z-DNA binding protein in Saccharomyces cerevisiae. *EMBO J.* **1992**, 10, 3787-3796.

[3] Zhang S. Emerging biological materials through molecular self-assembly. *Biotechnol Adv.* **2002**, 5, 321-339.
[4] Zhang S. Fabrication of novel biomaterials through molecular self-assembly. *Nat Biotechnol.* **2003**, 10, 1171-1178.
[5] Yokoi, H., Kinoshita, T., Zhang S. Dynamic reassembly of peptide RADA16 nanofiber scaffold. *Proc. Natl. Acad. Sci. USA* **2005**, 102, 8414-8419.
[6] Davide M., Marini, Wonmuk H., Douglas A., Zhang S., Roger D. Left-Handed Helical Ribbon Intermediates in the Self-Assembly of a β-Sheet Peptide. *Nano Lett.* **2002**, 4, 295–299.
[7] Mi K., Wang G., Liu Z., Feng Z., Huang B., Zhao X. Influence of a Self-Assembling Peptide, RADA16, Compared with Collagen I and Matrigel on the Malignant Phenotype of Human Breast-Cancer Cells in 3D Cultures and in vivo. *Macromol Biosci.* **2009**, 9, 437–443.
[8] Zhang S., Gelainb F., Zhao X. Designer self-assembling peptide nanofiber scaffolds for 3D tissue cell cultures. *Seminars in Cancer Biology* **2005**, 5, 413-440.
[9] Yuan Y., Cong C., Zhang J., Wei L., Li S., Chen Y., Tan W. , Cheng J., Li Y., Zhao X., Lu Y. Self-assembling peptide nanofiber as potential substrates in islet transplantation. *Transplantation Proceedings* **2008**, 40, 2571–2574.
[10] Ellis-Behnke R., Liang Y., You S., Tay D., Zhang S., So K., Schneider G Nano neuro knitting: peptide nanofiber scaffold for brain repair and axon regeneration with functional return of vision. *Proc. Natl. Acad. Sci. USA* **2006**, 103, 5054-5059.
[11] Qiu F., Chen Y., Zhao X., Comparative studies on the self-assembling behaviors of cationic and catanionic surfactant-like peptides. *J Coll & Inter Sci.* **2009**, 1, 477–484.
[12] Qiu F., Chen Y., Tang C., Zhou Q., Wang C., Shi Y., Zhao X. De Novo Design of a Bolaamphiphilic Peptide with Only Natural Amino Acids. *Macromol Biosci.* **2008**, 8, 1053–1059.
[13] Santoso S. Self-assembly of surfactant-like peptides with variable glycine tails to form nanotubes and nanovesicles. *Nano Lett.* **2002**, 2, 687–691.
[14] Zhao X.,Yusuke N.,Philip J., Patrick K., H. Gobind K., Zhang S., Designer short peptide surfactants stabilize G protein-coupled receptor bovine rhodopsin. *Proc. Natl. Acad. Sci. USA* **2006**, 47, 17707-17712.
[15] Von M. Positive charged surfactant-like peptides self-assemble into nanostructures. Langmuir **2003**, 19, 4332–4337.
[16] Wallin E., Von Heinje G. Genome-wide analysis of integral membrane protein from eubacterial, archean and eukaryotic organisms. *Protein Science* **1998**, 7, 1029–1038.
[17] Loll P. Membrane protein structural biology: the high throughput challenge. *J Struct Biol.* **2003**, 142, 144–153.
[18] Patrick K., Zhao X., Michael V., Marc A B., Barry D., Zhang S. Self-Assembling Peptide Detergents Stabilize Isolated Photosystem Ion a Dry Surface for an Extended Time. *PLoS Biol.* **2005**, 7, e230.
[19] Whitesides G., Mathias J., Seto C. Molecular self-assembly and nanochemistry: a chemical strategy for the synthesis of nanostructures. *Science* **1991**, 5036, 1312-1319.
[20] Mrksich M., Whitesides G. Using self-assembled monolayers to understand the interactions of man-made surfaces with proteins and cells. *Annu Rev Biophys Biomol Struct.* **1996**, 25, 55-78.

[21] Chen C., Mrksich M., Huang S., Whitesides G., Ingber D. Geometric control of cell life and death. *Science* **1997**, 5317, 1425-1428.

[22] Holmes T., Sonsoles de L., Su X., Liu G., Alexander R., Zhang S. Extensive neurite outgrowth and active synapse formation on self-assembling peptide scaffolds. *Proc. Natl. Acad. Sci. USA* **2000**, 6, 6728-6733.

[23] Ruan L., Zhang H., Luo H., Liu J., Tang F., Shi Y., Zhao X. Designed amphiphilic peptide forms stable nanoweb, slowly releases encapsulated hydrophobic drug, and accelerates animal hemostasis. *Proc. Natl. Acad. Sci. USA* **2009**, 13, 5105-5110.

[24] Hartgerink J., Beniash E., Stupp S., Self-assembly and mineralization of peptide-amphiphile nanofibers. *Science* **2001**, 5547, 1684-1688.

[25] Hartgerink J., Beniash E., Stupp S. Peptide-amphiphile nanofibers: a versatile scaffold for the preparation of self-assembling materials. *Proc. Natl. Acad. Sci. USA* **2002**, 8, 5133-5138.

[26] Reches M., Gazit E. Casting metal nanowires within discrete self-assembled peptide nanotubes. *Science* **2003**, 5619, 625-627.

[27] Scheibel T., Parthasarathy R., Sawicki G., Lin X., Jaeger H., Lindquist S. Conducting nanowires built by controlled self-assembly of amyloid fibers and selective metal deposition. *Proc. Natl. Acad. Sci. USA* **2003**, 8, 4527-4532.

[28] Whaley S., English D., Hu E., Barbara P., Belcher A.. Selection of peptides with semiconductor binding specificity for directed nanocrystal assembly. Nature **2000**, 6787, 665-668.

[29] Lee S., Mao C., Flynn C., Belcher A. Ordering of quantum dots using genetically engineered viruses. *Science* **2002**, 5569, 892-895.

[30] Mao C., Flynn C., Hayhurst A., Sweeney R., Qi J., Georgiou G., Iverson B, Belcher A. Viral assembly of oriented quantum dot nanowires. *Proc. Natl. Acad. Sci. USA* **2003**, 12, 6946-6951.

CHAPTER 4

MICROPATTERNED POLYMER STRUCTURES FOR CELL AND TISSUE ENGINEERING

Kyung-Jin Jang[1], Deok-Ho Kim[2], Sun-Min Kim[3], Andre Levchenko[2] and Kahp-Yang Suh[1*]

[1]*School of Mechanical and Aerospace Engineering, Seoul National University, Seoul 151-742, Korea*

[2]*Department of Biomedical Engineering and Institute of Cell Engineering, Johns Hopkins University, Baltimore, MD 21218, USA*

[3]*Department of Mechanical Engineering, Inha University, 253 Young Hyun-dong, Nam-gu, Incheon, 402-751, Republic of Korea*

[*]*E-mail: sky4u@snu.ac.kr*

1. Introduction

There has been great interest in the development of engineering methods for generating cellular microenvironments with biomaterials [1, 2]. Living tissues which maintain a well-organized three dimensional architecture *in vivo* are composed of various cell types, embedded in optimized hierarchical structures of extracellular matrix (ECM). ECM is a complex assembly of many fiber proteins forming large-scale matrix with micro/nanoscale topography. Cellular behavior can be affected by ECM in biological and mechanical ways and thus fundamental understanding of this active cell microenvironment is essential in advancing the field of cellular and tissue engineering [3-7]. To better elucidate the mechanism involved in cellular behavior and function in a microenvironment, cells have been cultured on a variety of micropatterned substrates of natural biomaterials or synthetic biomaterials [8]. Through precise control of mechanical, structural and chemical properties of biomaterial surfaces, such platforms can provide an insight into how surface properties and culture conditions can affect cell behavior and function [9-12].

The spatial distribution of each cell type can be controlled via soft lithography based micropatterning techniques, thus allowing one to precisely manipulate cell–cell interactions [9]. Photolithography is the conventional patterning technique of choice, but this lithographic technique has a number of limitations when applied to curved, nonplanar surfaces and involves multiple and cell-unfriendly processing steps to create the patterns. Other approaches, such as microcontact printing, microfluidic channels and elastomeric stencils, are limited in the pattern geometry and size. Simply, the patterned substrate was made of self-assembled monolayers [9, 13], polymers [14], ECM proteins [15, 16], cell adhesive peptides [17], or a combination thereof. In particular, polymeric biomaterials enable the fabrication of regular patterns or topographical features, thereby controlling the size, shape, and spatial position of cells anchored to a surface. In addition, polymers offer several advantages that are not readily available in silicon and glass, including a wide range of material characteristics, biological compatibility, ease of processing and prototyping, and lower costs. Thus, simple fabrication technologies for polymers would find uses in a wide range of biological and biomedical applications including cell and tissue engineering.

In this chapter, we describe the use for micropatterned polymeric biomaterials for application in cell and tissue engineering. This chapter is comprised of two major parts; first, we describe the techniques using polymeric microstructures for cell patterning towards controlling the cellular microenvironment such as cell-protein, cell-cell, and cell-topography interactions; second, we discuss how these techniques can be used to create more complex multicellular architecture for tissue engineering applications using patterned co-culture and microfabricated 3D scaffolds.

2. Applications of Micropatterned Polymers in Cell Patterning

In this section, we introduce a number of microfabrication-based cell patterning techniques using polymeric microstructures such as microcontact printing, stencil-based patterning, microfluidic patterning, and microtopographic patterning.

2.1. *Microcontact printing*

Microcontact printing (μCP), one of the soft lithography techniques, was developed to print self-assembled monolayer, organic polymers, cell adhesion proteins, lipid bilayers, and complex biomolecules. μCP has been successfully applied in generating patterns with contrasted chemical functionalities [18-20] and protein patterns for the study of cell attachment [21, 22]. These techniques are based on the contact-transfer of the desired molecules from an elastomeric stamp (usually polydimethylsiloxane, PDMS) for the pattern in the range of

1–100 μm (Fig. 1A) [18]. Briefly, a PDMS stamp, fabricated in desired pattern (Fig. 1A), is inked with a patterning solution and contacted onto a substrate after solvent evaporation, resulting in a printed pattern. The hydrophobic nature of PDMS can be changed to hydrophilic by exposing it to an oxygen plasma [23]. Some parameters such as humidity, pressure, time, and hydration should be considered to control the surface chemistry and to inhibit the aggregation and denaturation of proteins. μCP eliminates the use of cytotoxic photoresists, sophisticated clean-room facilities and achieves a good balance between simplicity, low cost, reproducibility due to high fidelity, compatibility and high filling efficiency of the treated surface [18, 24, 25].

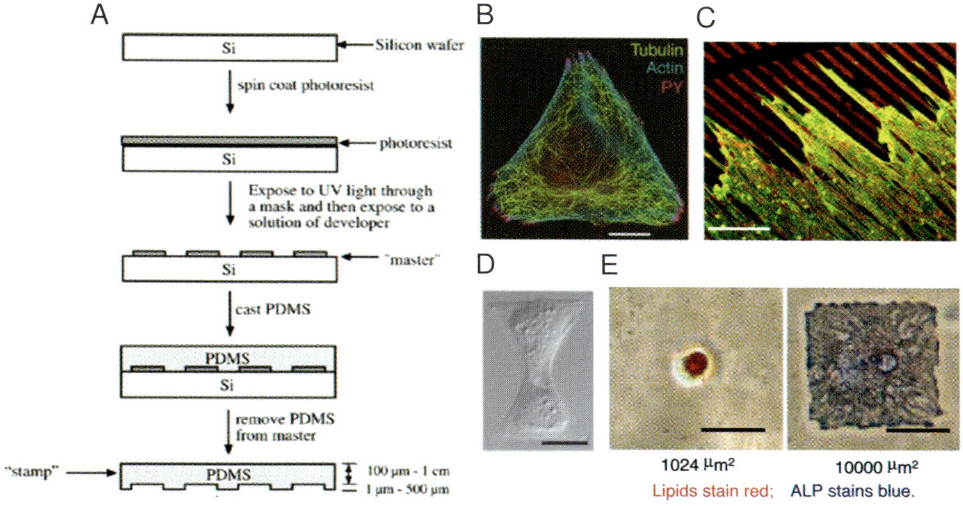

Fig. 1. Microcontact printing for selective adhesion of cells to patterned substrate. (A) A schematic diagram illustrating the generation of a lithographically defined master and a PDMS stamp with replica molding: prepolymer PDMS is cast onto the master, cured and peeled to create a stamp with relief features. Reprinted from [32]. (B) Immunofluorescent staining for phosphotyrosine (PY), microtubules (tubulin) and phalloidin-Alexa488 staining for actin in B16F1 cells on a triangular microetched island. Reprinted from [31]. (C) Cardiac cell sheet was stained for actin (green) and fibronectin (red), and scratched using a thin needle to expose underlying fibronectin lines. Reprinted from [37]. (D) Differential interference contrast images of endothelial cell pairs confined to bow-tie-shaped patterns. Reprinted from [29]. (E) Human mesenchymal stem cells on small and large fibronectin islands after 1 week of culture. The images indicate that cells on the small islands stained for lipids, thus differentiating into adipogenic fate, whereas cells on large islands stained for alkaline phosphatase and differentiated into osteoblasts. Reprinted from [38]. Scale bars: 10 μm in (B), 200 μm in (C), 25 μm in (D), and 50 μm in (E).

μCP has been employed to investigate complex cellular processes such as adhesion, migration, growth, cell-cell interactions and gene expressions by engineering the cellular architecture [26]. For instance, micropatterned substrates fabricated by μCP-based techniques have been successfully used to guide migration of fibroblasts [27], to control growth, apoptosis and differentiation of capillary endothelial cells [9, 28, 29], and to study spreading of melanoma mouse cells [30]. Combined with live-cell time-lapse imaging with fluorescent proteins, μCP-based cell patterning techniques can also enable visualization of dynamic cellular responses in high spatiotemporal resolutions for wide applications in tissue engineering and cell biology. For instance, Kandere-Grzybowska *et al.* [31] recently developed an anisotropic solid microetching (ASOMIC)-based technique that can enable molecular dynamics imaging of living mammalian cells by platinum replica electron microscopy (Fig. 1B). Contact-printed surfaces have been also applied to guide directed neurite growth [32, 33] and neural stem cells [34] to evaluate respiratory activities of HeLa cells [35], to activate mast cells in the presence of lipid bilayers [36], and to create engineered anisotropic cardiac tissue (Fig. 1C) [37].

Furthermore, μCP-based cell patterning approach also allows precise control and measurements of cell-cell interactions on a single cell level. Nelson *et al.* [29] demonstrated the use of μCP technique in controlling pairwise cell interactions using bow-tie-shaped agarose well pattern, allowing to study the role of cell-cell adhesion in cell proliferation (Fig. 1D). Cell culture on micropatterned ECM islands of various sizes enabled by using μCP technique may be also used for directing stem cell fate for tissue engineering applications. For example, McBeath *et al.* [38] recently demonstrated that human mesenchymal stem cells differentiate into osteoblasts when they were allowed to flatten and spread, and into adipocytes when they were kept unspread and round (Fig. 1E).

2.2. *Stencil-based patterning*

Micropatterning using an elastomeric stencil, a thin layer of material containing holes, can be used to pattern cells to the specific regions of a substrate. In the past, metallic stencils, such as nickel stencil [39] and a stainless-steel stencil [40], were used to generate cellular micropatterns. However, metallic stencils do not seal against the substrate and the fabrication of metallic stencils for the scale of single cell is challenging. Microfabricated elastomeric stencils can be sealed on a substrate and physically prevent from contacting with materials to substrate. As selective physical barriers, stencils allow the pattern on a substrate with features of any size or shape and leave the substrate exposed through the holes for adding or removing inorganic materials or living cells. It is easy and simple to use and has great benefits for engineering the cellular microenvironment [22, 26, 41-43]. The stencil can be applied with tweezers or hand repeatedly on cell culture surface, peeled off after cell attachment, applied to all cell types and substrates, and reused after an ethanol washing.

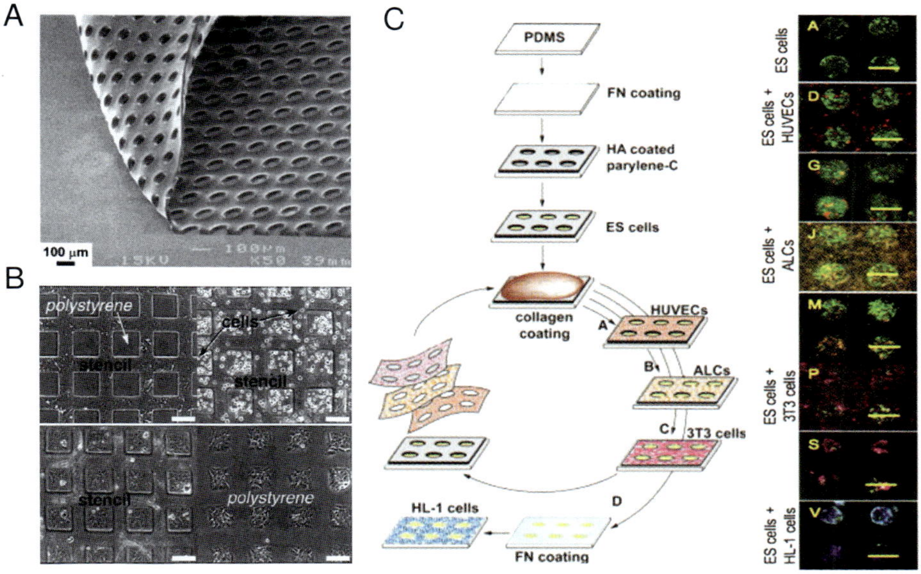

Fig. 2. Microfabricated stencil-based cell patterning. (A) SEM image of a 50 μm thick PDMS stencil with 100 μm holes. Reprinted from [32]. (B) Microscopic image of patterned cells to a polystyrene surface using a ~100 μm thick stencil containing 140 μm side squares separated by 100 μm. Reprinted from [41]. (C) A schematic representation of the dynamic co-culture system using HA-coated parylene-C stencils (left) and fluorescent images of the formation of dynamic co-cultures (right). Reprinted from [46].

Using these stencils, micropatterns of proteins and cells were generated for various biological and biomedical applications. For example, Ostuni *et al.* generated cell pattern onto the various surfaces to study cell spreading using a PDMS stencil-based lift-off methods [42]. Folch *et al.* described two fabrication methods to make elastomeric membrane with PDMS to allow for making living cell microarrays using stencil with controlled height and shape of the holes (Fig. 2B) [41] Recently, microfabricated parylene membranes, which are robust and biocompatible, were also used for micropatterning method to pattern cells and proteins [44-46], allowing for patterned co-cultures in tissue engineering applications. or example, Jinno *et al.* [46] demonstrated the potential of parylene-C technology for generating five temporally controlled patterned co-cultures of murine embryonic stem cells (ES) in culture with various secondary cell types, suggesting that dynamic co-cultures generated by using parylene-C stencils may be applicable in studying the role of cellular interactions in ES cell differentiation (Fig. 2C).

2.3. *Microfluidic patterning*

Microfluidic patterning provides tools to spatially control cells and materials with appropriately designed configurations. This method uses an elastomeric microchannel as a guide to pattern polymers, proteins, and cells onto selected regions [15, 24, 26, 32, 42, 47-49]. The major advantage of microfluidic patterning is its straightforward fabrication process and generation of patterns by restricting fluid flow to the desired regions of a substrate. For example, Kim *et al.* [50] presented micromolded polymer patterns by allowing a low-velocity polymer precursor to fill the microchannels spontaneously by capillary action, namely micromolding in capillaries (MIMIC). Using this method, deeper and wider microchannels can be generated by pressure-driven flow over large areas.

Most of the microchannel systems have been fabricated using PDMS polymer due to the easy handling. Inside the microchannels fabricated with PDMS, fluids are blocked from wetting the substrate in the areas where the PDMS contacts the surface due to a unique property of PDMS, allowing for a highly conformal contact. Fluid can be either cured into a solid itself or used to remove underlying material depending on its composition. Although this approach can be used for short-term biological control and template-based patterning, it can be merely applied to a few, metabolically slow cell types, because the flow must be arrested, while the energy-consuming processes of anchorage and spreading take place [51].

Using microfluidic patterning, proteins and cells can be immobilized and delivered selectively to desired areas of a substrate. Takayama *et al.* presented microfluidic cell patterning techniques using multiple laminar flow of liquids in capillary systems, controlling the characteristics of the surface for the selective cell adhesion (Fig. 3A) [47] or allowing partial treatment of single cells with pharmacological inhibitor (Fig. 3B) [52]. Ten *et al.* [53] presented that hierarchical multi-layered microstructure of cells and biopolymer, such as collagen or collagen-chitosan matrix, can be formed using microchannels. Hydrogels can be fabricated with control over the spatial properties of the materials by embedding a gradient of functional materials, such as RGD peptide, directly into the material for cell and tissue engineering applications (Fig. 3C) [54]. Khademhosseini *et al.* [55] demonstrated an approach to fabricate multiphenotype cell arrays, such as hepatocytes, fibroblasts, and embryonic stem cells, on two dimensional substrates or within reversibly sealed individual microfluidic channels (Fig. 3D). This method was performed by a multi-step process using reversible sealing of PDMS molds and each cell was immobilized in the microwells within channel of low shear stress regions.

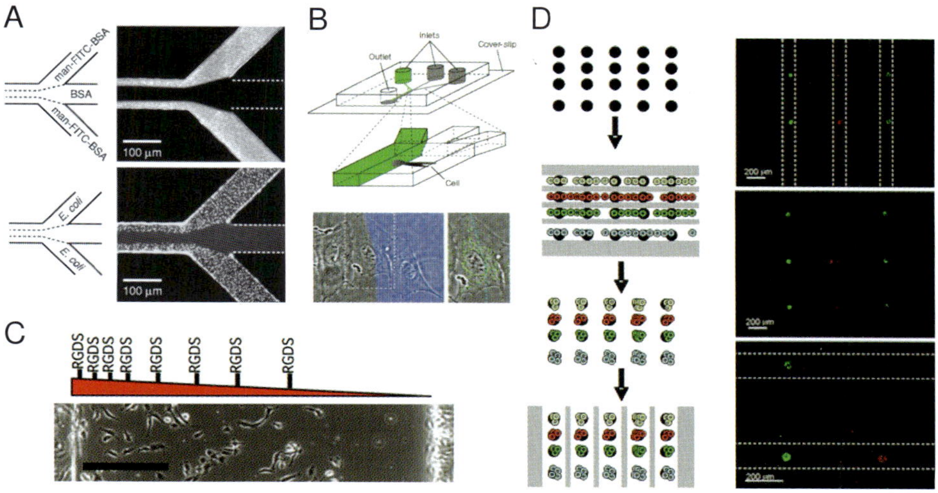

Fig. 3. Microfluidic approaches for cell patterning. (A) Laminar flow patterning using microfluidic channels. A PDMS microfluidic device was used to pattern man-FITC-BSA and E.coli. Reprinted from [47]. (B) Experimental set-up for partial treatment of cells using laminar flows (top). The blue region (Dextran-70,000 Cascade Blue stain) reveals the flow of medium containing latrunculin A (bottom left). Enlarged view of the middle cell and its mitochondria (green) (bottom right). Reprinted from [52]. (C) Endothelial cells attached to the regions of the hydrogel that contained high RGDS concentrations. Scale bar: 200 µm. Reprinted from [54]. (D) Schematic image (left) and fluorescent image (right) of the formation of multiphenotype cell arrays within PDMS microchannels containing microwells. Reprinted from [55].

2.4. *Microtopographic patterning*

Microtopographic patterning is a technique to generate surface roughness using a variety of microlithography and microfabrication moulding techniques, in which a polymer layer is moulded into the features of the polymer mould, to study cell behaviors in 3D environments [56-59]. Topographic patterns are useful for describing cell behaviors due to the guided alignment, elongation, and movement of cells on the designed pattern. The behavior of different cells has been examined using a large variety of microtopographic substrates such as columns, dots, pits, pores, gratings, and random surface roughness [60-66]. Thus, the use of surfaces with patterned topologies and adhesiveness to control morphology and behavior of cells has become a common strategy in tissue engineering.

Cell alignment and elongation are related to the probability of cell protrusion to a given direction, as following the theory of contact guidance [3, 67]. Cell spreading and exploration are restricted on the topographic surface, due to limited flexibility of the cytoskeleton [68]. It has been reported that microtopographic surfaces provide physical cues that guide the migration of several cell types, including fibroblasts, endothelial cells, and neuritis [69, 70]. Also, several studies have been dealing with systematic analysis of the combined effects of surface topography and rigidity on cell behavior [71, 72]. Lenhert *et al.*

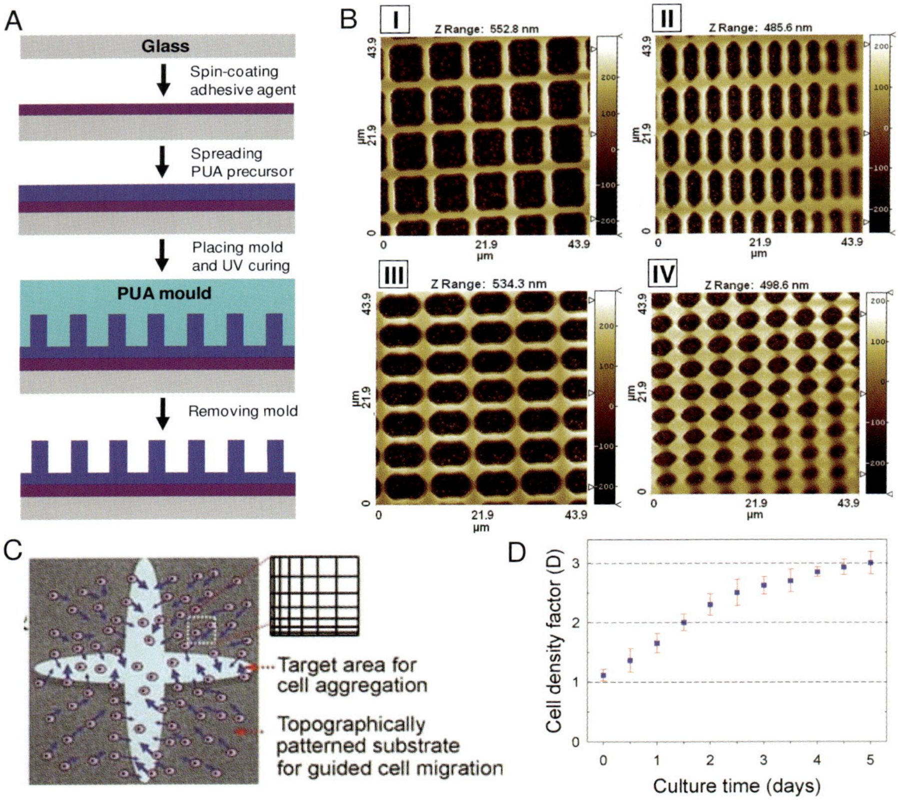

Fig. 4. (A) Schematic illustration of the microfabrication process used to generate PUA micropattern arrays. (B) AFM images of four distinct regions of different local densities. (C) The strategy for cell aggregation inside the 2D target area by using topographically tailored substratum. (D) Time-dependent change in the cell density factor in the central target area over a culture for 5 days after seeding. Reprinted from [80].

demonstrated that a capillary force-induced cell alignment and elongation extended from contact guidance using anisotropic roughness with cell behavior [58]. Ball *et al.* [59] showed that osteoblast-like cells respond differently to similar surface roughness with ordered (aligned grooves) and disordered (random) features. On ordered pillars and gratings, despite having similar surface roughness, cells responded differently. Crouch *et al.* [73] showed the anisotropic behaviors of cell adhesion to well controlled gratings with various widths and depths to investigate topographic effects on cell behaviors. The aspect ratio of the gratings is a useful factor to characterize topographic effects on cell alignment and elongation. Human foreskin fibroblast (HFF) cells and smooth muscle cells were aligned if the angle of their long axis with respect to the grating direction is ±15°; while endothelial cells and human colonic epithelial (HCEC) cells were aligned with angle of ±20° and ±10°, respectively [58, 65, 67, 68, 73-77].

To generate microtopographic patterns, capillary force lithography (CFL) techniques offer a number of advantages in fabricating geometry-controllable, robust microstructures over a large area [78, 79]. Capillarity is a simple and useful concept by one step patterning process with polymer materials and generated when a liquid wets a capillary tube and moves with lowering of the free energy. A recent study demonstrated that microtextured substrates with variable local density and anisotropy fabricated by CFL-based molding techniques can guide the organization and migration of fibroblasts in spatially desirable locations [80].

3. Microengineering of Cellular Interaction by Polymeric Biomaterials

3.1. *Patterned co-cultures for controlling cell-cell interactions*

The generation of co-culture system is crucial to understanding intricate cellular mechanisms and cell-cell interactions for cell and tissue engineering. An important aspect in tissue formation and function is the interaction between multiple types of cells within the tissue [81]. Despite this need, most commonly used *in vitro* studies lack the multicellular functionality and the organization that parallels the *in vivo* cellular microenvironment. In traditional co-culture techniques, multiple cells were seeded randomly and thus it is difficult to control the degree of various homotypic and heterotypic cell-cell interactions. To overcome this limitation, patterned co-cultures have been developed using various microfabrication technologies, including photolithography, microfluidics, membrane lift-off, switchable surfaces, [6, 16, 26, 47, 82-88]. Briefly, stencils of

PDMS [41] and parylene-C [45, 88] were used to pattern cells on a variety of substrates. Furthermore, patterned co-cultures have been generated by changing the surface properties from cell repulsive to cell-adhesive by electroactive and thermally responsive polymers [89, 90], magnetic forces [91], oxygen plasma treatment [85]. Some types of microfluidic systems enable novel approaches for generating co-culture cellular constructs [92]. These approaches use the ability to produce robust, patterned networks of microchannels for specific cell types, followed by disassembly of the construct, realignment with a different superimposed channel network, and culturing of another cell type.

For the simple and reproducible fabrication methods, layer-by-layer deposition is used for coculture system with specialized materials and extensive expertise. Khademhosseini *et al.* [86] demonstrated a moulding-assisted layer-by-layer deposition of ionic biopolymers of HA (negatively charged) and poly-L-lysine (PLL) (positively charged). In this method, micropatterns of non-biofouling HA were used to immobilize one cell type and ionic adsorption of PLL to HA patterns was used to switch the HA surfaces from cell repulsive to adherent, thereby facilitating the adhesion of a second cell type. This simple moulding-assisted layer-by-layer deposition approach is a valuable tool to control cell-cell interactions, maintain cells in culture, and engineer organs for tissue engineering [86, 92].

As a coculture model, liver cell cocultures have been examined to achieve physiologically significant functions of hepatocyte. A challenge in liver tissue engineering using coculture system is to maintain cell anchorage environment and to identify essential environmental signals required to maintain hepatic functions for long periods [93]. The unique property of primary hepatocytes is a higher selectivity in their cell attachment and spreading on tissue culture substrate and collagen than that of many other cell types. Hepatocyte functions are enhanced when co-cultured with fibroblasts, endothelial cells, stellate cells, and liver epithelial cells [84, 94-98], whereas isolated cells de-differentiate and lose their hepato-specific function. Moreover, microfabricated substrates can be used to induce variations in the degree of cell–cell interactions. First, Bhatia *et al.* [83] developed a patterned co-culture system of primary hepatocytes using photolithography. This method was effective in controlling cell contact and adhesion on the collagen patterned surface. As a more biocompatible technique, μCP-based methods were used to overcome some drawbacks of photolithography process [24, 99, 100]. A more dynamic, 3D microfabricated interdigitating system to control various cell-cell interactions has recently been demonstrated by Bhatia and coworkers [6, 87]. Their system employed a microfabricated silicon platform with moving parts or dielectrophoresis (DEP) to bring cells in close proximity to each other and could be used for improved dynamic and temporal regulation of cellular structures.

Khademhosseini *et al.* [101] presented a technique to culture human embryonic stem (hES) cells with controlled size of cluster for maintenance and subsequent differentiation. To maintain their undifferentiated state, hES cells are commonly cultured as cell cluster with feeder layer of murine embryonic fibroblasts (MEFs). Therefore, an approach controlling the size of hES cell clusters in co-culture with MEF feeder cells using micropatterning techniques may be beneficial for controlling the homogeneity of the cultures. The results of co-cultures of MEFs and hES cells generated on microwell-patterned PDMS surfaces reveals that cells are maintained in an undifferentiated condition homogeneously. In addition, the cell clusters can be restored to generate homogenous cell aggregates for the research of stem cell differentiation.

3.2. *Microfabricated 3D polymeric scaffolds for tissue engineering*

Living tissues are composed of highly organized ensembles of various cell types embedded in ECM with complex 3D topographical features [102, 103]. In native tissue, the ECM is composed of specific proteins, signaling molecules, growth factors, and many tropic agents and possesses hierarchically arranged topography that influences various cellular functions, such as adhesion, proliferation, migration, and differentiation [9, 10, 13-17, 82, 104-108]. Therefore, it is essential to generate defined scaffolds serving to mimic the structure and functions of ECM and guide the dynamic organization of cells into tissues. Tissue engineering has emerged to replace a wide range of dysfunctional tissues and regenerate tissues using cells, scaffolds, and growth factors alone or in combination.

Cells on 3D architectures with a complex set of mechanical forces and biochemical signals behave similar with *in vivo* conditions that cannot be replicated in standard 2D cell culture. For instance, breast cancer cells cultured in 3D in the presence of antibodies for specific integrin receptors become non-cancerous as opposed to 2D culture systems [109]. A 3D self assembling peptide scaffold has been shown to promote tissue-like function and further to provide a microenvironment capable of differentiating stem cells into mature liver cells acquiring a spheroidal morphology [110]. This matrix has also been applied to neural cell cultures and numerous other cell types providing a better physiological approach [111]. Also, many approaches on hepatic-tissue engineering involve seeding isolated hepatocytes on surfaces, biodegradable polymer films [112], three dimensional porous polymeric scaffolds [113-115], ligand modification polymers [116, 117], natural ECM components [118, 119], and collagen foams [120], which have been shown to enhance hepatocyte adhesion.

As scaffold materials, polymers enable the fabrication of regular patterns or topographical features and microfabrication techniques had led to produce highly organized networks of microenvironments for mimicking 3D tissue constructs for multiple cell types [121-123]. Microfabrication technology has been successfully applied to biodegradable polymers, such as polyglycolic acid (PGA) [124], polyglycerol sebacate (PGS) [125], poly(lactic co-glycolic) acid (PLGA) [126], and hydrogel [127]. Also, scaffolds containing microvascular networks have been produced in biocompatible non-degradable polymers [122] and biodegradable polymers [126]. Compartments containing hepatocytes have been constructed in a biodegradable elastomer [125]. In the case of stepwise use of photolithography and microsyringe deposition, it has been used to produce scaffolds in PLGA [128] and polyurethane (PU). Also, a microfluidic network of vascular channels has been produced in 3D by bonding together 5 to 35 layers of degradable or non-degradable polymer films containing networks of trenches [125, 126]. For better mimicking tissue architecture, it can be possible to combine photolithography and soft lithography to generate high-aspect ratio structures for the embedded 3D cell culture.

4. Conclusions and Perspective

In the past decade, advances in microfabrication techniques have shown much potential in generating patterned biomaterials interface for cell and tissue engineering. These capabilities enable in-depth investigation of cell responses in controlled microenvironment, which will expand our knowledge in cell-cell and cell-material interactions. A next step is to explore the use of microfabrication techniques to create biomimetic materials for clinical applications such as tissue regeneration. Future developments with nanoscale control of patterned polymers would allow more biomimetic control of cell-material interactions, arising from a rapid accumulation of evidence on the importance of controlling cellular processes on multiple length scales.

Acknowledgements

This work was supported by grants (R21-EB008562) from National Institute of Health.

References

[1] G. M. Whitesides, E. Ostuni, S. Takayama, X. Y. Jiang, and D. E. Ingber, "Soft lithography in biology and biochemistry," *Annual Review of Biomedical Engineering*, vol. 3, pp. 335-373, 2001.

[2] S. Raghavan and C. S. Chen, "Micropatterned environments in cell biology," *Advanced Materials*, vol. 16, pp. 1303-1313, 2004.

[3] A. Curtis and C. Wilkinson, "Topographical control of cells," *Biomaterials*, vol. 18, pp. 1573-1583, 1997.

[4] M. P. Lutolf and J. A. Hubbell, "Synthetic biomaterials as instructive extracellular microenvironments for morphogenesis in tissue engineering," *Nature Biotechnology*, vol. 23, pp. 47-55, 2005.

[5] N. Sniadecki, R. A. Desai, S. A. Ruiz, and C. S. Chen, "Nanotechnology for cell-substrate interactions," *Annals of Biomedical Engineering*, vol. 34, pp. 59-74, 2006.

[6] E. E. Hui and S. N. Bhatia, "Micromechanical control of cell-cell interactions," *Proceedings of the National Academy of Sciences of the United States of America*, vol. 104, pp. 5722-5726, 2007.

[7] D. H. Kim, P. K. Wong, J. Park, A. Levchenko, and Y. Sun, "Microengineered Platforms for Cell Mechanobiology," *Annu Rev Biomed Eng*, vol. 11, pp. 203-233, 2009.

[8] A. Khademhosseini, R. Langer, J. Borenstein, and J. P. Vacanti, "Microscale technologies for tissue engineering and biology," *Proceedings of the National Academy of Sciences of the United States of America*, vol. 103, pp. 2480-2487, 2006.

[9] C. S. Chen, M. Mrksich, S. Huang, G. M. Whitesides, and D. E. Ingber, "Geometric control of cell life and death," *Science*, vol. 276, pp. 1425-1428, 1997.

[10] D. Falconnet, G. Csucs, H. M. Grandin, and M. Textor, "Surface engineering approaches to micropattern surfaces for cell-based assays," *Biomaterials*, vol. 27, pp. 3044-3063, 2006.

[11] J. Fink, M. Thery, A. Azioune, R. Dupont, F. Chatelain, M. Bornens, and M. Piel, "Comparative study and improvement of current cell micro-patterning techniques," *Lab on a Chip*, vol. 7, pp. 672-680, 2007.

[12] D. B. Weibel, W. R. DiLuzio, and G. M. Whitesides, "Microfabrication meets microbiology," *Nature Reviews Microbiology*, vol. 5, pp. 209-218, 2007.

[13] R. Singhvi, A. Kumar, G. P. Lopez, G. N. Stephanopoulos, D. I. C. Wang, G. M. Whitesides, and D. E. Ingber, "Engineering Cell-Shape and Function," *Science*, vol. 264, pp. 696-698, 1994.

[14] C. H. Thomas, J. B. Lhoest, D. G. Castner, C. D. McFarland, and K. E. Healy, "Surfaces designed to control the projected area and shape of individual cells," *Journal of Biomechanical Engineering-Transactions of the Asme*, vol. 121, pp. 40-48, 1999.

[15] A. Folch and M. Toner, "Cellular micropatterns on biocompatible materials," *Biotechnology Progress*, vol. 14, pp. 388-392, 1998.

[16] S. N. Bhatia, U. J. Balis, M. L. Yarmush, and M. Toner, "Microfabrication of hepatocyte/fibroblast co-cultures: Role of homotypic cell interactions," *Biotechnology Progress*, vol. 14, pp. 378-387, 1998.

[17] C. B. Herbert, T. L. McLernon, C. L. Hypolite, D. N. Adams, L. Pikus, C. C. Huang, G. B. Fields, P. C. Letourneau, M. D. Distefano, and W. S. Hu, "Micropatterning gradients and controlling surface densities of photoactivatable biomolecules on self-assembled monolayers of oligo(ethylene glycol) alkanethiolates," *Chemistry & Biology*, vol. 4, pp. 731-737, 1997.

[18] A. Bernard, E. Delamarche, H. Schmid, B. Michel, H. R. Bosshard, and H. Biebuyck, "Printing patterns of proteins," *Langmuir*, vol. 14, pp. 2225-2229, 1998.

[19] G. Csucs, R. Michel, J. W. Lussi, M. Textor, and G. Danuser, "Microcontact printing of novel co-polymers in combination with proteins for cell-biological applications," *Biomaterials*, vol. 24, pp. 1713-1720, 2003.

[20] J. C. Love, L. A. Estroff, J. K. Kriebel, R. G. Nuzzo, and G. M. Whitesides, "Self-assembled monolayers of thiolates on metals as a form of nanotechnology," *Chemical Reviews*, vol. 105, pp. 1103-1169, 2005.

[21] A. Bernard, D. Fitzli, P. Sonderegger, E. Delamarche, B. Michel, H. R. Bosshard, and H. Biebuyck, "Affinity capture of proteins from solution and their dissociation by contact printing," *Nature Biotechnology*, vol. 19, pp. 866-869, 2001.

[22] K. Y. Suh, J. Seong, A. Khademhosseini, P. E. Laibinis, and R. Langer, "A simple soft lithographic route to fabrication of poly(ethylene glycol) microstructures for protein and cell patterning," *Biomaterials*, vol. 25, pp. 557-563, 2004.

[23] M. Morra, E. Occhiello, R. Marola, F. Garbassi, P. Humphrey, and D. Johnson, "On the Aging of Oxygen Plasma-Treated Polydimethylsiloxane Surfaces," *Journal of Colloid and Interface Science*, vol. 137, pp. 11-24, 1990.

[24] Y. N. Xia and G. M. Whitesides, "Soft lithography," *Angewandte Chemie-International Edition*, vol. 37, pp. 551-575, 1998.

[25] S. A. Ruiz and C. S. Chen, "Microcontact printing: A tool to pattern," *Soft Matter*, vol. 3, pp. 168-177, 2007.

[26] A. Folch and M. Toner, "Microengineering of cellular interactions," *Annual Review of Biomedical Engineering*, vol. 2, pp. 227-+, 2000.

[27] G. Kumar, C. C. Ho, and C. C. Co, "Guiding cell migration using one-way micropattern arrays," *Advanced Materials*, vol. 19, pp. 1084-1090, 2007.

[28] L. E. Dike, C. S. Chen, M. Mrksich, J. Tien, G. M. Whitesides, and D. E. Ingber, "Geometric control of switching between growth, apoptosis, and differentiation during angiogenesis using micropatterned substrates," *In Vitro Cellular & Developmental Biology-Animal*, vol. 35, pp. 441-448, 1999.

[29] C. M. Nelson and C. S. Chen, "VE-cadherin simultaneously stimulates and inhibits cell proliferation by altering cytoskeletal structure and tension," *J Cell Sci*, vol. 116, pp. 3571-81, 2003.

[30] D. Lehnert, B. Wehrle-Haller, C. David, U. Weiland, C. Ballestrem, B. A. Imhof, and M. Bastmeyer, "Cell behaviour on micropatterned substrata: limits of extracellular matrix geometry for spreading and adhesion," *Journal of Cell Science*, vol. 117, pp. 41-52, 2004.

[31] K. Kandere-Grzybowska, C. Campbell, Y. Komarova, B. A. Grzybowski, and G. G. Borisy, "Molecular dynamics imaging in micropatterned living cells," *Nat Methods*, vol. 2, pp. 739-41, 2005.

[32] R. S. Kane, S. Takayama, E. Ostuni, D. E. Ingber, and G. M. Whitesides, "Patterning proteins and cells using soft lithography," *Biomaterials*, vol. 20, pp. 2363-2376, 1999.

[33] A. K. Vogt, L. Lauer, W. Knoll, and A. Offenhausser, "Micropatterned substrates for the growth of functional neuronal networks of defined geometry," *Biotechnology Progress*, vol. 19, pp. 1562-1568, 2003.

[34] A. Ruiz, L. Buzanska, D. Gilliland, H. Rauscher, L. Sirghi, T. Sobanski, M. Zychowicz, L. Ceriotti, F. Bretagnol, S. Coecke, P. Colpo, and F. Ross, "Micro-stamped surfaces for the patterned growth of neural stem cells," *Biomaterials*, vol. 29, pp. 4766-4774, 2008.

[35] M. Nishizawa, K. Takoh, and T. Matsue, "Micropatterning of HeLa cells on glass substrates and evaluation of respiratory activity using microelectrodes," *Langmuir*, vol. 18, pp. 3645-3649, 2002.

[36] M. Wu, R. N. Orth, D. A. Holowka, H. G. Craighead, and B. A. Baird, "Mast cell activation in response to microscale patterned lipid bilayer," *Biophysical Journal*, vol. 84, pp. 520a-521a, 2003.

[37] N. Bursac, K. K. Parker, S. Iravanian, and L. Tung, "Cardiomyocyte cultures with controlled macroscopic anisotropy: a model for functional electrophysiological studies of cardiac muscle," *Circ Res*, vol. 91, pp. e45-54, 2002.

[38] R. McBeath, D. M. Pirone, C. M. Nelson, K. Bhadriraju, and C. S. Chen, "Cell shape, cytoskeletal tension, and RhoA regulate stem cell lineage commitment," *Developmental Cell*, vol. 6, pp. 483-495, 2004.

[39] S. B. Carter, "Haptotactic Islands - a Method of Confining Single Cells to Study Individual Cell Reactions and Clone Formation," *Experimental Cell Research*, vol. 48, pp. 189-&, 1967.

[40] Y. Jimbo, H. P. C. Robinson, and A. Kawana, "Simultaneous Measurement of Intracellular Calcium and Electrical-Activity from Patterned Neural Networks in Culture," *Ieee Transactions on Biomedical Engineering*, vol. 40, pp. 804-810, 1993.

[41] A. Folch, B. H. Jo, O. Hurtado, D. J. Beebe, and M. Toner, "Microfabricated elastomeric stencils for micropatterning cell cultures," *Journal of Biomedical Materials Research*, vol. 52, pp. 346-353, 2000.

[42] E. Ostuni, R. Kane, C. S. Chen, D. E. Ingber, and G. M. Whitesides, "Patterning mammalian cells using elastomeric membranes," *Langmuir*, vol. 16, pp. 7811-7819, 2000.

[43] A. Khademhosseini, S. Jon, K. Y. Suh, T. N. T. Tran, G. Eng, J. Yeh, J. Seong, and R. Langer, "Direct Patterning of protein- and cell-resistant polymeric monolayers and microstructures," *Advanced Materials*, vol. 15, pp. 1995-2000, 2003.

[44] R. Pal, K. E. Sung, and M. A. Burns, "Microstencils for the patterning of nontraditional materials," *Langmuir*, vol. 22, pp. 5392-5397, 2006.

[45] D. Wright, B. Rajalingam, J. M. Karp, S. Selvarasah, Y. B. Ling, J. Yeh, R. Langer, M. R. Dokmeci, and A. Khademhosseini, "Reusable, reversibly sealable parylene membranes for cell and protein patterning," *Journal of Biomedical Materials Research Part A*, vol. 85A, pp. 530-538, 2008.

[46] S. Jinno, H. C. Moeller, C. L. Chen, B. Rajalingam, B. G. Chung, M. R. Dokmeci, and A. Khademhosseini, "Microfabricated multilayer parylene-C stencils for the generation of patterned dynamic co-cultures," *J Biomed Mater Res A*, vol. 86, pp. 278-88, 2008.

[47] S. Takayama, J. C. McDonald, E. Ostuni, M. N. Liang, P. J. A. Kenis, R. F. Ismagilov, and G. M. Whitesides, "Patterning cells and their environments using multiple laminar fluid flows in capillary networks," *Proceedings of the National Academy of Sciences of the United States of America*, vol. 96, pp. 5545-5548, 1999.

[48] A. Folch, A. Ayon, O. Hurtado, M. A. Schmidt, and M. Toner, "Molding of deep polydimethylsiloxane microstructures for microfluidics and biological applications," *Journal of Biomechanical Engineering-Transactions of the Asme*, vol. 121, pp. 28-34, 1999.

[49] P. Kim, D. H. Kim, B. Kim, S. K. Choi, S. H. Lee, A. Khademhosseini, R. Langer, and K. Y. Suh, "Fabrication of nanostructures of polyethylene glycol for applications to protein adsorption and cell adhesion," *Nanotechnology*, vol. 16, pp. 2420-2426, 2005.

[50] E. Kim, Y. N. Xia, and G. M. Whitesides, "Polymer Microstructures Formed by Molding in Capillaries," *Nature*, vol. 376, pp. 581-584, 1995.

[51] D. T. Chiu, N. L. Jeon, S. Huang, R. S. Kane, C. J. Wargo, I. S. Choi, D. E. Ingber, and G. M. Whitesides, "Patterned deposition of cells and proteins onto surfaces by using three-dimensional microfluidic systems," *Proceedings of the National Academy of Sciences of the United States of America*, vol. 97, pp. 2408-2413, 2000.

[52] S. Takayama, E. Ostuni, P. LeDuc, K. Naruse, D. Ingber, and G. Whitesides, "Laminar flows - Subcellular positioning of small molecules," *Nature*, vol. 411, pp. 1016-1016, 2001.
[53] W. Tan and T. A. Desai, "Microfluidic patterning of cells in extracellular matrix biopolymers: Effects of channel size, cell type, and matrix composition on pattern integrity," *Tissue Engineering*, vol. 9, pp. 255-267, 2003.
[54] J. A. Burdick, A. Khademhosseini, and R. Langer, "Fabrication of gradient hydrogels using a microfluidics/photopolymerization process," *Langmuir*, vol. 20, pp. 5153-6, 2004.
[55] A. Khademhosseini, J. Yeh, G. Eng, J. Karp, H. Kaji, J. Borenstein, O. C. Farokhzad, and R. Langer, "Cell docking inside microwells within reversibly sealed microfluidic channels for fabricating multiphenotype cell arrays," *Lab on a Chip*, vol. 5, pp. 1380-1386, 2005.
[56] L. Ponsonnet, V. Comte, A. Othmane, C. Lagneau, M. Charbonnier, M. Lissac, and N. Jaffrezic, "Effect of surface topography and chemistry on adhesion, orientation and growth of fibroblasts on nickel-titanium substrates," *Materials Science & Engineering C-Biomimetic and Supramolecular Systems*, vol. 21, pp. 157-165, 2002.
[57] K. Anselme, M. Bigerelle, B. Noel, A. Iost, and P. Hardouin, "Effect of grooved titanium substratum on human osteoblastic cell growth," *Journal of Biomedical Materials Research*, vol. 60, pp. 529-540, 2002.
[58] S. Lenhert, A. Sesma, M. Hirtz, L. F. Chi, H. Fuchs, H. P. Wiesmann, A. E. Osbourn, and B. M. Moerschbacher, "Capillary-induced contact guidance," *Langmuir*, vol. 23, pp. 10216-10223, 2007.
[59] M. Ball, D. M. Grant, W. J. Lo, and C. A. Scotchford, "The effect of different surface morphology and roughness on osteoblast-like cells," *Journal of Biomedical Materials Research Part A*, vol. 86A, pp. 637-647, 2008.
[60] D. C. Miller, A. Thapa, K. M. Haberstroh, and T. J. Webster, "Endothelial and vascular smooth muscle cell function on poly(lactic-co-glycolic acid) with nano-structured surface features," *Biomaterials*, vol. 25, pp. 53-61, 2004.
[61] E. K. F. Yim, R. M. Reano, S. W. Pang, A. F. Yee, C. S. Chen, and K. W. Leong, "Nanopattern-induced changes in morphology and motility of smooth muscle cells," *Biomaterials*, vol. 26, pp. 5405-5413, 2005.
[62] M. A. Wood, C. D. W. Wilkinson, and A. S. G. Curtis, "The effects of colloidal nanotopography on initial fibroblast adhesion and morphology," *Ieee Transactions on Nanobioscience*, vol. 5, pp. 20-31, 2006.
[63] A. V. Sapelkin, S. C. Bayliss, B. Unal, and A. Charalambou, "Interaction of B50 rat hippocampal cells with stain-etched porous silicon," *Biomaterials*, vol. 27, pp. 842-846, 2006.
[64] C. H. Choi, S. H. Hagvall, B. M. Wu, J. C. Y. Dunn, R. E. Beygui, and C. J. Kim, "Cell interaction with three-dimensional sharp-tip nanotopography," *Biomaterials*, vol. 28, pp. 1672-1679, 2007.
[65] J. L. Charest, A. J. Garcia, and W. P. King, "Myoblast alignment and differentiation on cell culture substrates with microscale topography and model chemistries," *Biomaterials*, vol. 28, pp. 2202-2210, 2007.
[66] A. Saez, M. Ghibaudo, A. Buguin, P. Silberzan, and B. Ladoux, "Rigidity-driven growth and migration of epithelial cells on microstructured anisotropic substrates," *Proceedings of the National Academy of Sciences of the United States of America*, vol. 104, pp. 8281-8286, 2007.
[67] P. Clark, P. Connolly, A. S. G. Curtis, J. A. T. Dow, and C. D. W. Wilkinson, "Cell Guidance by Ultrafine Topography Invitro," *Journal of Cell Science*, vol. 99, pp. 73-77, 1991.

[68] P. Clark, P. Connolly, A. S. G. Curtis, J. A. T. Dow, and C. D. W. Wilkinson, "Topographical Control of Cell Behavior .2. Multiple Grooved Substrata," *Development*, vol. 108, pp. 635-644, 1990.
[69] X. Y. Jiang, D. A. Bruzewicz, A. P. Wong, M. Piel, and G. M. Whitesides, "Directing cell migration with asymmetric micropatterns," *Proceedings of the National Academy of Sciences of the United States of America*, vol. 102, pp. 975-978, 2005.
[70] P. Gustavsson, F. Johansson, M. Kanje, L. Wallman, and C. E. Linsmeier, "Neurite guidance on protein micropatterns generated by a piezoelectric microdispenser," *Biomaterials*, vol. 28, pp. 1141-1151, 2007.
[71] S. Li, J. L. Guan, and S. Chien, "Biochemistry and biomechanics of cell motility," *Annual Review of Biomedical Engineering*, vol. 7, pp. 105-150, 2005.
[72] E. J. Semler, C. S. Ranucci, and P. V. Moghe, "Tissue assembly guided via substrate biophysics: Applications to hepatocellular engineering," *Tissue Engineering I: Scaffold Systems for Tissue Engineering*, vol. 102, pp. 1-46, 2006.
[73] A. S. Crouch, D. Miller, K. J. Luebke, and W. Hu, "Correlation of anisotropic cell behaviors with topographic aspect ratio," *Biomaterials*, vol. 30, pp. 1560-1567, 2009.
[74] E. T. denBraber, J. E. deRuijter, L. A. Ginsel, A. F. vonRecum, and J. A. Jansen, "Quantitative analysis of fibroblast morphology on microgrooved surfaces with various groove and ridge dimensions," *Biomaterials*, vol. 17, pp. 2037-2044, 1996.
[75] W. Hu, E. K. F. Yim, R. M. Reano, K. W. Leong, and S. W. Pang, "Effects of nanoimprinted patterns in tissue-culture polystyrene on cell behavior," *Journal of Vacuum Science & Technology B*, vol. 23, pp. 2984-2989, 2005.
[76] P. Uttayarat, G. K. Toworfe, F. Dietrich, P. I. Lelkes, and R. J. Composto, "Topographic guidance of endothelial cells on silicone surfaces with micro- to nanogrooves: Orientation of actin filaments and focal adhesions," *Journal of Biomedical Materials Research Part A*, vol. 75A, pp. 668-680, 2005.
[77] S. A. Fraser, Y. H. Ting, K. S. Mallon, A. E. Wendt, C. J. Murphy, and P. F. Nealey, "Sub-micron and nanoscale feature depth modulates alignment of stromal fibroblasts and corneal epithelial cells in serum-rich and serum-free media," *Journal of Biomedical Materials Research Part A*, vol. 86A, pp. 725-735, 2008.
[78] K. Y. Suh, Y. S. Kim, and H. H. Lee, "Capillary force lithography," *Advanced Materials*, vol. 13, pp. 1386-1389, 2001.
[79] K. Y. Suh and H. H. Lee, "Capillary force lithography: Large-area patterning, self-organization, and anisotropic dewetting," *Advanced Functional Materials*, vol. 12, pp. 405-413, 2002.
[80] D. H. Kim, C. H. Seo, K. Han, K. W. Kwon, A. Levchenko, and K. Y. Suh, "Guided cell migration on microtextured substrates with variable local density and anisotropy," *Adv. Funct. Mater.*, vol. 19, pp. 1579-1586, 2009.
[81] R. Langer and J. P. Vacanti, "Tissue Engineering," *Science*, vol. 260, pp. 920-926, 1993.
[82] S. N. Bhatia, M. L. Yarmush, and M. Toner, "Controlling cell interactions by micropatterning in co-cultures: Hepatocytes and 3T3 fibroblasts," *Journal of Biomedical Materials Research*, vol. 34, pp. 189-199, 1997.
[83] S. N. Bhatia, U. J. Balis, M. L. Yarmush, and M. Toner, "Probing heterotypic cell interactions: Hepatocyte function in microfabricated co-cultures," *Journal of Biomaterials Science-Polymer Edition*, vol. 9, pp. 1137-1160, 1998.
[84] S. N. Bhatia, U. J. Balis, M. L. Yarmush, and M. Toner, "Effect of cell-cell interactions in preservation of cellular phenotype: cocultivation of hepatocytes and nonparenchymal cells," *Faseb Journal*, vol. 13, pp. 1883-1900, 1999.

[85] A. Tourovskaia, T. Barber, B. T. Wickes, D. Hirdes, B. Grin, D. G. Castner, K. E. Healy, and A. Folch, "Micropatterns of chemisorbed cell adhesion-repellent films using oxygen plasma etching and elastomeric masks," *Langmuir*, vol. 19, pp. 4754-4764, 2003.

[86] A. Khademhosseini, K. Y. Suh, J. M. Yang, G. Eng, J. Yeh, S. Levenberg, and R. Langer, "Layer-by-layer deposition of hyaluronic acid and poly-L-lysine for patterned cell co-cultures," *Biomaterials*, vol. 25, pp. 3583-3592, 2004.

[87] D. R. Albrecht, G. H. Underhill, T. B. Wassermann, R. L. Sah, and S. N. Bhatia, "Probing the role of multicellular organization in three-dimensional microenvironments," *Nature Methods*, vol. 3, pp. 369-375, 2006.

[88] D. Wright, B. Rajalingam, S. Selvarasah, M. R. Dokmeci, and A. Khademhosseini, "Generation of static and dynamic patterned co-cultures using microfabricated parylene-C stencils," *Lab on a Chip*, vol. 7, pp. 1272-1279, 2007.

[89] M. N. Yousaf, B. T. Houseman, and M. Mrksich, "Using electroactive substrates to pattern the attachment of two different cell populations," *Proceedings of the National Academy of Sciences of the United States of America*, vol. 98, pp. 5992-5996, 2001.

[90] W. S. Yeo, M. N. Yousaf, and M. Mrksich, "Dynamic interfaces between cells and surfaces: Electroactive substrates that sequentially release and attach cells," *Journal of the American Chemical Society*, vol. 125, pp. 14994-14995, 2003.

[91] A. Ito, Y. Takizawa, H. Honda, K. I. Hata, H. Kagami, M. Ueda, and T. Kobayashi, "Tissue engineering using magnetite nanoparticles and magnetic force: Heterotypic layers of cocultured hepatocytes and endothelial cells," *Tissue Engineering*, vol. 10, pp. 833-840, 2004.

[92] J. Fukuda, A. Khademhosseini, J. Yeh, G. Eng, J. J. Cheng, O. C. Farokhzad, and R. Langer, "Micropatterned cell co-cultures using layer-by-layer deposition of extracellular matrix components," *Biomaterials*, vol. 27, pp. 1479-1486, 2006.

[93] R. N. B. Bhandari, L. A. Riccalton, A. L. Lewis, J. R. Fry, A. H. Hammond, S. J. B. Tendler, and K. M. Shakesheff, "Liver tissue engineering: A role for co-culture systems in modifying hepatocyte function and viability," *Tissue Engineering*, vol. 7, pp. 345-357, 2001.

[94] L. Agius, "Metabolic Interactions of Parenchymal Hepatocytes and Dividing Epithelial-Cells in Co-Culture," *Biochemical Journal*, vol. 252, pp. 23-28, 1988.

[95] M. T. Donato, M. J. Gomezlechon, and J. V. Castell, "Drug-Metabolizing-Enzymes in Rat Hepatocytes Cocultured with Cell-Lines," *In Vitro Cellular & Developmental Biology*, vol. 26, pp. 1057-1062, 1990.

[96] R. F. Menzeleev, A. I. Bozhkov, E. N. Zvonkova, Y. M. Krasnopolskyii, and V. I. Shvets, "Enhancement of Liver-Cell Proliferation by Gm(3) Ganglioside," *Bulletin of Experimental Biology and Medicine*, vol. 119, pp. 414-417, 1995.

[97] M. Harimoto, M. Yamato, M. Hirose, C. Takahashi, Y. Isoi, A. Kikuchi, and T. Okano, "Novel approach for achieving double-layered cell sheets co-culture: overlaying endothelial cell sheets onto monolayer hepatocytes utilizing temperature-responsive culture dishes," *Journal of Biomedical Materials Research*, vol. 62, pp. 464-470, 2002.

[98] M. A. Nandkumar, M. Yamato, A. Kushida, C. Konno, M. Hirose, A. Kikuchi, and T. Okano, "Two-dimensional cell sheet manipulation of heterotypically co-cultured lung cells utilizing temperature-responsive culture dishes results in long-term maintenance of differentiated epithelial cell functions," *Biomaterials*, vol. 23, pp. 1121-1130, 2002.

[99] S. R. Quake and A. Scherer, "From micro- to nanofabrication with soft materials," *Science*, vol. 290, pp. 1536-1540, 2000.

[100] S. Kidambi, L. F. Sheng, M. L. Yarmush, M. Toner, I. Lee, and C. Chan, "Patterned co-culture of primary hepatocytes and fibroblasts using polyelectrolyte multilayer templates," *Macromolecular Bioscience*, vol. 7, pp. 344-353, 2007.

[101] A. Khademhosseini, L. Ferreira, J. Blumling, J. Yeh, J. M. Karp, J. Fukuda, and R. Langer, "Co-culture of human embryonic stem cells with murine embryonic fibroblasts on microwell-patterned substrates," *Biomaterials*, vol. 27, pp. 5968-5977, 2006.

[102] C. G. Galbraith and M. P. Sheetz, "Forces on adhesive contacts affect cell function," *Current Opinion in Cell Biology*, vol. 10, pp. 566-571, 1998.

[103] B. Geiger, A. Bershadsky, R. Pankov, and K. M. Yamada, "Transmembrane extracellular matrix-cytoskeleton crosstalk," *Nature Reviews Molecular Cell Biology*, vol. 2, pp. 793-805, 2001.

[104] C. Oneill, P. Jordan, P. Riddle, and G. Ireland, "Narrow Linear Strips of Adhesive Substratum Are Powerful Inducers of Both Growth and Total Focal Contact Area," *Journal of Cell Science*, vol. 95, pp. 577-586, 1990.

[105] D. A. Stenger, J. H. Georger, C. S. Dulcey, J. J. Hickman, A. S. Rudolph, T. B. Nielsen, S. M. Mccort, and J. M. Calvert, "Coplanar Molecular Assemblies of Aminoalkylsilane and Perfluorinated Alkylsilane - Characterization and Geometric Definition of Mammalian-Cell Adhesion and Growth," *Journal of the American Chemical Society*, vol. 114, pp. 8435-8442, 1992.

[106] B. M. Gumbiner, "Cell adhesion: The molecular basis of tissue architecture and morphogenesis," *Cell*, vol. 84, pp. 345-357, 1996.

[107] W. Tan, R. Krishnaraj, and T. A. Desai, "Evaluation of nanostructured composite collagen-chitosan matrices for tissue engineering," *Tissue Engineering*, vol. 7, pp. 203-210, 2001.

[108] E. Engel, A. Michiardi, M. Navarro, D. Lacroix, and J. A. Planell, "Nanotechnology in regenerative medicine: the materials side," *Trends in Biotechnology*, vol. 26, pp. 39-47, 2008.

[109] V. M. Weaver, O. W. Petersen, F. Wang, C. A. Larabell, P. Briand, C. Damsky, and M. J. Bissell, "Reversion of the malignant phenotype of human breast cells in three-dimensional culture and *in vivo* by integrin blocking antibodies," *Journal of Cell Biology*, vol. 137, pp. 231-245, 1997.

[110] C. E. Semino, J. R. Merok, G. G. Crane, G. Panagiotakos, and S. G. Zhang, "Functional differentiation of hepatocyte-like spheroid structures from putative liver progenitor cells in three-dimensional peptide scaffolds," *Differentiation*, vol. 71, pp. 262-270, 2003.

[111] T. C. Holmes, S. de Lacalle, X. Su, G. S. Liu, A. Rich, and S. G. Zhang, "Extensive neurite outgrowth and active synapse formation on self-assembling peptide scaffolds," *Proceedings of the National Academy of Sciences of the United States of America*, vol. 97, pp. 6728-6733, 2000.

[112] L. G. Cima, D. E. Ingber, J. P. Vacanti, and R. Langer, "Hepatocyte Culture on Biodegradable Polymeric Substrates," *Biotechnology and Bioengineering*, vol. 38, pp. 145-158, 1991.

[113] D. J. Mooney, K. Sano, P. M. Kaufmann, K. Majahod, B. Schloo, J. P. Vacanti, and R. Langer, "Long-term engraftment of hepatocytes transplanted on biodegradable polymer sponges," *Journal of Biomedical Materials Research*, vol. 37, pp. 413-420, 1997.

[114] S. S. Kim, H. Utsunomiya, J. A. Koski, B. M. Wu, M. J. Cima, J. Sohn, K. Mukai, L. G. Griffith, and J. P. Vacanti, "Survival and function of hepatocytes on a novel three-dimensional synthetic biodegradable polymer scaffold with an intrinsic network of channels," *Annals of Surgery*, vol. 228, pp. 8-13, 1998.

[115] U. Kneser, P. M. Kaufmann, H. C. Fiegel, J. M. Pollok, D. Kluth, H. Herbst, and X. Rogiers, "Long-term differentiated function of heterotopically transplanted hepatocytes on three-dimensional polymer matrices," *Journal of Biomedical Materials Research*, vol. 47, pp. 494-503, 1999.

[116] L. G. Griffith and S. Lopina, "Microdistribution of substratum-bound ligands affects cell function: hepatocyte spreading on PEO-tethered galactose," *Biomaterials*, vol. 19, pp. 979-986, 1998.

[117] K. Bhadriraju and L. K. Hansen, "Hepatocyte adhesion, growth and differentiated function on RGD-containing proteins," *Biomaterials*, vol. 21, pp. 267-272, 2000.

[118] D. J. Mooney, R. Langer, and D. E. Ingber, "Cytoskeletal Filament Assembly and the Control of Cell Spreading and Function by Extracellular-Matrix," *Journal of Cell Science*, vol. 108, pp. 2311-2320, 1995.

[119] Y. M. Elcin, V. Dixit, and G. Gitnick, "Hepatocyte attachment on biodegradable modified chitosan membranes: *In vitro* evaluation for the development of liver organoids," *Artificial Organs*, vol. 22, pp. 837-846, 1998.

[120] C. S. Ranucci, A. Kumar, S. P. Batra, and P. V. Moghe, "Control of hepatocyte function on collagen foams: sizing matrix pores toward selective induction of 2-D and 3-D cellular morphogenesis," *Biomaterials*, vol. 21, pp. 783-793, 2000.

[121] S. Kaihara, J. Borenstein, R. Koka, S. Lalan, E. R. Ochoa, M. Ravens, H. Pien, B. Cunningham, and J. P. Vacanti, "Silicon micromachining to tissue engineer branched vascular channels for liver fabrication," *Tissue Engineering*, vol. 6, pp. 105-117, 2000.

[122] J. T. Borenstein, H. Terai, K. R. King, E. J. Weinberg, M. R. Kaazempur-Mofrad, and J. P. Vacanti, "Microfabrication technology for vascularized tissue engineering," *Biomedical Microdevices*, vol. 4, pp. 167-175, 2002.

[123] K. Seunarine, N. Gadegaard, M. Tormen, D. O Meredith, M. O Riehle, and C. D. W. Wilkinson, "3D polymer scaffolds for tissue engineering," *Nanomedicine*, vol. 1, pp. 281-296, 2006.

[124] L. E. Freed, G. Vunjaknovakovic, R. J. Biron, D. B. Eagles, D. C. Lesnoy, S. K. Barlow, and R. Langer, "Biodegradable Polymer Scaffolds for Tissue Engineering," *Bio-Technology*, vol. 12, pp. 689-693, 1994.

[125] C. J. Bettinger, E. J. Weinberg, K. M. Kulig, J. P. Vacanti, Y. D. Wang, J. T. Borenstein, and R. Langer, "Three-dimensional microfluidic tissue-engineering scaffolds using a flexible biodegradable polymer," *Advanced Materials*, vol. 18, pp. 165-+, 2006.

[126] K. R. King, C. C. J. Wang, M. R. Kaazempur-Mofrad, J. P. Vacanti, and J. T. Borenstein, "Biodegradable microfluidics," *Advanced Materials*, vol. 16, pp. 2007-+, 2004.

[127] M. Cabodi, N. W. Choi, J. P. Gleghorn, C. S. D. Lee, L. J. Bonassar, and A. D. Stroock, "A microfluidic biomaterial," *Journal of the American Chemical Society*, vol. 127, pp. 13788-13789, 2005.

[128] G. Vozzi, C. Flaim, A. Ahluwalia, and S. Bhatia, "Fabrication of PLGA scaffolds using soft lithography and microsyringe deposition," *Biomaterials*, vol. 24, pp. 2533-2540, 2003.

CHAPTER 5

SYNTHESIS AND *IN VITRO/IN VIVO* RESPONSE TO PEPTIDE-POLYMER CONJUGATES

Amy S. Chung and Weiyuan John Kao*

School of Pharmacy, Division of Pharmaceutical Sciences, University of Wisconsin-Madison, Madison, WI, 53705, USA

**E-mail: wjkao@pharmacy.wisc.edu*

1. Introduction

As new biomaterials and the reformulation of existing materials continue to advance, evaluation and intervention of the host response to these materials through extensive material and biological characterization remains imperative. Host response to materials can range from acute inflammation that eventually becomes resolved as the material integrates into the body, to fibrosis and fibrous capsule development to rejection of the material. The shift from passively observing material interaction with the host to actively tailoring and guiding the host response at the implant-tissue interface has been steady, but with our currently limited mechanistic understanding of the host-material interaction, active guidance of the material's biocompatibility remains a critical challenge. This chapter highlights the current studies that aim to direct the host response to peptide conjugated polymer systems and the *in vitro* and *in vivo* biocompatibility assessments. Much of the chapter's focus will lie on the host and its response rather than the fate of the material in the host. Frequently applied chemistry to conjugate bioactive molecules onto polymeric systems will also be discussed and highlighted in the case studies. Case studies will demonstrate the effect of peptide conjugated substrates on the host response as modulated specifically by peptide and substrate. This chapter highlights representative studies, and does not describe all peptide-polymer conjugates and does not discuss peptide adsorbed/coated or entrapped materials. In addition, this chapter discusses implantable peptide-polymer scaffolds and not nanoscale materials or those intended to circulate the blood. However, through the evaluation of peptide conjugated materials on a macro scale, insight into the nano realm, which is even less understood, may be gained.

2. Host Response to Biomaterials

2.1. *Overview: Process and progression*

Host response to materials remains a developing area of study and is a highly complex process comprised of finely orchestrated cascade of overlapping and interrelated events. Upon injury, including the introduction of a biomaterial to the host, the body begins a wound healing response to the foreign entity. Wound healing is divided into three major phases: inflammation, tissue formation, and remodeling. When there are biomaterials involved, the progression of wound healing is modified to compensate for the persistent presence of the material in the host. Thus, the progression of wound healing response in the presence of a biomaterial can be divided into the following phases: injury, blood-material

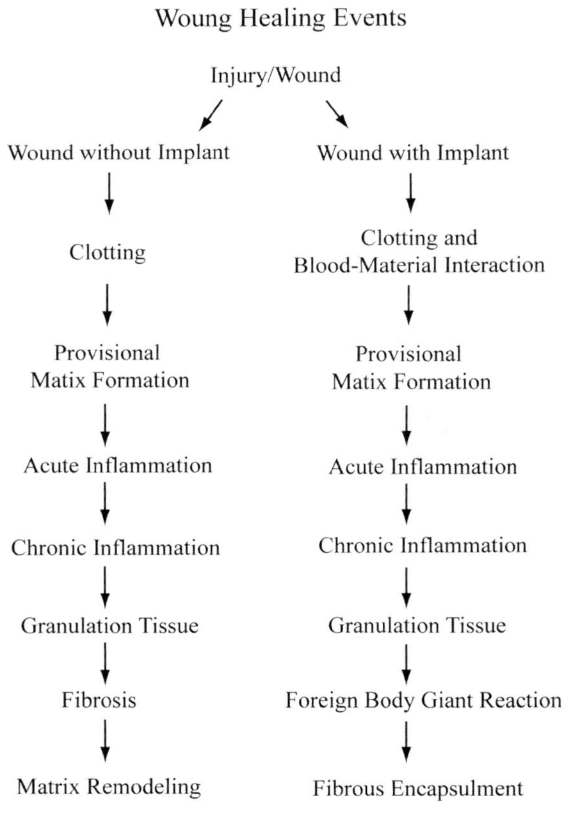

Fig. 1. Wound healing process with and without implant in the host. In the presence of an implant, the cascade of events that occur include the foreign body giant reaction in the host's attempt to wall off the foreign material.

interactions, provisional matrix formation, acute inflammation, chronic inflammation, granulation tissue, foreign-body reaction, and fibrous encapsulment.

Figure 1 highlights the cascade of host response events depending on the presence of the implant. The phases during wound healing without implant versus with implant materials do not completely differ and often overlap. For example, granulation tissue is not a response unique to wounds with implants and can occur during normal tissue healing without implant.

Host interaction with biomaterials begins with the Vroman effect, where blood protein adsorption on the biomaterial surface starts the development of the provisional matrix. With the highly dynamic protein adsorption on the material surface begins the host's coagulation and inflammation events. Clotting and blood-material interaction involve the formation of bulk fibrin around the injured site and the implant while inflammation brings the recruitment of cells including platelets, leukocytes such as neutrophils and other white blood cells. Inflammatory response to material serves as a normal event to wall off and locally contain the material at the injury site. In acute inflammation, neutrophils and monocytes enter the wound site as a part of exudation and begin to degrade the material and release a myriad of proteases, cytokines and oxygen-derived free radicals. However, depending on the physical and chemical properties of the material, the acute inflammatory phase may be prolonged (i.e. beyond 1 week) and lead to chronic inflammation. If wound healing proceeds normally, acute inflammation leads into granulation tissue, a phase that is marked by a soft, pink, granular appearance on the wound healing surface as well as signs of neovascularization. The lysosomal agents and chemical mediators produced during acute inflammation activate and trigger growth factor upregulation by endothelial cells and fibroblasts, and these cells also lay down the matrix bed of collagen and proteoglycans to resolve the tissue repair process.

When the persistent presence of the biomaterial in the host and the incompatibility lead to chronic inflammation however, much of the cells recruited during the acute inflammatory phase (i.e. monocytes, macrophage, lymphocytes) remain and a foreign body reaction ensues. Chronic inflammation can be a part of a foreign body reaction, which is characterized by the presence of foreign body giant cells and the encapsulation of the foreign object at the local implant site in the host's attempt to wall off the material. Macrophages attempt to phagocytose the material and the material is too large to be phagocytosed, they undergo "frustrated phagocytosis" and macrophages fuse to form foreign body giant cells. When foreign body reaction leads to fibrous encapsulation, densely packed avascular collagen around the material forms to locally contain the foreign body from the rest of the host. Host tolerance of the material will result in matrix remodeling processes as fibroblasts and endothelial cells that infiltrate the site produce extracellular matrix (ECM) components such as collagen, fibronectin and hyaluronic acid and form the new ECM, scar tissue. While the matrix bed is laid down, matrix degrading agents such as matrix metalloproteases and collagenases help rearrange and organize a structured ECM.

These delicately orchestrated complex events described above comprise the host response that is often determined by the chemistry of the material's surface. Controlling each host response event and achieving complete restoration of normal tissue structure and function is a difficult task given our currently limited mechanistic understanding of host response. However, rather than a relatively passive approach of implanting a material and monitoring the host response, an active approach of tailoring host response through the presentation of biofunctional peptides may prove to be one significant stride toward avoiding host rejection of the material.

2.2. *In vitro response to biomaterials*

In vitro assays allow the assessment of material cytotoxicity on cells and are invaluable in screening biomaterials to gain insight into material degradation, mechanical strength over time and whether the materials leach toxic substances that affect the viability of cells. Three major assays for testing material biocompatibility and toxicity *in vitro* include agar diffusion, extraction, and direct cell-biomaterial contact method. Material toxicity can be investigated through the agar diffusion method by covering a confluent layer of cells with agar containing a viability stain, then placing the biomaterial on the agar surface and examining the extent of the viable cells under and around the material after an incubation period. Thus agar diffusion assays are useful in evaluating material toxicity, and the method is often applied to highly dense materials [1,2]. Extraction studies (i.e., elution, extract dilution) are also employed to observe any linear relationship between cell cytotoxicity and the concentration of extracted biomaterial. The threshold concentration of the material extract on minimal and maximal cytotoxicity can be investigated with a confluent layer of cells being exposed to serially diluted material extract and assessing cell viability after the incubation period. Usually, the cells in the targeted implant area are candidates for the extract dilution test and how much of the material extract is absorbed by these cells can also be determined [3].

Direct contact is the most widely applied test in cell-material *in vitro* analysis, and it involves placing the material directly on top of a confluent layer of cells or directly placing cells on top of the material. After incubation, cells are microscopically evaluated for toxicity (through viability staining), adherent density and morphology. Direct cell-material contact studies are the most prevalent in testing material biocompatibility and can reveal the intermediate zone of damaged cells. Especially when testing for cell response to peptide conjugated materials, the assessment of the cells in direct interaction with the peptide presented on the material surface is imperative. Cell adhesion and spreading as modulated by various peptides are central to the study of biologically responsive peptide conjugated materials. Since its discovery by Pierschbacher and Ruoslahti in 1984, the arginine-glycine-aspartic acid (RGD) sequence has been the most effective peptide sequence for enhanced integrin-mediated cell adhesion and has been applied to a myriad of materials and assessed for enhanced cell adhesion and wound repair [4]. The tripeptide sequence has been shown to enhance osteoblast adhesion *in vivo* and a myriad of cells *in vitro*, including osteoblasts, chondrocytes, human umbilical vein endothelial cells, fibroblasts and monocytes [5-13]. Table 1 shows increased monocyte adherent cell density on RGD-PEG grafted on a semi-interpenetrating network (sIPN) of gelatin and PEGdiacrylate (PEGdA) compared to that on sIPNs grafted with control ligands triglycine (GGG) or methoxy [13].

Table 1. Adherent monocyte density on RGD-PEG grafted sIPN and control ligand-PEG grafted sIPN (adapted from [13]).

	Adherent Monocyte Density (cells/mm^2)			
Ligand-PEG grafted onto gelatin of sIPN	**Culture Time: 2 h**	**24 h**	**96 h**	**168 h**
GGG	328 ± 69	444 ± 16	207 ± 52	74 ± 40
Methoxy	145 ± 18	233 ± 14	106 ± 2	95 ± 12
RGD	1321 ± 74*	1071 ± 190*	350 ± 42*	157 ± 8*

* Significantly higher than all other ligand-PEG grafted sIPN ($p<0.001$)

Table 2. Synthetic peptides derived from ECM components and biological activities of peptide-chitosan membranes (adapted from [14]).

Peptide	**Sequence**	**Protein Source (Residues)**	**Fibroblast Attachment**	**Neurite Outgrowth**	**Ref**
531	GEFYFDLRLKGDKY	Human collagen alpha1, type IV	++	–	25,26
AG73	RKRLQVQLSIRT	Murine laminin alpha1 chain	++	+	23

Direct cell-biomaterial *in vitro* testing and high throughput assays have been coupled in current studies to screen biomaterials more rapidly while testing for cell adhesion and material influence on cell morphology and proliferation. Figure 2 below outlines a study by Mochizuki and others where two biologically active peptides derived from ECM components were conjugated to chitosan membranes and microscopically observed using a 96 well plate as a high throughput system [14]. Table 2 outlines the peptides used and Figure 2 shows cell response to each peptide-grafted chitosan membrane.

Though *in vitro* studies offer the advantage of providing information on a specific cell type response to the biomaterial, *in vitro* work has the limitation of being too simple of a system compared to the highly complex and dynamic *in vivo* system with all the physiologically relevant players present interacting with the material of interest. Recent direct cell-biomaterial contact studies have been

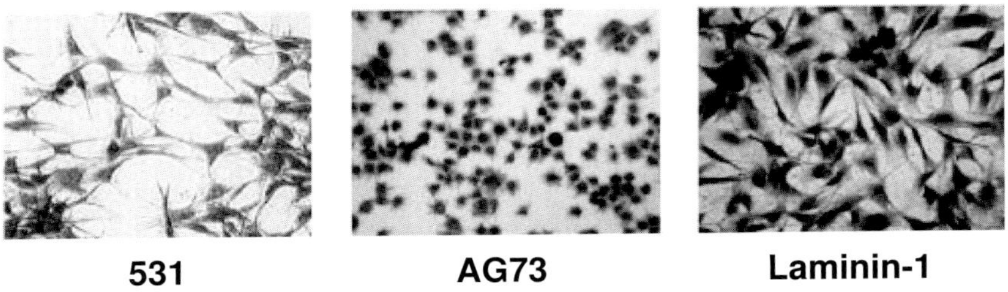

Fig. 2. Human foreskin fibroblasts adhered to chitosan membranes conjugated with different bioadhesive peptide sequences. 531 conjugated chitosan membranes and laminin support cell adhesion and spreading while AG73 supports cell adhesion but not spreading. Cells are stained with crystal violet [14].

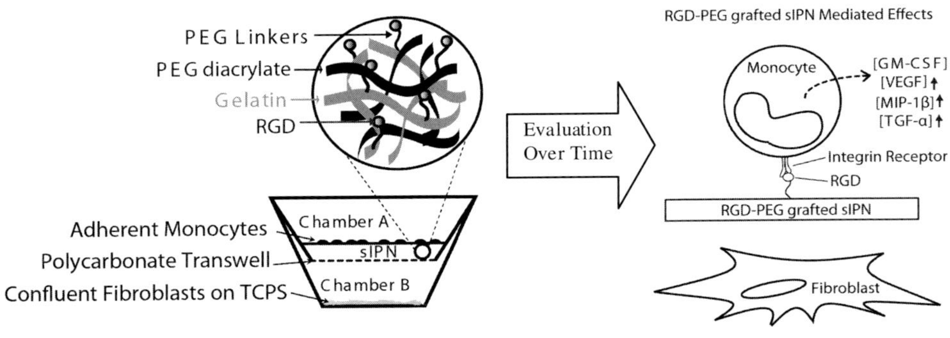

Fig. 3. A schematic of a co-culture of monocytes and fibroblasts with RGD-PEG grafted sIPN wound healing scaffold. Monocyte response to the RGD presenting sIPN and the communication between monocytes and fibroblasts in the presence of the RGD presenting sIPN scaffold were evaluated. Key wound healing factor expression in response to RGD-PEG grafted sIPN over time in the presence of fibroblasts could be evaluated [15].

developed to accommodate higher complexity and closer physiological relevance, such as the addition of a cell type to create a co-culture environment. In a work by Chung and Kao, monocyte interaction with an RGD-PEG conjugated hydrogel was examined in the presence of a confluent layer of fibroblasts [15]. Figure 3 below shows the co-culture schematic where monocyte response to the RGD presenting sIPN as perturbed by fibroblasts could be evaluated and key wound healing proteins could be profiled over time.

The co-culture setting allowed the evaluation of cell-material interaction in an environment closer to physiological conditions as well as the assessment of the biomaterial as a communicative barrier between two key wound healing cell types. Key wound healing factors including vascular endothelial growth factor (VEGF), monocyte inflammatory protein-1beta (MIP-1β), and tumor growth factor-alpha (TFG-α) were upregulated in a ligand specific response to RGD-PEG grafted sIPN in the presence of fibroblasts while granulocyte-macrophage colony-stimulating factor (GM-CSF) was downregulated. Other approaches to making the *in vitro* system more advanced have included the addition of dynamic components such as flow of media and nutrients on the system and making the cell culture 3D [16]. Although this type of work adds to the already challenging task of parsing out specific causal effects and the source of each response, it allows the system to more closely mimick the tissue environment.

2.3. *In vivo response to biomaterials*

In vivo testing of materials for tissue compatibility offers the obvious advantage over *in vitro* systems of having all the appropriate physiological components (cells, matrix, tissue structure and function, soluble proteins, etc.) present. *In vivo* investigations are intended to simulate end-use applications and thus the direct application of the biomaterial is used to assess biocompatibility in the clinical use setting. Where the assessment can vary is the duration, frequency, and the location of exposure, as well as the physicochemical stability and compatibility of the biomaterial itself. *In vivo* tests can reveal critical information on the biomaterials' compatibility at the tissue site, as well as on the function and the stability of the material in the host. *In vivo* analyses can reveal much information on host response including blood material interactions, matrix formation, inflammation, fibrous encapsulment and the other events as outlined in Figure 1. In addition, *in vivo* assays can also yield information on local and system toxicity, genotoxicity and local and systemic immune response.

In the case of biomaterial implantation, histological examination of the implant site after a given duration has remained a widely applied analysis of host tissue response. The presence and the abundance of certain cell types at the tissue-implant interface are examined for tissue compatibility by immunohistochemical staining or immunofluorescent labeling the histological sections. For example, polymorphonuclear leukocytes at the implant site indicate acute inflammation, the presence of mononuclear cells such as plasma cells and lymphocytes indicates chronic inflammation, lymphocytes and monocytes in high numbers suggest possible infection. Other indications of pathology include the examination of granulation tissue with key markers such as infiltrating fibroblasts, soft granular appearance of the healing site as well as collagen deposition and small capillary development. Foreign body giant cells and fibrous capsule of densely packed collagen indicate foreign body reaction and fibrous encapsulment, respectively. Figure 4 highlights key wound healing events in a dermal wound repair of a full thickness wound treated with a collagen implant in a mouse model [17]. Reepithelization and the newly formed epidermis along with granular tissue that mark the late stages of wound repair are shown along with the resorbed collagen implant (Figure 4B). Thus, the biocompatibility of the material at the tissue level and the incorporation of the implant material and the host tolerance of the material can be gauged by histology.

In addition to histological evaluations, host response is also analyzed by the use of various biomarkers. Tissue homogenate and exudates are often collected and analyzed for biomarkers including inflammatory biomarker proteins such as interleukins and tumor necrosis factors and matrix remodeling matrix metalloproteases often to be screened at the implant site [18]. Biomarkers can be identified in many ways, western blotting, enzyme linked immunosorbant assay (ELISA) can identify markers at the protein level and current applications of

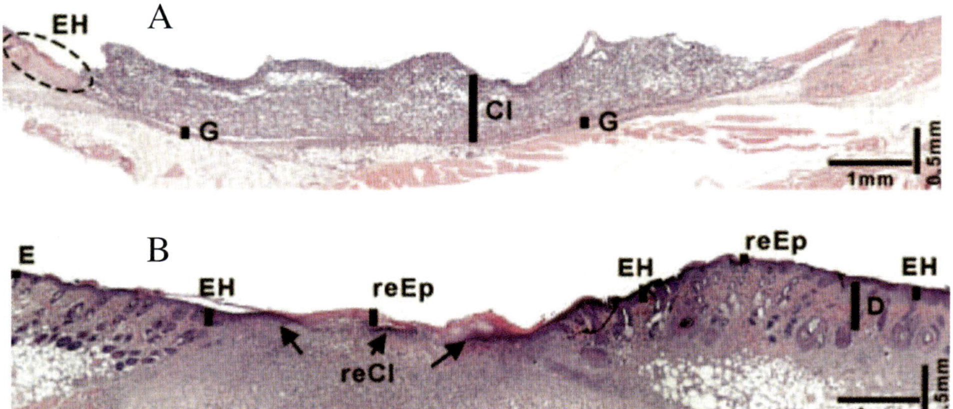

Fig. 4. Wound healing assessments at day 3 (A) and at day 14 (B) post collagen implantation. reEp: early re-Reepithelization; E: epidermis; D: dermis; EH; epidermal hyperplasia (new grown epidermis); reCI: resorption of collagen implant; G: granular tissue [17].

mass spectroscopy to profile the tissue and analyze host response to biomaterials is rapidly developing [19]. Consistent with trends in *in vitro* analyses, high throughput approaches are becoming rapidly incorporated into *in vivo* analyses. Thus, protein microarray chips and multiplexed cytokine assays can be employed to analyze tissue homogenate or wound exudates to provide reproducible and global protein analysis rapidly.

Genetic analysis of the tissue site can be carried out by northern blot analysis of the tissue homogenate or wound exudates, similar to western blot analysis for proteins. In situ hybridization can be applied to the tissue section to localize DNA or RNA of interest with probes, similar to immunohistochemistry that localizes proteins. Reverse transcriptase or real time polymerase chain reaction (RT-PCR and qRT-PCR, respectively) and ribonuclease protection assays can analyze mRNA at the tissue site. However, both northern blot analysis and in situ hybridization require a larger amount of sample and polymerase chain reactions are time consuming and cannot target many genes per assay. Analysis of tissue lysate or exudates employing cDNA microarrays can also provide a global gene expression at the wound site and can uncover cell signaling and transcription genes critical to wound healing that were not targeted with the other assays [20].

The protein and genetic analysis of tissue homogenates or exudates described above can be coupled within *in vivo* analyses, as well as with *in vitro* analyses. For example, analysis of inflammatory interleukins can be analyzed *in vitro* by investigating the protein levels through ELISA or western blot and the genetic interleukin expression by PCR. *In vivo*, ELISA or western blot can also be applied to analyze the tissue homogenate or exudates to observe interleukin protein levels, and PCR or ribonuclease protection assay can reveal genetic interleukin regulation *in vivo*. Microarrays can also be useful in coupling *in vitro* and *in vivo* host response analyses.

2.4. *Enhancing biological response: Host interaction with peptide-polymer conjugates*

Peptide sequences can enhance adhesion and elicit specific intracellular signaling events upon peptide-cell interaction. Due to their relatively robust stability compared to the whole protein and their ability to direct specific downstream effects upon interaction with the cell, peptide conjugated materials are emerging as a new class of materials that combine unique advantages from both the natural and synthetic world to yield a material with unique biological properties compared to conventional therapies.

Peptides have been conjugated to natural and synthetic polymers for tissue repair applications. Directing the host response by presenting biofunctional peptides on the material surface is one approach to improving host biocompatibility while simultaneously taking advantage of the mechanical and structural properties of the natural or synthetic polymer scaffold. Natural polymers possess highly ordered and complex quaternary structures that have excellent aqueous solubility, *in vivo* compatibility and controlled degradation, and break down into natural amino acids that can be metabolized in the host with minimal immune response and cytotoxicity. Thus, peptide conjugated natural polymers can offer a complex yet highly biocompatible platform that also has biofunctional sequences to direct cell response and tissue function. Peptides can also be grafted onto synthetic polymers and though they cannot provide the level of complexity that natural polymers can, synthetic polymers offer better availability, stability, chemical control and innateness in the host. Synthetic polymers are readily available at often lower cost than natural polymers and offer practicality as well as control over the physicochemical properties including chain length, functional groups, degree of crosslinking, chain architecture, and subsequently the elasticity, tensile strength and rheological properties and others. In addition, polymers such as polyethylene glycol have been established as a nonfouling polymer that resists nonspecific protein adsorption, and polymers such as polydimethoxysilane do not support bacterial growth [21]. Depending on the targeted tissue, the polymer can be tailored to provide the structural template close to the tissue site, and by conjugating critically active portions of the naturally derived material to synthetic polymers, specific signaling from the natural material and the inertness of the synthetic material can be combined to yield a controlled biomaterial with predictable and desired host response.

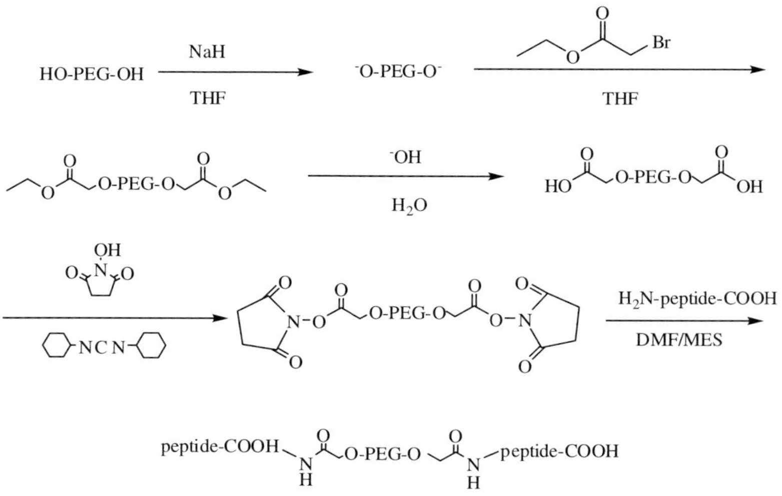

Fig. 5. Schematic of peptide conjugation onto polyethylene glycol by first activating the carboxy group with DCC and using N-hydroxysuccinimide as a leaving group adapted from [22].

3. Peptide-Polymer Conjugate Systems: Synthesis and Interaction with the Host

3.1. *Overview: Conjugation chemistry and properties*

The most common method used to conjugate bioactive peptides to polymers is with thiol or succinimide ester groups to create a covalent amide bond. This linkage is created by the activation of a carboxylic group on the material to react with the peptide's amine-terminus. Carboxylic acids can be activated by carbodiimide peptide coupling reagents, most commonly dicyclohexylcarbodiimide (DCC) or diisopropylcarbodiimide (DIC), and sometimes ethyl-(N', N'-dimethylamino)propylcarbodiimide hydrochloride (EDC). Outlined in Figure 5 is a reaction scheme demonstrating the conjugation of peptides onto polyethylene glycol by activating the carboxy groups with DCC, then conjugating N-hydroxysuccinimide (NH-Su) to ultimately serve as a leaving group for peptide conjugation [22]. More examples of these chemistries will be highlighted in the case studies to follow.

3.2. *Peptide conjugated natural polymers*

The ideal treatment for wounds is the application of natural tissue. However, as tissue sources are limited, components of the natural tissue can be used to substitute as a tissue repair scaffold to achieve maximal biocompatibility. Natural polymers include many of the ECM proteins such as collagen, fibronectin, laminin, chitosan, hyaluronic acid, and others. These polymers can provide multiple functions, for example, collagen provides structural function, but also contains biofunctional peptide sequences that have been demonstrated to enhance the stability and differentiation of encapsulated cells [23-25]. By conjugating bioactive peptide sequences onto these ECM-derived scaffolds, ligand-specific activity and signaling can be achieved to enhance cell attachment and support cell proliferation. As the scaffold onto which the peptide is conjugated is a naturally derived material, the biomaterial platform will be better incorporated into the injured tissue and subsequently cleared from the body in a non-inflammatory manner. This section outlines two case studies where the effects of peptide conjugated natural polymers on the *in vitro* and *in vivo* host response are described.

3.2.1. *Peptide conjugated natural polymers*

An adhesive peptide sequence Arg-Gly-Asp-Ser-Gly-Gly-Cys (RGDSGGC) was conjugated onto a chitosan membrane with reactive thiol groups incorporated

(Figure 6) [26]. RGD, an adhesive sequence, was conjugated to chitosan, as chitosan has shown to be promising polysaccharides for biocompatible and wound healing materials [27-30]. Reactive thiol groups were incorporated into the chitosan membrane by reacting it with 2-iminothiolane, as it has been demonstrated that the 2-iminothiolane undergoes a ring opening reaction with primary amines, including N-terminal α-and ε-amino groups of peptides or proteins [31].

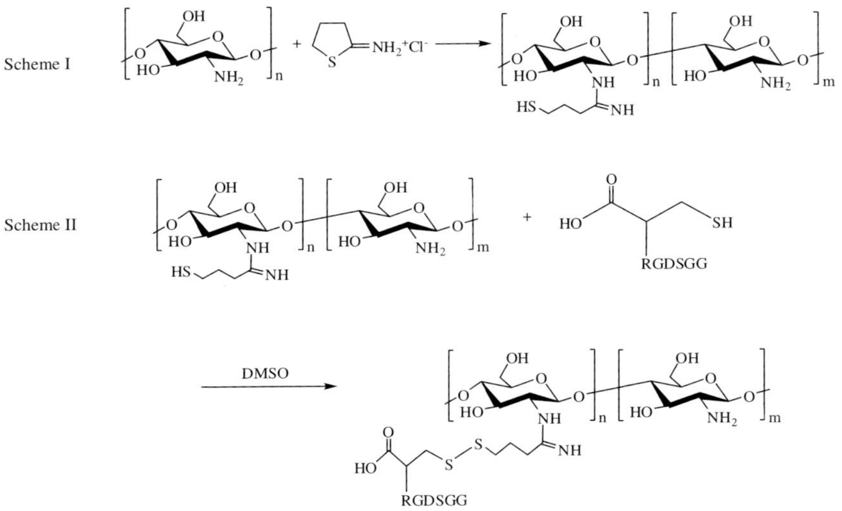

Fig. 6. Scheme I outlines incorporation of a thiol group through a ring opening reaction of 2-iminothiolane with chitosan and scheme II shows the coupling reaction of SH-chitosan with RGDSGGC (adapted from [26]).

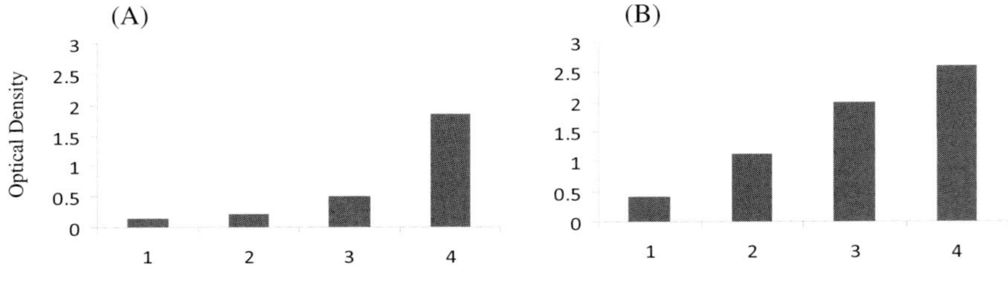

Fig. 7. Adhesivity of (A) chondrocytes and (B) fibroblasts: (1) Control (2) 0.0012% RGDSGGC-chitosan (3) 0.012% RGDSGGC-chitosan (4) 0.12% RGDSGGC-chitosan (adapted from [26]).

The resulting effect of the RGDSGGC peptide presented on the chitosan membrane was markedly enhanced affinity of both chondrocytes and fibroblasts onto this peptide conjugated polymer scaffold when compared to that on a plate coated with RGDSGGC. In addition, the authors showed enhanced affinity of both chondrocytes and fibroblasts in a peptide-concentration dependent manner. With increased RGDSGGC-chitosan concentration coated onto a microtiter plate, chondrocyte and fibroblast cell adhesivity, as measured by optical density of the crystal violet dye, was proportionally increased (Figure 7A, B), and fibroblast proliferation also increased proportionally (Figure 7A, B).

3.2.2. *Case study: Peptide complexed hyaluronic acid*

Another example of a peptide conjugated to a natural polymer material is the RGD containing peptide sequence covalently linked to hyaluronic acid as

(A)

(B)

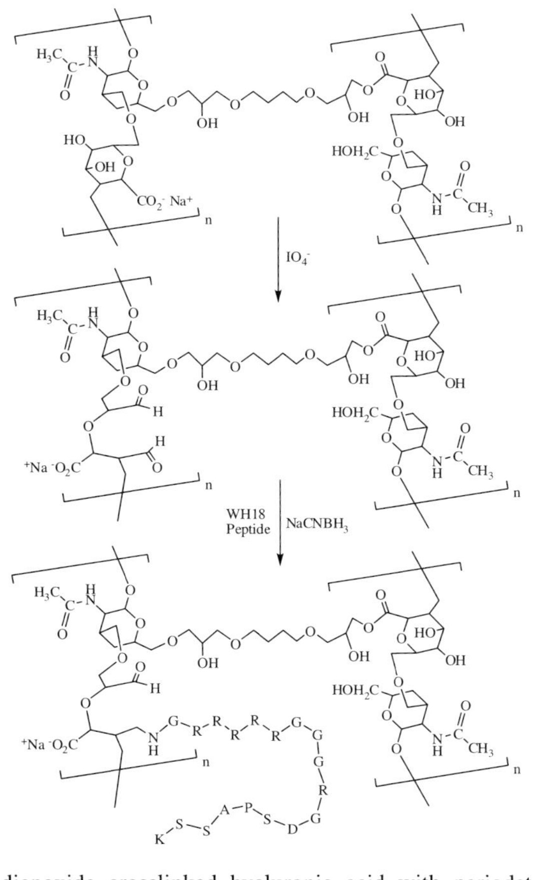

Fig. 8. Reaction of (A) diepoxide crosslinked hyaluronic acid with periodate to oxidize the polyhydroxyls of the glucuronic acid to create reactive aldehydes and of (B) activated aldehydes of the hyaluronic acid with the peptide sequence, followed by a reduction with sodium cyanoborohydride to form a stable amine on the conjugation site [32].

demonstrated by Glass and others [32]. Hyaluronic acid, a non-immunogenic polysaccharide found in many human tissues, is upregulated during repair and naturally cleared by the host. Though hyaluronic acid modifications with synthetic polymers have been commonly reported, studies on peptide conjugation on the polysaccharide are to date elusive. Hyaluronic acid crosslinked with a diepoxide is reacted with periodate to create reactive aldehydes by peroxidate oxidation of the polyhydroxyls of glucuronic acid (Figure 8A). A RGD containing 18 amino acid peptide sequence, Gly-Arg-Arg-Arg-Arg-Arg-Gly-Gly-Gly-Arg-Gly-Asp-Ser-Pro-Ala-Ser-Ser-Lys ($GR_5G_3RGDSPASSK$, or WH18), was then conjugated to hyaluronic acid through sodium cyanoborohydride reduction. Primary amines of the peptide sequence serve as nucleophiles to form secondary amine bonds, which are reduced by sodium cyanoborohyride, creating a more stable primary amine, and covalently linking the peptide to the carbonyl chains on hyaluronic acid (Figure 8B). The WH18 peptide sequence, while designed to present the RGD sequence recognized by the integrin receptors, was also designed with the D-isomer or arginine to protect it against a number of serine proteases known to be present in wounds.

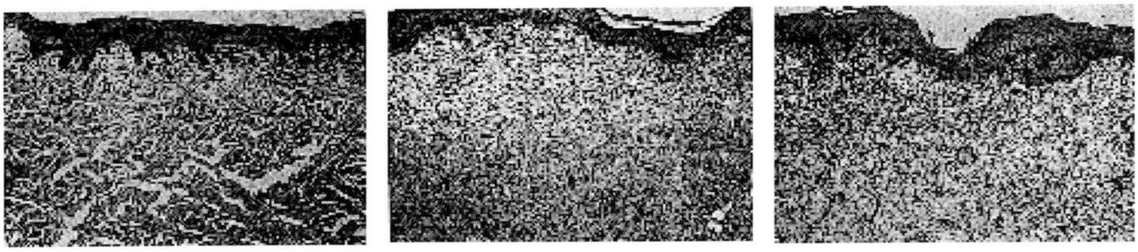

(A) (B) (C)

Fig. 9. Photomicrograph of 8-day-old burn wound (A) no treatment, air-exposed control, (B) treated with hyaluronic acid, and (C) treated with RGD-hyaluronic acid matrix. Note the very thin layer of loose edematous connective tissue subepidermally in the air-exposed controls, the wider subepidermal zone with some cellular infiltrate in the hyaluronic acid treated wound, and the majority of the dermis appearing as granulation tissue with marked cellular infiltrate in the RGD-hyaluronic matrix treated wound. (Hematoxylin and eosin, original magnification x100) [32].

In vitro, the conjugation of the RGD containing WH18 peptide sequence onto hyaluronic acid resulted in a 90% or greater attachment and subsequently supported spreading of human osteosarcoma cells (MG63). On surfaces that were treated with periodate in the absence of peptide, or that were not treated with periodate resulted in very little attachment of the osteosarcoma cells and no cell spreading on the material. They also described enhanced attachment of human colon fibroblasts, primary bovine epithelial cells and human gingival fibroblasts.

Thus, by conjugating an adhesive peptide sequence onto a naturally occurring polysaccharide material, cell adhesion and proliferation could be supported.

In a simultaneously reported study, the GR_5G_3RGDSPASSK conjugated hyaluronic acid matrix was tested for healing response of second-degree burn wounds in pigs. The RGD-hyaluronic acid matrix (with Tegaderm™ as outer secondary dressing) treated wounds showed significantly increased rates of epithelization compared to air exposed control and the hyaluronic acid treated wounds after one week. Along with enhanced epithelization, the RGD-hyaluronic acid matrix treated wounds showed marked cellular infiltrate compared to the air exposed control and the hyaluronic acid without peptide conjugation (Figure 9). In addition, increased granulation tissue was also observed with RGD-hyaluronic acid treated burns compared to the air exposed control.

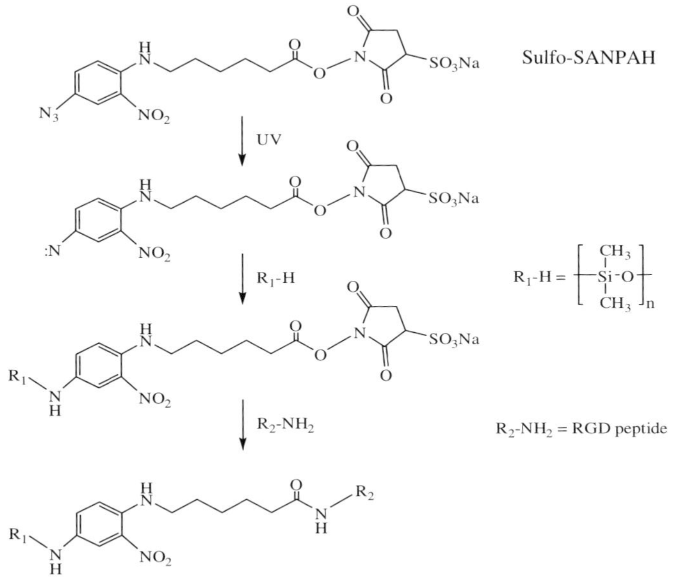

Fig. 10. A two-step succinimide based process for conjugating RGD peptide onto PDMS surfaces [36].

Hyaluronic acid has been tested in several models for wound healing applications, but with varying results. With the RGD-hyaluronic acid matrix, Glass and others demonstrated enhanced osteosarcoma cell adhesion and proliferation *in vitro* while Mertz and others showed significantly improved epithelization rate, cellular infiltration and granulation of tissue, complex processes that lead to the total repair of second degree burns *in vivo* [33].

3.3. *Peptide conjugated synthetic polymers*

Polymers can offer a practical and chemically and mechanically controllable option for biomedical applications, and polymers such as poly(dimethylsiloxane) (PDMS) have been widely used in the clinical setting, including surgical implants and catheters [34,35]. PDMS elastomers, with good compatibility with the human tissue and biological innertness, and excellent elasticity and transparency, are widely applied as surgical implants and catheters. However, though they are biocompatible and resist bacterial growth, these silicone elastomers do not support cell adhesion, a critical process in wound healing.

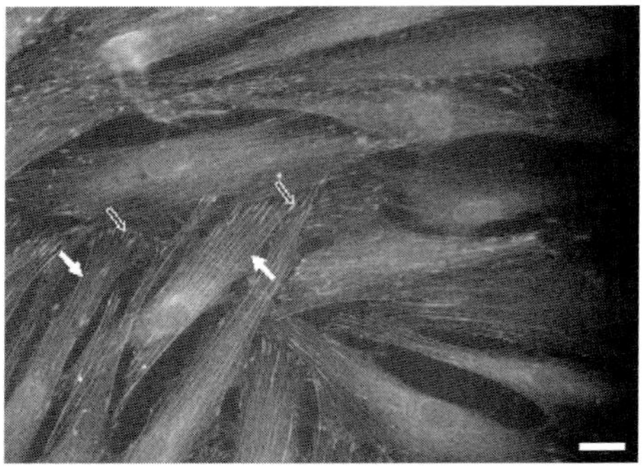

Fig. 11. Fluorescence microscopy images of human skin fibroblasts cultured on a RGD-conjugated PDMS substrate. The cells contain bundles of stress fibers (solid arrows), and their focal adhesions are also clearly seen (blank arrows). The cells were fixed and stained after 2 days in culture; Scale bar, 20μm [36].

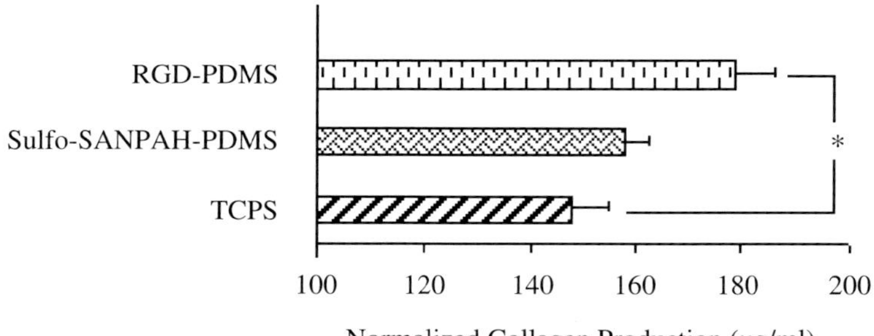

Fig. 12. Total soluble collagen production by human skin fibroblasts cultured on RGD-conjugated PDMS, sulfo-SANPAH activated PDMS surface (without RGD conjugation) and TCPS. Collagen concentrations are normalized to cell number *p<0.01 (adapted from [36]).

Li and others attempted to merge the excellent elasticity of the material with cell adhesion promoting properties by conjugating the bioadhesive peptide sequence RGD peptide onto the PDMS [36]. The conjugation of RGD onto PDMS was carried out through a succinimide based chemistry, using sulfosuccinimidyl 6-(4'-azido-2'-nitro-phenylamino) hexanoate (sulfo-SANPAH) (Figure 10). Unique to this photochemical, succinimide based conjugation of peptides onto a polymer surface is the ultimate peptide conjugation achieved through covalent amide bonds unlike coating or adsorption techniques that lead to ionic non-covalent interactions such as ionic, van der waals forces and hydrogen bonding. Figure 10 outlines the two step photochemical based conjugation of the RGD peptide onto the PDMS surface.

The RGD conjugated PDMS surfaces promoted adhesion, proliferation, and collagen secretion of human skin fibroblasts (HSFs). While few cells attached onto the PDMS surface, RGD-peptide conjugation on to the PDMS surface resulted in an enhanced adhesion and rapid proliferation of HSFs. RGD conjugated surfaces yielded a well spread and elongated fibroblasts that showed

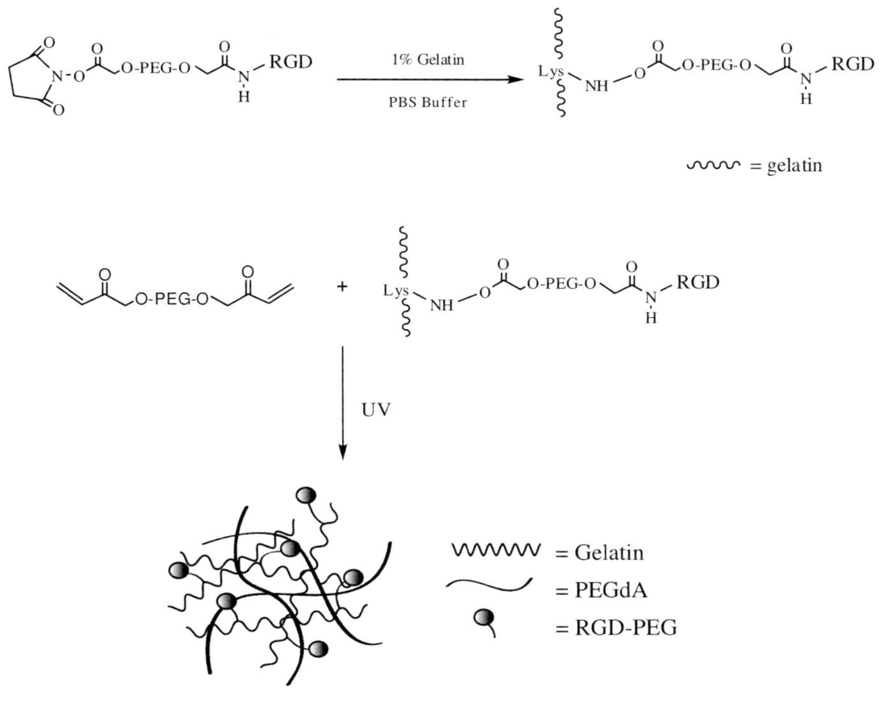

Fig. 13. Chemical schematic of the RGD-PEG grafted gelatin and PEGdA interpenetrating network scaffold. The RGD peptide is grafted onto a PEG linker via a succinimide based conjugation and the RGD-PEG grafted gelatin is polymerized with PEGdA to create a natural and synthetic polymer hybrid scaffold that presents a biofunctional peptide (adapted from [22]).

increased formation of actin microfilament bundles and focal adhesions, indicating strong cell-substrate interaction (Figure 11). Furthermore, the RGD conjugated PDMS surface promoted fibroblast collagen production when compared with that produced on sulfo-SANPAH activated PDMS surfaces and TCPS (Figure 12).

3.3.1. *Case study: Poly(ethylene glycol)*

Polyethylene glycol (PEG), which is a widely applied polymer that has been established in biocompatibility, is commonly found in biomedical devices and materials and is also found in food, cosmetics and drugs [37]. In a work by Waldeck and others, a wound healing scaffold composed of polyethylene glycol diacrylate (PEGdA) and gelatin semi-interpenetrating network (sIPN) was constructed to present the RGD peptide on a PEG linker [38]. Gelatin, a denatured form of collagen, has been widely accepted as biocompatible and is often found in food products and applied in bridging nerves and nerve tissue engineering [39,40]. The peptide conjugation chemistry was carried out similar to the succinimide based chemistry shown in Figure 5, except with one functional group of the polyethylene glycol used for the RGD peptide conjugation and the remaining functional group used to covalently link the RGD-PEG onto the lysyl group of the gelatin backbone to yield RGD-PEG grafted gelatin (Figure 13). When the RGD-PEG grafted gelatin was polymerized with PEGdA, the resulting hybrid sIPN presented the RGD peptide on the matrix surface on a PEG tether.

The RGD-PEG grafted sIPN with keratinocyte growth factor (KGF) incorporated into the matrix was applied onto a full-thickness wound on a rat model to investigate wound healing response *in vivo*. The resulting *in vivo* analysis revealed enhanced cell recruitment and granulation of tissue along with higher extracellular matrix organization, neovascularization and rate of

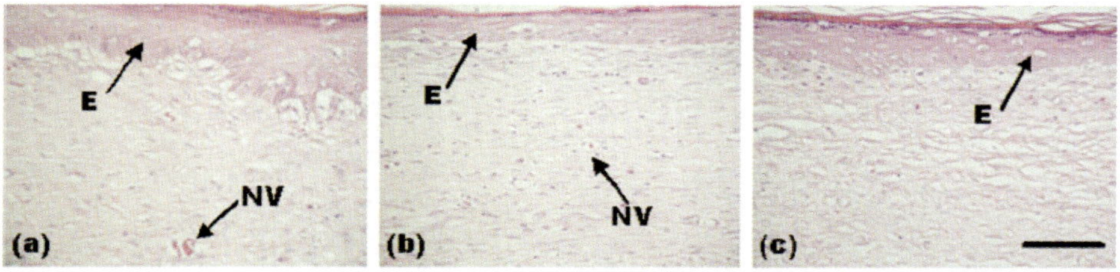

Fig. 14. Photomicrographs (x20) of (a) RGD modified sIPN + Keratinocyte growth factor interface at 3 weeks. (b) unmodified gelatin sIPN interface area at 3 weeks. (c) conventional dressing interface area at 3 weeks. Areas identified include neovascularization (NV) and epidermis (E) [38].

contraction was observed (Figure 14). Shown in Figure 14 are the effects of RGD-PEG sIPN + KGF, unmodified sIPN (i.e., unmodified gelatin and PEGdA only, and no RGD-PEG), and conventional dressing, Silverlon®. While the conventional dressing resulted in a visible depression in the healing wound, both the unmodified sIPN and the RGD-PEG sIPN + KGF supported the formation of tissue with no visible depression, demonstrating its structural effectiveness as a scaffold. In addition, the RGD-PEG sIPN + KGF resulted in high levels of macrophages and fibroblasts that were similar to undamaged tissue by three weeks, suggesting granulation of tissue at the later stages of wound healing for RGD-PEG sIPN + KGF treated wounds. The epidermis was restored to a thicker degree with more ridges for the RGD-PEG sIPN + KGF treated wounds as well as a basket-weave patterned ECM developing toward the epidermis. There were also larger occurrences of neovascularization as well as thicker and more dense collagen bundles in the RGD-PEG + KGF treated wounds when compared to unmodified sIPN or conventional dressing treated wounds.

4. Host Response to Peptide-Polymer Conjugate Systems: Future Directions and Challenges

Peptide conjugated polymer systems are a newly emerging class of biomaterials that can combine select advantages from biological and synthetic components to create a uniquely functionalized material. Advances in peptide conjugated materials have been exponential and a wealth of knowledge has been gained about the effect of peptide conjugated materials on the host response. Peptides offer stability and specific induction of cell events, but there remains much to be understood about the impact of these peptides' selectivity and presentation on the biomaterial surface and how that impacts cell behavior. For example, while some report the importance of $\alpha v\beta 3$ integrin-mediated fibroblast focal adhesion and stress fiber formation in fibroblasts to a RGD presenting surface, others have demonstrated the key role of $\beta 2$ containing integrins on monocyte adhesion onto a RGD presenting surface [41-43]. It is also becoming clearer that the density of peptides on the material plays a critical role in host response. For example, while Massia and Hubbell reported that a RGD density of 1 fmol/cm^2 grafted on a glass surface induced maximal fibroblast adhesion and spreading while Rowley and Mooney showed a 30 fmol/cm^2 RGD density on an alginate surface induced maximum myoblast adhesion and proliferation [41,44]. In addition, Sawyer and others have demonstrated a threshold for RGD density's impact on mesenchymal stem cells (MSC), where a high RGD concentration coated on the hydroxyapatite surface actually deterred MSC binding and spreading [45]. However, these studies report *in vitro* findings and the impact of the complex and dynamic interaction between blood proteins and a variety of host cells on the RGD presenting surface is even less understood. Even in *in vitro* systems the cause and effect based mechanisms behind cell-material interaction (i.e. enhance adhesion, proliferation and ECM production, etc.) are yet to be clearly deciphered and remain critical to the ultimate goal of directed host response. And though peptides are more stable than the whole protein, they are not exempt from thermal instability and hydrolysis and are thus subject to short shelf lives. Peptides can also be costly to synthesize and may be impractical for large scale treatments, but with rapid developments in recombinant DNA technologies that allow the synthesis of these sequences, overcoming the hurdle of high scale up cost is becoming more plausible. The biggest challenge will still be controlling the dynamic and spatial arrangement of multiple signals and ultimately translating this controlled surface into directed host response.

With current developments in our increasingly sophisticated understanding of protein structure-function through technologies such as crystallography, the trend in peptide conjugated systems is shifting toward peptide conjugated natural polymers. Natural biopolymers such as chitosan, collagen and hyaluronic acid are rapidly gaining interest, and the literature on peptide conjugated natural polymers is growing at a faster rate than peptide conjugated synthetic polymer systems. However, synthetic polymers are more robust than natural polymers and continue to be a more prevalent application in the clinical setting, and thus the endeavor to impart biological activity onto polymer surfaces to create uniquely advantageous biomaterials will continue.

References

1. C. Hendrich, M. Geyer D. Sheddin, N. Schutze, J. Eulert, R. Thull. "A new osteoblast culture system for standardized testing of biomaterials." *Biomed Tech (Berl)*, vol. 41, pp.278-283, 1996.
2. Tsuchiya, T. "Studies on the standardization of cytotoxity tests and new standard reference materials useful for evaluating the safety of biomaterials." *J Biomat App*, vol. 9, pp.138-157, 1994.
3. A. Huhtala, T. Pohjonen, L. Salminen, A. Salminen, K. Kaarniranta, H. Uusitalo. "*In vitro* biocompatibility of degradable biopolymers in cell cultures from various ocular tissues: extraction studies." *J Mater Sci Med,* vol.19, pp. 645-649, 2008.
4. M.D. Pierschbacher and E. Ruoslahti, "Cell attachment activity of fibronectin can be duplicated by small synthetic fragments of the molecule." *Nature*, vol. 309, pp.30-33, 1984.
5. H.S Shin, S.B, Jo, A.G. Mikos, "Modulation of marrow stromal osteoblast adhesion on biomimetic oligo[poly(ethylene glycol) fumarate] hydrogels modified with Arg-Gly-Asp peptides and a poly(ethylene glycol) spacer." *J Biomed Mater Res*, vol. 61, pp.169-179, 2002.

6. M. Kantlehner, P. Schaffner, D. Finsinger, J. Meyer, A. Jonczyk, B. Diefenbach, B. Nies, G. Holzemann, S.L. Goodman, H. Kessler. "Surface coating with cyclic RGD peptides stimulates osteoblast adhesion and proliferation as well as bone formation." *Chembiochem*, vol. 1, pp. 107-114, 2000.
7. A. Rezania and K.E. Healy, "Integrin subunits responsible for adhesion of human osteoblast-like cells to biomimetic peptide surfaces. *J Orthop Res*, vol. 1999, pp. 615-623, 1999.
8. S.P. Massia and J. Stark, "Immobilized RGD peptides on surface-grafted dextran promote biospecific cell attachment." *J Biomed Mater Res*, vol. 56, pp. 390-399, 2001.
9. S. Verrier, S. Pallu, R. Bareille, A. Jonczyk, J. Meyer, M. Dard, J. Amedee. "Function of linear and cyclic RGD-containing peptides in osteoprogenitor cells adhesion process." *Biomaterials*, vol. 23. pp. 585-596, 2002.
10. J. Yu, Y. Gu, K.T. Du, S. Mihardja, R.E. Sievers, R.J. Lee, "The effect of injected RGD modified alginate on angiogenesis and left ventricular function in a chronic rat infarct model." *Biomaterials*, vol. 30, pp. 751-756, 2009.
11. B. Zhao, Z. Yi, W. Tian, F. Cui, H. Feng, H. Hu, T. Kawakami, T. Tagaki, N. Nagai, "Improvement of adhesion and spreading of human gingival fibroblasts to RGD-grafted titanium surface," *J Hard Tissue Biol*, vol.15, pp. 65-68, 2006.
12. A.G. Karakecili, T.T. Dermirtas, C. Satriano, M. Gumusderelioglu, G. Marletta. "Evaluation of L292 fibroblast attachment and proliferation on Arg-Gly-Asp-Ser (RGDS)-immobilized chitosan in serum-containing /serum-free cultures." *J Biosci and Bioeng*, vol. 104, pp. 69-77, 2007.
13. A.S. Chung, H.M. Waldeck, D.R. Schmidt, W.J. Kao. "Monocyte inflammatory and matrix remodeling response modulated by grafted ECM-derived ligand identity and concentration." *J Biomed Mater Res*, published online Dec 2, 2008.
14. M. Mochizuki, N. Yamagata, D. Philp, K. Hozymi, T. Watanabe, Y. Kikkawa, Y. Kadoya, H.K. Kleinman, M. Nomizu, "Integrin-dependent cell behavior on ECM peptide conjugated chitosan membranes." *Pept Sci*, vol. 88, pp.122-130, 2007.
15. A.S. Chung and W.J Kao, "Fibroblasts regulate monocyte response to ECM-derived matrix: The effects on monocyte adhesion and the production of inflammatory, matrix remodeling and growth factor proteins. *J Biomed Mater Res,* In Press.
16. J.S. Stephens, J.A. Cooper, F.R. Phelan, Jr., J.P. Dunkers, "Perfusion flow bioreactor for 3D in situ imaging: investigating cell/biomaterials interactions." *Biotechnol Bioeng*, vol. 97, pp.952-961, 2006.
17. X. Wang, X. Yu, Y. Yan, R. Zhang. "Liver tissue responses to gelatin and gelatin/chitosan gels." *J Biomed Mater Res*, vol. 87, pp.62-68, 2008.
18. M. Kalltorp, S. Oblogina, S. Jacobsson, A. Karlsson, P. Tengvall, P. Thomsen. "*In vivo* recruitment, cytokine release and chemiluminescence response at gold, and thiol functionalized surfaces." *Biomaterials*, vol. 20, pp.736-742, 1999.
19. R.K. Caldwell, S.R. Opalenik, J.M. Davidson, R.M. Caprioli, L.B. Nanney, "Tissue profiling MALDI mass spectrometry reveals prominent calcium binding proteins in the proteome of regenerative MRL mouse wounds." *Wound Repair Regen*, vol. 16, pp. 442-449, 2008.
20. N.S. Gibran and F.F. Isik, "Use of high-throughput microarray membranes for cDNA analysis of cutaneous wound repair," *Methods in Molecular Medicine: Wound Healing Methods and Protocols,* vol. 78, pp.425-432, 2008. (Ed. Luisa A DiPietro and Aime L. Burns) Humana Press Inc., Totowa, NJ

21. J.M. Harris, "Poly(ethylene glycol) chemistry and biotechnical and biomedical applications.: *App Biochem Biotechnol*, vol. 41, 1992.
22. A.S. Chung, Q. Gao, W.J. Kao WJ, "Either integrin subunit β1 or β3 is involved in mediating monocyte adhesion, IL-1β protein and mRNA expression in response to surfaces functionalized with fibronectin-derived peptides." *J Biomater Sci Polym Ed*, vol. 18, pp. 713-729, 2007.
23. T. Aigner and J. Stove, "Collagens—major component of the physiological cartilage matrix, major target of cartilage degeneration, major tool in cartilage repair." *Adv Drug Deliv Rev*, vol.55, pp.1569-1593, 2003.
24. D.G. Wallace and J. Rosenblatt, "Collagen gel systems for sustained delivery and tissue engineering." *Adv Drug Deliv Rev*, vol. 55, pp.1631-1639, 2003.
25. C.R. Lee, A.J. Grodzinsky, M. Spector, "Biosynthetic response of passaged chondrocytein a type II collagen scaffold to a mechanical compression." *J Biomed Mater Res A*, vol. 64, pp.560-569, 2003.
26. T. Masuko, N. Iwasaki, S. Yamane, T. Funakoshi, T. Majima, A. Minami, N. Ohsuga, T. Ohta, S.I. Nishimura, "Chitosan-RGDSGGC conjugate as a scaffold material for musculoskeletal tissue engineering." *Biomaterials*, vol. 26, pp. 5339-5347, 2005.
27. S.V. Madihally and H.W.T. Matthew, "Porous chitosan scaffold for tissue engineering." *Biomaterials*, vol. 20, pp. 1133-1142, 1999.
28. J.K.F. Suh and H.W.T. Matthew, "Application of chitosan based polysaccharide biomaterials in cartilage tissue engineering: a review." *Biomateirals,* vol. 21, pp.2589-2598, 2000.
29. Z. Degim, N. Celebi, H. Sayan, A. Babul, D. Erdogan, G. Take, "An investigation on skin wound healing in mice with a taurine-chitosan gel formation." *Amino Acids*, vol.22, pp.187-198, 2002.
30. K. Peh, T. Kahn, H. Ching, "Mechanical, bioadhesive strength and biological evaluations of chitosan films for wound dressing." *J Pharm Sci*, vol.3, pp.303-311, 2000.
31. Q. Fu and D.C. Gowda, "Carbohydrate-directed conjugation of cobra venom factor to antibody by selective derivatization of the terminal galactose residues." *Bioconjugate Chem*, vol. 12, pp. 271-279, 2001.
32. J.R. Glass, K.T. Dickerson, K. Stecker, J.W. Polarek, "Characterization of a hyaluronic acid-Arg-Gly-Asp peptide cell attachment matrix" *Biomaterials*, vol. 17, pp. 1101-1108, 1996.
33. P.M. Mertz, S.C. Davis, L. Franzen, F.D. Uchima, M.P. Pickett, M.P., M.D. Pierschbacher, J.W. Polarek, "Effects of an arginine-glycine-aspartic acid peptide-containing artificial matrix on epithelial migration *in vitro* and experimental second-degree burn wound healing *in vivo*." *J Burn Care Rehabil*, vol. 17, pp.199-206, 1996.
34. S.P. Gorman and A.D. Woolfson, "Novel biomimetic and bioactive silicones." *Med Device Technol,* vol.13, pp.14-15, 2002.
35. K.Z. Gumargalieva, G.E. Zaikov, Y.V. Mioseev, "Quantitative foundations of polymer biocompatibility and biodestructibility," *Int J Polym Mater*, vol. 31, pp. 183-214, 1996.
36. B. Li, J. Chen, J.H.C. Wang, "RGD peptide conjugated poly(dimethylsiloxane) promotes adhesion, proliferation, and collagen secretion of human fibroblasts." *J Biomed Mater Res*, vol. 79, pp.989-998, 2006.
37. Hooftman G, Herman E, Schacht. Review: poly(ethylene glycol)s with reactive endgroups. II. Practical consideration for the preparation of protein-PEG conjugates. *J Bioact Compat Polymers*, vol. 11, pp. 135-159, 1996.

38. H. Waldeck, A. Chung, W. Kao. Interpenetrating polymer networks containing gelatin modified with PEGylated RGD and soluble KGF: Synthesis, characterization, and application in in vivo critical dermal wound. *J Biomed Mater Res*, vol. 82, pp. 861-871, 2007.
39. J. Li, F. Wang, L. Zhou, J. Cui, "Application of gelatin tube in bridge repair of sciatic nerve defect." *Zhongguo Linchuang Kangfu*, vol. 9, pp. 158-159, 2005.
40. B. Wu, Z. Luo, H. Meng, H. Hu, Y. Zhang, M. Li, "Preparation of crosslinked collagen-gelatin biomaterial and experiment of its cytotoxicity." *Shengwu Yixue Gongcheng Yu Linchuang*, vol. 11, pp. 420-425, 2007.
41. S.P. Massia and J.A. Hubbell, "An RGD spacing of 440 nm is sufficient for integrin alphaVbeta3 mediated fibroblast spreading and 140 nm for focal contact and stress fiber formation." *J Cell Biol*, vol. 14, pp. 1089-1100, 1991.
42. D. Yahalom, A. Wittelsberger, D.F. Mierke, M. Rosenblatt, J.M. Alexander, M. Chorey, "Identification of the principal binding site for RGD-containing ligand in the alphaVbeta3 integrin: a photoaffinity cross-linking study." *Biochem*, vol. 41, pp. 8321-8331, 2002.
43. A.K. McNally and J.M. Anderson, "Beta1 and beta2 integrins mediate adhesion during macrophage fusion and multinucleated foreign body giant cell formation." *Am J Path*, vol. 160, pp. 621-630, 2002.
44. J.A. Rowley and D.J. Mooney, "Alginate type and RGD density control myoblast phenotype," *J Biomed Mater Res*, vol. 60, pp. 217-223, 2001.
45. A.A. Sawyer, K.M. Hennessy, S.L. Bellis, "The effect of adsorbed serum proteins, RGD and proteoglycan-binding peptides on the adhesion of mesenchymal stem cells to hydroxyapatite." *Biomaterials*, vol. 28, pp. 383-392, 2007.

Section 2

Hybrid Biomaterials in Drug Delivery and Molecular Recognition

CHAPTER 6

SYNTHESIS OF MULTI-EPITOPIC GLYCOPEPTIDE-BASED CANCER VACCINES

Olivier Renaudet*, Isabelle Bossu and Pascal Dumy

Departement de Chimie Moléculaire, UMR-CNRS 5250 & ICMG FR 2607
Université Joseph Fourier, 38041 Grenoble Cedex 9 (France)
**E-mail: olivier.renaudet@ujf-grenoble.fr*

1. Introduction

The development of synthetic molecules that trigger a robust immune response against tumors remains a crucial challenge in cancer immunotherapy. Until now, most therapeutic vaccines are designed to eradicate circulating tumors after surgery or radiotherapy by targeting a tumoral specific molecular signature. Indeed, the glyco-patterning of the extracellular membrane is one major difference between malignant and normal cells. Tumors are characterized by altered or over-expressed carbohydrate moieties displayed by proteins and lipids, namely Tumor Associated Carbohydrate Antigens (TACAs) which results from a deregulation of the glycosylation pathways in the Golgi compartment [1-2]. The structural identification of these carbohydrate markers [3] have prompted several attempts to use them as a unique target for cancer vaccine, however only a low immune response is induced due to their inability to activate helper T lymphocytes. Taking advantage of the spectacular advances in the chemistry of oligosaccharides and conjugation methods, pioneering studies in the early 90's at the Sloan Kettering Institute for Cancer Research showed that the design of vaccine prototypes comprising TACAs conjugated to a suitable immunogenic delivery system is a key element to circumvent this drawback [4]. To this end, sophisticated molecular constructions such as semi-synthetic vaccines based on immunogenic protein and lipid carriers, fully synthetic TACA-based glycoconjugates or more recently nanoparticules were intensively investigated. Instead of giving a complete overview of each approach – that is discussed in details in excellent reviews [4,5,6,7,8] – this chapter rather covers the synthesis of homogeneous multi-epitopic TACA-based cancer vaccines. These lines indeed focus on efficient synthetic strategies to access low molecular weight, antigen delivery systems and are illustrated by selected well-defined constructions based on linear, dendrimeric type glycoconjugates.

2. Design of Synthetic Antigen Delivery Systems as Cancer Vaccine Prototypes

In contrast to some anti-bacterial vaccines based on fragments of capsular polysaccharides [9] – for instance, a vaccine against infections caused by *Haemophilus influenza* type b is now commercially available – the development of cancer vaccine prototypes capable of inducing an immediate, reproducible and long lasting immunity is far from being trivial. Numbers of TACAs are now well characterized as specific markers associated with cancer cells and can be classified in two distinct classes [10-11]. Being anchored by a lipid tail on the cancer cell surface, Le^y, Globo-H or gangliosides (*e.g.* GM_2, fucosyl GM_1) are large glycostructures which belong to the glycolipids family, whereas mucins (*e.g.* Tn, STn or TF) are generally attached as characteristic dense repeated clusters through serine or threonine residues of *O*-glycoproteins on epithelial cells (Figure 1). Cancer cells expressing TACAs can induce specific antibodies, but the immune system failed to eradicate tumors due to their poor immunogenicity [12]. This observation suggests that not only the production of antibodies by stimulating B-cell, but also the activation of helper T lymphocytes ($CD4^+$), and ideally of cytotoxic T lymphocytes ($CD8^+$), are required to trigger an efficient immune response and memory effect against tumors expressing the same carbohydrate markers [4-7]. In consequence, the current challenges for the development of vaccine prototypes consist in tuning both structure and composition to optimize the immunological response.

Besides the presence of TACAs that appears as prerequisite targets for synthetic vaccines, the ideal vaccine prototype should allow the activation of both humoral and cytotoxic response by recruiting B and T-cells help. To achieve this purpose, a traditional approach consists of coupling TACA – or a short unnatural peptide backbone bearing clustered carbohydrate antigens – to a carrier protein such as keyhole limpet hemocyanin (KLH) [4] or bovine serum albumin (BSA) (Figure 2, strategy A) [13]. After co-administration with QS-21 immunoadjuvant, several constructions were shown to induce efficient B-cell and helper T-cell response through an improved production of antibodies specific for TACAs, some of them being studied in advanced

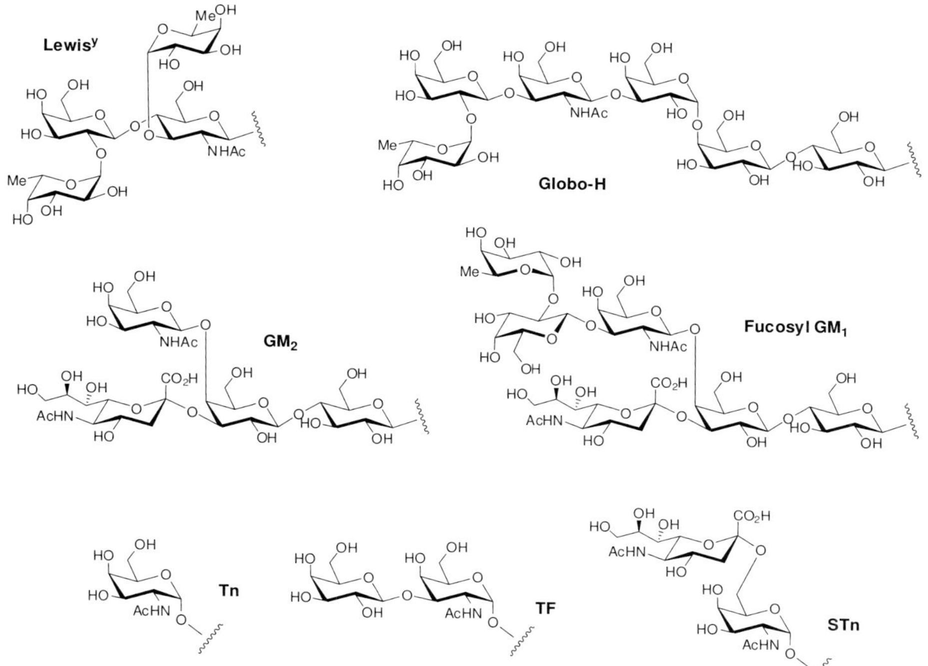

Fig. 1. Structures of several tumor-associated carbohydrate antigens.

pre-clinical and even clinical trials [4,10-11]. However, the utilization of such vaccine candidates remains unsatisfactory in cancer therapy for diverse reasons. In most cases, these constructions induce only a low level of the desired antibodies against TACAs, because the limited carbohydrate content over the carrier protein results in a high titer of antibodies against the carrier itself. In some cases, a carrier-induced complete suppression of the immune response towards the hapten can also be observed. In addition, the synthetic difficulties in coupling carbohydrate moieties to the protein lead to glycoconjugates with uncertain molecular composition and structure which remains a major drawback to a reproducible immune response.

Therefore, the administration of both the carbohydrate marker and relevant immunogenic T-cell epitope – usually a short peptide fragment from tetanus toxin or ovalbumin – in vaccination appears as an ideal alternative to circumvent these problems. Rather than mixing both counterparts in the same vaccine formulation, their covalent attachment within the same well-defined molecule and most importantly in a reproducible manner is preferable. This point is indeed crucial to ensure a safe delivery of the multiantigenic vaccine to the antigen presenting cells (APC) and the further internalization and antigen processing resulting in the activation of the immune response. It should also be mentioned that another additional approach for antigen delivery would consist in using, instead of carbohydrate antigens, a polymannosyl cluster that efficiently targets mannose receptors expressed on the surface of APC but this strategy won't be discussed in this chapter (for significant examples, see references [14-15]). To date, several molecular constructions combining a T-cell immunostimulant peptide epitope and TACAs have been developed on the basis of various low molecular weight scaffolds with accurate chemical definition such as linear peptides and dendrimer like structures (Figure 2, strategy B). The following parts of this chapter focus on the synthesis of these different classes of glycopeptides that are currently used either for coupling to a protein carrier or as full synthetic vaccine candidate.

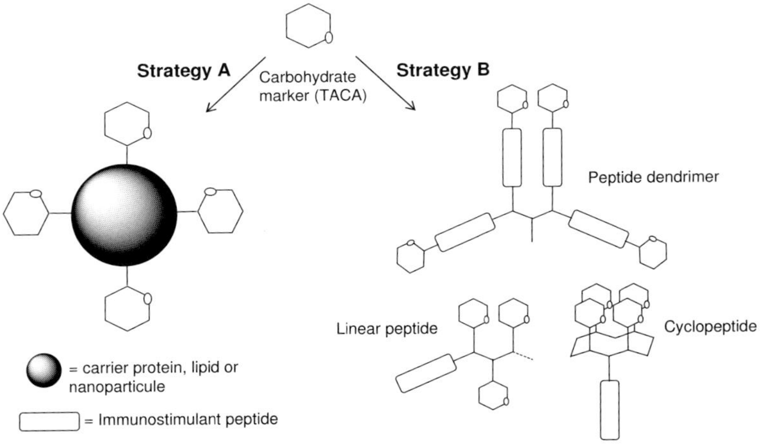

Fig. 2. Representation of the two main approaches for the design of synthetic vaccines.

3. Synthesis of Linear Glycopeptide-based Conjugates and Linkers

Glycopeptide and neoglycopeptide synthesis is an extremely vast topic as shown by the large number of related reviews (for excellent reviews, see [16-17]). Whereas the elongation of orthogonally protected peptidic structures by standard solid phase strategy rarely presents synthetic difficulties, the synthesis of complex carbohydrate structures, for which extraction from natural sources is not providing enough material for the construction of homogeneous glycoconjugates, reveals however more tedious. Although spectacular progress has been made in oligosaccharide chemistry [18-19], the control of the anomer stereoselectivity in each glycosylation step and *a fortiori* in the final conjugation of the full carbohydrate moiety to a pre-defined position in the peptide sequence, remains delicate. Taking these difficulties into account, glycoconjugates with T-cell epitopes and glycopeptide linkers are rather prepared following two other strategies for the construction of anticancer vaccines (Figure 3).

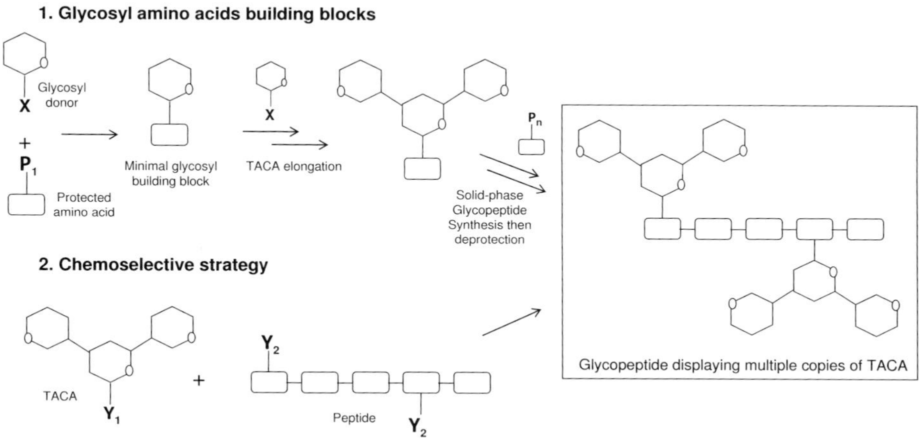

Fig. 3. Two main strategies for the synthesis of glycopeptides components or full antitumoral vaccines, X = leaving group, P = orthogonal protecting group, Y = mutually reactive groups.

The first one consists in the preparation of protected glycosyl amino acid building blocks beforehand, either composed of a αGalNAc unit linked to a serine/threonine moiety as minimal a building block or a full carbohydrate antigen bearing an unnatural amino acid linker at the reducing end, followed by their incorporation in the peptide framework during the solid phase glycopeptide synthesis. In a second convergent approach, highly efficient chemoselective ligation procedures were developed to conjugate unprotected carbohydrate and peptide containing highly mutually reactive chemical functions under mild aqueous conditions.

3.1. *Utilization of glycosyl amino acid building blocks*

3.1.1. *Synthesis of mucin antigen-T cell peptide conjugates*

The use of pre-assembled glycosyl amino acid building blocks for the preparation of glycopeptides comprises a suitable synthetic alternative to enable a stronger control of the glycosidic linkage, or at least to make the purification steps easier. Among the first examples of this strategy [20-21], Kunz has reported the synthesis of several extracellular peptide sequences from the tandem repeat domains of the native epithelial mucin glycoproteins. The synthesis starts from a galactosyl bromide which was coupled to the hydroxyl side chain of the Fmoc-protected threonine residue that is readily usable in Fmoc solid phase peptide synthesis [22]. Due to the presence of azide non-participating group at carbon 2, the α-glycosidic linkage was recovered in moderate yield. After subsequent azide reduction and deacetylation, the Fmoc protected Tn building block **1** was obtained (Figure 4).

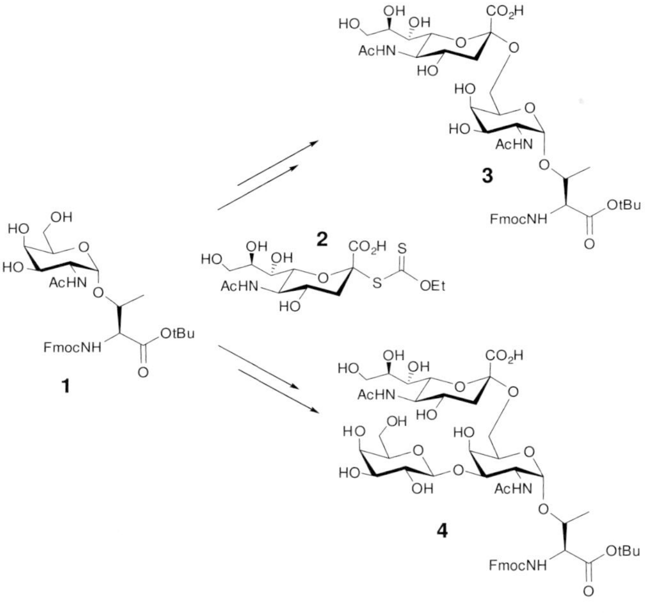

Fig. 4. Synthesis of 2,6-sialyl Tn and 2,6-sialyl TF building blocks.

From this minimal key building block **1**, further extensions can be realized to access more complex antigenic carbohydrates motifs. Taking advantage of the difference in reactivity of hydroxyl functional groups, a regioselective sialylation was performed on the galactosyl moiety with sialyl-xanthogenate **2** to afford α2,6-sialyl-Tn **3** [22-23] which was converted successively into α2,6-sialyl-TF antigen **4** [24]. The same group further developed an efficient synthesis of the MUC-1 glycopeptide antigen **5** containing the immunodominant PDTRP motif [23]. The incorporation of **3** into the sequence was performed on solid support using a resin containing the allylic HYCRON linker with HATU/HOAt coupling reagents, whereas other amino acids were coupled with HBTU/HOBt. As it was shown that MUC1 is not suitable to induce a tumor-selective response, the authors suggested the insertion of a T-helper peptide epitope by fragment condensation (Figure 5).

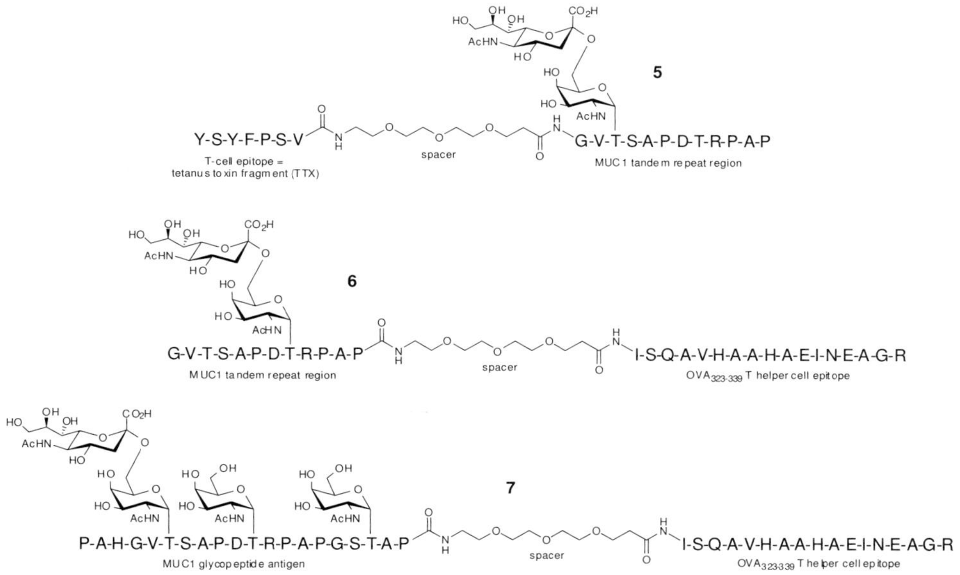

Fig. 5. Structure of MUC 1-T helper peptide conjugates.

The resulting resin bound STn-glycododecapeptide from MUC1 was finally linked by amide coupling to the tetanus toxin (YSYFPSV) containing a triethylene glycol spacer at the *N*-terminal end. After final cleavage then deprotection steps in solution, the full T-helper-spacer-MUC1 glycopeptide **5** was isolated by preparative HPLC in a satisfactory yield (47%) and suitable purity for immunological assays. Using a similar synthetic strategy, more recent studies by the same group report on the synthesis of several other constructions containing up to three STn motifs on a MUC1 peptide conjugated to the ovalbumin fragment $OVA_{323-339}$ as T-helper peptide epitopes **6-7** [25-26].

3.1.2. *Synthesis of linear peptide linker bearing clustered carbohydrate antigens*

While being developed for the conjugation to carrier proteins rather than as complete immunoactive structures, the clustered peptide linkers developed by Danishefsky have to be undeniably mentioned in this part. Denoted as the "Cassette Approach" by Danishefsky, the concept discussed above was explored to insert natural or unnatural amino acid functionality into carbohydrate motifs. The resulting glycosyl amino acid building blocks were then incorporated into peptide linkers displaying either single or clusters of carbohydrate antigens. It has to be noted that the final conjugation of glycopeptide linkers to the protein carrier is ensured by reductive amination or thio-maleimide chemoselective ligation but this aspect won't be further discussed in this part.

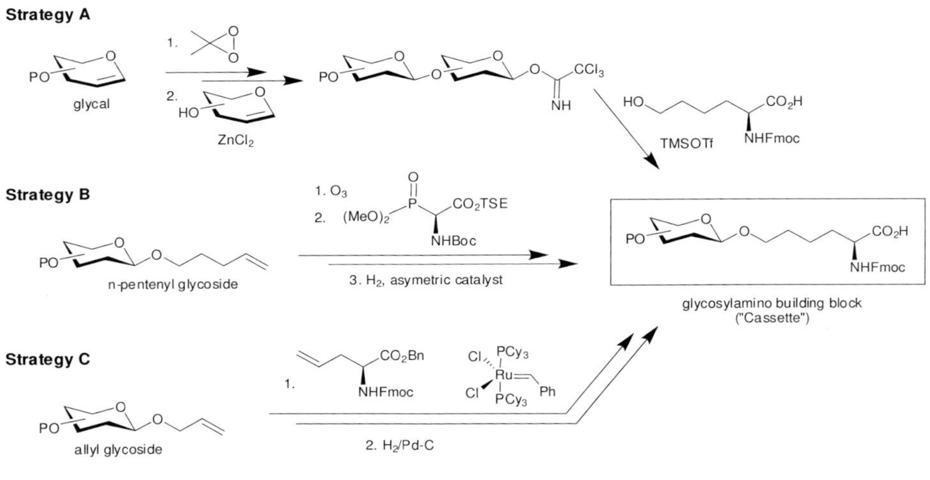

Fig. 6. Several "Cassette" strategies developed by Danishefsky and co-workers.

The major advancements of the Cassette Approach relies on previous development of the modular glycal approach which revealed extremely efficient to prepare the full carbohydrate domain both in solution [27] and on solid phase [28] before the amino acid coupling. It relies on the use of 1,2-anhydrosugars, namely glycals, as glycosyl donors and acceptors (Figure 6, strategy A). By treatment with dimethyldioxirane, the resulting highly reactive epoxide was proved to be excellent β-glycosyl donor in the presence of Lewis acid catalysts such as zinc chloride. If the reaction is performed with other suitably differentiated glycal acceptors, the procedure can be repeated iteratively to obtain the full carbohydrate antigen. This strategy allowed the preparation of sialylated structures such as sialylTF epitope [29] or the first total synthesis of the Globo-H antigen [30]. The last coupling step with protected amino acid building blocks is realized using glycal activation, or alternatively under classical glycosylation reaction with halide or trichloroacetimidate activation. The direct coupling of a trichloroacetimidate glycosyl donor bearing non-participating azide group with Fmoc-L-hydroxynorleucine benzyl ester using TMSOTf as promoter [31] providing the α-*O*-linked product in 71% yield, whereas glycal epoxide donor leads to the β-*O*-linked product in 60-80% yield. Both complementary strategies were followed to prepare glycosylamino acids building blocks containing the Tn, TF, STn, Le^y or Globo-H antigens.

The same group proposed a three steps synthetic methodology comprising the ozonolysis of *n*-pentenyl glycosyls, an Horner-Emmons olefination using tetramethylguanidine and a protected glycine-derived phosphonate, then a catalytic asymetric hydrogenation (Figure 6, strategy B) [32]. This protocol was proved efficient to prepare unnatural glycosylamino acids containing the Tn, the Globo-H and the Le^y antigens with excellent diastereomeric selectivity.

In addition, Gb3, GM2, and fucosyl GM1 glycosylamino acid building blocks were synthesized by olefin cross-metathesis reactions followed by hydrogenation (Figure 6, strategy C) [33]. This strategy was explored starting from allyl glycosides and Fmoc-L-allylglycine benzyl ester and by varying the catalyst nature. The structure of both substrates was finally optimized by adding a methyl group on the terminal olefin to prevent side product formation. Clusters of Gb3 antigen displayed by a MUC5AC associated with breast and gastric cancers peptide epitope was thus obtained from a Gb3 glycosylamino acid building block [34].

More recently, a new generation of peptide linker presenting multiple carbohydrate antigens was reported to reflect the degree of heterogeneity of the tumor surface glycopattern [35-36]. The authors postulated that the association of several TACAs associated with a particular cancer type within the same polyantigenic clustered vaccine could improve the immune response.

3.2. *Chemoselective methods*

From a synthetic point of view, the glycopeptide assembly still suffers from difficulties as it requires the preparation of large quantities of often complex glycosyl amino acids building blocks for their incorporation during peptide synthesis. In addition, each glycopeptide requires a specific and adapted synthetic route. Therefore, this strategy remains illusory to follow in a scale-up perspective. By contrast, chemoselective ligation strategies revealed an elegant alternative for the convergent assembly of complex biomolecules [37-38], firstly because the coupling procedure is usually quantitative, requiring neither protection nor activation steps and secondly because the synthesis of different building blocks is generally easier. Such strategies result from the condensation of fully deprotected polyfunctional building blocks bearing mutually highly reactive functions. Despite the presence of other reactive chemical functions, the coupling reaction occurs generally in aqueous conditions to provide the full molecular construction without additional chemical manipulation. Moreover, the resulting conjugate contains unnatural linkages which can be advantageous to improve immunogenicity as well as stability against enzymatic degradation.

3.2.1. *Convergent assembly by oxime ligation*

Among other chemoselective methods, oxime ligation has found increasing applications over the last decade, particularly for the glycoconjugate preparation [39]. It requires the prior introduction in both partners of either an aldehyde or a keto group and an aminooxy function. In the context of synthetic vaccine preparation, this strategy ensures a controlled molecular assembly as shown by Bertozzi with the synthesis of oxime-linked mucin mimics [40]. In this study, two tumor related Tn **8** and STn **9** antigens bearing aminooxy function at the anomer position were first prepared (Figure 7). The key step of this procedure is the glycosylation with *N*-hydroxysuccinimide from glycosyl chloride **10** using a phase transfer catalysis protocol [41], which leads to the α-glycoside intermediate **11** in moderate yield (57%). The subsequent azide reduction and hydrazinolysis afford aminooxy carbohydrate **8** with a defined anomer configuration which can be readily engaged in oxime coupling. A similar procedure was followed for the aminooxy STn **9** synthesis.

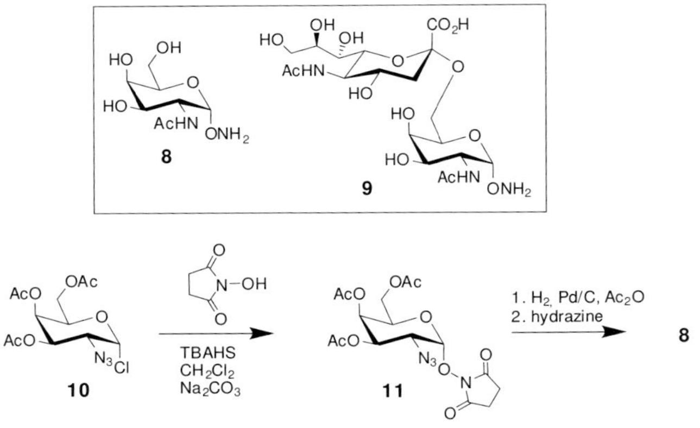

Fig. 7. Synthesis of aminooxy carbohydrate epitopes using phase transfer catalysis.

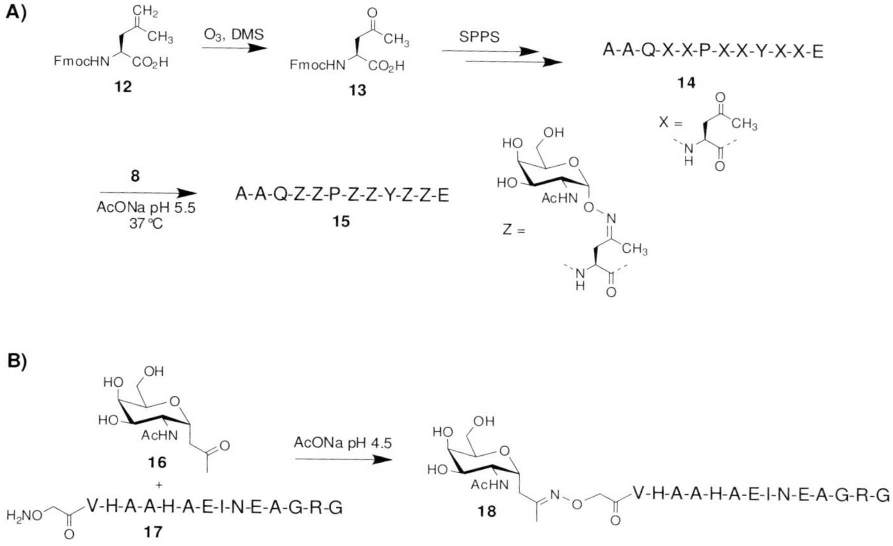

Fig. 8. Oxime ligation with: (A) aminooxy carbohydrate; (B) C-glycosyl ketone.

For the construction of the mucin mimic, the authors selected peptide fragments of endothelial mucin GlyCAM-1 with 12- and 17- residues containing several unnatural keto amino acids **13** – prepared by reductive ozonolysis of the commercially available Fmoc-dehydroleucine **12** – in place of serine or threonine (Figure 8). The final oxime assembly between the aminooxy carbohydrate and the peptide displaying clustered ketone **14** occurred in sodium acetate buffer pH 5.5 at 37°C until completeness of the reaction (24h). After RP-HPLC purification, homogenous oxime-linked multivalent glycopeptide **15** was recovered in 70% yield. A comparable ligation strategy using C-glycoside analogues of the Tn antigen was described. This carbohydrate moiety bearing α-C-glycosyl ketone **16** rather than aminooxy function was introduced either in single [42] or double [43] copies into an aminooxy containing peptide fragment of ovalbumin as T-cell epitope **17** (Figure 8). As above, the final oxime ligation proved efficient but revealed cis-trans isomerism of the oxime linkage in the glycopeptide **18**.

3.2.2. *Native chemical ligation*

A previous report with liposome-based constructs showed that the use of dimeric TACA coupled to a Pam_3Cys moiety derived from the *N*-terminal sequence of a lipoprotein of *E. coli* resulted in a promising immune response against TACAs without protein carrier or immunoadjuvant [44]. Later, the incorporation of T-cell epitope peptide into a three-component vaccine candidate was suggested by Boons and co-workers to enhance to production of IgG antibodies [45-46]. In order to improve the synthetic access to such lipoglycopeptide conjugate, Boons developed for the first time a methodology based on a sequential Native Chemical Ligation (NCL) process [47]. NCL results generally from the condensation between two peptides, one bearing *N*-terminal cysteine residue and the second a *C*-terminal thioester [48]. In a first reversible step, a trans-thioesterification occurs between the thioester and the thiol group to provide a thioester-linked intermediate. This intermediate undergoes an irreversible rearrangement to form a native amide bond at the ligation site. In Boons strategy, a Tn containing MUC1 was first prepared as B-cell epitope, using a glycosylated Fmoc-protected amino acid building block to be incorporated to the MUC1 peptide sequence containing a free cysteine at *N*-terminal end **19** (Figure 9). A helper T-epitope (YAF sequence) **20** bearing Acm-protected cystein and benzyl thioester on both sides was simultaneously synthesized on safety-catch linker and conjugated in sodium phosphate buffer containing guanidinium hydrochloride and thiophenol as catalyst. A first B- and T-cell bi-conjugate was thus obtained after 18h in a modest 48% yield. After Acm removal, attempts to couple B/T conjugate with Pam_3CysSK_4 α-thioester **21** using a similar procedure failed due to the low solubility of the lipopeptide. To circumvent this problem, the authors

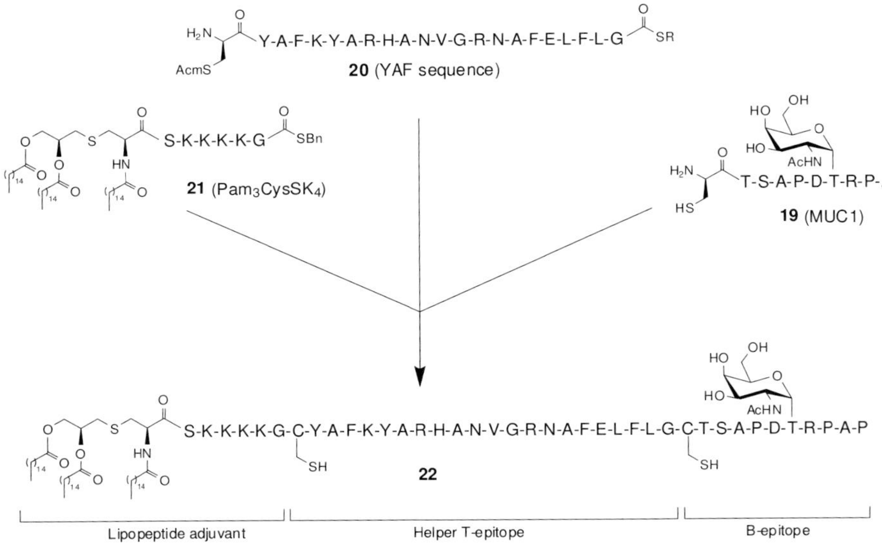

Fig. 9. Synthesis of three-component vaccine by sequential NCL.

suggested the incorporation of both peptides into liposomes. This procedure using dodecylphosphocholine film and sodium 2-mercaptoethane sulfonate instead of thiophenol as catalyst was successful as **22** was obtained in 2h in 83% yield. More recently, a similar liposome-mediated NCL was used to assemble more sophisticated lipoglycopeptide constructions which showed optimised immunological activity [49].

3.2.3. *Click-like cycloaddition*

A last promising chemoselective strategy can be briefly mentioned in this part. A preliminary study reports a copper-catalyzed version of the Huisgen 1,3-dipolar cycloaddition for the construction of clustered glycopeptide linker [50]. This procedure requires the introduction of an azide-containing linker into the carbohydrate antigen **23** and a peptide fragment **24** bearing several copies of acetylenic functional groups (Figure 10). A combination of copper wire and $CuSO_4$ was found to give the tris-triazole conjugate **25** quantitatively after 40h in water/acetonitrile mixture. As confessed however by the authors, this procedure still remains to be improved for further coupling of this glycopeptide to a carrier protein.

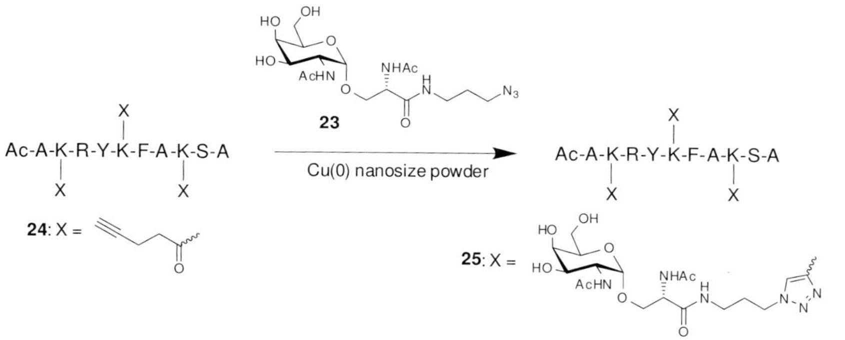

Fig. 10. Click-like procedure for multivalent glycopeptide linker synthesis.

4. Construction of Multi-epitopic Glycosylated Dendrimeric Type Structures

To prevent irrelevant immune response and ambiguous composition of semi-synthetic carrier protein-based vaccines, Leclerc and co-workers proposed an original approach which opened a new area in this field [51]. Expecting a significant immunity improvement, they showed that fully synthetic vaccine candidates having low molecular weight and based on well-defined dendrimeric-type structures are attractive scaffolds for assembling multiple epitopes. The essential feature of this new generation of vaccine model consists in combining both immunostimulant peptide fragments and TACAs as T-cell and B-cell epitopes respectively. In addition, mucin carbohydrate markers should preferentially be presented in a multivalent form to mimic the native structures expressed on the tumor cell surface. By comparison with monovalent conjugates, the multivalent presentation of mucin antigens, indeed favours the efficient delivery of the vaccine prototype to APCs by virtue of cell receptor cross-linking and endocytosis [52]. Secondly, the cluster formation also results in a high density of carbohydrate antigens at the surface of a small peptidic scaffold, thus eliciting the production of high titre of antibodies that are specific to tumors expressing the same carbohydrate antigens. Moreover, unlike the few methods available for carbohydrate conjugation to proteins and despite their relative structural complexity, the synthesis of homogenous branched glycoconjugates in good quantities relies on reproducible methods comparable to those described in paragraph 3.

4.1. *Multiple Antigen Glycopeptide (MAG) using a polylysine core*

On the basis of the multiple antigen peptides described earlier by Tam [53], Leclerc and co-workers designed multiple antigen glycopeptide (MAG) [51,54]. This MAG is composed of a polylysine core which was assembled on the Wang resin **26** pre-loaded with a βAla linker using the Fmoc strategy (Figure 11).

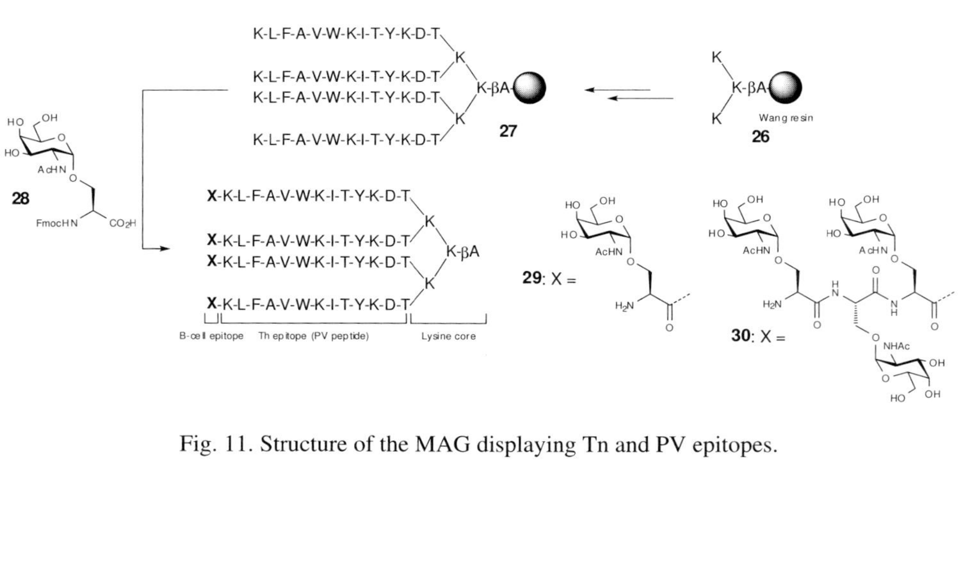

Fig. 11. Structure of the MAG displaying Tn and PV epitopes.

Successive coupling of FmocLys(Fmoc)OH residue provides four anchoring sites which were used for simultaneous elongation of four copies of a poliovirus peptide fragment KLFAVWKITYKDT. To the four *C*-terminal ends of the resulting dendrimer **27** were finally coupled four copies of the αGalNAc building block **28** attached to a serine side chain as the mucin-related Tn epitope. Interestingly, the amide bond formation was achieved using unprotected sugars to prevent side reactions which could occur during the final deacetylation. Further immunological studies with the resulting MAG **29** conjugated with four copies of Tn and PV epitopes confirmed that the polylysine carrier avoids undesired immune responses unlike the protein carrier. More importantly, other complex molecules such as MAG combining four copies of the PV epitope in line with the tri-Tn glycotope **30** and administrated with an immunoadjuvant presented high immunogenicity in prophylactic and therapeutic vaccinations in mice and in non-human primates [55]. Indeed, these authors observed an efficient IgG antibodies production, clearly confirming the induction of the expected T-cell dependent response.

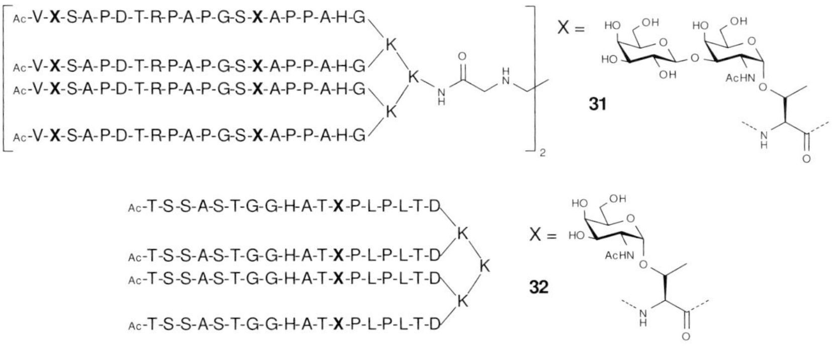

Fig. 12. Recent multiantigenic vaccines candidates based on lysine core.

These pioneering studies inspired further intensive research from the same group [56] and others who proposed similar promising constructions which were not being tested so far. For example, a pure glycopeptide dendrimer **31** containing eight peptide chains of the tandem repeat region of MUC1 displaying two cancer related TF antigens was synthesized on a tri-lysine core (Figure 12). The authors proposed an elegant sequential segment coupling strategy using *N*-alkyl cysteine-assisted thioesterification that revealed efficient to produce the glycodendrimer **31** in good yield and purity [57].

Another solid-phase strategy was followed to prepare multivalent glycopeptides of mucin MUC1 and MUC4 which display Tn antigens [58]

(Figure 12). A tetramer glycopeptide antigen **32**, consisting of the 16 amino acids tandem repeat of mucin MUC4 was prepared using a peptide synthesizer on a Tentagel resin bearing a lysine core through a Wang linker and with the Fmoc-ThrGalNAc building block. The glycopeptide **32** was obtained in 68% yield after acidic cleavage and HPLC purification. This strategy was further extended to prepare a more complex octameric MUC1 tandem repeat glycopeptide with similar success.

A simpler model based on a single lysine core was also proposed (Figure 13). In this study, oxime chemoselective ligation was used for the convergent assembly of a multiantigenic tri-branched glycopeptide mimicking the MUC1 glycoprotein and containing the universal Pan DR (PADRE) T helper epitope [59]. In this study, the authors first prepared two MUC1 repeat units **33-34** containing either the Tn or T antigen on the threonine residue, and an aminooxy acetic acid linker at *N*-terminal end (Figure 13). The PADRE peptide epitope **35** was next synthesized in line with a MUC1 repeat unit bearing a Lys-Ala dipeptide at the *C*-terminal end. The lysine side chain was used for incorporation of a serine residue as masked aldehyde whereas a protected aldehyde was introduced during the peptide cleavage by aminolysis with aminoacetaldehyde-dimethylacetal [60]. After successive aldehyde formations and oxime ligations, the final multiantigenic MUC1 glycopeptide **36** was obtained and evaluated in mice. Immunological assays showed that their construction induce antibodies that recognized native MUC1 expressed on human breast tumors.

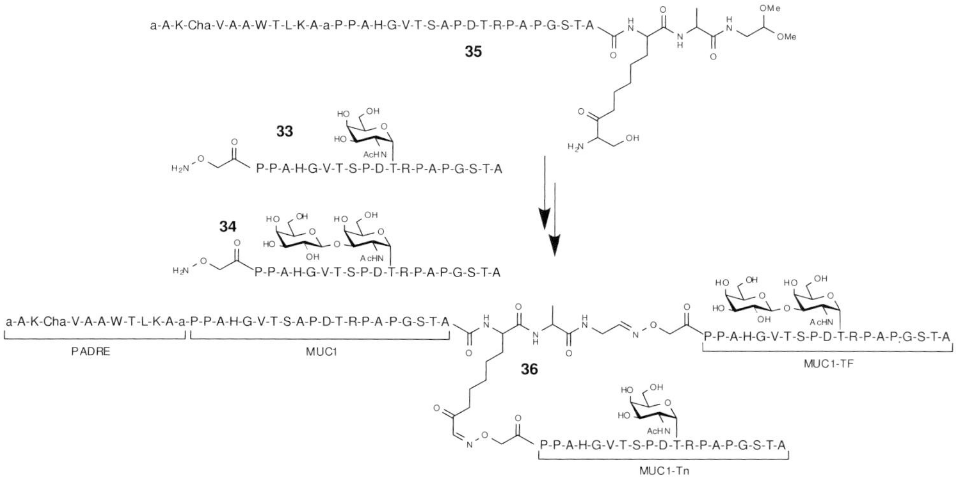

Fig. 13. Oxime assembly of multiantigenic vaccines candidates based a single lysine core.

4.2. Multi-epitopic cyclo-glycopeptide

In the late 80's, Mutter and co-workers proposed a new concept for the design of artificial proteins [61] based on a conformationally restricted cyclopeptide core. This scaffold was more recently exploited as Regioselectively Addressable Functionalized Template (RAFT) [62] for the assembly of various ligands and functional units that confer both recognition and effector properties [63]. It is commonly composed of two proline-glycine (Pro-Gly) β turns that stabilize its conformation into an antiparallel β sheet and up to six amino acid residues containing regioselectively functionalizable side chains directed on two independent domains. The large diversity of commercial orthogonally protected amino acids makes this scaffold easy to handle. This template revealed particularly useful for the chemoselective preparation of glycoconjugates using oxime ligation [64]. Instead of using the stereoselective PTC procedure (see paragraph 3.2.1), the authors have proposed another efficient route using glycosyl fluoride donors to introduce the *N*-hydroxyphthalimide moiety as the masked aminooxy group [65]. This reaction was performed with boron trifluoride etherate as promoter and the final deprotection with methylhydrazine, providing aminooxy carbohydrates. Several biologically relevant carbohydrates with either α or β anomer configuration and tumor-associated antigens such as Tn **8** and TF **37** analogues [66] were thus prepared (Figure 14).

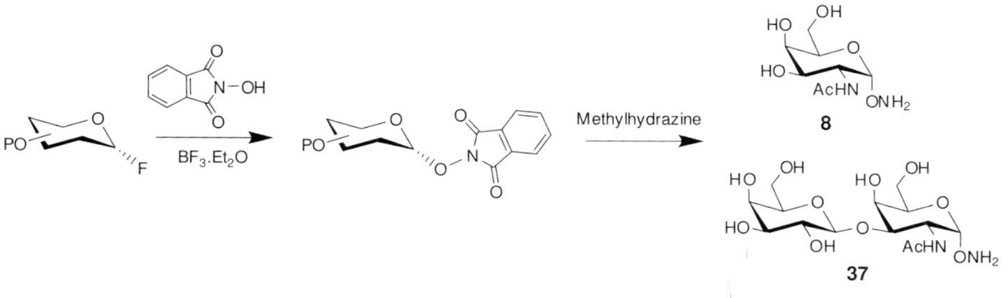

Fig. 14. Synthetic strategy for aminooxy carbohydrates using fluoride activation.

In our laboratory, we showed that such aminooxy carbohydrates can be efficiently incorporated into cyclodecapeptides containing aldehydes or ketones to provide well-defined glycoclusters in solution [67-68] as well as on solid support [69-70]. More sophisticated glycosylated constructions were also prepared using an iterative oxime-based strategy [71-72].

On the model of the MAG vaccines [54], we investigated the use of the cyclopeptide scaffold for the construction of multi-epitopic vaccines [73]. We thus designed vaccine prototypes **38** combining a cluster of Tn antigen on the upper domain of the template and helper T-cell peptide epitope from the type I-poliovirus protein (PV) on the second addressable domain (Figure 15). A linear orthogonally protected decapeptide was first prepared using an automated peptide synthesizer on an acido-labile support such as the SASRIN resin. After cleavage of the linear peptide, the head-to-tail cyclization was achieved by treatment with PyBOP (benzotriazol-1-yl-oxytripyrrolidinophosphonium hexafluorophosphate) under high dilution to prevent intermolecular side reactions. The protecting groups were next removed regioselectively, then protected serine residues as masked aldehydes [74] and aminooxy acetic acid were incorporated to the lysine side chain pointing on the upper and lower addressable domains respectively. The full deprotection of the template by acidolysis provides **39** on which PV peptide functionalised with aldehyde at *N*-terminus can be coupled by oxime ligation. This coupling reaction was performed in sodium acetate buffer pH 4. Further oxidative cleavage of serines by treatment with sodium periodate liberates four glyoxo-aldehyde functions that were finally used for linking aminooxy Tn. The final glycocluster **38** displaying PV and Tn was thus obtained in excellent yield and purity. Biological investigations clearly showed that the cyclopeptide template revealed an efficient non-immunological carrier molecule. Moreover, this multi-epitopic construction elicited a specific immune response towards tumors expressing the human form of Tn antigen, highlighting his potential for the design of more elaborated tumor vaccine prototypes.

A new generation of TACA-based vaccine prototype was indeed optimised recently [75-76]. For the first time, four essential components for immune activation were assembled within the same molecular construction **40** (Figure 15). This molecule contains: a cluster of carbohydrate antigens to elicit a B-cell response and trigger high affinity tumor-specific antibodies; T helper and T cytotoxic epitopes to ensure both humoral and cellular eradication of tumors; a palmitic acid rather than potentially toxic external immunoadjuvants to provide self-adjuvanting properties. Therefore, a chimeric CTL-Th peptide with a cysteine at *C*-terminus, composed of a T-cell epitope from ovalbumin ($OVA_{257-264}$) in line with a universal T helper epitope (PADRE) and bearing a palmitic acid moiety at the *N*-terminal end was prepared. This lipopeptide was inserted to a cyclopeptide template **41** displaying oxime-linked clustered Tn analogues using disulfide bond formation. The resulting glycolipopeptide **40** was finally purified by RP-HPLC and charaterized by mass spectroscopy. Immunological investigations with OVA-expressing mouse B16 melanoma

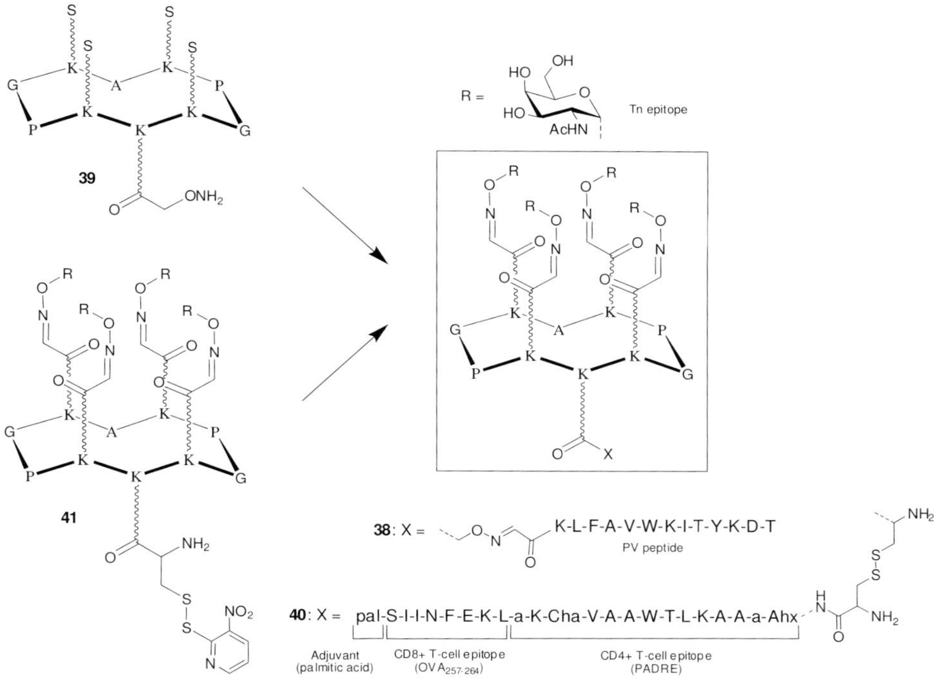

Fig. 15. Multi-epitopic anticancer synthetic vaccines based on cyclodecapeptide scaffold.

showed a strong production of antibodies that recognized human tumor cell lines and stimulation of T-cells without administration of an external adjuvant. More interestingly, an improved survival and a significant reduction of tumor size in mice inoculated with MO5 carcinoma cells were also observed, suggesting the promising potential of four-component vaccine prototypes for human immunotherapy against cancers. It should be noted that similar cyclic glycopeptide models were used as multi-epitopic scaffolds for the preparation of vaccine against HIV using either click chemistry [77] or Lansbury aspartylation [78] for the attachment of carbohydrate epitope, which strengthens the interest of cyclopeptide scaffolds as tool for immunotherapy.

4.3. *Other multivalent scaffolds*

Other diverse other multivalent scaffolds were also described and have shown interesting potential for an immunological purpose. For example a poly(aminoamine) dendrimer was decorated with 4 to 32 copies of the carbohydrate TF antigen as breast cancer marker by amide coupling [79] or tetrameric comb-like dendrimers containing Tn antigens and influenza virus hemaglutinin fragments which were assembled by maleimide/thiol chemoselective ligation [80]. Other non-peptidic scaffolds such as calixarene macrocycle bearing 4 copies of the Tn analogue and one P3CS immunoadjuvant moiety were also prepared by sequential amide coupling [81].

5. Conclusion

Surfing on the spectacular advancements of synthetic methods, the development of anticancer vaccines has found major evolutions in the past few years. As described above, more sophisticated but fully synthetic homogenous antigen delivery systems, combining a suitable arrangement of cluster of cancer carbohydrate markers and peptide epitopes within the same molecular scaffold were reported, showing both specific and improved immunogenicity against human tumors. More remarkably, this effect was strengthened by recent covalent incorporation of adjuvant moiety into the vaccine construction which provides novel self-adjuvanting properties [45-47,75-76]. Together with the clustered heterogenic display of diverse carbohydrate antigens [35-36], these last results certainly mark a further step for structural optimisations toward selective human cancer immunotherapy.

References

[1] Hakomori, S., "Tumor-Associated Carbohydrate Antigens," *Annual Review of Immunology*, Vol. 2, 1984, pp. 103–126.

[2] Feizi, T., and Childs, R. A., "Carbohydrate Structures of Glycoproteins and Glycolipids as Differentiation Antigens, Tumor-Associated Antigens and Components of Receptor Systems," *Trends in Biochemical Sciences*, Vol. 10, No. 1, 1985, pp. 24–29.

[3] Springer, G. F., "T and Tn, General Carcinoma Auto-Antigens," *Science*, Vol. 224, No. 4654, 1984, pp. 1198–1206.

[4] Danishefsky, S. J., and Allen, R. J., "From the Laboratory to the Clinic: a Retrospective on Fully Synthetic Carbohydrate-Based Anticancer Vaccines," *Angewandte Chemie-International Edition*, Vol. 39, No. 5, 2000, pp. 836–863.

[5] Roy, R., "New Trends in Carbohydrate-Based Vaccines," *Drug Discovery Today: Technologies*, Vol. 1, No. 3, 2004, pp. 327–336.

[6] Slovin, S. F., Keding, S. J., and Ragupathi, G, "Carbohydrate Vaccines as Immunotherapy for Cancer" *Immunology and Cell Biology*, Vol. 83, No. 4, 2005, pp. 418–428.

[7] Pietersz, G. A., Pouniotis, D. S., and Apostolopoulos, V., "Design of Peptide-Based Vaccines for Cancer," *Current Medicinal Chemistry*, Vol. 13, No. 14, 2006, pp. 1591-1607.

[8] Couvreur, P., and Vauthier, C., "Nanotechnology: Intelligent Design to Treat Complex Disease," *Pharmaceutical Research*, Vol. 23, No. 7, 2006, pp. 1417–1450.

[9] Verez-Bencomo, V. et al. "A Synthetic Conjugate Polysaccharide Vaccine Against Haemophilus influenzae Type b," *Science*, Vol. 305, No. 5683, 2004, pp. 522–525.

[10] Dube, D. H., and Bertozzi, C. R., "Glycans in Cancer and Inflammation – Potential for Therapeutics and Diagnostics," *Nature Reviews Drug Discovery*, Vol. 4, No. 6, 2005, pp. 477–488.

[11] Hakomori, S., and Zhang, Y.M., "Glycosphingolipid Antigens and Cancer Therapy," *Chemistry & Biology*, Vol. 4, No. 2, 1997, pp. 97-104.

[12] Fukuda, M., "Possible Roles of Tumor-Associated Carbohydrate Antigens." *Cancer Research*, Vol. 56, No. 10, 1996, pp. 2237–2244.

[13] Kunz, H., and Birnbach, S., "Synthesis of Tumor Associated Tn- and T-antigen Type *O*-Glycopeptides and Their Conjugation to Bovine Serum Albumin," *Angewandte Chemie-International Edition*, Vol. 25, No. 4, 1986, pp. 360–362.

[14] Grandjean, C., et al., "One-pot Synthesis of Antigen-Bearing, Lysine-Based Cluster Mannosides using Two Orthogonal Chemoselective Ligation Reactions," *Angewandte Chemie-International Edition*, Vol. 39, No. 6, 2000, pp. 1068–1072.

[15] Adams, E. W., et al., "Carbohydrate-Mediated Targeting of Antigen to Dendritic Cells Leads to Enhanced Presentation of Antigen to T Cells," *ChemBioChem*, Vol. 9, No. 2, 2008, pp. 294–303.

[16] Herzner, H., et al., "Synthesis of Glycopeptides Containing Carbohydrate and Peptide Recognition Motifs," *Chemical Reviews*, Vol. 100, No. 12, 2000, pp. 4495–4537.

[17] Bertozzi, C. R., and Kiessling, L. L., "Chemical Glycobiology," *Science*, Vol. 291, No. 5512, 2001, pp. 2357–2364.

[18] Seeberger, P. H., and Haase, W.-C., "Solid-Phase Oligosaccharide Synthesis and Combinatorial Carbohydrate Libraries," *Chemical Reviews*, Vol. 100, No. 12, 2000, pp. 4349–4393.

[19] Galonic, D. P., and Gin, D. Y., "Chemical Glycosylation in the Synthesis of Glycoconjugate Antitumor Vaccines," *Nature*, Vol. 446, No. 7139, 2007, pp. 1000–1007.

[20] Mathieux, N., et al. "Synthesis of Glycopeptide Sequences of Repeating Units of the Mucins MUC 2 and MUC 3 Containing Oligosaccharide Side-Chains with Core 1, Core 2, Core 3, Core 4 and Core 6 Structure," *Journal of the Chemical Society-Perkin Transactions 1*, No. 16, 1997, pp. 2359–2368.

[21] Phaedria, M. et al., "Synthesis of T-Antigen-Containing Glycopeptides as Potential Cancer Vaccines," *Journal of the Chemical Society-Perkin Transactions 1*, No. 24, 1999, pp. 3559–3564.

[22] Liebe, B., and Kunz, H., "Solid-Phase Synthesis of a Tumor-Associated Sialyl-Tn Antigen Glycopeptide with a Partial Sequence of the Tandem Repeat of the MUC-1 Mucin," *Angewandte Chemie-International Edition*, Vol. 36, No. 6, 1997, pp. 618–620.

[23] Keil, S., et al., "Towards the Development of Antitumor Vaccines: A Synthetic Conjugate of a Tumor-Associated MUC1 Glycopeptide Antigen and a Tetanus Toxin Epitope," *Angewandte Chemie-International Edition*, Vol. 40, No. 2, 2001, pp. 366–369.

[24] Brocke, C., and Kunz, H., "Synthetic Glycopeptides of the Tandem Repeat Sequence of the Epithelial Mucin MUC4 with Tumour-associated Carbohydrate Antigens," *Synlett*, No. 13, 2003, pp. 2052–2056.

[25] Westerlind, U., et al., "Synthetic Vaccines Consisting of Tumor-Associated MUC1 Glycopeptide Antigens and a T-Cell Epitope for the Induction of a Highly Specific Humoral Immune Response," *Angewandte Chemie-International Edition*, Vol. 47, No. 39, 2008, pp. 7551–7556.

[26] Dziadek, S., et al., "A Fully Synthetic Vaccine Consisting of a Tumor-Associated Glycopeptide Antigen and a T-Cell Epitope for the Induction of a Highly Specific Humoral Immune Response," *Angewandte Chemie-International Edition*, Vol. 44, No. 46, 2005, pp. 7630–7635.

[27] Danishefsky, S. J., and Bilodeau, M. T., "Glycals in Organic Synthesis: The Evolution of Comprehensive Strategies for the Assembly of Oligosaccharides and Glycoconjugates of

Biological Consequence," *Angewandte Chemie-International Edition*, Vol. 35, No. 13-14, 2005, pp. 1380–1419.

[28] *Seeberger, P. H., and Danishefsky, S. J., "Solid-Phase Synthesis of Oligosaccharides and Glycoconjugates by the Glycal Assembly Method: A Five Year Retrospective,"* Account of Chemical Research, *Vol. 31, No. 10, 1998, pp. 685–695.*

[29] Schwarz, J. B., et al., "A Broadly Applicable Method for the Efficient Synthesis of α-O-Linked Glycopeptides and Clustered Sialic Acid Residues," *Journal of the American Chemical Society*, Vol. 121, No. 12, 1999, pp. 2662–2673.

[30] Bilodeau, M. T., et al., "Total Synthesis of a Human Breast Tumor Associated Antigen," *Journal of the American Chemical Society*, Vol. 117, No. 29, 1995, pp. 7840–7841.

[31] Keding, S. J., Endo, A., and Danishefsky, S. J., "Synthesis of Non-Natural Glycosylamino Acids Containing Tumor-Associated Carbohydrate Antigens," *Tetrahedron*, Vol. 59, No. 35, 2003, pp. 7023–7031.

[32] Allen, J. R., Harris, C. R., and Danishefsky, S. J., "Pursuit of Optimal Carbohydrate-Based Anticancer Vaccines: Preparation of a Multiantigenic Unimolecular Glycopeptide Containing the Tn, MBr1, and Lewis(y) Antigens," *Journal of the American Chemical Society*, Vol. 123, No. 9, 2001, pp. 1890–1897.

[33] Wan, Q., et al., "Olefin Cross-Metathesis: A Powerful Tool for Constructing Vaccines Composed of Multimeric Antigens," *Journal of Carbohydrate Chemistry*, Vol. 24, No. 4-6, 2005, pp. 425–440.

[34] Zhu, J., et al., "Biologics through Chemistry: Total Synthesis of a Proposed Dual-Acting Vaccine Targeting Ovarian Cancer by Orchestration of Oligosaccharide and Polypeptide Domains," *Journal of the American Chemical Society*, Vol. 131, No. 11, 2009, pp. 4151–4158.

[35] Keding, S. J., and Danishefsky, S. J., "Natural Product Synthesis Special Feature: Prospects for Total Synthesis: a Vision for a Totally Synthetic Vaccine Targeting Epithelial Tumors," *Proceedings of the National Academy of Sciences of the United States of America*, Vol. 101, No. 33, 2004, pp. 11937-11942.

[36] Ragupathi, G., et al., "Preparation and Evaluation of Unimolecular Pentavalent and Hexavalent Antigenic Constructs Targeting Prostate and Breast Cancer: A Synthetic Route to Anticancer Vaccine Candidates," *Journal of the American Chemical Society*, Vol. 128, No. 8, 2006, pp. 2715–2725.

[37] Hang, H. C., and Bertozzi, C. R., "Chemoselective Approaches to Glycoprotein Engineering," *Accounts of Chemical Research*, Vol. 34, No. 9, 2001, pp. 727–736.

[38] Kimmerlin, T., and Seebach, D., "100 Years of Peptide Synthesis: Ligation Methods for Peptide and Protein Synthesis with Applications to beta-Peptide Assemblies," *Journal of Peptide Research*, Vol. 65, No. 2, 2005, pp. 229–260.

[39] Langenhan, J. M., and Thorson, J. S., "Recent Carbohydrate-Based Chemoselective Ligation Applications," *Current Organic Synthesis*, Vol. 2, No. 1, 2005, pp. 59–81.

[40] Marcaurelle, L. A., et al., "Synthesis of Oxime-Linked Mucin Mimics Containing the Tumor-Related Tn and Sialyl Tn Antigens," *Organic Letters*, Vol. 3, No. 23, 2001, pp. 3691–3694.

[41] Cao, S., Tropper, F. D., Roy, R., "Stereoselective Phase Transfer Catalyzed Syntheses of Glycosyloxysuccinimides and their Transformations into Glycoprobes," *Tetrahedron*, Vol. 51, No. 24, 1995, pp. 6679–6686.

[42] Peri, F., et al., "Synthesis and Biological Evaluation of an Anticancer Vaccine Containing the C-glycoside Analogue of the Tn Epitope," *Bioconjugate Chemistry*, Vol. 12, No. 3, 2001, pp. 325–328.

[43] Cipolla, L., et al., "Novel Tn Antigen-Containing Neoglycopeptides: Synthesis and Evaluation as Anti Tumor Vaccines," *Bioorganic & Medicinal Chemistry*, Vol. 10, No. 5, 2002, pp. 1639–1646.

[44] Toyokuni, T., et al., "Synthetic Vaccines: Synthesis of a Dimeric Tn Antigen-Lipopeptide Conjugate that Elicits Immune Responses Against Tn-Expressing Glycoproteins," *Journal of the American Chemical Society*, Vol. 116, No. 1, 1994, pp. 395–396.

[45] Buskas, T., Ingale, S., Boons, G.-J., "Towards a Fully Synthetic Carbohydrate-Based Anticancer Vaccine: Synthesis and Immunological Evaluation of a Lipidated Glycopeptide Containing the Tumor-Associated Tn Antigen," *Angewandte Chemie-International Edition*, Vol. 44, No. 37, 2005, pp. 5985–5988.

[46] Ingale, S, et al., "Robust Immune Responses Elicited by a Fully Synthetic Three-Component Vaccine," *Nature Chemical Biology*, Vol. 3, No. 10, 2007, pp. 663–667.

[47] Ingale, S., Buskas, T., and Boons, G.-J., "Synthesis of Glyco(lipo)peptides by Liposome-Mediated Native Chemical Ligation," *Organic Letters*, Vol. 8, No. 25, 2006, pp. 5785–5788.

[48] Dawson, P. E., et al., "Synthesis of Proteins by Native Chemical Ligation," *Science*, Vol. 266, No. 5186, 1994, pp. 776–779.

[49] Ingale, S., et al., "Increasing the Antigenicity of Synthetic Tumor-Associated Carbohydrate Antigens by Targeting Toll-Like Receptors," *ChemBioChem*, Vol. 10, No. 3, 2009, pp. 455–463.

[50] Wan, Q., et al., "A Potentially Valuable Advance in the Synthesis of Carbohydrate-Based Anticancer Vaccines through Extended Cycloaddition Chemistry," *Journal of Organic Chemistry*, Vol. 71, No. 21, 2006, pp. 8244–8249.

[51] Bay, S, et al., "Preparation of a Multiple Antigen Glycopeptide (MAG) Carrying the Tn Antigen - a Possible Approach to a Synthetic Carbohydrate Vaccine," *Journal of Peptide Research*, Vol. 49, No. 6, 1997, pp. 620–625.

[52] Ota, S., et al., "Cellular Processing of a Multibranched Lysine Core with Tumor Antigen Peptides and Presentation of Peptide Epitopes Recognized by Cytotoxic T Lymphocytes on Antigen-Presenting Cells," *Cancer Research*, Vol. 62, No. 5, 2002, pp. 1471–1476.

[53] Tam, J. P., "Synthetic Peptide Vaccine Design: Synthesis and Properties of a High-Density Multiple Antigenic Peptide System," *Proceedings of the National Academy of Sciences of the United States of America*, Vol. 85, No. 15, 1988, pp. 5409–5413.

[54] Lo-Man, R., et al., "A Fully Synthetic Immunogen Carrying a Tumor-Associated Carbohydrate for Active Immunotherapy," *Cancer Research*, Vol. 59, No. 7, 1999, pp. 1520–1524.

[55] Lo-Man, R., et al., "A Fully Synthetic Therapeutic Vaccine Candidate Targeting Carcinoma-Associated Tn Carbohydrate Antigen Induces Tumor-Specific Antibodies in Nonhuman Primates," *Cancer Research*, Vol. 64, No. 14, 2004, pp. 4987–4994.

[56] Freire, T., et al., "Carbohydrate Antigens: Synthesis Aspects and Immunological Applications in Cancer," *Mini-Reviews in Medicinal Chemistry*, Vol. 6, No. 12, 2006, pp. 1357–1373.

[57] Ozawa, C., et al., "Efficient Sequential Segment Coupling Using *N*-Alkylcysteine-Assisted Thioesterification for Glycopeptide Dendrimer Synthesis," *Organic Letters*, Vol. 10, No. 16, 2008, pp. 3531–3533.

[58] Becker, T., Kaiser, A., Kunz, H., "Synthesis of Dendrimeric Tumor-Associated Mucin-Type Glycopeptide Antigens," *Synthesis*, No. 7, 2009, pp. 1113–1122.

[59] Cremer, G.-A., et al., "Synthesis and Biological Evaluation of a Multiantigenic Tn/TF-Containing Glycopeptide Mimic of the Tumor-Related MUC1 Glycoprotein," *ChemMedChem*, Vol. 1, No. 9, 2006, pp. 965–968.

[60] Cremer, G.-A., et al., "Synthesis of Branched Oxime-Linked Peptide Mimetics of the MUC1 Containing a Universal T-Helper Epitope," *Chemistry, a European Journal*, Vol. 10, No. 24, 2004, pp. 6353–6360.

[61] Mutter, M., et al., "Strategies for the De Novo Design of Proteins," *Tetrahedron*, Vol. 44, No. 3, 1988, pp. 771-785.

[62] Dumy, P., et al., "A Convenient Synthesis of Cyclic-Peptides as Regioselectively Addressable Functionalized Templates (RAFT)," *Tetrahedron Letters*, Vol. 36, No. 8, 1995, pp. 1255–1258.

[63] Renaudet, O., "Recent Advances on Cyclopeptide-Based Glycoclusters," *Mini-Reviews in Organic Chemistry*, Vol. 5, No. 4, 2008, pp. 274–286.
[64] Boturyn, D., et al., "RAFT Nano-constructs: Surfing to Biological Applications," *Journal of Peptide Science*, Vol. 14, No. 2, 2008, pp. 224–240.
[65] Renaudet, O., and Dumy, P., "Expedient Synthesis of Aminooxylated-Carbohydrates for Chemoselective Access of Glycoconjugates," *Tetrahedron Letters*, Vol. 42, No. 43, 2001, pp. 7575–7578.
[66] Renaudet, O., and Dumy, P., "Synthesis of Multivalent Chemoselectively Template-Assembled Glycopeptide Presenting the Cancer Related T-Antigen," *Tetrahedron Letters*, Vol. 45, No. 1, 2004, pp. 65–68.
[67] Renaudet, O., and Dumy, P., "Chemoselectively Template-Assembled Glycoconjugates as Mimics for Multivalent Presentation of Carbohydrates," *Organic Letters*, Vol. 5, No. 3, 2003, pp. 243–245.
[68] Renaudet, O., and Dumy, P., "Synthesis of Multitopic Neoglycopeptides Displaying Recognition and Detection Motifs," *Bioorganic & Medicinal Chemistry Letters*, Vol. 15, No. 15, 2005, pp. 3619–3622.
[69] Renaudet, O., and Dumy, P., "On-bead Synthesis and Binding Assay of Chemoselectively Template-Assembled Multivalent Neoglycopeptides," *Organic & Biomolecular Chemistry*, Vol. 4, No. 13, 2006, pp. 2628–2636.
[70] Renaudet, O., and Dumy, P., "A Fully Solid-Phase Synthesis of Biotinylated Glycoclusters," *Open Glycoscience*, Vol. 1, No. 1, 2008, pp. 1–7.
[71] Singh, Y., et al., "Preparation of a Multitopic Glycopeptide Oligonucleotide Conjugate," *Organic Letters*, Vol. 7, No. 7, 2005, pp. 1359–1362.
[72] Renaudet, O., Boturyn, D., and Dumy, P., "Biomolecular Assembly by Iterative Oxime Ligations," *Bioorganic & Medicinal Chemistry Letters*, Vol. 19, 2009, in press.
[73] Grigalevicius, S., et al., "Chemoselective Assembly and Immunological Evaluation of Multiepitopic Glycoconjugates Bearing Clustered Tn Antigen as Synthetic Anticancer Vaccines," *Bioconjugate Chemistry*, Vol. 16, No. 5, 2005, pp. 1149–1159.
[74] Geoghegan, K. F., and Stroh, J. G., "Site-Directed Conjugation of Nonpeptide Groups to Peptides and Proteins via Periodate-Oxidation of a 2-Amino Alcohol - Application to Modification at N-Terminal Serine," *Bioconjugate Chemistry*, Vol. 3, No. 2, 1992, pp. 138–146.
[75] Renaudet, O., et al., "Towards Self-Adjuvanting Multivalent B and T cell Epitopes Synthetic Glyco-Lipopeptide Cancer Vaccine," *ChemMedChem*, Vol. 3, No. 5, 2008, pp. 737–741.
[76] Bettahi, I., et al., "Antitumor Activity of a Self-Adjuvanting Glyco-Lipopeptide Vaccine Bearing B Cell, CD4+ and CD8+ T Cell Epitopes," *Cancer Immunology Immunotherapy*, Vol. 58, No. 2, 2009, pp. 187–200.
[77] Wang, J., et al., "Novel Template-Assembled Oligosaccharide Clusters as Epitope Mimics for HIV-Neutralizing Antibody 2G12. Design, Synthesis, and Antibody Binding Study," *Organic & Biomolecular Chemistry*, Vol. 5, No. 10, 2007, pp. 1529–1540.
[78] Krauss, I. J., et al., "Fully Synthetic Carbohydrate HIV Antigens Designed on the Logic of the 2G12 Antibody," *Journal of the American Chemical Society*, Vol. 129, No. 36, 2007, pp. 11042–11044.
[79] Baek, M.-G., Roy, R., and Rittenhouse-Olson, K., "Synthesis and Antibody Binding Properties of Glycodendrimers Bearing the Tumor Related T-Antigen," *Chemical Communication*, No. 3, 2001, pp. 257–258.
[80] Vepřek, P., et al., "Comblike Dendrimers Containing Tn Antigen Modulate Natural Killing and Induce the Production of Tn Specific Antibodies," Journal of Medicinal Chemistry, Vol. 49, No. 21, 2006, pp 6400–6407.
[81] Geraci, C., et al., "Calix[4]arene Decorated with Four Tn Antigen Glycomimetic Units and P_3CS Immunoadjuvant: Synthesis, Characterization, and Anticancer Immunological Evaluation," Bioconjugate Chemistry, Vol. 19, No. 3, 2008, pp. 751–758.

CHAPTER 7

STIMULI-SENSITIVE PARTICLES FOR DRUG DELIVERY

Stephanie J. Grainger and Mohamed E. H. El-Sayed*

University of Michigan, Department of Biomedical Engineering, 1101 Beal Avenue Lurie Biomedical Engineering Building, Room 2150, Ann Arbor, MI 48109, USA
E-mail: melsayed@umich.edu

1. Introduction

Natural and synthetic polymers have been used to fabricate different types of particles that vary in shape, size (micro- or nano-sized), degradability, and type of surface groups. [1] These particles have been routinely used as vehicles for delivery of therapeutic agents due to their ability to protect the encapsulated drug coupled with their ease of fabrication, tunable degradation kinetics, and high surface to volume ratio, which allows the display of a large number of targeting agents and/or imaging probes. [2-4] The first generation of polymeric particles released the encapsulated drug via degradation of the polymer matrix regardless of where these particles are located within the body. [5] However, there is a significant interest in delivering therapeutic drug molecules selectively to

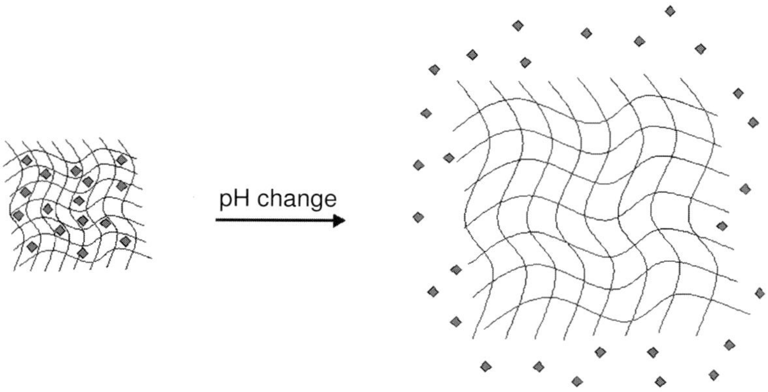

Fig. 1. A schematic drawing of "smart" pH-sensitive polymers cross-linked to form a drug-loaded hydrogel that senses the change in environment pH, swells, and releases the encapsulated drug.

diseased tissues by utilizing certain cues that are specific to the targeted tissue/cell to trigger the release of the encapsulated drug from the particulate carriers. This need catalyzed the development of "smart" particles, which are fabricated using stimuli-sensitive polymers that can sense and respond to small changes in environment conditions such as pH, temperature, light, and ionic strength. [6] We are particularly interested in pH-sensitive polymers, which are characterized by their unique ability to sense small changes in environment pH that trigger a corresponding change in the polymer's physical properties such as size, shape, hydrophobicity, and/or degradation rate. [2, 7, 8] Earlier studies showed that cross-linkage of pH-sensitive polymers yields "smart" hydrogels with tunable swelling behavior, which have been used as carriers for controlled drug delivery (Figure 1). In this chapter, we discuss the potential of "smart" particles developed using pH-sensitive polymers as carriers for delivery of a wide range of therapeutic molecules. [9-16]

1.1. *pH-sensitive polymers with acidic functional groups*

One class of pH-sensitive polymers is known as polyelectrolytes or polyanions, which is characterized by a large number of ionizable acidic groups such as carboxylic or sulfonic acid groups (Figure 2). Examples of common polyanions

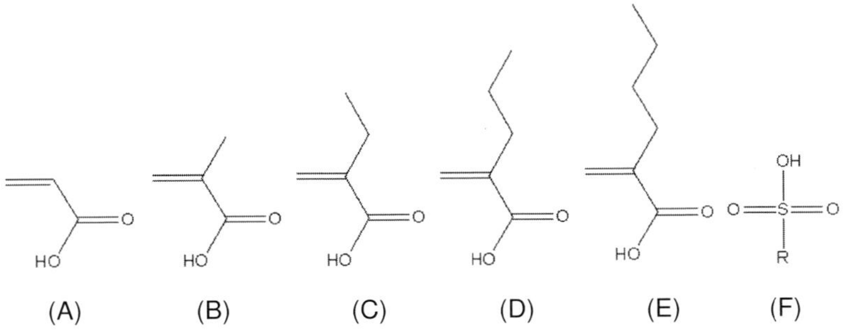

Fig. 2. The chemical structures of: (A) acrylic acid, (B) methyl acrylic acid, (C) ethyl acrylic acid, (D) propyl acrylic acid, (E) butyl acrylic acid, and (F) sulfonic acid monomers used to synthesize "smart" pH-sensitive polymers.

used in drug delivery include poly(acrylic acid) and poly(sulfonic acid) polymers. The pendant acidic groups of these polymers are typically ionized in neutral and alkaline solutions and their electrostatic repulsion affects the physical properties of the polymer. The pH at which the pendant acidic groups become ionized depends on the pKa (the log value of the acid dissociation constant) of the polymer, which in turn depends on the polymer's composition and molecular weight. [17]

Hoffman, Stayton and coworkers characterized the pH-dependent membrane-destabilizing activity of poly(acrylic acid) (PAA), poly(methyl acrylic acid) (PMAA), poly(ethyl acrylic acid) (PEAA), poly(propyl acrylic acid) (PPAA), and poly(butyl acrylic acid) (PBAA) polymers. Their results showed that the systematic increase in the length of the hydrophobic alkyl group by one methylene unit (CH_2) results in an increase in the polymer's pKa value and consequently affects the pH at which this polymer switches from a hydrophilic conformation to a hydrophobic and membrane-destabilizing one. This was evident by the increase in the polymer's pKa from 6.3 for PEAA to 6.7 for PPAA to 7.4 for PBAA, which limited the utility of PBAA as a carrier for drug delivery because of its non-specific membrane-destabilizing activity at physiologic pH. [18, 19] Duncan *et al.* showed that the pH-dependent membrane-destabilizing activity of these polymers decreases with the decrease in polymer concentration, which indicates that it is a concentration-dependent effect. [20] Poly(acrylic acid) polymers have been formulated into drug-loaded particles for oral drug delivery where they retain their therapeutic cargo in the acidic environment of the stomach but release the encapsulated drug in the alkaline environment of the

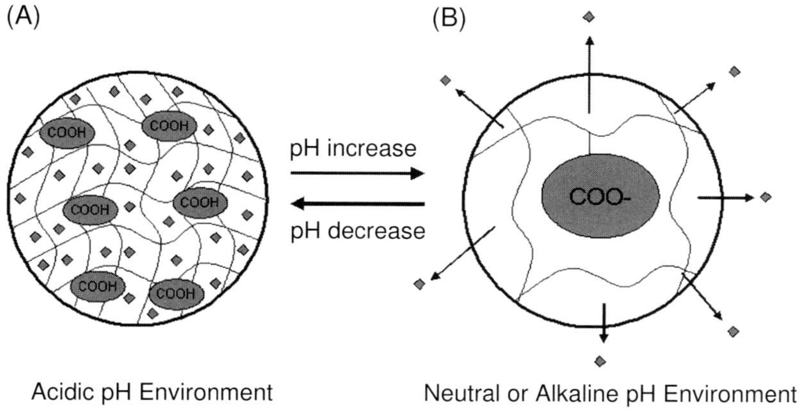

Fig. 3. A schematic drawing of a drug-loaded particle formulated using poly(acrylic acid) polymers. (A) The pendant carboxylic acid groups are unionized in the acidic environment of the stomach and the particle retains the loaded drug. Whereas, in neutral and alkaline environments of the small intestine (B), the pendant carboxylic acid groups become ionized, the particle swells due to electrostatic repulsion of the ionized groups and release the loaded drug molecules into the surrounding medium.

small intestine due to ionization of the carboxylic acid groups and swelling of the polymer matrix (Figure 3).

Poly(acrylic acid) copolymers incorporating hydrophobic methyl methacrylate (MMA) or butyl methacrylate (BMA) monomers were synthesized where the chemical structure and percentage of the hydrophobic monomer influenced the polymer's pKa value. For example, Barba *et al.* synthesized a range of poly(MMA-*co*-AA) copolymers with an increasing volumetric ratio of MMA monomer (0, 25, 30, 40, 50, 60, 70, 75, 100%) and examined their dissolution at different pH values. Her results showed that the increase in MMA content in a given polymer increased the pH necessary to dissolve this polymer (pH 4.0 – 6.8; co-polymers with 75% and higher MMA content were not soluble), which indirectly indicates the increase in the polymer's pKa with the increase in MMA content. [7]

Another study by Licea-Claverie *et al.* showed that the insertion of a variable number of methylene groups in a poly(MMA) polymer increases the polymer's pKa (1 – 10 CH_2 spacers; MW range: 43 – 90 KDa; pKa range: 3.8 – 7.3) due to the formation of hydrophobic microdomains that act as a cross-linker that minimizes the polymer's dissolution and swelling. [21] One example that clearly indicates the effect of solution pH on poly(acrylic acid) polymers is reported by Guan *et al.* who utilized poly(acrylic acid-9-aminoacridine-*co*-acrylamide) as a pH sensor in biological applications. This application depends on the polymer's (MW 3.5 KDa) ability to change its fluorescence intensity as it transitions from double to single protonation to amino and finally imino forms as a function of environment pH (pH 0 – 13.71). [22]

The second group of pH-sensitive polymers with acidic functional groups includes poly(sulfonic acid) polymers and their derivatives. These polymers have pendant sulfonate groups (–SO_3H) with pKa values of 2-3 thus become ionized over a wide pH range. [23] Polysulfonates are often used as cross-linking agents of other polymers such as styrene and vinyl-based polymers to tune the pKa of the formulated particles for a specific application. For example, McCormick *et al.* synthesized hydrogel-based particles using 3-[*N*-(2-methacroyloyethyl)-*N,N*-dimethylammonio] propanesulfonate (MW 49 KDa; polydispersity index (PDI) = 1.04) via controlled polymerization techniques. These particles were synthesized using an aqueous salt solvent system, which is an unconventional method for synthesis of acrylic-based polymers that typically require an organic solvent. These particles are attractive for drug delivery applications due to their biocompatibility, ease of production in aqueous salt solvent systems, and narrow distribution of molecular weight. [24]

1.2. *pH-sensitive polymers wth basic functional groups*

This class of pH-sensitive polymers include poly[2-(dimethylamino)ethyl methacrylate] (PDMAEMA) and poly(vinylamine) (PVAm) polymers, which display basic functional groups such as primary, secondary, and tertiary amine groups that become ionized at low pH values (Figure 4). [25-30]

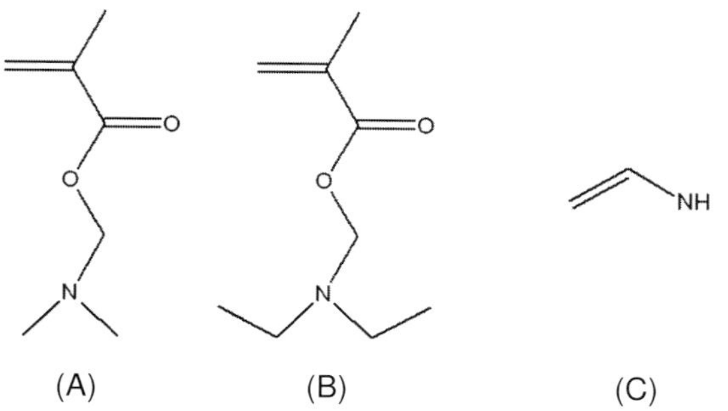

Fig. 4. The chemical structures of: (A) *N,N'*-dimethylaminoethyl methacrylate, (B) *N,N'*-diethylaminoethyl methacrylate, and (C) vinyl amine monomers, which are commonly used to prepare "smart" pH-sensitive cationic polymers.

Unlike anionic polymers, which exhibit pH-induced transitions in their physical conformation around pH 4-6, these cationic polymers display the change in their conformation at pH 8 or higher based on their pKa values (Figure 5) [31-33] Several investigations focused on modifying these cationic polymers to reduce their pKa values to match the physiologic pH to become useful in biological and pharmaceutical applications. [34] One approach is to incorporate hydrophobic monomers into the cationic polymer backbone to shift the polymer's overall pKa towards the neutral pH range. [35, 36] For example, Kang and Bae modified the sulfonamide homopolymer (pKa 6.10) by copolymerization with 10-50 mol% of sulfadimethoxine to reduce the degree of ionization necessary for dissolution from 85% for the homopolymer to 18% for the copolymer (MW: 112.3 – 81.4 KDa; pKa 6.25). [31] Another example involves the grafting of hydrophobic *N*-isopropyl acrylamide (NIPAM) to cationic chitosan polymer (MW of 21.6 KDa; 10.5 – 48% grafted NIPAM) to prepare pH-sensitive hydrogel particles. The degree of swelling of these particles was influenced by the charge and the pKa of the chitosan, the cross-linking density, and the environment's pH and ionic strength. [37] Modulating the degree of NIPAM grafting proved to modulate the degree of particle swelling and the associated release kinetics of the incorporated drug. [38]

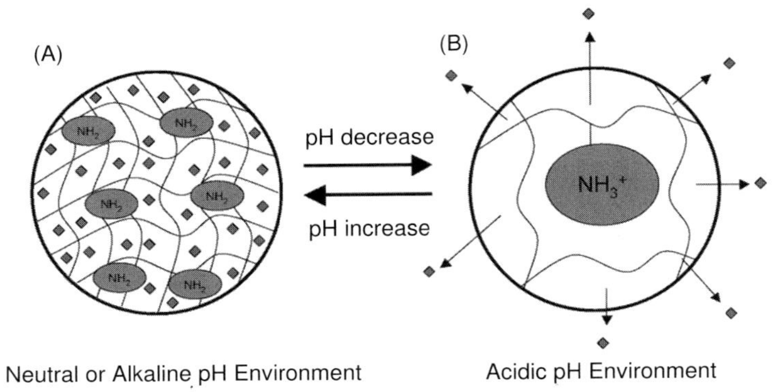

Fig. 5. A schematic drawing of a drug-loaded particle formulated using poly(vinyl amine) polymers. (A) In a neutral or alkaline environment, the pendant amine groups remain unionized and the particle entraps the loaded drug. However, as the pH drops below the pKa value of these NH_2 groups (B), they become protonated and the particle swells due to electrostatic repulsion between the positively charged groups and releases the loaded drug molecules into the surrounding medium.

2. Synthesis Strategies for pH-Sensitive Polymers

Random free radical polymerization has been used to synthesize several groups of pH-sensitive polymers. [39] However, this technique suffers multiple limitations including limited control over the polymerization process and the exact composition of the resulting homo- and co-polymers, the limited ability to synthesize branched or three dimensional structures, the broad distribution of the polymer's molecular weight, and diminished versatility in the type of incorporated functional groups. [40, 41] The emergence of controlled free radical polymerization techniques has accelerated the development of well-defined polymer compositions with a narrow distribution of molecular weight, customized architectures, and versatile functional groups that proved to be successful in the area of drug delivery. These controlled polymerization techniques include reversible addition-fragmentation chain transfer (RAFT), atom transfer radical polymerization (ATRP), and nitroxide-mediated polymerization (NMP) techniques, which have been used to synthesize several pH-sensitive polymers. [37, 42]

2.1. *Reversible addition-fragmentation chain transfer (RAFT) technique*

RAFT polymerization requires the presence of a reagent that reacts by reversible addition-fragmentation chain transfer mechanism (Figure 6). The effectiveness of these reagents depends on their transfer constant, which is determined by the nature of the X, Z, and R groups. Certain thiocarbonylthio compounds where X is sulfur, R is a free radical leaving group that is capable of reinitiating polymerization, and Z is a group that modifies the activity of the transfer constant proved to be the most effective reagents in RAFT polymerization. [43] Initiation of RAFT polymerization starts with cleavage of the initiator (e.g. azobisisobutyronitrile; AIBN) to yield reactive free radicals (I·) that react with the monomer (M) to form a growing polymer chain (P_n·). Subsequently, the growing chain adds to the RAFT agent followed by fragmentation and release of a free radical leaving group (R·), which re-initiates the polymerization reaction. The ratio of monomer to RAFT reagent determines the molecular weight of the resulting polymer and its distribution. Given the fact that this reaction involves the formation of free radical intermediates, radical-radical termination reactions

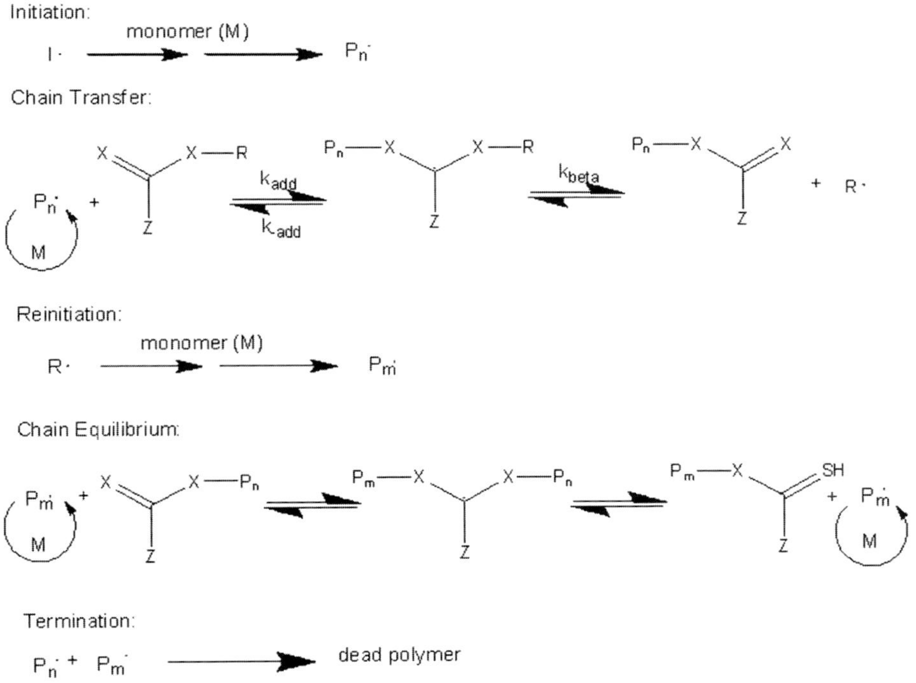

Fig. 6. Schematic drawing showing the mechanism of reversible addition-fragmentation chain transfer (RAFT) polymerization.

may occur, yielding dead polymers. One key advantage of RAFT polymerization is that the polymer retains the active functionality, the thiocarbonylthio group, which can be reactivated and used to build block, star-shaped, or more complex polymer architectures. [44-46] For example, Covertine *et al.* synthesized a series of diblock co-polymers composed of a positively-charged block of DMAEMA and a second endosomolytic block composed of DMAEMA and PAA in roughly equimolar ratios together with BMA as carriers for model nucleic acids using RAFT polymerization techniques. These polymers proved to be sharply hemolytic at endosomal pH values particularly those with high BMA content. They successfully condensed siRNA into 80-250 nm particles with slightly positive Zeta potentials that proved to knock down GAPDH expression in Hela cells in a trend that followed their hemolytic activity. [47] This clearly demonstrates the potential of RAFT polymerization in developing well-controlled polymer compositions for drug delivery.

2.2. *Atom transfer radical polymerization (ATRP) technique*

The term "atom transfer radical polymerization" was coined by Matyjeszewski in 1995 to describe the use of metal catalysts in combination with aromatic ligands to yield well-controlled polymer structures with narrow molecular weight distributions [48]. This mechanism of reaction involves the transfer of a halogen atom (X) from the dormant polymer chain to a metal catalyst yielding an active chain end (a radical; P·) that can add monomer units to the polymer chain through the propagation step (Figure 7). The selected catalyst in this reaction consists of a transition metal and a halogen. The transition metal (e.g. copper) has two oxidation states separated by one electron step and can strongly bind to a multidentate ligand forming a complex. The halogen, typically bromine or chlorine, should be able to migrate rapidly between the growing polymer chain and the catalyst [48]. One of the limitations of ATRP is the reaction intolerance to carboxylic acid and other ionic groups that can react with the catalyst and

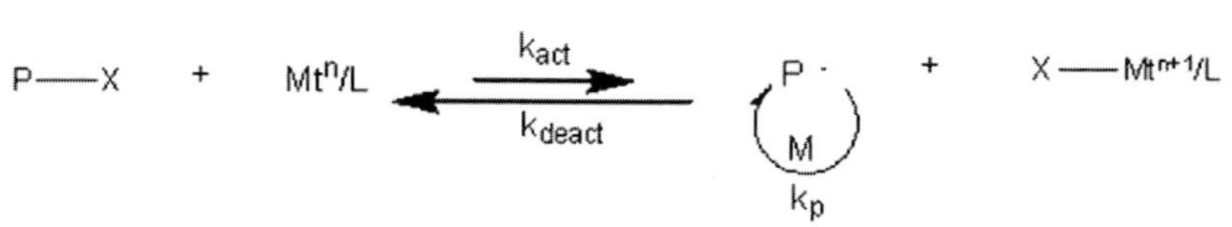

Fig. 7. Schematic drawing showing the mechanism of atom transfer radical polymerization (ATRP).

impede the achievement of equilibrium. A key advantage of the ATRP technique is that the resulting polymer retains the halogen moiety in the growing chain end, which allows reactivation of the chain end and use as a macroinitiator for a second polymerization reaction. ATRP is typically used to synthesize higher molecular weight polymers compared to the RAFT technique. One example is the synthesis of PMMA (MW 180 kDa) by ATRP using sulfonyl chloride initiator and copper as a catalyst yielding a polymer with a PDI of 1.1 compared to a PDI of 1.5 when synthesized using random free radical polymerization. [48]

2.3. *Nitroxide-mediated polymerization (NMP) technique*

The rationale behind nitroxide-mediated polymerization is to use the nitroxide group to efficiently cap the end of the growing polymer chains by a reversible termination reaction to ensure equal growth of all polymer chains while suppressing undesirable termination reactions. NMP reactions utilize alkoxyamines to function as both an initiator and end-capping group, which gives full control over the concentration of initiating radicals in the reaction mixture. This polymerization reaction starts with hemolytic cleavage of the alkoxyamine upon heating to produce the initiating radical (R3·) and the stabilized (·ONR1R2) that should be present long enough for a monomer unit (M) to react with the initiating radical before recombination takes place (Figure 8). Originally, NMP reactions were carried out at elevated temperatures (> 100°C), but have also been recently carried out in aqueous media at lower temperatures (<100°C). [49] It is important to note that the alkoxyamine group can withstand reaction conditions of other controlled radical polymerizations such as RAFT and ATRP, which makes it possible to synthesize block co-polymers by combining NMP with other techniques. [48]

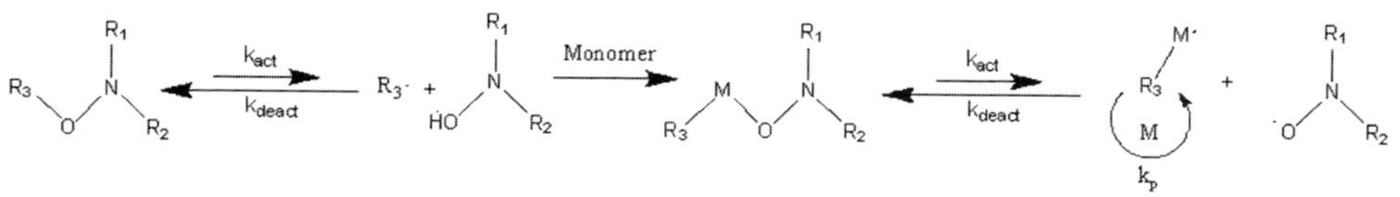

Fig. 8. Mechanism of nitroxide-mediated polymerization (NMP) technique.

3. "Smart" Particles

3.1. *Role of "smart" particles in delivery of therapeutic nucleic acids*

Several nucleic acid molecules including plasmid DNA (pDNA), antisense oligodeoxynucleotides (ASODN), and silencing RNA (siRNA) show potential therapeutic activity against cancer, inflammation, and neurodegenerative diseases. Activity of these molecules depends on their ability to reach their intracellular targets commonly present in the cytoplasm of the diseased cell. However, the systemic administration of therapeutic nucleic acids results in their degradation by nuclease enzymes, non-specific distribution throughout the body, rapid elimination into the urine, and limited cellular uptake via endocytosis, which collectively result in degradation of the administered dose and loss of therapeutic activity. [50-53]

Cationic polymers proved to be efficient carriers for delivery of nucleic acids into targeted cells. [26] They complex negatively-charged DNA molecules through electrostatic interactions forming polyplexes/particles that encapsulate the nucleic acids in their cores "shielding it" from serum proteins, nucleases, and other denaturing factors present in the systemic circulation. These particles typically carry a net positive charge which allows them to interact with the negatively-charged cell surface, trigger adsorptive-mediated endocytosis, and gain access into the cell. However, for these particles to be therapeutically effective, they have to escape the endosomal-lysosomal trafficking pathway, enter the cytoplasm, and release the encapsulated therapeutic cargo to interact with its desired intracellular target(s). [50, 54-57]

The endosomal compartment has a membrane-bound ATP-dependent proton pump that acidifies the endosome down to pH 5.0. Certain cationic polyamidoamine polymers such as poly(ethyleneimine) (PEI) have primary and secondary amine groups with a pKa of 5.5-7.2 distributed on the polymer's backbone. Endocytosis of PEI-based particles results in buffering of the endosomal pH, which triggers further transport of hydronium ions into the endosome and the influx of counter ions such as chloride, which increases the endosomal osmotic pressure. The osmotic gradient causes water influx into the endosome, which eventually ruptures the endosomal membrane and releases its contents into the cytoplasm in a process known as the "proton sponge" effect. [58] Boussif and Richardson tested the transfection efficiency of PEI (9 – 13.5 PEI nitrogen groups per single phosphate group of the DNA), which produced a 10^4-fold higher transfection efficiency compared to the control. [59, 60]

Some cationic polymers such as poly(L-lysine) (PLL) proved to be effective in forming polyplexes that shield the DNA but are not effective in disrupting the endosomal membrane. Other cationic polymers with pKas that match the endosomal pH value such as poly(L-histidine) are used to achieve endosomal escape via the proton sponge mechanism. [61] For example, *N*-Ac-poly(L-histidine)-graft-poly(L-lysine) polymer was used to achieve effective condensation of model DNA and effective transfection into human embryonic kidney 293 cells, which is attributed to the shift in carrier pKa from 8.0 for PLL to pKa 6.0 for the PLH co-polymer. This shift in carrier pKa allows for buffering of the endosomal pH, which triggers the endosomal disruption cascade via the proton sponge mechanism. [62]

"Smart" anionic polymers have also been used to enhance the delivery of nucleic acids past the endosomal membrane and into the cytoplasm of the target cell, but through a different mechanism compared to the cationic ones. "Smart" anionic polymers are characterized by their ability to switch from a hydrophilic, stealth-like conformation at physiologic pH to a hydrophobic, membrane-destabilizing one in response to acidic pH gradients. Consequently, these anionic polymers have been used as carriers for nucleic acids where they are physically

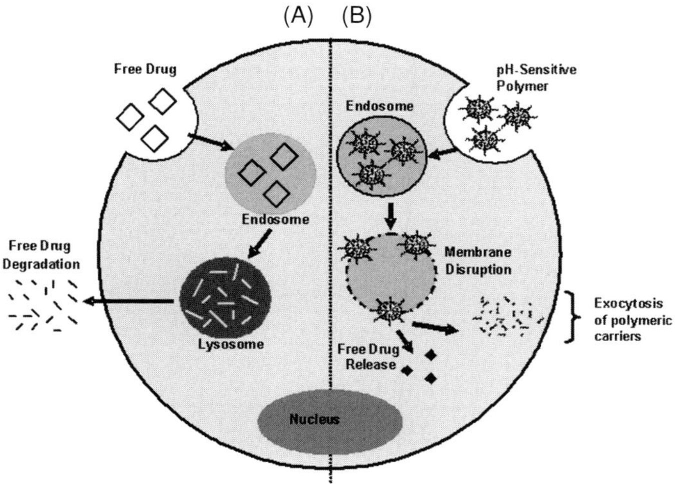

Fig. 9. A schematic drawing comparing the cellular uptake of free nucleic acid (A) and "smart" particles loaded with the desired nucleic acid (B) into targeted cells. Free nucleic acid is trapped in the endosomal-lysosomal trafficking pathway, which results in its degradation and loss of therapeutic activity. Whereas, "smart" particles "sense" the drop in endosomal pH, which triggers a change in the polymer conformation that ruptures the endosomal membrane and delivers the encapsulated particles into the cytoplasm to slowly release the nucleic acid cargo to produce the desired therapeutic activity.

mixed or chemically conjugated to the desired DNA to form a particle that may also incorporate additional cationic polymers for better condensation of the nucleic acid. [63-70] The ratio of the "smart" polymer's anionic functional groups (COOH or SO_3H), the phosphate group of the DNA, and the cationic group of the adjuvant polymer are adjusted so the +/- ratio is sufficient to form a stable cationic particle. [71] Once these particles are internalized by endocytosis into the target cell, the pH-sensitive anionic polymer will sense the drop in endosomal pH and switch to the hydrophobic conformation, which ruptures the endosomal membrane and delivers the encapsulated particles into the cytoplasm to slowly release the nucleic acid cargo to produce the desired therapeutic activity (Figure 9).

Tirrell and co-workers were the first to show that anionic PEAA (20 KDa; pKa 5.9) causes disruption of lipid membranes at acidic pH values. [19, 72-74] Cheung *et al.* capitalized on these initial observations and evaluated the ability of another anionic polymer, PPAA, to improve the *in vitro* transfection efficiency of pDNA and improve complex stability against serum proteins. His results showed that the incorporation of PPAA (61 KDa) in the DOTAP/DNA complexes increased their stability against a range of serum proteins and produced a 20-fold increase in DNA transfection compared to the complexes prepared without PPAA. [18, 19, 75, 76] Subsequent *in vivo* studies showed that DOTAP/PPAA/ASODN complexes targeted against the thrombospondin-2 (TSP2) gene can successfully knock down the desired gene and improved would healing.

To achieve better control over the membrane-destabilizing activity of these anionic activities, several co-polymers that incorporate EAA and PAA monomers with hydrophobic BMA monomers were synthesized. [77, 78] An interesting new approach was to incorporate the pyridyldisulfide acrylate (PDSA) monomers in these co-polymer compositions, which allows direct conjugation of thiolated nucleic acids or cationic peptides via a simple disulfide exchange. [77, 78]. Several co-polymer compositions incorporating a pH-sensitive monomer (EAA or PAA), a hydrophobic monomer (BMA), and PDSA were synthesized and conjugated to cationic PLL. [78] These polymer-PLL conjugates proved to condense model ASODN into stable particles that retained the pH-dependent membrane-destabilizing activity of the parent polymer. [78]

Encrypted polymers are another class of acid-sensitive carriers that proved effective in delivery of therapeutic nucleic acids. [18, 79] Murthy *et al.* prepared a hydrophobic random co-polymer incorporating DMAEMA, BA, BMA, and styrene benzaldehyde (SBA), which was masked by hydrophilic PEG chains anchored to the polymer backbone via acid-sensitive acetal linkages. [18, 80]

The PEG chains were conjugated to cationic PLL chains for condensation of nucleic acids via electrostatic interactions forming stable complexes. In the endosome, the acetal linkage will be hydrolyzed in response to the acidic environment thus unmasking the hydrophobic polymer backbone, which ruptures the endosomal membrane and releases the condensed nucleic acid into the cytoplasm. These encrypted polymers proved 9 times more effective at endosomal disruption compared to PPAA homopolymers and were effective in delivery of model ASODN into macrophage-like cells *in vitro*. [17, 81]

3.2. *Role of "smart" particles in delivery of peptides and proteins*

The route of administration of peptide and protein drugs dictates the formulation parameters required to achieve efficient drug delivery. Oral and parenteral delivery routes have distinctive sets of challenges. Orally-administered peptide and protein drugs have to survive the acidity of the stomach, withstand the hydrolytic activity of the metabolizing enzymes in the small intestine, permeate across the intestinal epithelium and reach the systemic circulation to become therapeutically effective. [82, 83] However, the enzymatic susceptibility of peptide and protein drugs coupled with their large size and hydrophilicity result in poor oral bioavailability and diminished therapeutic activity. [82-84] "Smart" cationic and anionic polymers have been used as carriers to enhance oral absorption of peptide and protein drugs across the gastrointestinal tract (GIT). [85-87] These pH-sensitive carriers shield the encapsulated drug from the metabolizing enzymes and harsh environment of the GIT while providing a mechanism to tune the site and rate of drug release in response to changes in the environment pH (Figure 10).

Several anionic polymers such as methyl acrylic acid (Eudragit L-100; MW 135 KDa), methyl methacrylate (S-100; MW 135 KDa), and hydroxypropyl methylcellulose phthalate (HP-55) have been commercially used as enteric coatings for oral delivery of peptide and protein drugs, where they release the encapsulated drug molecules into the small intestine in response to the alkaline pH. [88-91] Earlier research focused on optimizing the polymer composition and consequently its pKa to tune the site of release of the encapsulated peptide/protein drug in the small intestine. For example, Serres *et al.* loaded calcitonin hydrogel particles prepared using NIPAM, BMA, and AA monomers where the molar ratio of the hydrophilic AA monomer varied from 0-10%. Results showed that the particles prepared using a higher AA content had a higher drug loading capacity, were more stable, and released the encapsulated

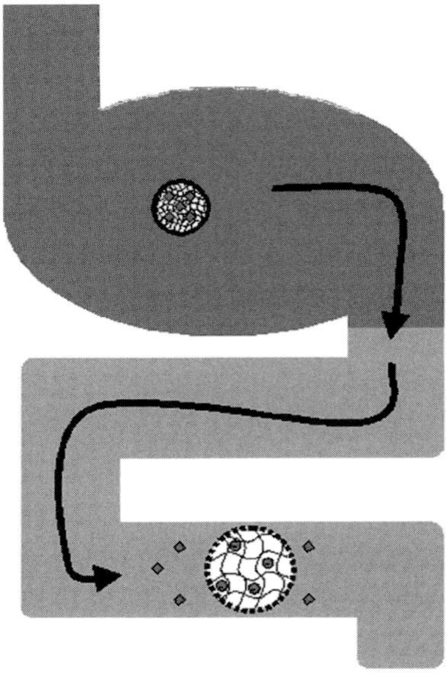

Fig. 10. A schematic drawing showing a "smart" particle fabricated using an anionic polymer (e.g. poly(acrylic acid)) to encapsulate a peptide/protein drug. In the acidic environment of the stomach, the carboxylic acid groups of the polymer are unionized and the particle retains its therapeutic cargo. However, once this particle reaches the small intestine, the carboxylic acid group becomes ionized and the particle swells due to the electrostatic repulsion between the ionized groups, thus releasing the encapsulated drug into the intestine to be absorbed.

drug into the duodenum compared to those with a higher content of the hydrophobic NIPAM monomer. [92]

To achieve efficient delivery of peptide/protein drug molecules to the ileum, the encapsulating carrier should have a higher pKa value than the ileum pH (6.0). Dowding and co-workers developed a gel mixture of NIPAM with N-N'-methylenebisacrylamide (BA) using 2% w/w of MAA as a cross-linking agent. The MAA units in this gel have a pKa of 6.7, which caused the hydrogel to swell in the ileum in response to environment pH. [85] Eaimtrakam *et al.* was the first to develop a four-layer carrier system that incorporated water-insoluble ethylcellulose and an enteric coating composed of each of the Eudragit copolymers, which are anionic acrylic-based polymers. Results showed that the S-100 polymer coat with the pKa of 6.8 (1:2 carboxyl:ester groups) swelled and adhered to the ileum wall for up to three hours after administration, which shielded the encapsulated drug molecules from the hydrolytic enzymes commonly present in the duodenum. [93] Venkatesh *et al.* compared the release profile of 15 mg of pindolol coated with either ethylcellulose (0.5% w/v) or a mixture of Eudragit S-100 (1.5-3% w/v) and HP-55 (1.5-3% w/v) with a pKa of 5.4. Results showed that enteric coatings slowed the drug release at low pH (< 4.5), but did not affect drug release at neutral pH (7.2), which allowed for site-specific release of the encapsulated drug into the ileum and escaping the acidic environment of the stomach and upper sections of the small intestine where the environment pH will reduce the drug's solubility. [87]

4. Future Directions

Stimuli-sensitive polymers play an important role in the development of advanced delivery vehicles that can effectively deliver a wide range of therapeutic molecules including nucleic acids, peptides, and proteins. There is a growing interest in developing stimuli-sensitive polymers that can recognize and respond to biologically-relevant stimuli so they can be used as carriers for tissue- and cell-specific drug delivery. The rapid advancement in the area of polymer synthesis and the increasing popularity of controlled polymerization techniques will further accelerate the development of new sophisticated carriers with well-defined compositions that can exploit physiological signals to trigger the release of their therapeutic cargo in a controlled fashion. Further, it is expected that the next generation of stimuli-sensitive carriers will have a hybrid composition that combines polymeric structures with natural biological motifs to further exploit natural transport mechanisms to reach their target tissue/cell as well as natural elimination pathways after the delivery of their cargo.

LIST OF ABBREVIATIONS

AIBN	azobisisobutyronitrile
ASODN	antisense oligodeoxynucleotide
ATRP	atom transfer radical polymerization
BA	butyl acrylate
BMA	butyl methacrylate
GIT	gastrointestinal tract
MMA	methyl methacrylate
NIPAM	*N*-isopropyl acrylamide
NMP	nitroxide-mediated polymerization
PAA	poly(acrylic acid)
PBAA	poly(butyl acrylic acid)
PDI	polydispersity index
PDMAEMA	poly[*N,N'*-(dimethylamino) ethyl methacrylate]
pDNA	plasmid DNA

PDSA	pyridyldisulfide acrylate
PEAA	poly(ethyl acrylic acid)
PEI	poly(ethyleneimine)
PLL	poly(L-lysine)
PMAA	poly(methyl acrylic acid)
PPAA	poly(propyl acrylic acid)
PVAm	poly(vinylamine)
RAFT	reversible addition-fragmentation chain transfer polymerization
siRNA	silencing RNA
TSP2	thrombospondin-2

References

[1] RC Thomson, SL Ishaug, AG Mikos, R Langer, Polymers for biological systems. in: R. Meyers (Ed.), Molecular biology and biotechnology, VCH Publishers, Inc., New York, NY, 1995.

[2] AS Hoffman, PS Stayton, Bioconjugates of smart polymers and proteins: Synthesis and applications, Macromolecular Symposia 207(Fundamentals and Applications of Polymer Gels) (2004) 139-151.

[3] A Schlossbauer, J Kecht, T Bein, Biotin-avidin as a protease-responsive cap system for controlled guest release from colloidal mesoporous silica, Angewandte Chemie International Edition in English 48(17) (2009) 3092-3095.

[4] A Schlossbauer, D Schaffert, J Kecht, E Wagner, et al., Click chemistry for high-density biofunctionalization of mesoporous silica, Journal of the American Chemical Society 130(38) (2008) 12558-12559.

[5] NA Peppas, C Donini, Protein delivery systems. in: G. Wnek and G. Bowlin (Eds.), Encyclopedia of Biomaterials and Biomedical Engineering, Vol. 4, Informa Healthcare U.S.A. Inc., New York, NY, 2008.

[6] MEH El-Sayed, AS Hoffman, PS Stayton, Smart polymeric carriers for enhanced intracellular delivery of therapeutic macromolecules, Expert Opinion on Biological Therapy 5(1) (2005) 23-32.

[7] AA Barba, A Dalmoro, F De Santis, G Lamberti, Synthesis and characterization of p(MMA-AA) copolymers for targeted oral drug delivery, Polymer Bulletin (2009).

[8] RA Siegel, BA Firestone, Ph-dependent equilibrium swelling properties of hydrophobic polyelectrolyte copolymer gels, Macromolecules 21(11) (1988) 3254-3259.

[9] PS Stayton, AS Hoffman, Immobilization of "smart" polymer-protein conjugates. in: T Cass, FS Ligler (Eds.), Immobilized biomolecules in analysis: a practical approach, Oxford University Press, New York, NY, 1998.

[10] JP Chen, AS Hoffman, Polymer-protein conjugates. Ii. Affinity precipitation separation of human immunogammaglobulin by a poly(n-isopropylacrylamide)-protein a conjugate, Biomaterials 11(9) (1990) 631-634.

[11] A Chilkoti, Site-specific conjugation of a temperature-sensitive polymer to a genetically engineered protein, Bioconjugate Chemistry 5(6) (1994) 504-507.

[12] PS Stayton, T Shimoboji, C Long, A Chilkoti, et al., Control of protein-ligand recognition using a stimuli-responsive polymer, Nature 378(6556) (1995) 472-474.

[13] JE Morris, AS Hoffman, Affinity precipitation of proteins by polyligands, Biotechnology and Bioengineering 41(10) (1993) 991-997.

[14] Z Ding, RB Fong, CJ Long, PS Stayton, et al., Size-dependent control of the binding of biotinylated proteins to streptavidin using a polymer shield, Nature 411(6833) (2001) 59-62.
[15] H Maeda, SMANCS and polymer-conjugated macromolecular drugs: Advantages in cancer chemotherapy, Advanced Drug Delivery Reviews 6(2) (1991) 181-202.
[16] R Duncan, J Kopecek, Soluble synthetic polymers as potential drug carriers, Advances in Polymer Science 57 (1984) 51-101.
[17] AS Hoffman, PS Stayton, O Press, N Murthy, et al., Design of "Smart" Polymers that can direct intracellular drug delivery, Polymers for Advanced Technologies 13 (2002) 992-999.
[18] AS Hoffman, PS Stayton, O Press, N Murthy, et al., Bioinspired polymers that control intracellular drug delivery, Biotechnology and Bioprocess Engineering 6 (2001) 205-212.
[19] N Murthy, JR Robichaud, DA Tirrell, PS Stayton, et al., The design and synthesis of polymers for eukaryotic membrane disruption, Journal of Controlled Release 61 (1999) 137-143.
[20] R Duncan, P Ferruti, D Sgouras, A Tuboku-Metzger, et al., A polymer-Triton X-100 conjugate capable of pH-dependent red blood cell lysis: A model system illustrating the possibility of drug delivery within acidic intracellular compartments, Journal of Drug Targeting 2 (1994) 341-347.
[21] A Licea-Claverie, E Rogel-Hernandez, R Salgado-Rodriguez, JA Lopez-Sanchez, et al., The use of hydrophobic spacers in the development of new temperature- and pH-sensitive polymers, Macromolecular Symposia 207(Fundamentals and Applications of Polymer Gels) (2004) 193-215.
[22] X Guan, Z Liu, Z Su, Synthesis and photophysical behaviors of temperature/pH-sensitive polymeric materials, European Polymer Journal 43(7) (2007) 3094-3105.
[23] MG Neumann, IA Pastre, AM Chinelatto, OA El Seoud, Effects of the structure of anionic polyelectrolytes on surface potentials of their aggregates in water, Colloid and Polymer Science 274(5) (1996) 475-481.
[24] MS Donovan, BS Sumerlin, AB Lowe, CL McCormick, Controlled/living polymerization of sulfobetaine monomers directly in aqueous media via raft, Macromolecules 35 (2002) 8663-8666.
[25] SI Kang, YH Bae, pH-Induced volume-phase transition by reversible crystal formation, Macromolecules 34 (2001) 8173-8178.
[26] T Traitel, R Goldbart, J Kost, Smart polymers for responsive drug-delivery systems, Journal of Biomaterial Sciences, Polymer Edition 19(6) (2008) 755-767.
[27] O Korostynska, K Arshak, E Gill, A Arshak, Review on state-of-the-art in polymer based pH sensors, Sensors 7 (2007) 3027-3042.
[28] A Benrebouh, D Avoce, XX Zhu, Thermo- and pH-sensitive polymers containing cholic acid derivatives, Polymer 42 (2001) 4031-4038.
[29] HC Chiu, AT Wu, YF Lin, Synthesis and characterization of acrylic acid-containing dextran hydrogels, Polymer 42 (2001) 1471-1479.
[30] EEL Kathmann, LA White, CA McCormick, Water-soluble polymers 73. Electrolyte- and pH-responsive zwitter ionic copolymers of 4-[2-acrylamido-2-methylpropyl)-dimethylammonio]butanoate with 3-[(acrylamio-2-methylpropyl)dimethylammonio]propanesulfonate, Macromolecules 30 (1997) 5297-5304.
[31] SI Kang, YH Bae, pH-Induced solubility transition of sulfonamide-based polymers, Journal of Controlled Release 80 (2002) 145-155.
[32] M Sakata, M Todokoro, T Kai, M Kunitake, et al., Effect of cationic polymer adsorbent pKa on the selective removal of endotoxin from an albumin solution, Chromatographia 53 (2001) 619-623.
[33] SH Yuk, SH Cho, SH Lee, pH/Temperature-responsive polymer composed of poly(*N,N*-dimethylamino)ethyl methacrylate-co-ethylacrylamide, Macromolecules 30 (1997) 6856-6859.

[34] X Chen, Y Wang, R Pelton, pH-Dependence of the properties of hydrophobically modified polyvinylamine, Langmuir 21(25) (2005) 11673-11677.
[35] OE Philippova, D Hourdet, R Audebert, A Khokhlov, pH-Responsive gels of hydrophobically modified poly(acrylic acid), Macromolecules 30 (1997) 8278-8285.
[36] H Feil, YH Bae, J Feijen, SW Kim, Mutual influence of pH and temperature on the swelling of ionizable and thermosensitive hydrogels, Macromolecules 25 (1992) 5528-5530.
[37] SY Kim, SM Cho, YM Lee, SJ Kim, Thermo- and pH-responsive behaviors of graft copolymer and blend based on chitosan and *N*-isopropylacrylamide, Journal of Applied Polymer Science 78(7) (2000) 1381-1391.
[38] S Mima, M Miya, R Iwamoto, Y Susumu, Highly deacetylated chitosan and its properties, Journal of Applied Polymer Science 28(6) (1983) 1909-1917.
[39] Y Miura, N Nakamura, I Taniguchi, A Ichikawa, Radical polymerization of butyl acrylate and random copolymerization of styrene and butyl acrylate and styrene and methyl methacrylate mediated by monospiro- and dispiropiperidinyl-*N*-oxyl radicals, Polymer 44(12) (2003) 3461-3467.
[40] K Matyjaszewski, J Xia, Atom transfer radical polymerization, Chemical Reviews 101 (2001) 2921-2990.
[41] CJ Hawker, E Elce, J Dao, W Volksen, et al., Well-defined random copolymers by a "living" free-radical polymerization process, Macromolecules 29 (1996) 2686-2688.
[42] SY Park, YH Bae, Novel pH-sensitive polymers containing sulfonamide groups, Macromolecular Rapid Communication 20 (1999) 269-273.
[43] J Chiefari, YK Chong, F Ercole, J Krstina, et al., Living free-radical polymerization by reversible addition–fragmentation chain transfer: the RAFT process, Macromolecules 31 (1998) 5559–5562.
[44] G Moad, YK Chong, A Postma, E Rizzardo, et al., Advances in RAFT polymerization: The synthesis of polymers with defined end-groups, Polymer 46 (2005) 8458-8468.
[45] G Moad, J Chiefari, YK Chong, J Krstina, et al., Living free radical polymerization with reversible addition-fragmentation chain transfer (the life of RAFT), Polymer International 49 (2000) 993-1001.
[46] H Mori, AHE Muller, New polymeric architectures with (meth)acrylic acid segments, Progress in Polymer Science 28 (2003) 1403-1439.
[47] AJ Convertine, DSW Benoit, CL Duvall, AS Hoffman, et al., Development of a novel endosomolytic diblock copolymer for siRNA delivery, Journal of Controlled Release 133 (2009) 221-229.
[48] MF Zambaux, F Bonneaux, R Gref, Influence of experimental parameters on the characteristics of poly(lactic acid) nanoparticles prepared by double emulsion method, Journal of Controlled Release 50 (1998) 31-40.
[49] B Grassi, G Clisson, A Khoukh, L Billon, Nitroxide-mediated radical polymerization of acrylamide in water solution, European Polymer Journal 44(1) (2008) 50-58.
[50] ME Davis, Non-viral gene delivery systems, Current Opinion in Biotechnology 13 (2002) 128-131.
[51] S Dorudi, JM Northover, RG Vile, Gene transfer therapy in cancer, British Journal of Surgery 80 (1993) 566-572.
[52] C Plank, K Zatloukal, M Cotten, K Mechtler, et al., Gene transfer into hepatocytes using asialoglycoprotein receptor mediated endocytosis of DNA complexed with an artificial tetra-antennary galactose ligand, Bioconjugate Chemistry 3 (1992) 533-539.
[53] HC Chiou, MV Tangco, SM Levine, D Robertson, et al., Enhanced resistance to nuclease degradation of nucleic acids complexed to asialoglycoprotein-polylysine carriers, Nucleic Acid Research 22 (1994) 5439-5446.
[54] SC De Smedt, J Demeester, WE Hennink, Cationic polymer-based gene delivery systems, Pharmaceutical Research 17 (2000) 113-126.

[55] NA Jones, IRC Hill, S Stolnik, F Bignotti, et al., Polymer chemical structure is a key determinant of physicochemical and colloidal properties of polymer-DNA complexes for gene delivery, Biochemica et Biophysica Acta 1517(1-18) (2000).
[56] S Hwang, N Bellocq, ME Davis, Effects of structure of beta-cyclodextrin-containing polymers on gene delivery, Bioconjugate Chemistry 12 (2001) 280-290.
[57] DV Schaffer, NA Fidelman, N Dan, DA Lauffenburger, Vector unpacking as a potential barrier for receptor-mediated polyplex gene delivery, Biotechnology and Bioengineering 67 (2000) 598-606.
[58] DW Pack, AS Hoffman, S Pun, PS Stayton, Design and development of polymers for gene delivery, Nature Reviews Drug Discovery 5 (2005) 581-593.
[59] O Boussif, F Lezoualc'h, MA Zanta, MD Mergny, et al., A versatile vector for gene and oligonucleotide transfer into cells in culture and *in vivo*: polyethylenimine, Proceedings of the National Academy of Sciences USA 92(16) (1995) 7297-7301.
[60] SCW Richardson, NG Pattrick, YK Stella Man, P Ferruti, et al., Poly(amidoamine)s as potential nonviral vectors: ability to form interpolyelectrolyte complexes and to mediate transfection *in vitro*, Biomacromolecules 2 (2001) 1023-1028.
[61] CY Wang, L Huang, Polyhistidine mediates an acid-dependent fusion of negatively charged liposomes, Biochemistry 23 (1984) 4409-4416.
[62] JM Benns, JS Choi, RI Mahato, JS Park, et al., pH-Sensitive cationic polymer gene delivery vehicle: *N*-AC-poly(L-histidine)-*graft*-poly(L-lysine) comb shaped polymer, Journal of Bioconjugate Chemistry 11 (2000) 637-645.
[63] FM Hughson, Structural characterization of viral fusion proteins, Current Biology 5 (1995) 265-274.
[64] J Ren, JC Sharpe, RJ Collier, E London, Membrane translocation of charged residues at the tips of hydrophobic helices in the t domain of diphtheria toxin, Biochemistry 38 (1999) 976-984.
[65] AE Smith, Viral vectors in gene therapy, Annual Review of Microbiology 49 (1995) 807-838.
[66] SA Rosenberg, P Aebersold, K Cornetta, A Kasid, et al., Gene transfer into humans - immunotherapy of patients with advanced melanoma, using tumor-infiltrating lymphocytes modified by retroviral gene transduction, New England Journal of Medicine 323 (1990) 570-578.
[67] K Shimotohno, HM Temin, Formation of infectious progeny virus after insertion of herpes simplex thymidine kinase gene into DNA of an avian retrovirus, Cell 26 (1981) 67-77.
[68] CJ Tabin, JW Hoffman, SP Goff, RA Weinberg, Adaptation of a retrovirus as a eukaryotic vector transmitting the herpes simplex virus thymidine kinase virus, Molecular Cell Biology 2 (1982) 426-436.
[69] Z Debyser, A short course on virology/vectorology/gene therapy, Current Gene Therapy 3 (2003) 495-499.
[70] P Mitchell, Vector problems still thwart gene-therapy promise, Lancet 351(9099) (1998) 346.
[71] W Guo, RL Lee, Receptor-targeted gene delivery via folate-conjugated polyethylenimine, American Association of Pharmaceutical Scientists: PharmSci 1(4) (1999).
[72] JL Thomas, DA Tirrell, Polyelectrolyte-sensitized phosholipid vesicles, Accounts of Chemical Research 25(8) (1992) 336-342.
[73] JL Thomas, SW Barton, DA Tirrell, Membrane solubilization by a hydrophobic polyelectrolyte: Surface activity and membrane binding, Biophysical Journal 67 (1994) 1101-1106.
[74] N Murthy, I Chang, PS Stayton, AS Hoffman, pH-Sensitive hemolysis by random copolymers of alkyl acrylates and acrylic acid, Macromolecular Symposia 172 (2001) 49-55.
[75] CY Cheung, N Murthy, PS Stayton, AS Hoffman, A pH-sensitive polymer that enhances cationic lipid-mediated gene transfer, Bioconjugate Chemistry 12 (2001) 906-910.

[76] TR Kyriakides, CY Cheung, N Murthy, P Bornstein, et al., pH-Sensitive polymers that enhance intracellular drug delivery *in vivo*, Journal of Controlled Release 78 (2001) 295-303.
[77] V Bulmus, M Woodward, L Lin, N Murthy, et al., A new pH-responsive and glutathione-reactive endosomal membrane-disruptive polymeric carrier for intracellular delivery of biomolecular drugs, Journal of Controlled Release 93 (2003) 105-120.
[78] MEH El-Sayed, AS Hoffman, PS Stayton, Rational design of composition and activity correlations for pH-sensitive and glutathione-reactive polymer therapeutics, Journal of Controlled Release 101 (2005) 47-58.
[79] H Ringsdorf, Structure and properties of pharmacologically active polymers, Journal of Polymer Science, Symposium 51 (1975) 135-153.
[80] N Murthy, J Campbell, N Fausto, AS Hoffman, et al., Design and synthesis of pH-responsive polymeric carriers that target uptake and enhance the intracellular delivery of oligonucleotides, Journal of Controlled Release 89 (2003) 365-374.
[81] RW Taft, MM Kreevoy, The evaluation of inductive and resonance effects on reactivity. I. Hydrolysis rates of acetals and non-conjugated aldehydes and ketones, Journal of the American Chemical Society 77 (1955) 5590-5595.
[82] UB Kompella, VHL Lee, in: V. Lee (Ed.), Peptide and protein drug delivery, Pharmacokinetics of peptide and protein drugs, Marcel Dekker, New York, 1991, pp. 391-484.
[83] R Rabkin, DC Dahl, in: K. Audus and T. Raub (Eds.), Biological barriers in protein delivery, Renal uptake and disposal of proteins and peptides, Plenum Press, New York, 1993, pp. 299-338.
[84] XH Zhou, Overcoming enzymatic and absorption barriers to non-parenterally administered protein and peptide drugs, Journal of Controlled Release 29 (1994) 239-252.
[85] PJ Dowding, B Vincent, E Williams, Preparation and swelling properties of poly(NIPAM) "minigel" particles prepared by inverse suspension polymerization, Journal of Colloid and Interface Science 221 (2000) 268-272.
[86] Z Hu, G Kimura, Y Ito, S Mawatari, et al., Technology to obtain sustained release characteristics of drugs after delivered to the colon, Journal of Drug Targeting 6(6) (1998) 439-448.
[87] H Venkatesh, NM Sanghavi, Controlled drug delivery of pH-dependent soluble drug-pindolol, Drug Development and Industrial Pharmacy 20(1) (1994) 111-118.
[88] BK Davis, Control of diabetes with polyacrylamide implants containing insulin, Experientia 28 (1972) 348.
[89] BK Davis, Diffusion in polymer gel implants, Proceedings of the National Academy of Sciences USA 71 (1974) 3120-3123.
[90] R Langer, J Folkman, Polymers for the sustained release of proteins and other macromolecules, Nature 263(797-800) (1976).
[91] MV Sefton, E Nishimura, Insulin permeability of hydrophilic polyacrylate membranes, Journal of Pharmaceutical Sciences 69 (1980) 208-209.
[92] A Serres, M Baudys, SW Kim, Temperature and pH-sensitive polymers for human calcitonin delivery, Pharmaceutical Reseasrch 13(2) (1996) 196-201.
[93] S Eaimtrakarn, Y Itoh, J Kishimoto, Y Yoshikawa, et al., Retention and transit of intestinal mucoadhesive films in rat small intestine, International Journal of Pharmaceutics 224 (2001) 61-67.

CHAPTER 8

DESIGN AND SYNTHESIS OF ENDOSOMOLYTIC CONJUGATED POLYASPARTAMIDE FOR CYTOSOLIC DRUG DELIVERY

Kwangwon Seo and Dukjoon Kim*

Department of Chemical Engineering, Sungkyunkwan University, 300 Chunchun-dong, Jangan-gu, Suwon, Kyungki-do, 440-746, Korea
E-mail: djkim@skku.edu

1. Introduction

As interest in intracellular delivery of macromolecular therapeutics such as plasmid DNA, oligonucleotides (ODNs), ribozymes, anticancer drugs, and immunotoxins have increased through development of biotechnology and nanotechnology, various drug carriers for efficient delivery have been extensively studied.[1-4] When the drug carriers are internalized into cells *via* specific (receptor-mediated) or non-specific (adsorptive) endocytosis, they are trafficked to the endosome and eventually degraded by acid-catalyzed lysosomal enzymes or recycled back to the plasma membrane; this intracellular pathway is shown in Figure 1. It was well known that the internal pH of the compartments decreases from 7.2 to 5.5 from endosome to lysosome. Therefore, it is required to release the drug into the cytosol after endosomal escape by membrane fusion or disruption using the acidic pH in the endosome to achieve an enhanced therapeutic effect.[5, 7]

A variety of endosomolyic polymers, especially pH-sensitive polymers, have been studied as intracellular drug delivery carriers for the past decades; representatively, they are: poly(ethylene imine)s (PEI)[8]; imidazole-related polymers[9]; poly(amidoamine)s and related polymers [10, 11]; poly[2-(dimethylaminoethyl) methacrylate (pDMAEMA)-based polymers[12] as cationic polymer systems and poly(acrylic acid) [13, 14] as anionic polymer systems. Nevertheless, these polymer carriers have some drawbacks regarding their drug delivery applications, such as difficult syntheses, toxicity, low transfection efficiency, and non-biodegradability. Though the mechanism of this membrane destabilization is poorly understood, it is triggered by a fall in pH following endocytic internalization of the polymer.

Poly(amino acid)s and their derivatives have become the focus of prospective biomaterials given their superior biocompatibility and biodegradability and low toxicity. Instead of synthesis by *N*-carboxyamino acid anhydride (NCA) polymerization, a convenient synthetic method can be applied by using poly(succinimide) (PSI) as an intermediate product for their preparation. PSI can be feasibly converted to hydrophilic biodegradable poly(amino acid) or poly(aspartamide)s such as poly(L-aspartic acid), poly(asparagine), and poly[(2-hydroxyethyl)aspartamide] by simple hydrolysis or aminolysis, to which various molecules can be conjugated since the succinimide ring in the PSI is readily reacted with primary amines. A variety of biodegradable poly(aspartamide)s have been studied for application as drug delivery carriers, especially after introducing a convenient synthesis of high molecular weight poly(succinimide) by acid-catalyzed polycondensation of L-aspartic acid [15]. In this chapter, synthesis and characteristics of poly(aspartamide), along with their derivatives and application as cytosolic drug delivery carriers, are discussed.

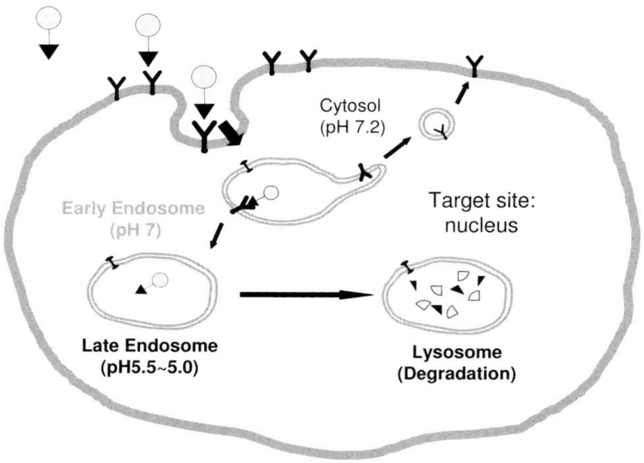

Fig. 1. The intracellular pathway of drug carrier after endocytosis.

2. Synthesis of Poly(aspartamide)s

For the rational design of synthetic poly(aspartamide)s, as drug carriers, the feasibility of their synthesis, subsequent conjugation with therapeutic compounds, and enzymatic degradability should be considered. The synthetic method of poly(aspartamide)s, by polymerization of NCA monomers can not only produce high molecular weight polymers but also control molecular weight, while it is very difficult due to several complicated reaction and purification steps for the synthesis.[16, 17] Another synthetic approach is by aminolysis of PSI, where PSI is prepared by acid-catalyzed polycondensation of L-aspartic acid and used as an intermediate material for the preparation of synthetic poly(aspartamide)s. Though high molecular weight PSI was conventionally prepared by polycondensation of L-aspartic acid in a large amount of phosphoric acid as the catalyst and solvent under reduced pressure, it is too difficult to remove considerable amount of phosphoric acid.[18] In 1997, a new synthesis was developed by polycondensation of L-aspartic acid using a catalytic amount of phosphoric acid in a mixed solvent of mesitylene and sulforane, where the

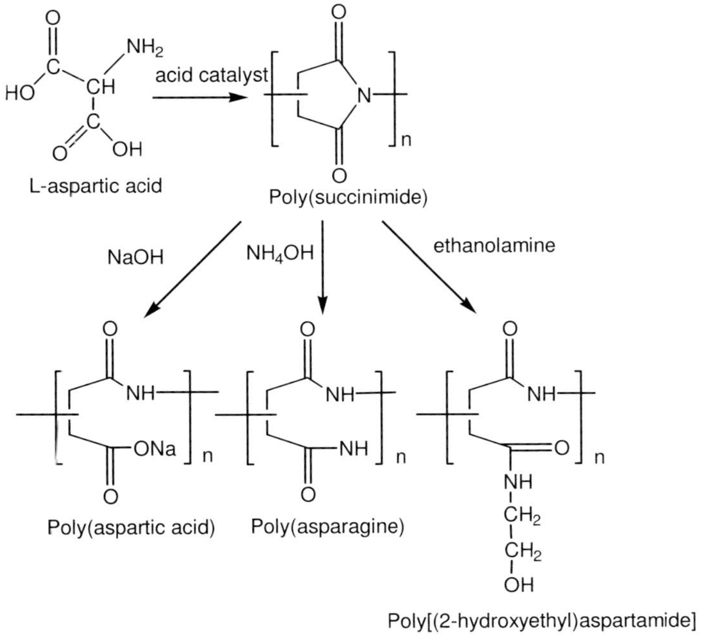

Fig. 2. Synthetic scheme of poly(aspartic acid), poly(asparagines), and poly[(2-mydroxyethyl)aspartamide] from L-aspartic acid.

molecular weight of PSI was 64,000 g/gmol.[15] As shown in Figure 2, PSI can be converted into poly(aspartic acid) (PASP) by alkali-hydrolysis and poly(asparagine) through simple aminolysis with ammonia, where the ratio of *α*-opening and *β*-opening was approximately 30:70 (Figure 3), indicating that the *β*-opening occurred predominantly over *α*-opening.

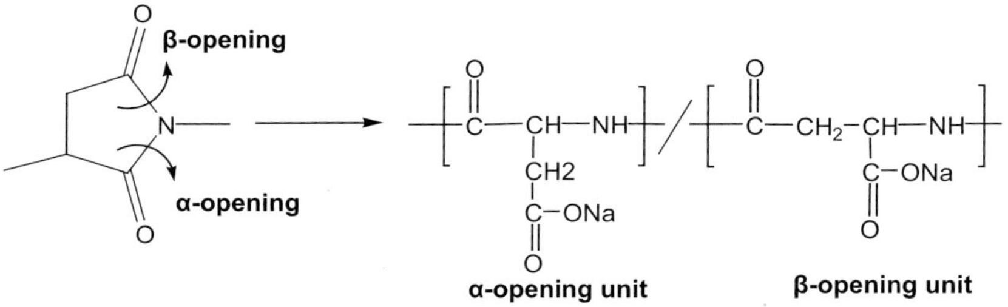

Fig. 3. α- and β- ring-opening of PSI.

α, β-poly(*N*-2-hydroxyethyl)-D, L-aspartamides (PHEA) is a synthetic water-soluble polymer investigated as a plasma expander.[18] This polymer was developed by aminolysis of PSI with excess ethanolamine (Figure 2) and has many advantages such as good biocompatibility, high water solubility, low cost for preparation, and feasible modification using the hydroxyl groups of PHEA for biomedical application.

3. Conjugation of Hydrophobic and Hydrophilic Macromers

PSI is susceptible to ring-opening graft reactions by aminolysis with nucleophiles since it is composed of a succinimide ring and conveniently converted into a conjugated-poly(aspartamide). In addition, a secondary reaction through the hydroxyl or carboxylic groups of PASP and PHEA can provide various poly(aspartamide) derivatives with specific functions. Figure 4 shows the successive graft reaction of PSI and many kinds of hydrophobic or hydrophilic molecules, ligands, drugs, and ionic groups containing primary amine group are allowed by aminolysis under conditions of low temperature using *N,N*-dimethylformamide (DMF) as the solvent.

In this ring-opening reaction, the reactivity increased with the nucleophilicity of amine functions and decreased with molecular weight of conjugated molecules. The amine function for conjugation was introduced into the polyaspartamide by the reaction with diamines such as ethylene diamine, hexamethylene diamine, and polyethylene glycol diamine; however, if the graft reaction goes beyond a certain time, the PSI will be cross-linked to form a gel. In PHEA, various ligands or molecules can be conjugated by an ester reaction of the hydroxyl groups with carboxy acid or acrylate.

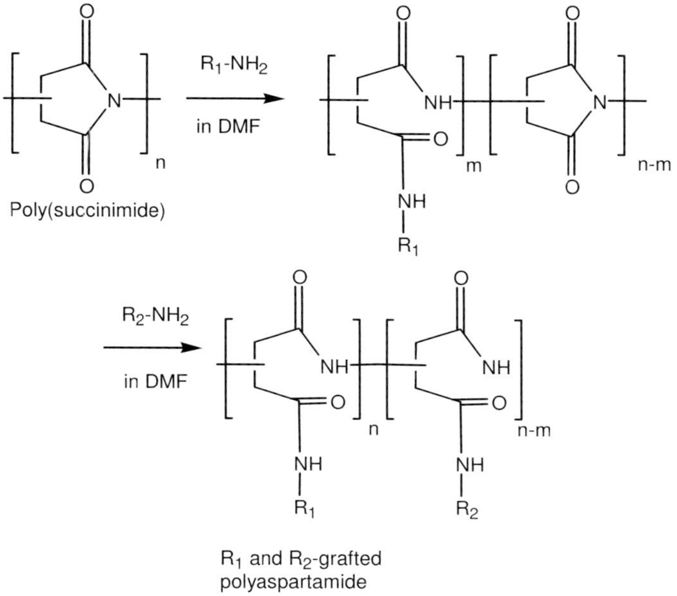

Fig. 4. Successive ring-opening reactions of PSI with R_1-NH_2 and R_2-NH_2.

Generally, the molecular weight of the graft copolymers is lower than that of the starting PSI, since the graft reaction of PSI with primary amine causes a partial hydrolysis of PSI chains as well as the aminolysis of succinimide rings.[19] The final molecular weight of the poly(aspartamide) graft copolymers is in the range of 25,000 ~ 55,000 g/gmol. Until now, various conjugated-polyaspartamide derivatives have been reported by the graft reaction of PSI with poly(caprolactone) (PCL), poly(L-lactic acid) (PLA), cholesterols, octaceylamine (C18), *O*-(2-aminoethyl)-*O*'-methylpolyethylene glycol (MPEG), ethyleneimide oligomer, spermine, glycidyltrimethylammonium chloride (GTA), 1-(3-aminopropryl)imidazole(API) for biomedical applications.

4. Self-aggregation

Amphiphilic polyaspartamides composed of hydrophobic and hydrophilic groups form nano-sized micellar aggregates, which have the structure of a hydrophobic inner core and a hydrophilic shell, by self-assembly in aqueous solutions. The driving force of aggregation is strong hydrophobic interactions with almost all polymer aggregates having microdomains over one another. Either primary small aggregates below 100 nm or secondary large aggregates over 100 nm can be formed by self-assembly of amphiphilic graft copolymers based on poly(aspartamide)s, given their stiff amide backbone structure, where the secondary aggregate formation is caused by a kinetically-controlled process.[20] Comb-type amphiphilic polymers with a flexible backbone favor primary

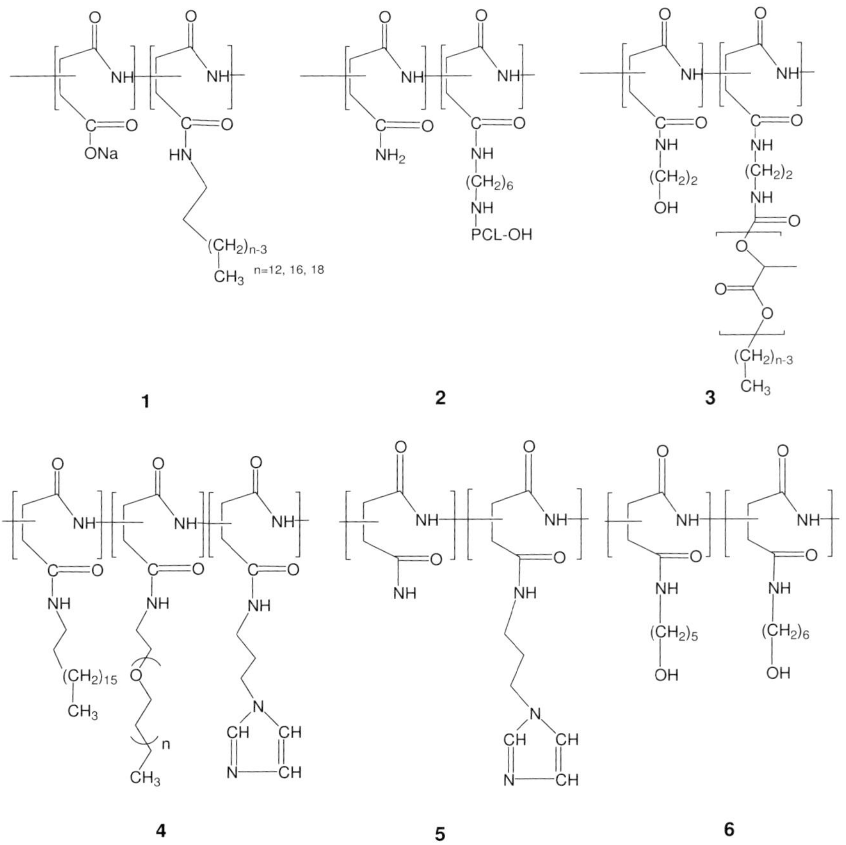

Fig. 5. Chemical structure of various amphiphilic polyaspartamides (1: akylchain-g-poly(aspartic acid); 2: PCL-g-poly(asparagine); 3: PLA-g-PHEA; 4: C18/MPEG/API-g-polyaspartamide; 5: API-g-poly(asparagine); 6: poly(*N*-subsituted α/β asparagines).

aggregate formation by the intramolecular interaction between neighboring hydrophobic side chains in the same backbone, whereas polymers with stiff backbones may be associated with secondary aggregation by the intermolecular interaction of surfaces between the polymers. The critical concentration to form self-aggregates is generally called "critical aggregation concentration (cac)". The shape and character of the self-aggregates by amphiphilic polyaspartamides is mainly affected by molecular weight and the T_g of the graft copolymers, length and degree of substitution (DS) of the hydrophobic or hydrophilic moiety, and their crystallinity. Various amphiphlic polyaspartamides, which can form nano-aggregates in aqueous solution, have been developed by aminolysis reaction of PSI with various hydrophobic molecules [20-26] and some of them are shown in Figure 5.

Self-aggregates of amphiphilic alkyl chain-grafted polyaspartic acids and polycaprolactone-grafted polyasparagines were prepared by Kim and coworkers.[20, 21] As shown in Figure 6, CAC decreased with increasing length or DS of the alkyl chains and PCL. Nano-aggregates of PCL-g-PASNs were formed by a precipitation and dialysis method. Their size decreased from 160 to 60 nm with more stable aggregates forming upon increase of the DS of PCL

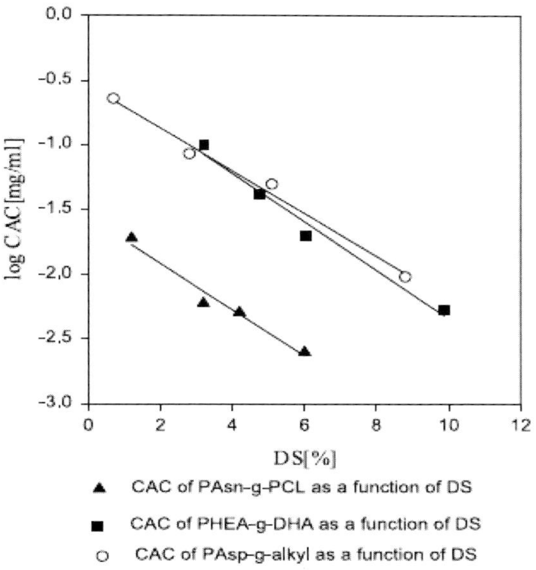

Fig. 6. CAC of polyaminoacids grafted with hydrophobic moieties determined by emission fluorescence of pyrene. (Jeong, J. H., et al., "Polymer Micelle-like Aggregates of Novel Amphiphilic Biodegradable Poly(asparagines) Grafted with Poly(caprolactone)", *Polymer,* Vol. 44, 2003, pp. 583-591. With permission).

from 1 to 5%. This is due to the reinforced interactions with PCL chains by an increase in hydrophobicity and crystallinity.

Kim and coworkers also prepared amphiphilic poly(2-hydroxyethyl)aspartamides (PHEA) by grafting lactic acid oligomers onto PHEA, which showed the transition from a micelle to vesicle structure with a DS of the lactic acid and formed nano-sized vesicles, nanosomes. [22] Our research group developed novel imidazole-containing polyaspartamides by successive graft reaction of MPEG and API on PSI. [23] Their aggregate size in aqueous solution decreased from 250 to 130 nm upon increasing the DS of the hydrophilic MPEG chains from 1.5 to 3.1%, as shown in Figure 7.

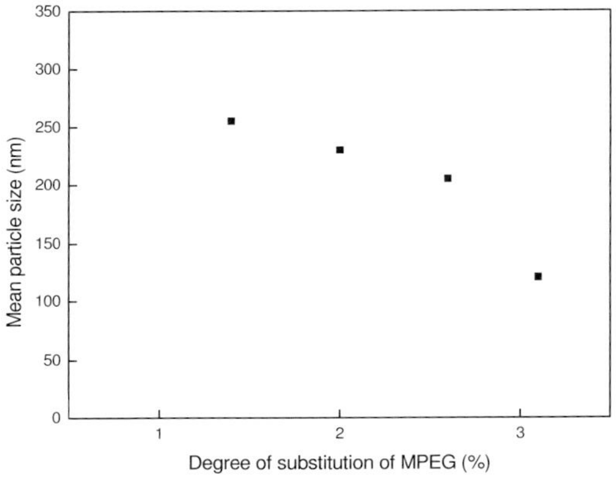

Fig. 7. Mean particle size of MPEG/API-g-polyaspartamide as a function of degree of substitution of MPEG.

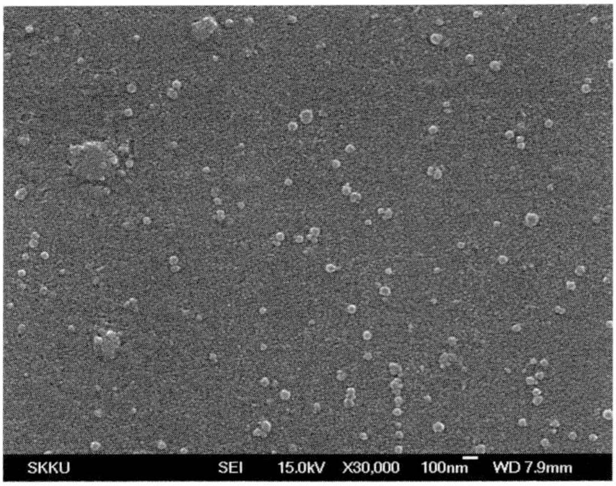

Fig. 8. SEM image of the C18/MPEG/API-grafted polyaspartamide.

Amphiphilic polyaspartamides grafted by C18, MPEG, and API were also prepared by us, which formed spherical nano-aggregates of 88 nm in phosphate buffered saline (PBS, Ph 7.4) and their SEM picture is shown in Figure 8. Conjugation of C18 chains reinforced the hydrophobic interaction between the long alkyl chains, and thus small size of aggregates below 100 nm could be formed by self-assembly.

5. Phase Transition Behaviors

The phase transition behavior of polyaspartamides centers around ionic or hydrophobic groups and their DS in the polymer chain. The pH of the phase transition is controlled by the pK_a and DS of the ionic groups grafted to the polymers. When the hydrophobic and hydrophilic balance is well defined, polyaspartamides could present lower critical solution temperatures (LCST) due to hydrogen bonding between amide groups in the polymer backbone and water molecules.

Novel polyaspartamides grafted with 1-(3-aminopropyl)imidazole, whose pK_a was 6.5, were prepared for drug delivery application by our research group. [27] As shown in Figure 9, they showed sharp pH-responsive phase transition

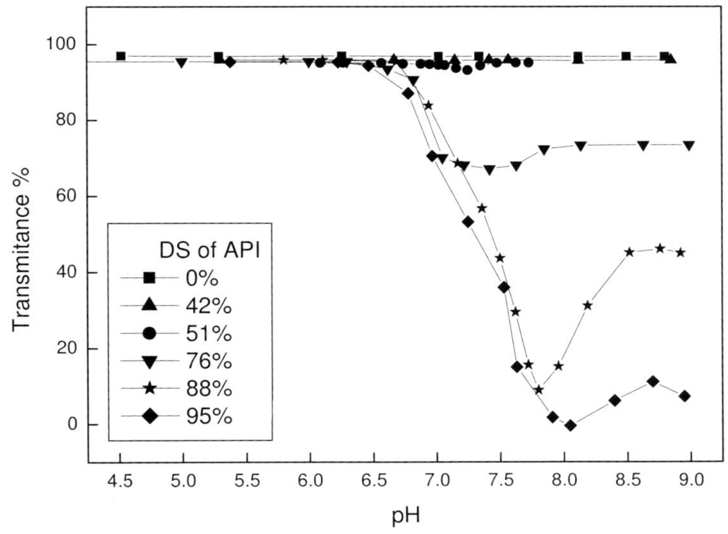

Fig. 9. Light transmittance of API-g-polyasparagine as a function of pH.

behavior between pH 6.4 and 6.8 with DS of API by protonation of imidazole groups, which was in the range of endosomal pH.

Thermoresponsive poly(α-*N*-substituted γ-glutamine)s and poly(*N*-substituted α/β-asparagine)s were developed by Kobayashi an coworkers by grafting 5-aminopentanol and 6-aminohexanol onto poly(γ-glutamic acid) and PSI. [28, 29] As shown in Figure 10, the LCST increased from 23 °C to 44 °C with the content of 5-aminopentanol increased from 50% to 80%. This sharp LCST of poly(amino acid) derivatives similar to poly(*N*-isopropylacrylamide) (PNIPAM) is caused by hydrogen bonding between the amide bond in polymer backbone and water molecules.

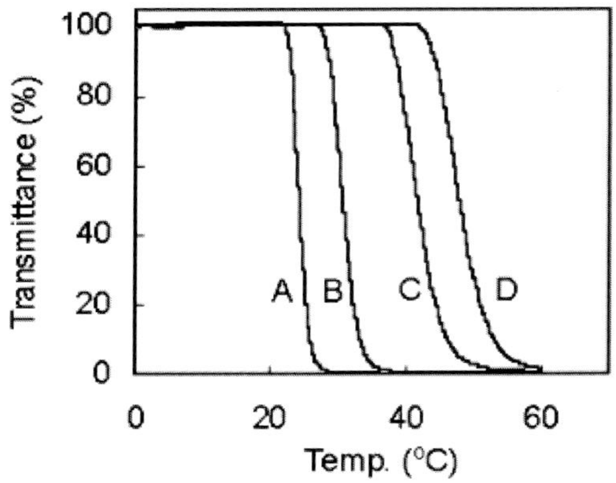

Fig. 10. Effect of temperature on light transmittance of 1 wt% aqueous solution of thermoresponsive poly(amino acid)s. The content of 5-5-aminopentanol is 50% (A), 60% (B), 70% (C), and 80% (D). (Tachibana, Y., et al., "Biodegradable Thermoresponsive Poly(amino acid)s", *Chem. Comm.*, 2003, 106-107. With permission).

6. pH-Sensitive Properties

A variety of pH-sensitive polymers have found wide applications in biomedical and pharmaceutical fields, as they enhance drug release responses to pH changes in the physiological environment such as the intestine, stomach, endosome, and tumor. A pH-sensitive polyaspartamide derivative can conveniently be prepared by grafting various cationic or anionic function groups to a polymer backbone. Among the many ionic functional groups, the imidazole group with a pK_a value of 6.0 ~ 6.5 has an electron lone pair on the unsaturated nitrogen, and is easily protonated in a slightly acidic environment. Thus, imidazole-containing pH-sensitive polymers have attracted a great deal of attention in intracellular drug delivery field due to their amphoteric, low-toxic, and ionic properties associated with such pH sensitivity.[30, 31] Recently, a series of novel pH-sensitive polyaspartamide derivatives with various DS of C18, MPEG and API were prepared by successive graft reactions of C18, MPEG, and API onto PSI and their pH-sensitive properties were investigated. They showed stable nano-aggregates in PBS 7.4 and their size changed according to pH. These behaviors were controlled by the DS of C18 and API. The polymers with a low DS of 8% formed nano-aggregates above pH 6.8, while they were completely dissociated at pH below 6.8. This aggregation behavior of C18/MPEG/API-g-polyaspartamides is reversible. As shown in Figure 11, polymers with a high DS of 15% formed stable nano-aggregates between pH 5 and pH 8. Their size slightly increased with decreasing pH as the hydrophobic interactions with the octadecyl chains were stronger than the repulsive interactions with the protonated imidazole groups under acidic pH in the polymer system with low DS of octadecylamine. This was contrary to the polymer system with a high DS of octadecylamine. These aggregation behaviors of pH-sensitive polyaspartamides should have a correlation with endosome lysis and drug release properties of polymers, controlled by the DS of the ionic and hydrophobic groups.

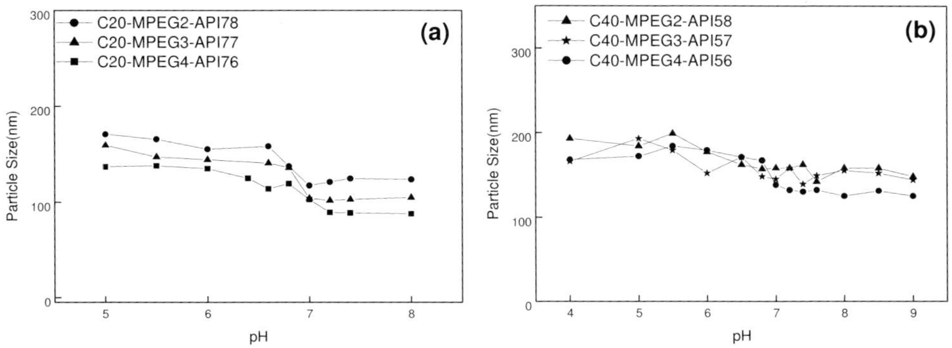

Fig. 11. Particle size changes of C18/MPEG/API-grafted polyaspartamides with (a) 15% and (b) 32% of DS of C18.

Histidine- and octadecylamine-conjugated poly(2-hydroxylethyl)aspartamides (PHEA-g-C18-His) were synthesized by Kim and coworkers via an ester linkage using *N*-Boc-L-histidine, followed by deprotection of Boc groups as an endosomolytic carrier for delivery of doxorubicin [32] and the chemical structure is shown in Figure 12. The doxorubicin release from these polymer aggregates was accelerated by decreasing the pH through ionization of the histidine groups, and the existence of histidines in the polymers enhanced the cytosolic delivery of doxorubicin by endosome lysis.

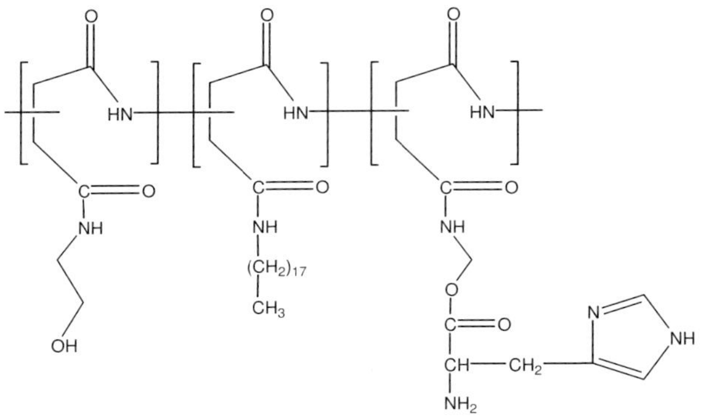

Fig. 12. Molecular structure of PHEA-g-C18-histidine.

7. Hemolytic and Agglutination Properties

The pH-dependent hemolysis property of polymers has some correlation with endosome lysis and would serve as a preliminary test to evaluate the endosomolytic ability of polymers [33, 34], though the hemolysis tests does not completely present the endosomolytic abilities of polymers. In our research group, two types of pH-sensitive endosomolytic polymers based on imidazole-g-polyaspartamides were prepared: MPEG and API-grafted polyaspartamide (MPEG/API-g-PASPAM); C18, MPEG, and API-grafted polyaspartamide

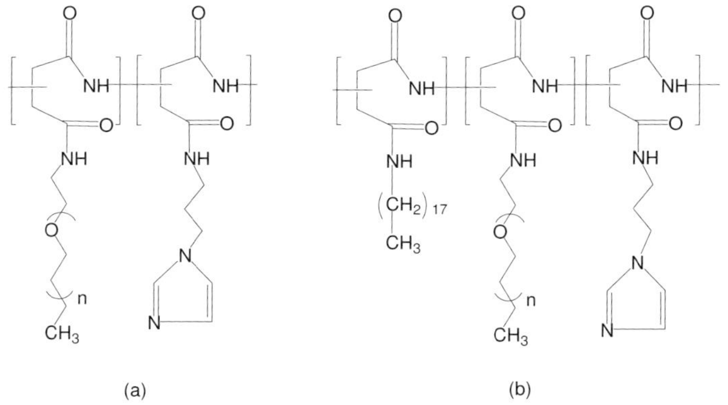

Fig. 13. Chemical structures of (a) MPEG/API-g-polyaspartamide and (b) C18/MPEG/API-g-polyaspartamide.

(C18/MPEG/API-g-PASPAM) and their hemolysis behavior were investigated to evaluate their ensodomolytic ability. The structures of the two polymers are shown in Figure 13 (a) and (b), respectively.

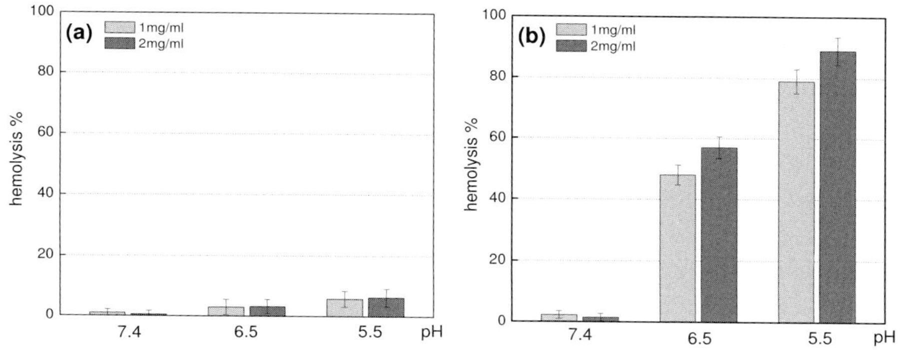

Fig. 14. Hemolysis by (a) MPEG/API-g-polyaspartamide and (b) C18/MPEG/API-g-polyaspartamide as a function of pH after 1 hour incubation with 2w/v% red blood cell suspension.

Figure 14 (a) and (b) shows the results of hemolysis by (a) MPEG/API-g-PASPAM and (b) C18/MPEG/API-g-PASPAM at various pHs. MPEG/API-g-PASPAM showed no hemolysis activity with pH, but the agglutination of red blood cells (RBCs) by polymers was observed and their agglutinate size increased with decreasing pH from 7.4 to 5.5, as shown in Figure 15 (a) and (b).

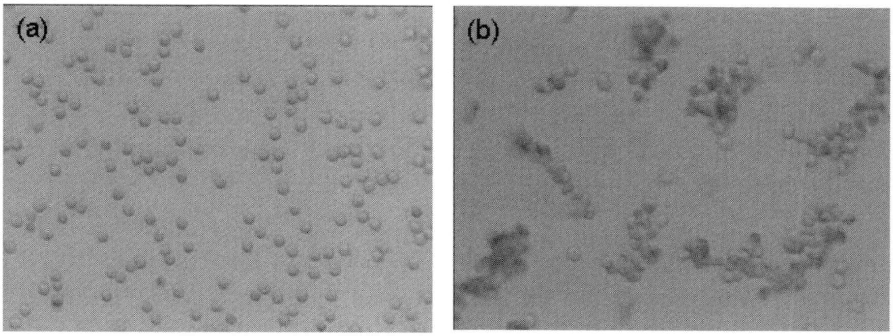

Fig. 15. Images of RBC suspensions after incubation for 30 min in the presence of MPEG3-API97 at (a) pH 7.4 and (b) pH 5.5.

This agglutination phenomenon occurs due to the interaction between negatively charged RBC membranes and positively charge polyaspartamides in acidic environments and is related to the unique properties of the polymeric system, since the cationic monomers do not agglutinate even at high concentrations. Erythrocytes are often agglutinated by surrounding polycations within minutes, even at very low concentrations. For C18/MPEG/API-g-PASPAM, no hemolysis occurred above pH 7, while they considerably lysed the red blood cells at pH 5.5. This result indicates that only the C18/MPEG/API-g-PASPAM, composed of both imidazole and C18 groups, can cause hemolysis in API-containing systems. This is because the hydrophobic interaction between the lipid core and C18 chain played a critical role in membrane fusion, after polymer binding to the outer shell, by electrostatic interactions between the positively-charged imidazole groups and negatively-charged lipid bilayers. This membrane lysis involved two steps: linkage of positively-charged polymers with the negatively-charged membrane; penetration and rupturing of lipid cores by hydrophobic interactions.

The blood compatibility is one of the most important properties of drug delivery carriers, as the blood is the first biological environment they encounter after intravenous administration. Both poly(aspartamide) systems did not cause any hemolysis or agglutination at normal pHs, indicating that polyaspartamides have good blood compatibility under physiological conditions.

8. Endosomal Escape and Cytosolic Delivery of Therapeutic Agents

As mentioned in the introduction, one of the most significant barriers for cytosolic delivery of therapeutics that work inside the cell is the endosomal barrier. For therapeutics such as plasmid DNA, anticancer drugs, oligonucleotides (ODNs), ribozymes, and immunotoxins, their ability to reach their intracellular target depends on their ability to escape the endosome and into the cytoplasm.[35-37]

Polycations that have considerable secondary or tertiary amines can provide buffering effect in an endo/lysosomal pH range and destabilize the endosome by "proton sponge" effect. The so-called "proton sponge" hypothesis was first reported by Behr and coworkers [38] and the mechanism is shown in Figure 16.

After macromolecules are trafficked to the endosome *via* endocytosis, the endosomal compartmen is acidified through the activity of the membrane-bound V-ATPase proton pumps. Once cationic polymers bearing unprotonated amino groups are present in the endosome, they absorb protons that are pumped and buffer the internal pH of the endosome. Due to repulsion between the protonated amine groups, the polymer swells and an influx of Cl^- counterions occurs in order to maintain electroneutrality. The influx of protons and Cl^- ions increases the osmolarity inside the endosome, which eventually induce abrupt swelling and rupture of the endosome.

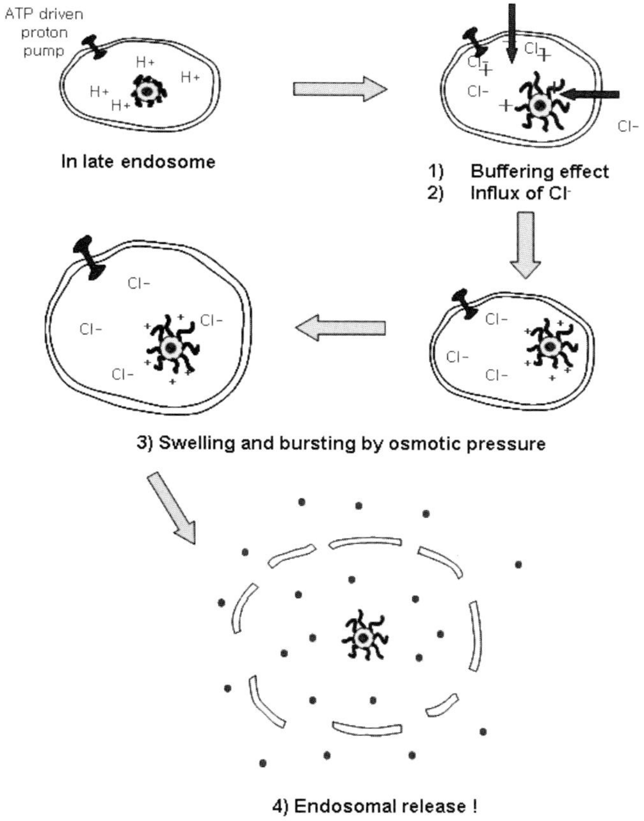

Fig. 16. Proton sponge mechanism of cationic polymers in endosome.

Recently, cationic polymers such as histidylated chitosan, histidylated poly(lysine), polyhistidine-based polymers, poly(4-vinylimidazole), and imidazole-containing polymers have shown considerable promise as nonviral vectors for DNA delivery, given their endosomolytic ability by imidazole groups.[39-44] The first use of histidine-containing polymers for DNA delivery was reported in 1998 by Midoux and coworkers [45]. Histidine-rich peptide (H5WYG) is a variant of the HA-2 subunit of the influenza virus hemaglutin, designed by substituting lysine with histidyl residues. This histidine-rich peptide did not disrupt the membrane at neutral pH, but showed a powerful membrane disruption ability at pH 6.4.

The cationic polyaspartamides conjugated with plenty of bufferable amine groups such as histidine, imidazole, and spermine are promising candidates for cytosolic drug delivery by endosome destabilization due to their convenient conjugation of various molecules and branched structure as well as biocompatibility and biodegradability. Our research group has designed endosomolytic polyaspartamides grafted with C18, MPEG, and API, with superior pH-dependent membrane fusion properties (9.7). Zhuo and coworkers prepared polyaspartamide-based, oligo-ethyleneimine brushes (PASP-EDA, PASP-TEPAm PASP-PEHA, and PASP-PEI423) from PSI *via* a ring-opening reaction with *N*-Boc-protected ethyleneimine, tetraethylenepentamine, pentaethylenehexamine, and linear polyethyleneimine for DNA delivery, respectively, [46] and their structures are shown in Figure 17.

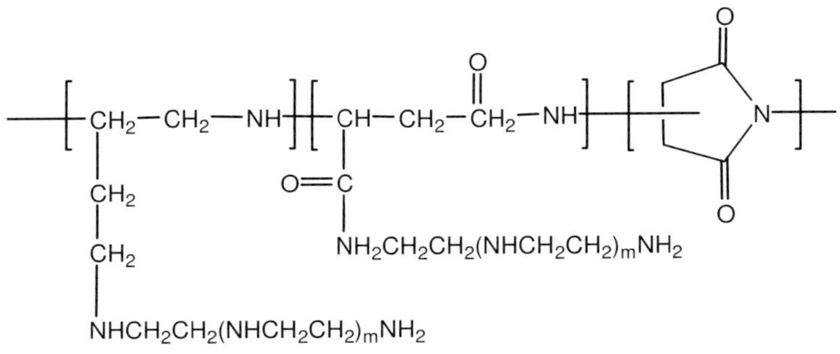

PASP-TEPA: m=3
PASP-PEHA: m=4
PASP-PEI 423:m=9

Fig. 17. Chemical structure of polyaspartamide-based oligo-ethyleneimine brushes.

These polymers possessed high buffer capacity and condensed plasmid DNA to small sized polymer/DNA complexes in the range of 160-400 nm. As shown in Figure 18, the transfection efficiencies of polycation/DNA complexes in HEK 293 cells are greatly dependent on the structure of the polymer side chains. PASP-EDA/pRE Luc and PASP-TEPA/pRE Luc complexes showed very low luciferase expression in HEK 293 cells at various *N*/*P* ratios, while the luciferase expression in HEK 293 cells by PASP-PEHA/pRE Luc and PASP-PEI 423/pRE Luc complexes at various *N*/*P* ratios was as high as that of branched PEI 25000 when *N*/*P* ratio was 10:1.

Giammona and coworkers prepared PHEA-spermine (PHEA-Spm) and PHEA-spermine-butyramide (PHEA-Spm-C4) by subsequent reaction of the hydroxyl groups in the polymeric side chains with spermine.[47] These protonable copolymers having polyaspartamide backbone can form complexes with plasmid DNA even at low polycation/DNA weight ratios ranging from 0.75/1 to 2/1. The size of the polycation/DNA complexes decreased with increasing polycation/DNA weight ratio, until nano-sized dimensions were reached. They also indicated higher transfection efficiency than PEI in luciferase transfection assay with both cell lines tested at C/P ratio of 10. However partial hydrophobization of PHEA-Spm with C4 portion did not increase transfection efficiency, although DNA interaction with polymers was strengthened to give smaller polyplex sizes. The high transfection efficiency of these highly bufferable polymers demonstrates that polyplexes can efficiently escape endosome by the proton sponge mechanism as described for PEI.

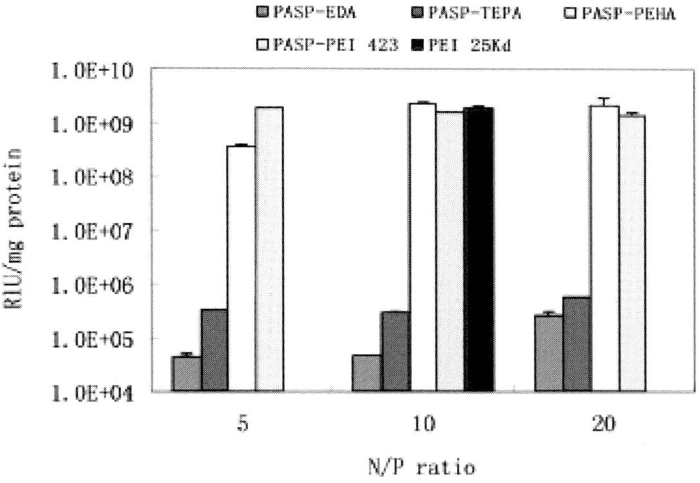

Fig. 18. Transfection efficiencies of polyaspartamide-based oligoethyleneimine brushes/pRE Luc complexes in HEK293 cells. Branched PEI (M.W. 25000) was used as a control. Data represent the mean and standard deviation (n=2). (Zhang, M., et al., "Polyaspartamide-Based Oligo-ethylenimine Brushes with High Buffer Capacity and Low Cytotoxicity for Highly Efficient Gene Delivery", *Bioconjug. Chem.*, Vol. 20, No. 3, 2009, pp. 440-446. With permission).

9. Biocompatibility

The biocompatibility of polymeric drug carriers is a critical factor for biomedical applications. Many polymer systems such as PEI, poly-L-lysine, and poly(amido amide) have difficulties such as cytotoxicity of the cationic polymers derived from the charge density, non-biodegradability, and elimination by the reticuloendothelial system or other organs when introduced into the blood stream.

Polypeptides and related artificial poly(amino acid)s are well-known to be biodegradable and biocompatible.[48] Because polyaspartamides having main chains composed of peptide links (amide bonds) are synthetic poly(amino acid) derivatives, they can undergo biodegradation by enzymes, being broken into amino acids essential to the body. Generally, polyaspartamides by themselves are not cytotoxic to many types of cells [25, 32] and that polyaspartamide-based oligo-ethylenimine brushes and spermine-g-PHEA showed much lower toxicity than PEI [46, 47].

10. Summary

Poly(aspartamides), which are derivatives of poly(amino acids), have received considerable attention due to their superior biocompatibility and biodegradability for biomedical and pharmaceutical applications. Because there is a convenient method to prepare poly(aspartamide)s by using PSI as an intermediate, various functional molecules can be conjugated to poly(aspartamide)s by a simple aminolysis reaction. A variety of amphiphilic polyaspartamides have been prepared by introducing hydrophobic moieties such as PCL, PLA, and alkylamines into hydrophilic polyaspartamides to form stable nano-aggregates with low CAC in aqueous media. Moreover, imidazole-containing polyaspartamides show pH-dependant phase transitions and size changes while thermosensitive polyaspartamides show LCST similar to PNIPAM. The structures and properties of these polymers are significantly affected by the DS and molecular weight of the functional molecules in the side chains. Especially, endosomolytic, imidazole-containing polyaspartamides have been developed and showed to have pH-dependent membrane fusion properties and enhanced cytosolic delivery. Cationic polyaspartamides designed for DNA delivery present superior DNA compression properties and transfection efficiencies higher than PEI. In addition, most of the polyaspartamide derivatives are non-toxic and biocompatible. Based on these properties, endosomolytic polyaspartamides have many advantages as carriers for intracellular therapeutic delivery and will be the focus of further research.

References

[1] Drummond, D. C., Zignani, M., and Leroux, J. C., "Current Status of pH-Sensitive Liposome in Drug Delivery", *Progress in Lipid Research*, Vol. 39, 2000, pp. 409-460.
[2] Panyam, J. and Labhasetwar, V., "Biodegradable Nanoparticles for Drug and Gene Delivery to Cells and Tissue", *Adv. Drug Deliv. Rev.*, Vol. 55, 2003, pp. 329-347.
[3] Zuber, G., et al., "Towards Synthetic Viruses", *Adv. Drug Deliv. Rev.*, Vol. 52, 2001, pp. 245-253.
[4] Nishiyama, N. and Kataoka, Kazunori, "Current State, Achievements, and Future Prospects of Polymeric Micelles as Nanocarriers for Drug and Gene Delivery", *Pharmacol. Ther.*, Vol. 112, 2006, pp. 630-648.
[5] Sheff, D., "Endosomes as a Route for Drug Delivery in the Real World", *Adv. Drug Deliv. Rev.*, Vol. 56, 2004, pp. 927-930.
[6] Watson, P., Jones, A. T., and Stephens, D. J., "Intracellular Trafficking Pathways and Drug Delivery: Fluorescence Imaging of Iiving and Fixed cells", *Adv. Drug Deliv. Rev.*, Vol. 57, 2001, pp. 43-61.
[7] Lechardeur, D., Verkman, A. S., and Lukacs, G. L., "Intracellular Routing of Plasmid DNA During Non-viral Gene Transfer", *Adv. Drug Deliv. Rev.*, Vol. 57, 2005, pp. 755-767.
[8] Godbey, W. T., Wu, K. K., and Mikos, A. G., "Poly(ethylenimine) and Its Role in Gene Delivery", *J. Control. Rel.*, Vol. 60, 1999, pp. 149-160.
[9] Pichon, C., Goncalves, C., and Midoux, P., "Histidine-rich Peptides and Polymers for Nucleic Acids Delivery", *Adv. Drug Deliv. Rev.*, Vol. 53, 2001, 75-94.
[10] Ferruti, P., et al., "Amphoteric Linear Poly(amido-amine)s as Endosomolytic Polymers: Correlation Between Physicochemical and Biological Properties", *Macromolecules*, Vol. 33, 2000, pp. 7793-7800.
[11] Ferruti, P., Marchisio, M. A., and Duncan, R., "Poly(anido-amine)s: Biomedical Applications", *Macrol. Rapid Commun.*, Vol. 23, 2003, pp. 332-355.
[12] Zuidam, N. J., et al., "Effects of Physicochemical Characteristics of Poly [2-(dimethylamino)ethyl methacrylate]-based Polyplexes on Cellular Association and Internalization", *J. Drug. Target.*, Vol. 8, 2000, pp. 51-66.
[13] Murthy, N., et al., "The Design and Synthesis of Polymers for Eukaryotic Membrane Disruption", *J. Control. Rel.*, Vol. 61, 1999, pp. 137-143.
[14] Bulmus, V., et al., "A New pH-responsive and Glutathione-reactive, Endosomal Membrane-disruptive Polymeric Carrier for Intracellular Delivery of Biomolecular Drugs", *J. Control. Rel.*, Vol. 93, 2003, pp. 105-120.
[15] Tomida, M. and Nakato, T., "Convenient Synthesis of High Molecular Weight Poly(succinimide) by Acid-catalysed Polycondensation of L-Aspartic Acid", *Polymer*, Vol. 38, 1997, pp. 4733-4736.
[16] Cha, J .N., et al., "Biomimetic Synthesis of Ordered of Silica Structures Mediated by Block Copolypeptides", *Nature*, Vol. 403, 2000, pp. 289–292.
[17] Poland, D. and Scheraga, H.A., *Theory of Noncovalent Structure in Polyamino acids, in: Poly- α -amino acids*, Marcel Dekker, NY, 1967, pp. 391–398.
[18] Neri, P., et al., "Synthesis of *α, β*-Poly(*N*-2-hydroxyethyl)-D, L-aspartamides, A New Plasma Expander", *J. Med. Chem.*, Vol. 16, 1973, pp. 893-897.
[19] Mendichi, R., et al., "Molecular Characterization of *α, β*-Poly(*N*-2-hydroxyethyl)-D, L-aspartamide Derivatives as Potential Self-assembling Copolymers Forming Polymeric Micelles", *Polymer*, Vol. 44, 2003, pp. 4871-4879.

[20] H. S. Kang, et al., "Effects of Grafted Alkyl Groups on Aggregation Behavior of Amphiphilic Poly(aspartic acid)", *Langmuir*, Vol. 17, 2001, pp. 7501-7506.
[21] Jeong, J. H., et al., "Polymer Micelle-like Aggregates of Novel Amphiphilic Biodegradable Poly(asparagines) Grafted with Poly(caprolactone)", *Polymer,* Vol. 44, 2003, pp. 583-591.
[22] Lee, H. J., et. al., "Biodegradable Polymersomes from Poly(2-hydroxyethyl aspartamide) Grafted with Lactic Acid Oligomers in Aqueous Solution", *Macromolecules*, Vol. 39, 2006, pp. 4938-4940.
[23] Seo, K. and Kim, D., "pH-Dependent Self-assembling Behavior of Imidazole-containing Polyaspartamide Derivatives", *J. Biomed. Mater. Res. A*, early view in online.
[24] Caliceti, P., et al. "Synthesis and Biopharmaceutical Characterisation of New Poly(hydroxyethylaspartamide) Copolymers as Drug Carriers", *Biochimica et Biophysica Acta*, Vol. 1528, 2001, pp. 177-186.
[25] Cavallaro, G., et al. "Poly(hydroxyehylaspartamide) Derivatives as Colloidal Drug Carrier Systems", *J. Control. Rel.*, Vol. 89, 2003, pp. 285-295.
[26] M. Suwa, et al., "Self-Association Behavior of Hydrophobically Modified Poly(aspartic acid) in Water Studied by Fluorescence and Dynamic Light Scattering Techniques", *Macromolecules*, Vol. 33, 2000, pp. 7884-7892.
[27] Seo, K. and Kim, D. "Phase Transition Behavior of Novel pH-Sensitive Polyaspartamide Derivatives Grafted with 1-(3-Aminopropyl)imidazole", *Macromol. Biosci.*, Vol. 6, 2006, pp. 758-766.
[28] Tachibana, Y., et al., "Biodegradable Thermoresponsive Poly(amino acid)s", *Chem. Comm.*, 2003, 106-107.
[29] Tachibana, Y., et al., "Thermo- and pH-Responsive Biodegradable Poly(α-N-Substituted γ-Glutamine)s", *Biomacromolecules*, Vol. 4, 2003, pp. 1132-1134.
[30] Lee, E. S., et al., "Poly(L-histidine)–PEG Block Copolymer Micelles and pH-Induced Destabilization", *J. Controll. Rel.*, Vol. 90, 2003, pp. 363-374.
[31] Lee, E. S., Na, K., and Bae, Y. H., "Super pH-Sensitive Multifunctional Polymeric Micelle", *Nano letters*, Vol. 5, 2005, pp. 325-329.
[32] Yang, S. R., Lee, H. J., and Kim, J. –D., "Histidine-conjugated Poly(amino acid) Derivatives for The Novel Endosomolytic Delivery Carrier of Doxorubicin", *J. Control. Rel.*, Vol. 114, 2006, pp. 60-68.
[33] Plank, C., et al., "The Influence of Endosome-disruptive Peptides on Gene Transfer Using Synthetic Virus like Gene Transfer System", *J. Biol. Chem.*, Vol. 269, No. 17, 1994, pp. 12918-12924.
[34] Bulmus, V., et al., "A New pH-Responsive and Glutathione-reactive, Endosomal Membrane-disruptive Polymeric Carrier for Intracellular Delivery of Biomolecular Drug", *J. Controll. Rel.*, Vol. 93, 2003, pp. 105-120.
[35] Zauner, W., Ogris, M., and Wagner, E., "Polylysine-based Transfection Systems Utilizing Receptor-mediated Delivery", Adv. Drug Deliv. Rev., Vol. 30, 1998, 97-113.
[36] Han, S.-O., et al., "Development of Biomaterials for Gene Therapy", *Molecular Therapy*, Vol. 2, 2000, pp. 302-317.
[37] Godbey, W. T., et al., "Poly(ethylenimine)-mediated Transfection: A New Paradigm for Gene Delivery", J. Biomed. Mater. Res., Vol. 51, 2000, pp. 321-328.
[38] Behr, J. –P., "The Proton Sponge: A Trick to Enter Cells the Viruses Did Not Exploit, *Chimia*, Vol. 51, 1997, pp. 34-36.
[39] Midoux, P. and Monsigny, M., "Efficient Gene Transfer by Histidylated Polylysine/pDNA Complexes", *Bioconjuate Chem.*, Vol. 10, 1999, pp. 406-411.

[40] Park, J. S., et al., "*N*-Acetyl Histidine-Conjugated Glycol Chitosan Self-assembled Nanoparticles for Intracytoplasmic Delivery of Drugs: Endocytosis, Exocytosis and Drug Release", *J. Control. Rel.*, Vol. 115, 2006, pp. 37-45.

[41] Park, T. G., Jeong, J. H., and Kim, S. W., "Current Status of Polymeric Gene Delivery Systems", *Adv. Drug Deliv. Rev.*, Vol. 58, 2006, pp. 467-486.

[42] Yang, Y., et al., "Poly(imidazole/DMAEA)phosphazene/DNA self-assembled nanoparticles for gene delivery: Synthesis and in vitro transfection", *J. Control. Rel.*, Vol. 127, 2008, pp. 273-279.

[43] Putnam, et al., "Polyhistidine-PEG:DNA nanocomposites for gene delivery", *Biomaterials*, Vol. 24, 2003, pp. 4425-4433.

[44] Ihm, J. E., et al., "High Transfection Efficiency of Poly(4-vinylimidazole) as A New Gene Carrier", *Bioconjug. Chem.*, Vol. 14, 2003, pp. 707-708.

[45] Midoux, P., et al., "Membrane Permeabilization and Efficient Gene Transfer by A Peptide Containing Several Histidines", *Bioconjugate Chem.*, Vol. 9, 1998, pp. 260-267.

[46] Zhang, M., et al., "Polyaspartamide-Based Oligo-ethylenimine Brushes with High Buffer Capacity and Low Cytotoxicity for Highly Efficient Gene Delivery", *Bioconjug. Chem.*, Vol. 20, No. 3, 2009, pp. 440-446.

[47] Cavallaro, G., et al., "Polyhydroxyethylaspartamide-spermine Copolymers: Efficient Vectors for Gene Delivery", *J. Control. Rel.*, Vol. 131, 2008, pp. 54–63.

[48] Naira, L. S. and Laurencin, C. T., "Biodegradable Polymers as Biomaterials", *Prog. Polym. Sci.*, Vol. 32, 2007, pp. 762–798.

CHAPTER 9

ENGINEERING OF CELL-PENETRATING PEPTIDE-CONJUGATED INTRACELLULAR DELIVERY SYSTEMS

Rupa R. Sawant and Vladimir P. Torchilin*

Department of Pharmaceutical Sciences and Center for Pharmaceutical Biotechnology and Nanomedicine, Northeastern University, Boston, MA 02115, USA

**E-mail: v.torchilin@neu.edu*

1. Introduction

Direct intracellular delivery of peptides and proteins, oligonucleotides and their derivatives, nanoparticles, such as liposomes, micelles and quantum dots, synthetic polymers, and other macromolecules and nanoparticles was difficult with pre-existing methodologies until the discovery of cell-penetrating peptides (CPPs). Many drugs should be delivered inside the cytoplasm or onto individual organelles, such as nuclei (target for gene and antisense therapy), lysososmes (target for the delivery of deficient lysosomal enzymes), and mitochondria (target for pro-apoptotic anticancer drugs) to exert their therapeutic action. After uptake, the drug/drug-loaded nanocarriers are challenged by acidic pH of endosomes/ lysosomes, the lysosomal enzymes and even they escape from endosomal/ lysosomal degradation, they should be stable in cytosol. It has been proven that CPPs are able to vehiculate variety of cargoes across the plasma membrane and deliver the payload intracellularly; the process termed as "protein transduction" [1, 2]. Protein transduction domains (PTDs) or CPPs include relatively short (up to approx. 20 residues) peptides that are rich in basic amino acids residues and bear a net positive charge at physiological pH.

CPPs can be divided into three classes: protein-derived peptides, model peptides, and designed peptides [3, 4]. Protein-derived peptides are the short stretches of the protein domain that are primarily responsible for the translocation ability, also called as PTDs, examples are TAT peptide (TATp) (48–60) derived from 86-mer Tat protein [5], penetratin_(43–58) derived from homeodomain of *Drosophilia* Antennapedia [6], pVEC derived from murine vascular endothelial cadherin [7] and signal sequence-based peptides or membrane translocating sequences (MTSs) [8]. Model peptides are CPPs that mimic the translocation properties of known CPPs; example is the model amphipathic peptide (MAP) [9]. Designed CPPs encompass the chimeric peptides that are produced by the fusion of hydrophilic and hydrophobic domains from different sources; examples are transportan, fusion of galanin and mastoparan [10]; and MPG, chimera of peptide from fusion sequence of HIV-1 gp41 protein and peptide from the nuclear localization sequence of SV40 T-antigen [11]. In addition, synthetic peptides such as polyarginines also show potential for translocation [12]. All the CPPs are highly positively charged, contributed by basic residues lysine or arginine; lysine is the primary contributor in transportan and MAP, while arginine contributes in TAT peptide, penetratin and pVEC. In terms of the cellular uptake and cargo delivery kinetics, MAP has the fastest uptake, followed by transportan, TATp (48–60), and penetratin. Similarly, MAP has the highest cargo delivery efficiency, followed by transportan, TATp (48–60), and penetratin.

TATp, the most frequently used CPP, is derived from the transcriptional activator protein encoded by human immunodeficiency virus type 1 (HIV-1) [13]. Green [14] and Frankel [15] demonstrated that the 86-mer trans-activating transcriptional activator, Tat, protein encoded by HIV-1, was efficiently internalized by cells *in vitro* when introduced in the surrounding media. Later it was shown that residues 49–57 were responsible for membrane translocation, with the positive charge contributing largely to transduction ability of TAT [16]. These CPPs have opened a new path in drug delivery, allowing the translocation of various cargo molecules into cells.

The mechanism of cellular translocation of CPPs is still subject to controversial discussion and in some cases, the mechanism is cell-type or cargo specific. Earlier it was concluded that CPPs enter cells very rapidly within minutes even at 4°C and thus involves energy-independent mechanism [5, 11, 17, 18]. This work relied on fluorescence imaging or flow cytometry analysis of chemically fixed cells. Then it was pointed out that certain fixation procedures may cause artifacts leading to an overestimation of cellular uptake [19, 20]. Richard et al. demonstrated that the distribution pattern of TAT (48–60) and R9 as well as their conjugates was different in living versus fixed cells [21]. It can be concluded that CPPs can enter the cells by two distinct routes: energy-dependent vesicular mechanisms, referred to as endocytosis, or via a direct process involving translocation of the lipid bilayer. Clathrin-mediated endocytosis was suggested in [22] where TATp showed co-localization with the classical endocytic marker, transferring. This was substantiated further in [23], where TAT PTD and Antp PTD showed uptake only at 37°C. Studies also suggested that the PTDs do not provoke a "real translocation" but are only responsible for cell-surface adherence, which subsequently results in their endocytosis and accumulation in endosomes [24]. In fact, direct electrostatic interaction between the positive residues of CPPs and the negative residues of the cell-surface proteoglycans or glycosaminoglycans (such as heparin sulfate, heparin) is required in internalization, regardless of the mechanism of cellular uptake [23, 25-27]. Another proposed mechanism for internalization is the clathrin, caveolae-independent endocytosis. This type of uptake was suggested in [12, 28]. Unlike the rapid uptake of transferrin, a marker for clathrin-mediated endocytosis, the internalization of TAT-cargo was very slow, reaching the plateau after several hours, with co-localization of TATp with the markers of caveolar uptake. The cellular uptake was affected in the presence of drugs that either disrupt lipid rafts or alter caveolar trafficking. Another mechanism proposed for CPP-conjugated to large cargoes (MW>30,000 Da) is macropinocytosis [29-31]. Recent studies have shown that increasing the peptide concentration (HIV-TAT and R8/9) above a certain threshold results in extensive cytosolic labeling that is unlikely to be attributable to any form of endocytosis [32, 33]. It has been also shown that a single CPP can simultaneously exploit multiple modes of uptake to enter cells [32, 34, 35]. Recently, this issue was explored in depth for cationic CPPs; in these detailed study it was found that penetratin equally exploits macropinocytosis, clathrin-mediated endocytosis, and caveolae/lipid-raft-mediated endocytosis to enter HeLa cells [32]. Yang, et al. reported successful translocation of poly(2-hydroxytethyl aspartamide) (PHEA) in both fixed and unfixed HeLa cells, when oligoarginine (Arg(8)) known as one of the CPPs was conjugated via a thioether linkage. It was suggested that an endocytosis was a key mechanism. The fluorescence spectra of PHEA-Arg(8) in liposome solutions showed that PHEA-Arg(8) was collectively adsorbed in the negative liposome membrane due to the high cationic property of a conjugated Arg(8), representing that a surface adsorption was a first step in the internalization of PHEA-Arg(8). The membrane leakage activity of PHEA-Arg(8) was much lower than that of Arg(8) own, meaning that PHEA-Arg(8) does not effectively disrupt the cell membrane integrity. It was also suggested that PHEA-Arg(8) could be internalized by an adsorptive-endocytosis [36].

In all cases, after the endocytic uptake, the internalized CPPs either alone or linked to cargoes should escape from the endocytic vesicles to the cytosol to avoid the lysosomal degradation. Escape from the endocytic vesicles is believed to be the most important step in the efficient intracellular delivery of functional macromolecules. Several studies have shown that CPPs linked to quantum dots [37], oligonucleotides [38], pDNA [39], peptides [34, 40] or proteins [41] remain trapped in endocytic vesicles after uptake, unless an endosomal escape device is included in the system. A variety of tools to enhance the endosomal escape of CPP-attached cargoes are reported in literature such as use of fusogenic lipids [42-44], membrane disruptive peptides [30, 45-47] and polymers [48, 49], and lysomotropic agents [30, 50, 51]. CPPs can also cross the membrane bilayer directly in an energy independent process [10, 52].

Thus, CPP may use different pathways to cross the cell membrane and the type of CPP and cargo attached play an important role in selecting translocation pathway. Also once internalized, efficient endosomal escape has to take place so as to allow the cargo to reach its sub cellular target. This review focuses on the use of CPPs, in particular TATp, for the intracellular delivery of variety of cargos.

2. CPP-modified Delivery Systems

The interest in CPP-modified systems is mainly due to variety of cargoes that can be transported by CPPs (such as small molecules, peptides and proteins, nanoparticles, DNA, liposomes and micelles) and low toxicity (Figure 1). A cargo can be bound to the CPP covalently or non-covalently. Covalent coupling can be achieved by either chemical coupling or by expression as a fusion construct [53]. Chemical conjugation of CPP to cargoes is the most common approach used for CPP-modified cargo delivery. Cargo molecules can be prepared so as to contain CPP segments from the beginning as a part of their structures [54]. CPPs can also be attached via disulfide cross-linking [55] and in this case the cargo molecules must have a free sulfhydryl moiety that has to be selectively cross-linked with CPPs. Also, various types of hetero/homobifunctional cross-linkers are commercially available. These are designed to have functional groups to form cross-links between amino moieties (e.g., succinimidyl esters) and/or thiol moieties (e.g., maleimides or alkyl halides). Amino moieties are usually found in proteins, as their N-terminus and the ε-position of lysine side chains rather than cysteines. However covalent modifications involve risks of altering the biological activity of cargo. This is especially important in the case of charged oligonucleotide or siRNA for which CPP coupling has led o restricted biological activities [56]. Non-covalent approach involves ionic interactions and was originally developed for gene delivery. Several CPPs have been reported in literature to form non-covalent complexes with biomolecules [11, 57-62].

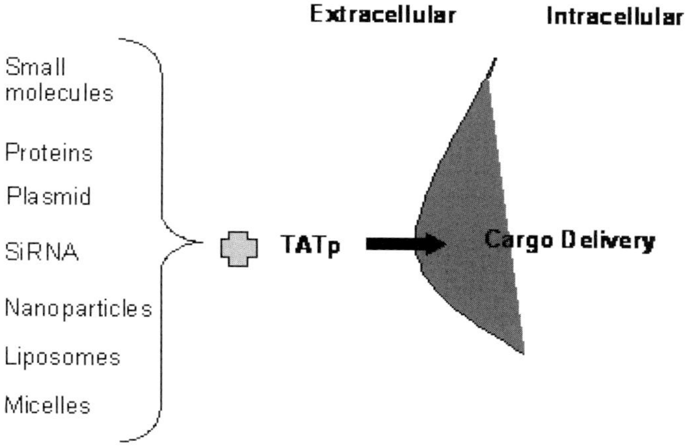

Fig. 1. Intracellular delivery of various cargos using TATp.

2.1. *Delivery of proteins and peptides*

Transport of proteins and peptides across the cell membrane is still a challenging task, primarily due to the impermeable nature of the cell membrane that restricts the cellular drug uptake to only small (<600 Da) and hydrophobic molecules. Since it was proved that TATp was able to transport various proteins across cell membranes [63], CPPs have shown to be effective for delivery of wide range of peptides and proteins [64-67] and also to target various diseases including cancer, asthma, ischemia, diabetes [68, 69]. The first proof of concept was shown in the case of delivery of the 120 kDa β-galactosidase coupled to TAT by Schwarze et al. [54]. It was shown that the TAT- β-galactosidase fusion protein can be delivered into almost all tissues, even crossing the blood-brain barrier in mice.

In the case of delivery of peptides and proteins for cancer therapy, TAT-mediated delivery of a peptide derived from C-terminus of p53 has shown to reduce tumor growth upon intra-peritoneal injection into mice with β-cell lymphoma [70]. CPPs have also been used to target B-cell lymphoma oncogene. A peptide for 'Epstein Barr Virus" associated with TATp has been reported to block proliferation [71].

Kwon et al. have developed a modified 'antibody targeted, triggered, electrically modified prodrug-type strategy' (ATTEMPTS) approach in delivery of macromolecular drugs, which integrates the cell-penetrating PTDs into a heparin/protamine-regulated delivery system (Figure 2) [72]. The system consists of the targeting component (such as antibody), coupled to a heparin molecule.

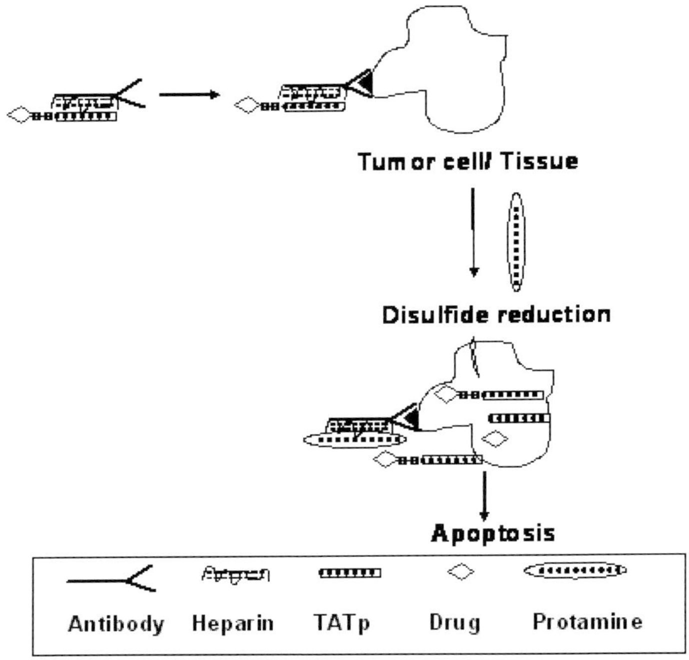

Fig. 2. Schematics of the CPP-modified ATTEMPTS system.

The drug component (such as the macromolecular drug) is covalently linked with a PTD peptide such as TAT via a disulfide bond. These two components spontaneously associate with each other through charge–charge interactions between the anionic heparin and the cationic TAT. The prodrug feature (i.e. due to inhibition of the cell-penetrating function by heparin) and targeting moieties can prevent interaction of the drug complex with normal tissues during tumor-targeting, thereby alleviating drug-associated toxic effects. Once the TAT-Drug/Ab-Heparin complexes reach the target, a competing agent such as protamine sulfate can be administered which binds to heparin with greater affinity than TAT and thus dissociating the TAT-Drug conjugate from its Hep-Ab counterpart. Then the TAT-Drug conjugates can be taken up by the targeted tumor cells. Once inside tumor cells, the drug molecule can be detached from

PTD through reduction of S–S linkage by the elevated level of glutathione in the cytosol, inducing tumor-specific apoptosis. *In vitro* findings using asparaginase (ASNase) as a model macromolecular anti-tumor agent were able to validate the feasibility of this delivery system. The chemically constructed TAT-ASNase conjugates not only were able to translocate into the MOLT-4 cells and elicit the cytotoxic effects, but also this PTD-mediated intracellular drug uptake could be regulated (with on/off control) by the addition of heparin and protamine. Later they also used a similar approach to permit antibody-directed administration of inactive protease drugs such as tissue-specific plasminogen activator (t-PA) and allow a subsequent triggered release of the active t-PA at the target site [73].

Recently it was found that fusion of TATp with elastin-like polypeptide (ELP) inhibited adhesion, spreading, invasion and migration of SKOV-3 ovarian cancer cells in cell culture. Furthermore, it was also confirmed that Tat-ELP has anti-metastatic potential in an experimental ovarian cancer metastasis model *in vivo*, causing approximately 80% reduction in the tumor burden [74].

TAT-mediated protein delivery showed potential as a therapeutic and prophylactic vaccine. Exogenous proteins can not enter the cytosol and access the MHC class I processing pathway. Therefore, it is difficult to design a protein-based vaccine that induces class I-restricted cytotoxic T-lymphocyte (CTL) response. However, after conjugating the antigen protein to TATp, such as TAT-ovalbumin conjugate, resulting in effective killing of the target cells by antigen-specific CTLs [75].

TAT PTD was also used to eradicate tumor by utilizing dendritic cell (DC)-based immunotherapy [76]. Immunization with DCs loaded with TAT PTD-TRP2 peptide resulted in complete protective immunity and significant inhibition of lung metastases in a 3-day tumor model. T cell response generated by DC/TAT-TRP2 was higher than that induced by DC/TRP2 [77].

TAT transduction domain also showed a potential for application in inflammatory conditions. Proinflammatory cytokines such as TNF-α and IL-1β mediate their action by activating NF-κB; therefore, methods to reduce NF-κB activity will be beneficial in chronic inflammatory conditions. The nonphosphorylatable, nondegradable suppressor Iκ-Bα mutant strongly inhibits NF-κB activity. The fusion of this mutant with TAT PTD resulted in rapid and efficient uptake in the cells, inhibition of TNF-α or IL-1β-incuced NF-κB activation in a dose-dependent manner and NF-κB-mediated transcription [78].

TAT PTD was also used to transducer a biologically active neuroprotectant Bcl-xL in cerebral ischemia. Death of neuronal cells following cerebral ischemia is associated with apoptosis, and TAT-Bcl-xL fusion protein (called PTD-HA-

Bcl-xL) resulted in robust protein transduction in cultures and also delivered the protein across the blood-brain barrier to decrease neuronal cell death [79].

Recently L- or D-forms of penetratin, or the L- or D-forms of octaarginine (L- or D-R8), was used for nasal insulin delivery. It was found that CPPs dramatically increased nasal insulin absorption, and it was more pronounced for L- and D-penetratin than L- or D-R8. L-penetratin was the most effective promoter of insulin absorption compared with others CPPs. The pharmacological availability and bioavailability of nasally administered insulin was up to 76.7 % and 50.7 % relative to the subcutaneous route, respectively [80].

Heat shock protein 70 (HSP70) is an intracellular stress protein that confers cytoprotection to a variety of cellular stressors. Weeler et al. generated a Tat-HSP70 fusion protein using recombinant methods and treated HSF –/– cells with either Tat-HSP70 or recombinant HSP70 prior to exposure to hyperoxia or lethal heat shock. They showed that biologically active, exogenous HSP70 can be delivered into cells using the HIV-1 Tat protein, and that the Tat-mediated delivery of HSP70 confers cytoprotection against thermal stress and hyperoxia and may represent a novel approach to augmenting intracellular HSP70 levels [81]. Superoxide dismutase fused to TAT or to Pep-1 has been shown to protect pancreatic beta cells against oxidative stress [82].

Morris et al. developed a new technique for protein delivery based on a peptide, Pep-1 [60]. This Pep-1 has the capability to deliver different peptides, proteins, and antibodies inside different cells, *in vivo* and *in vitro,* without any chemical coupling between the cargo and Pep-1 [64]. This approach has the significant advantage of not requiring any chemical modification of the CPP or protein cargo, thus simplifying the formulation process. This Pep-1 strategy has also been used to deliver therapeutic proteins *in vivo* across the blood-brain barrier [83].

Antibodies are usually the most difficult large proteins to deliver into cell and TATp has also enabled delivery of antibodies for radiotherapeutic application [84]. Thus ability of CPPs to delivery antibodies to cells proves their potential in the field of intracellular delivery.

2.2. *Delivery of nanoparticles*

The first example of use of TATp as a vector for nanoparticulate delivery was described in 1999 [85]. In this study, the functionalized iron oxide nanoparticles with TATp showed efficient labeling of cells, and thus might serve as a tool for magnetic resonance imaging (MRI) or magnetic separation of homed cells *in vivo*. TATp (48–57) was coupled to the dextran-coated superparamagnetic iron oxide particles (CLIO) (41nm). The peptide was attached to CLIO amine, activated with succinimidyl-iodoacetate. These particles enabled internalization into cell lines tested (mouse lymphocytes, human natural killer cells and HeLa cells) over 100-fold more efficiently when compared with TAT-free controls. Later in another study, T cells were magnetically labeled without affecting their normal responses to stimulation [86]. Upon the intravenous injection, the homing of T cells to the spleen could be detected by MRI and their biodistribution profile could be followed by MRI *in vivo*. Other studies observed the uptake of TATp-labeled iron oxide particles by T cells, B cells, and macrophages over 72 h and found that the uptake was quick with no loss in the cell viability [87]. However the TATp–iron oxide conjugates were accumulated primarily in the cytoplasm in contrast to nuclear localization observed by other authors. In general, the labeling with TATp–CLIO did not induce toxicity and did not alter the differentiation or proliferation pattern of CD34+ cells. The TATp–CLIO-labeled CD34+ cells and control cells were subsequently injected intravenously into the immunodeficient mice [88]. Around 4% of the injected dose of the cells migrated to the bone marrow (per gram of the tissue), and the labeled and control cells showed similar biodistribution profile. Nonetheless, it was possible to visualize the labeled cells by MRI within mouse bone marrow at the single-cell level. Also, such magnetically labeled cells could be recovered from the bone marrow after *in vivo* homing using magnetic separation columns. Work by Zhao et al. suggested that the cellular uptake of the TATp–CLIO increased nonlinearly upon increasing TATp-to-CLIO ratios, giving a 100- fold increase with 15 TATp per CLIO particle thus enhancing the sensitivity of imaging by MRI [89]. Work carried by Lewin et al. showed that TATp-functionalized superparamagnetic nanoparticles were able to track labeled cells *in vivo* using MRI and also could recover the cells using magnetic-separation column [55]. When the surface of CLIO was modified with D-polyarginyl peptide or TATp, the nanoparticles could traverse through the cell monolayers. Such nanoparticles can be used, for example, for labeling of immune cells for *in vivo* imaging purposes [90].

The same approach was applied to prepare octaarginine-coated liposomes to target airway cells by inhalation [91]. In another study, shell cross-linked (SCK) nanoparticles were prepared by the micellization of amphiphilic block copolymers of poly(epsilon–caprolactone–beta-acrylic acid) and conjugated to TATp that was independently built on a solid support, resulting in TATp-modified nanocage conjugate. Such a conjugate when analyzed by confocal microscopy with CHO and HeLa cells, showed binding and transduction inside the cells [92]. The authors then characterized the SCK nanoparticles for the optimum number of TATp per particle required to enhance the transduction efficiency [93]. The authors prepared the conjugates with 52, 104 and 210 CPP moieties per particle, which were then evaluated for biocompatibility *in vitro* and *in vivo* [94]. *In vitro* studies showed the inflammatory responses to the conjugates, but *in vivo* evaluation of the conjugates in mouse did not result in major incompatible responses. Thus, TAT peptide–SCK conjugate can be used as scaffolds for preparing antigen for immunization.

TATp (48–57) was also conjugated to FITC-doped silica nanoparticles (FSNPs) for bioimaging purposes. TATp– FSNPs were prepared by microemulsion system and showed labeling of human lung adenocarcinoma cells (A-549) *in vitro* unlike FSNPs that showed no effective labeling. TATp-modified nanoparticles have also been investigated for their capability to deliver the diagnostic and therapeutic agents across the blood brain barrier. For *in vivo* bioimaging potential, TATp– FSNPs were administered intra-arterially to the brain of rats. TATp-conjugated FSNPs labeled the brain blood vessels, showing the potential for delivering agents to the brain without compromising the blood brain barrier [95].

Gold particles are also intracellular delivery vectors of choice because of some important properties. They can be synthesized in sizes varying from 0.8 to 200 nm and can be further modified with a variety of small molecules, peptides, proteins, DNA, and polymers. Tkachenko et al. prepared peptide-gold particle complexes by conjugating peptides to bovine serum albumin (BSA) and then attaching BSA-peptide conjugates to gold nanoparticles. Initial studies found that the conjugates were internalized by endocytosis and did not localize into the nuclei of NIH3T3 or HepG2 cells [88]. Conversely, it was shown that smaller (3nm) gold particles functionalized with TATp traversed through the cell membrane of human fibroblast cells and accumulated within the nuclei [96]. The reason for this success could depend on method of gold nanoparticles synthesis, the difference in particle size or cell types used. Also here, the authors used transmission electron microscopy (TEM) to avoid the fixation induced artifacts. Recently Nativo et al., studied the uptake of *ca.* 16 nm surface-modified gold nanoparticles by human fibroblast cells (HeLa cells) by TEM [97]. They found that TATp- modified gold nanoparticles located in the endosomes, supporting the assumption that the predominant uptake mechanism enabled by TAT is endocytosis. Successful nuclear targeting was observed after surface modification with a cocktail of CPPs and a peptide acting as a nuclear localization signal (GGFSTSLRARKA).

To study the effect of nanoparticle shape/size on cellular uptake, Zhang et al. constructed a spherical and two cylindrical nanoparticles, with different lengths. It was found that when the nanoparticles were functionalized with the TAT PTD, the smaller, spherical nanoparticles had a higher rate of cell entry into Chinese hamster ovary (CHO) cells than did the larger, cylindrical nanoparticles. It was also found that nanoparticles were released after internalization and that the rate of cell exit was dependent on both the nanoparticle shape and the amount of surface-bound PTD [98].

Quantum dots (QDs) have received a great amount of interest for use as fluorescent labels in biological applications. QDs are brightly fluorescent and very photostable, satisfying even imaging applications that require single molecule detection at high repetition rates over long periods of time (minutes to hours) [99]. However they have little cellular uptake and modification with CPPs provides good solution. The functionalization of quantum dots with CPPs has been shown to improve biocompatibility. Attachment of CPPs to QDs has been carried out with techniques such as covalent binding between a cysteine and lysine residues [100], using biotin-conjugated peptides to streptavidin-coated nanoparticles [101-103], or via a polyhistidine peptide linker exhibiting affinity for the metals contained within nanocrystals [104]. Non-covalent delivery of QDs has also been achieved with Pep-1 [105]. TATp-modified CdS:Mn/ZnS QDs were delivered intra-arterially into rats and were able to efficiently label brain tissue within minutes [100].

Another well investigated drug carriers are liposomes. These are artificial phospholipids vesicles with the size varying from 50 to 1000 nm and greater, which can be loaded with a variety of drugs [106, 107]. Further, addition of polyethylene glycol (PEG) coating renders these liposomes long-circulating (ability to stay in the blood long time) [108] so as to accumulate in various pathological areas with compromised (leaky) vasculature, such as tumors. It has been proven that [109] the long-circulating liposomes can be made 'targeted', where antibodies or other specific binding molecules have been attached to the water-exposed tips of PEG chains [110].

Polymeric micelles, are widely gaining interest as pharmaceutical carrier due to their small size (10-100 nm), *in vivo* stability, ability to solubilize water insoluble anticancer drugs, and prolonged blood circulation times [111, 112]. The typical core shell structure of polymeric micelles is formed by self assembly of amphiphilic block-copolymers consisting of hydrophilic and hydrophobic monomer units in aqueous media [111]. The use of special amphiphilic molecules as micelle building blocks can also introduce the property of micelle extended blood half- life upon intravenous administration. The block copolymer micelles can also target their payload to specific tissues through either passive or active means. The passive targeting is due to the small micellar size which assists in spontaneous penetration into the interstitium in the body compartments with the leaky vasculature (tumors and infarcts) by the enhanced permeability and retention (EPR) effect [111-114]. The active targeting can be achieved by attachment of target-specific molecules to their surface [111, 112].

Micelles made of PEG-phosphatidyl ethanolamine (PEG-PE) can provide additional advantages for particle stability when compared with conventional amphiphilic polymer micelles due to the existence of two fatty acid acyls, which might contribute considerably to an increase in the hydrophobic interactions between the polymeric chains in the micelle core [115]. PEG-PE micelles demonstrate good stability, longevity, and ability to accumulate in the areas with damaged vasculature (EPR effect in leaky areas, such as infarcts and tumors) [115, 116]. Both liposomes and micelles can be easily modified with CPP. Some possible ways to attach CPP to micelles and liposomal surfaces is shown in Figure 3.

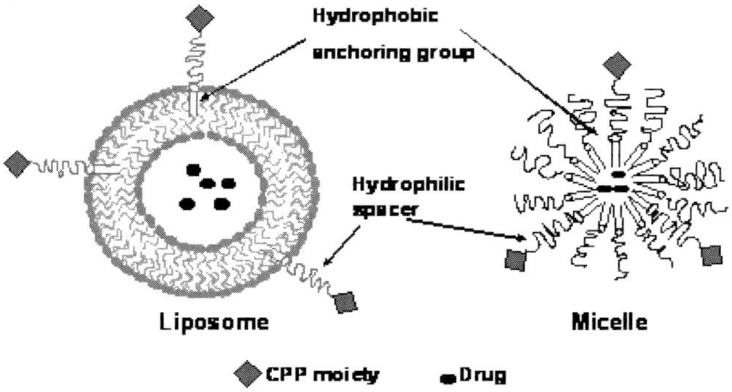

Fig. 3. CPP attached to liposomes and micelles by the insertion into the hydrophobic phase of liposome membrane or micelle inner core via spacer arm (linker) with hydrophobic "anchor".

TATp (47–57)-modified liposomes were delivered intracellularly in different cells, such as murine Lewis lung carcinoma (LLC) cells, human breast tumor BT20 cells, and rat cardiac myocyte H9C2 cells [117]. Liposomes were modified with TATp via *para*-nitrophenyl (pNP) groups at the distal ends of the liposome containing pNP-PEG-PE. The preparations of TATp-liposomes, which allowed for the direct contact of TATp residues with cells, displayed an enhanced uptake by the cells. This suggested that the translocation of TATp-liposomes into cells require direct free interaction of TATp with the cell surface. Further studies on the intracellular trafficking of rhodamine-labeled TATp-liposomes loaded with FITC-dextran, revealed that TATp-liposomes remained intact inside the cell cytoplasm within 1 h of translocation, after 2 h they migrated into the perinuclear zone, and at 9 h the liposomes disintegrated there [118]. It was found that the translocation of liposomes by TATp or penetratin was proportional to the number of peptide molecules attached to the liposomal surface and as few as five peptide number was already sufficient to enhance the intracellular delivery of liposomes. The kinetics of the uptake was peptide-and cell-type dependent [119]. Coupling of TATp to the outer surface of liposomes was also described that resulted in an enhanced binding and endocytosis of the liposomes in ovarian carcinoma cells [120]. Here, TATp was covalently coupled to the maleimide-derivatized PEG-DSPE present in the liposomal bilayer via a sulfhydryl-maleimide coupling reaction.

Antp (43-58) and TATp coupled to small unilamellar liposomes were accumulated in higher proportions within tumor cells and dendritic cells than unmodified control liposomes [121]. It was found that the uptake was time- and concentration dependent and at least 100 PTD molecules per small unilamellar liposomes were required for efficient uptake inside cells. The uptake of the modified liposomes was inhibited by the preincubation of liposomes with heparin, suggesting the role of heparin sulfate proteoglycans in CPP-mediated uptake.

Conventional liposomes have limited intracellular targeting capacity and are cleared rapidly by the lungs. Therefore, the modification of liposome aerosols for lung drug delivery was investigated. The effect of three CPPs – TATp, Antp, and octaarginine conjugated to neutral liposomes was studied. It was found that the modified liposomes were efficiently internalized by airway epithelial cells in culture and were able to deliver cargo (e.g. dextran) to the cytoplasm of the cells [91].

The requirement of direct unhindered contact of CPP with cells was also shown in case of TATp-modified micelles [122]. These micelles when loaded with anticancer drug paclitaxel demonstrated increased cytotoxicity with various cancer cells *in vitro*. This was considered as a result of increased interaction with cells of TATp-modified micelles compared to non-modified-micelles. Another application of CPPs is the labeling of cells with semiconductor nanocrystals or quantum dots (QDs). QDs are more popular than standard fluorophores for studying tumor pathophysiology since they are photostable, more robust and stable light emitters and relatively insensitive to the wavelength of the excitation. They are also capable of distinguishing tumor vessels form both the perivascular cells and the matrix, with concurrent imaging. QDs trapped within PEG-PE micelles bearing TATp-PEG-PE linker were successfully applied for labeling mouse endothelial cells *in vitro*. For *in vivo* tracking, bone marrow-derived progenitor cells were labeled with TATp-bearing QD-containing micelle *ex vivo*, and then injected in the mouse bearing tumor in a cranial window model. It was then possible to track the movement of labeled progenitor cell to tumor endothelium, introducing an attempt towards understanding fine details of tumor neovascularization.

2.3. *Delivery of nucleic acids*

Another exceptionally important yet challenging task is intracellular delivery of nucleic acids. Various methods used to deliver these highly negatively charged biomolecules are associated with cellular toxicity or poor efficiency in certain types of cells (e.g. lipofectamnine or microinjection). Currently, liposomes and cationic polymers are used for transfection but they are also less efficient and their use is often accompanied by high level of toxicity.

Due to size of plasmid and high number of negative charges, non-covalent approach has been mostly used. It has been reported that TATp binds to DNA to form complexes which can be internalized through endocytosis [25]. Ignatovich et al. has observed moderate reporter gene expression after incubation of cultured cells with TATp-plasmid complexes. However, after the intravenous injection into mice, it resulted in only low expression levels, mainly in liver [123]. This was mainly attributed to non-specific hepatic uptake of macromolecules as well as rapid clearance due to interactions with serum albumin.

CPPs have been used to enhance gene delivery by solid lipid nanoparticles (SLN, lipidic nanocarriers without inner aqueous space) [124]. SLN gene vector was modified with dimeric TATp (TAT2) and compared with polyethylenimine (PEI) for gene expression *in vitro* and *in vivo*. The presence of TAT2 in SLN gene vector enhanced the gene transfection compared to PEI both *in vitro* and *in vivo*. TATp-functionalized polymeric nanoparticles (complexes of polyethylenimine and DNA) effectively delivered gene vectors into undifferentiated and differentiated SH-SY5Y cells [49]. In a different approach, for improving the transfection and protecting DNA from degradation, thiocholesterol-based cationic lipids (TCL) were used in the formation of nanolipoparticles (NLPs). The NLPs were sequentially modified with TATp that resulted in TATp-NLPs with a zwitterionic surface and higher transfection efficiency than the cationic NLPs [125]. The conjugation of TATp to lipoplexes enhanced the gene transfection in primary cell cultures by the endocytic uptake [42]. It was also shown in [39] that TATp-modified lipoplexes are mainly internalized by cells *via* a cholesterol-dependent clathrin-mediated pathway.

There are many examples of combining CPPs with cationic liposomes for the delivery of DNA. TATp–liposomes prepared with the addition of a small quantity of a cationic lipid (DOTAP) were incubated with DNA which formed firm non-covalent complexes with DNA. Such TATp–liposome–DNA complexes when incubated with mouse fibroblast NIH 3T3 and cardiac myocytes H9C2 showed substantially higher transfection *in vitro*, with lower cytotoxicity than the commonly used Lipofectin®. NIH/3T3, BT20, or H9C2 cells were transfected by incubation with TAT peptide–liposome/plasmid complexes in serum-free media for 4 h at 37 °C under 6% CO_2. The flow cytometry data demonstrated that the treatment of NIH/3T3 cells with TATp–liposome/pEGFP-N1 complexes results in high fluorescence, i.e. high transfection outcome. Similar results were obtained with all cell lines tested. Confocal microscopy confirmed the transfection of various cells with TATp–liposome/DNA complexes. From 30 to 50% of both cell types in the field of view showed a bright green fluorescence, while lower fluorescence was observed in virtually all cells. Under *in vivo* conditions, the intratumoral injection of TATp–liposome–DNA complexes also resulted in an efficient transfection. Histologically, hematoxylin/eosin-stained tumor slices in both control and experimental animals showed a typical pattern of poorly differentiated carcinoma, however, under the fluorescence microscope, samples from control mice (non-treated mice or mice injected with TATp-free liposome/plasmid complexes) showed only a background fluorescence, while slices from tumors injected with TATp–liposome/plasmid complexes contained bright green fluorescence in tumor cells indicating an efficient TATp-mediated transfection [118]. The study thus implicated the usefulness of TATp–liposomes for *in vitro* and localized *in vivo* gene therapy.

We have also recently investigated the potential of TATp-modified liposomes to enhance the delivery of the model gene, plasmid encoding for the GFP (pEGFP-N1), to human brain tumor U-87 MG cells *in vitro* and in an intracranial model in nude mice [126]. The size distribution of DNA-loaded TATp–liposomes was narrow (around 250 nm) and the DNA complexation was firm at lipid/DNA (+/−) charge ratios of 5 and higher. TATp–lipoplexes had demonstrated an enhanced delivery of pEGFP-N1 to U-87 MG tumor cells *in vitro* at lipid/DNA (+/−) charge ratios of 5 and 10. *In vivo* transfection of intracranial brain tumors by intratumoral injections of TATp–lipoplexes showed an enhanced delivery of pEGFP-N1 selectively to tumor cells and subsequent effective transfection compared to plain plasmid-loaded lipoplexes. No transfection (green fluorescence of the GFP) was noted in the normal brain adjacent to tumor. Thus, TATp–lipoplexes can be used to augment the delivery of genes to tumor cells when injected intratumorally, without affecting the normal adjacent brain.

Another example is gene delivery into immunocompetent cells to modulate immune response. Antigen presenting cells (APC) are among the most important cells of the immune system since they link the innate and the adaptative immune responses, directing the type of immune response to be elicited. However, APC are very resistant to transfection. To increase the efficiency of APC transfection, we have used liposome-based lipoplexes additionally modified with cell-penetrating TATp for better intracellular delivery of a model plasmid encoding for the enhanced-green fluorescent protein (pEGFP). pEGFP-bearing lipoplexes made of a mixture of PC:Chol:DOTAP (60:30:10 molar ratio) with the addition of 2% mol of PEG-PE conjugate (plain-L) or TATp-PEG-PE (TATp-L) were shown to effectively protect the incorporated DNA from degradation. Uptake assays of rhodamine-labeled lipoplexes and transfections with the EGFP reporter gene were performed with APC derived from the mouse spleen. TATp-L-based lipoplexes allowed for significantly enhanced both, the uptake and transfection in APC [127].

We have recently reported a double –targeted delivery system simultaneously capable of extracellular accumulation and intracellular penetration for gene therapy for the treatment of myocardial ischemia. We have used low cationic liposomes–plasmid DNA complexes (lipoplexes) modified with TATp and/or with monoclonal anti-myosin monoclonal antibody 2G4 (mAb 2G4) specific toward cardiac myosin, for targeted gene delivery to ischemic myocardium. *In vitro* transfection of both normoxic and hypoxic cardiomyocytes was enhanced by the presence of TATp as determined by fluorescence microscopy and ELISA. The *in vitro* transfection was further enhanced by the additional modification with mAb 2G4 antibody in the case of hypoxic, but not normoxic cardiomyocytes. However, we did not observe a synergism between TATp and mAb 2G4 ligands under our experimental condition. In *in vivo* experiments, we have clearly demonstrated an increased accumulation of mAb 2G4-modified TATp lipoplexes in the ischemic rat myocardium and significantly enhanced transfection of cardiomyocytes in the ischemic zone. Thus, the genetic transformation of normoxic and hypoxic cardiomyocytes can be enhanced by using lipoplexes modified with TATp and/or mAb 2G4 [128].

Another delivery system reported in literature is the 'multifunctional envelope-type nano device' (MEND) [129]. This method involves three steps: (i) DNA condensation with a polycation such as poly-L -lysine (PLL), (ii) lipid film hydration for the electrostatic binding of the condensed DNA, and (iii) sonication to package the condensed DNA with lipids. Further MEND was surface-modified with octaarginine on the envelope as a device for membrane penetration to enhance cellular uptake, showed a 1000-fold higher transfection activity. This system can also be PEGylated. Helper lipids like dioleoylphosphatidylethanolamine (DOPE) and cholesteryl hemisuccinate (CHEMS) can be added to promote endosomal release and nuclear delivery of the cargo [43].

CPPs have also been used to enhance the intracellular delivery of DNA by PEI-based DNA complexes [130, 131] and by dendrimers [132-134].

RNAi technology has also been improved with CPP-mediated delivery of SiRNA [59, 135]. The first report about CPP-mediated delivery of siRNA was published in 2003 by Simeoni et al.[136]. SiRNA were non-covalently complexed with the MPG peptide leading to strong down regulation of the target protein. Davidson et al. has reported a string RNAi effect in hard to transfect primary neuronal cells [137]. Here, siRNA directed against several endogenous proteins were coupled to penetratin via a disulfide bond. We have described recently a novel approach for siRNA cellular delivery using siRNA encapsulated into liposomes additionally bearing arginine octamer (R8) molecules attached to their surface (R8-liposomes). The R8-liposomal siRNA demonstrated a very high stability against degradation by the blood serum and very high transfection efficiency into SK-MES-1 lung tumor cells resistant towards the Lipofectamine 2000-mediated transfection. siRNA in R8-liposomes effectively inhibited the targeted gene and significantly reduced the proliferation of cancer cells [138]. Arginine-9 (R9) was also investigated as a potential carrier for siRNAs [139]. Penetratin and transportan featuring terminal cysteines have been covalently attached to a 5'-thiol modified siRNA and produced expression knockdown for up to seven days [140]. Successful delivery of siRNA has also been reported using MEND technology [141].

Even though there are many examples of successful CPP-mediated internalization, several studies with CPP-siRNA revealed that TAT and penetratin alone affected gene expression and that penetratin-siRNA elicited an immunological response, challenging the use of these CPPs in delivery systems [142, 143].

2.4. *Stimuli-sensitive nanoparticulate drug delivery system*

Ideal nanoparticular drug delivery system should be able to (1) specifically accumulate in the required organ or tissue, and then (2) penetrate inside target cells delivering its load (drug or DNA) intracellularly. Organ or tissue (tumor, infarct) accumulation could be achieved by the passive targeting *via* the EPR effect [113, 114] assisted by prolonged circulation of such nanocarrier (for example, as a result of its coating with protecting polymer such as PEG); or by the antibody-mediated active targeting [144] and [145], while the intracellular delivery could be mediated by certain internalizable ligands (folate, transferrin) [146] and [147] or by CPPs [66]. Evidently, such drug delivery system (DDS) should simultaneously carry on its surface various active moieties, i.e. be multifunctional and possess the ability to "switch on" certain functions (such as intracellular penetration) only when necessary, for example under the action of local stimuli characteristic of the target pathological zone (first of all, increased temperature or lowered pH values characteristic of inflamed, ischemic, and neoplastic tissues). These "smart" DDS should be built in such a way that during the first phase of delivery, a non-specific cell-penetrating function is shielded by the function providing organ/tissue-specific delivery (sterically protecting polymer or antibody). Upon accumulating in the target, protecting polymer or antibody attached to the surface of the DDS *via* the stimuli-sensitive bond should detach under the action of local pathological conditions (abnormal pH or temperature) and expose the previously hidden second function allowing for the subsequent delivery of the carrier and its cargo inside cells (Figure 4).

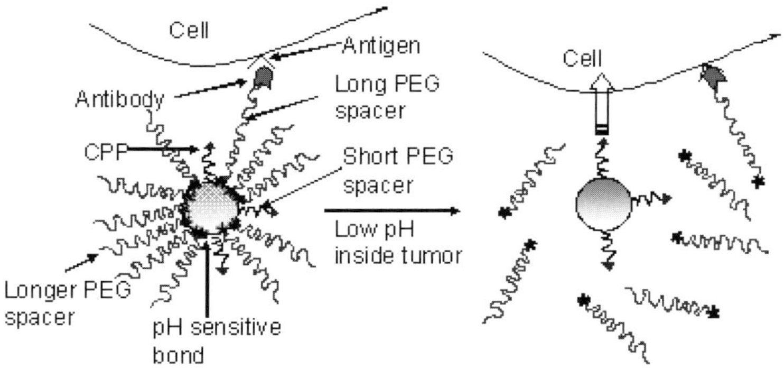

Fig. 4. The principle scheme of the action of stimuli-sensitive double-targeted nanaocarrier. The surface of the nanocarrier is modified with a CPP via a relatively short spacer; with longer PEG chains; and with even longer PEG chains decorated at distal termini with a target-specific ligand (antibody). CPP is shielded with longer chains, while these PEG chains and PEG–antibody chains are attached to the surface via pH-sensitive bonds. The whole system is stable in the blood and accumulates in the tumor via the PEG-mediated EPR effect and via antibody-mediated targeting. Inside the tumor, protective PEG chains and PEG–antibody conjugates are detached from the surface because of fast hydrolysis of pH-sensitive bonds at the lowered intratumors pH, CPP becomes exposed and allows for the intracellular delivery.

With this in mind, we have suggested and prepared targeted long-circulating PEGylated liposomes and PEG–PE-based micelles possessing several functionalities [148, 149]. First, such systems were capable of targeting a specific cell or organ by attaching the monoclonal antibody (infarct-specific antimyosin antibody 2G4 or cancer-specific antinucleosome antibody 2C5) to their surface *via* reactive pNP–PEG–PE moieties. Second, these liposomes and micelles were additionally modified with TATp moieties attached to the surface of the nanocarrier by using TATp-short PEG–PE derivatives. PEG–PE used for liposome surface modification or for micelle preparation was made degradable by inserting the pH-sensitive hydrazone bond between PEG and PE (PEG–Hz–PE). Under normal pH values, TATp functions on the surface of nanocarriers were "shielded" by long protecting PEG chains (pH-degradable PEG_{2000}–PE or PEG_{5000}–PE) or by long pNP–PEG–PE moieties used to attach antibodies to the nanocarrier (non-pH-degradable PEG_{3400}–PE or PEG_{5000}–PE). At pH 7.5–8.0, both liposomes and micelles demonstrated high specific binding with antibody substrates, but very limited internalization by NIH/3T3 or U-87 cells. However, upon brief incubation (15-to-30 min) at lower pH values (pH 5.0–6.0) nanocarriers lost their protective PEG shell because of acidic hydrolysis of PEG–Hz–PE and acquired the ability to be effectively internalized by cells *via* TATp moieties (Figure 5).

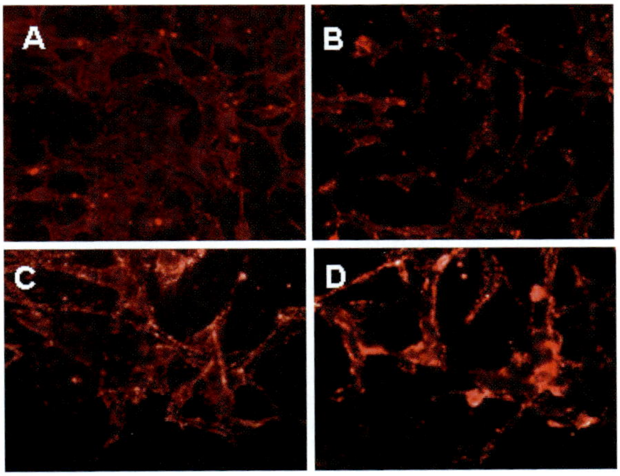

Fig. 5. Fluorescence microscopy showing internalization of Rh-PE-labeled-TATp containing micelles by NIH 3T3 fibroblast cells after incubating micelles at pH 8.0 (A), pH 5.0 (B)* for 30 min and RH-PE-labeled-TATp containing liposomes internalization by U87 MG astrocytoma using: 9 mol % pH-non-sensitive PEG-PE at pH 7.4 (C), 9 mol % pH-sensitive PEG-Hz-PE after incubation at pH 5.0 for 20 min (D)*. The cleavable (pH sensitive) PEG-PE-based TATp-containing liposomes/micelles kept at pH 7.4-8 show only marginal association with cells while those preincubated for 20-30 min at pH 5.0 demonstrated dramatically enhanced association with the cells (higher fluorescence), i.e., better accessibility of TATp moieties for cell interaction.*The pH of these formulations was raised back to pH 7.4 after their incubation at pH 5.0 and prior to incubation with cell.

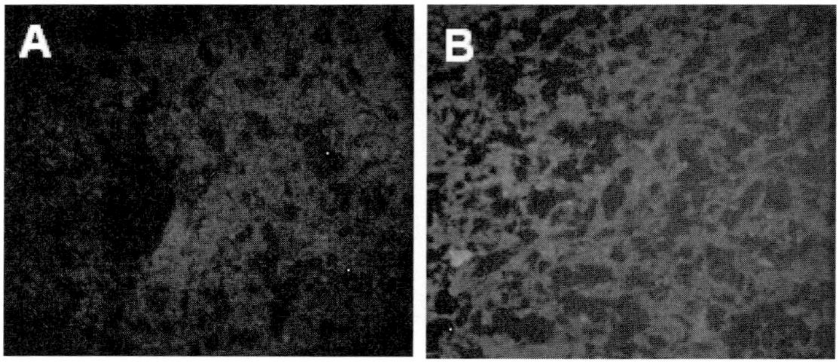

Fig. 6. Fluorescence microscopy images of LLC tumor sections from tumors injected with pGFP-loaded TATp-bearing liposomes with pH-non-cleavable PEG coat (A) and with pH-cleavable PEG coat (B).

In vivo, TATp-modified pGFP-loaded liposomal preparations have been administered intratumorally in tumor-bearing mice and the efficacy of tumor cell transfection was followed after 72 h. The administration of pGFP–TATp–liposomes with non-pH-sensitive PEG coating has resulted in only minimal transfection of tumor cells because of steric hindrances for the liposome-to-cell interaction created by the PEG coat, which shielded the surface-attached TATp. At the same time, the administration of pGFP–TATp–liposomes with the low pH-detachable PEG resulted in the highly efficient transfection since the removal of PEG under the action of the decreased intratumoral pH leads to the exposure of the liposome-attached TATp residues, enhanced penetration of the liposomes inside tumor cells and more effective intracellular delivery of the pGFP (Figure 6) [150].

TATp-modified stimuli-sensitive polymeric micelles with an enhanced ability to interact with cells under acidified conditions have also been described in [151]. These results can be considered as an important step in the development of tumor-specific stimuli-sensitive drug and gene delivery systems.

3. Problems with CPP-mediated Delivery and Ways to Overcome

Although there is still some controversy about the details of the mechanism of uptake of CPP, it is widely accepted that the CPP-cargo conjugates are internalized via endocytosis [21, 32, 152]. Some papers suggest that free CPPs can allow for the endosomal escape [153-156], however, this escape mechanism can not be generalized for peptides linked to bulky cargos. In the case of macromolecules, CPPs can facilitate the membrane translocation. Still, after the uptake, these macromolecules are generally subjected to acidic pH of endosomes/lysosomes and the digestive enzymes of the lysosomes. Thus, the endosomal escape is believed to be the rate limiting step for efficient intracellular delivery of cargos linked to CPPs.

One approach is the use of fusogenic lipids such as DOPE which is reported to transform from lamellar phase to inverted hexagonal phase at low pH. This transformation promotes fusion of lipid bilayers, resulting in endosomal escape [157]. Zhou et al. have shown that DOPE containing liposomes helped in fusion between the liposomes and the endosomal membrane after endocytosis resulting in the destabilization of this membrane and release of complexed DNA to the cytosol [158]. Kogure et al. used MEND as a gene delivery system consisting of DOPE as fusogenic lipid, to enhance release from endosomes [159, 160]. Here, the MEND consisted of condensed plasmid DNA core that is encapsulated in a lipid bilayer composed of DOPE and anionic CHEMS [129]. The system was further modified with octaarginine linked to stearyl moiety for insertion into lipid bilayer [43]. MEND was also used for delivery of oligodeoxynucleotides [161], siRNA [141] and proteins [162]. The fusogenic lipids and octaarginine have also been utilized to deliver protein to mitochondria [44] and to deliver an encapsulated antigen to cytosol of dendritic cells [163].

Wadia et al. have used the fusogenic segment of influenza HA2 protein to enhance endosomal escape of CPP-attached cargo [30]. However later it has been reported that more than 99 % of the TAT fusion protein was trapped in macropinosomes [164]. Another modified HA2 peptide has been used for cytosolic delivery of anticancer peptide shepherdin which exhibited more cytotoxicity *in vitro* [47]. Lao et al. showed that incorporation of histidine tail onto TATp resulted in significantly more increase in gene expression than unmodified TATp/pDNA complex [165]. The imidazole group of histidine has a pK_a of ~6.0, therefore allowing it to become protonated in the acidic environment of the endosome. At physiological pH the histidines will remain neutrally charged, thereby imparting selective membrane disruption in the acidic endosome [166].

Another strategy is to use PEI to attain endosomal release by buffering against the adenosine-5'-triphosphate (ATP)-dependent proton pump located in the membrane of endosomes. PEI contains several secondary amines that are easily protonated in the acidic environment of the endosome. As protons are pumped in, PEI absorbs the protons leading to endosomal swelling and membrane disruption [167]. The use of PEI/pDNA complexes with Antennapedia CPP has been reported to enhance the gene expression more that the unmodified particles in brain capillary endothelial primary cells [168]. Kleemann et al. used HIV-1 TAT covalently coupled to 25 kDa PEI through a heterobifunctional PEG spacer resulting in a TAT-PEG-PEI conjugate. This was used to complex DNA and significantly higher transfection efficiencies for TAT-PEG-PEI were detected in mice [130] due to the stabilizing effect of PEG *in vivo*.

Suk et al. attached RGD or HIV-1 TAT peptides to PEI/DNA nanocomplexes via PEG spacer molecules. Both RGD and TAT improved the cellular uptake of gene vectors and enhanced gene transfection efficiency of primary neurons up to 14-fold [49].

Use of lysomotropic agents such as chloroquine has been used in combination with PNA for efficient splice correction [45, 50, 51]. However this has no application *in vivo* due to its pharmacological effects.

In any case, it looks like CPPs are really becoming promising tools for the intracellular delivery of various drugs and drug-loaded pharmaceutical nanocarriers.

List of Acronyms and Abbreviations

Cell-penetrating peptides	CPPs
Protein transduction domain	PTDs
Membrane translocating sequences	MTSs
Model amphipathic peptide	MAP
Human immunodeficiency virus type 1	HIV-1
poly(2-hydroxytethyl aspartamide)	PHEA
Antibody targeted, triggered, electrically modified prodrug-type strategy	ATTEMPTS
Asparaginase	ASNase
Tissue-specific plasminogen activator	t-PA
Elastin-like polypeptide	ELP
Cytotoxic T-lymphocyte	CTL
Dendritic cell	DC
Heat shock protein 70	HSP70
Magnetic resonance imaging	MRI
Shell cross-linked	SCK
FITC-doped silica nanoparticles	FSNPs
Bovine serum albumin	BSA
Quantum dots	QDs

Polyethylene glycol	PEG
Enhanced permeability and retention	EPR
Phosphatidylethanolamine	PE
Polyethylenimine	PEI
Thiocholesterol-based cationic lipids	TCL
Nanolipoparticles	NLPs
Antigen presenting cells	APC
Multifunctional envelope-type nano device	MEND
Poly-L -lysine	PLL
Dioleoylphosphatidylethanolamine	DOPE
Cholesteryl hemisuccinate	CHEMS
Drug delivery system	DDS
para-nitrophenyl	pNP
Adenosine-5'-triphosphate	ATP
Transmission electron microscopy	TEM
Solid lipid nanoparticles	SLN

References

[1] Berry, C.C., "Intracellular delivery of nanoparticles via the HIV-1 tat peptide," *Nanomed*, Vol. 3, No. 3, 2008, pp. 357-65.

[2] Torchilin, V.P., "Tatp-mediated intracellular delivery of pharmaceutical nanocarriers," *Biochem Soc Trans*, Vol. 35, No. Pt 4, 2007, pp. 816-20.

[3] Lindgren, M., et al., "Cell-penetrating peptides," *Trends Pharmacol Sci*, Vol. 21, No. 3, 2000, pp. 99-103.

[4] Zorko, M., and Langel, U., "Cell-penetrating peptides: mechanism and kinetics of cargo delivery," *Adv Drug Deliv Rev*, Vol. 57, No. 4, 2005, pp. 529-45.

[5] Vives, E., Brodin, P., and Lebleu, B., "A truncated HIV-1 Tat protein basic domain rapidly translocates through the plasma membrane and accumulates in the cell nucleus," *J Biol Chem*, Vol. 272, No. 25, 1997, pp. 16010-7.

[6] Derossi, D., et al., "The third helix of the Antennapedia homeodomain translocates through biological membranes," *J Biol Chem*, Vol. 269, No. 14, 1994, pp. 10444-50.

[7] Elmquist, A., et al., "VE-cadherin-derived cell-penetrating peptide, pVEC, with carrier functions," *Exp Cell Res*, Vol. 269, No. 2, 2001, pp. 237-44.

[8] Rojas, M., et al., "Genetic engineering of proteins with cell membrane permeability," *Nat Biotechnol*, Vol. 16, No. 4, 1998, pp. 370-5.

[9] Oehlke, J., et al., "Cellular uptake of an alpha-helical amphipathic model peptide with the potential to deliver polar compounds into the cell interior non-endocytically," *Biochim Biophys Acta*, Vol. 1414, No. 1-2, 1998, pp. 127-39.

[10] Pooga, M., et al., "Cell penetration by transportan," *Faseb J*, Vol. 12, No. 1, 1998, pp. 67-77.

[11] Morris, M.C., et al., "A new peptide vector for efficient delivery of oligonucleotides into mammalian cells," *Nucleic Acids Res*, Vol. 25, No. 14, 1997, pp. 2730-6.
[12] Futaki, S., et al., "Arginine-rich peptides. An abundant source of membrane-permeable peptides having potential as carriers for intracellular protein delivery," *J Biol Chem*, Vol. 276, No. 8, 2001, pp. 5836-40.
[13] Jeang, K.T., Xiao, H., and Rich, E.A., "Multifaceted activities of the HIV-1 transactivator of transcription, Tat," *J Biol Chem*, Vol. 274, No. 41, 1999, pp. 28837-40.
[14] Green, M., and Loewenstein, P.M., "Autonomous functional domains of chemically synthesized human immunodeficiency virus tat trans-activator protein," *Cell*, Vol. 55, No. 6, 1988, pp. 1179-88.
[15] Frankel, A.D., and Pabo, C.O., "Cellular uptake of the tat protein from human immunodeficiency virus," *Cell*, Vol. 55, No. 6, 1988, pp. 1189-93.
[16] Park, J., et al., "Mutational analysis of a human immunodeficiency virus type 1 Tat protein transduction domain which is required for delivery of an exogenous protein into mammalian cells," *J Gen Virol*, Vol. 83, No. Pt 5, 2002, pp. 1173-81.
[17] Derossi, D., et al., "Cell internalization of the third helix of the Antennapedia homeodomain is receptor-independent," *J Biol Chem*, Vol. 271, No. 30, 1996, pp. 18188-93.
[18] Schwarze, S.R., and Dowdy, S.F., "In vivo protein transduction: intracellular delivery of biologically active proteins, compounds and DNA," *Trends Pharmacol Sci*, Vol. 21, No. 2, 2000, pp. 45-8.
[19] Lundberg, M., and Johansson, M., "Is VP22 nuclear homing an artifact?," *Nat Biotechnol*, Vol. 19, No. 8, 2001, pp. 713-4.
[20] Pichon, C., Monsigny, M., and Roche, A.C., "Intracellular localization of oligonucleotides: influence of fixative protocols," *Antisense Nucleic Acid Drug Dev*, Vol. 9, No. 1, 1999, pp. 89-93.
[21] Richard, J.P., et al., "Cell-penetrating peptides. A reevaluation of the mechanism of cellular uptake," *J Biol Chem*, Vol. 278, No. 1, 2003, pp. 585-90.
[22] Console, S., et al., "Antennapedia and HIV transactivator of transcription (TAT) "protein transduction domains" promote endocytosis of high molecular weight cargo upon binding to cell surface glycosaminoglycans," *J Biol Chem*, Vol. 278, No. 37, 2003, pp. 35109-14.
[23] Lundberg, M., Wikstrom, S., and Johansson, M., "Cell surface adherence and endocytosis of protein transduction domains," *Mol Ther*, Vol. 8, No. 1, 2003, pp. 143-50.
[24] Leifert, J.A., Harkins, S., and Whitton, J.L., "Full-length proteins attached to the HIV tat protein transduction domain are neither transduced between cells, nor exhibit enhanced immunogenicity," *Gene Ther*, Vol. 9, No. 21, 2002, pp. 1422-8.
[25] Sandgren, S., Cheng, F., and Belting, M., "Nuclear targeting of macromolecular polyanions by an HIV-Tat derived peptide. Role for cell-surface proteoglycans," *J Biol Chem*, Vol. 277, No. 41, 2002, pp. 38877-83.
[26] Mai, J.C., et al., "Efficiency of protein transduction is cell type-dependent and is enhanced by dextran sulfate," *J Biol Chem*, Vol. 277, No. 33, 2002, pp. 30208-18.
[27] Violini, S., et al., "Evidence for a plasma membrane-mediated permeability barrier to Tat basic domain in well-differentiated epithelial cells: lack of correlation with heparan sulfate," *Biochemistry*, Vol. 41, No. 42, 2002, pp. 12652-61.
[28] Rothbard, J.B., et al., "Role of membrane potential and hydrogen bonding in the mechanism of translocation of guanidinium-rich peptides into cells," *J Am Chem Soc*, Vol. 126, No. 31, 2004, pp. 9506-7.
[29] El-Andaloussi, S., et al., "A novel cell-penetrating peptide, M918, for efficient delivery of proteins and peptide nucleic acids," *Mol Ther*, Vol. 15, No. 10, 2007, pp. 1820-6.

[30] Wadia, J.S., Stan, R.V., and Dowdy, S.F., "Transducible TAT-HA fusogenic peptide enhances escape of TAT-fusion proteins after lipid raft macropinocytosis," *Nat Med*, Vol. 10, No. 3, 2004, pp. 310-5.
[31] Jones, A.T., "Macropinocytosis: searching for an endocytic identity and role in the uptake of cell penetrating peptides," *J Cell Mol Med*, Vol. 11, No. 4, 2007, pp. 670-84.
[32] Duchardt, F., et al., "A comprehensive model for the cellular uptake of cationic cell-penetrating peptides," *Traffic*, Vol. 8, No. 7, 2007, pp. 848-66.
[33] Fretz, M.M., et al., "Temperature-, concentration- and cholesterol-dependent translocation of L- and D-octa-arginine across the plasma and nuclear membrane of CD34+ leukaemia cells," *Biochem J*, Vol. 403, No. 2, 2007, pp. 335-42.
[34] Maiolo, J.R., Ferrer, M., and Ottinger, E.A., "Effects of cargo molecules on the cellular uptake of arginine-rich cell-penetrating peptides," *Biochim Biophys Acta*, Vol. 1712, No. 2, 2005, pp. 161-72.
[35] Nakase, I., et al., "Cellular uptake of arginine-rich peptides: roles for macropinocytosis and actin rearrangement," *Mol Ther*, Vol. 10, No. 6, 2004, pp. 1011-22.
[36] Yang, S.R., et al., "Intracellular delivery enhancement of poly(amino acid) drug carriers by oligoarginine conjugation," *J Biomed Mater Res A*, Vol. 86, No. 1, 2008, pp. 137-48.
[37] Ruan, G., et al., "Imaging and tracking of tat peptide-conjugated quantum dots in living cells: new insights into nanoparticle uptake, intracellular transport, and vesicle shedding," *J Am Chem Soc*, Vol. 129, No. 47, 2007, pp. 14759-66.
[38] Youngblood, D.S., et al., "Stability of cell-penetrating peptide-morpholino oligomer conjugates in human serum and in cells," *Bioconjug Chem*, Vol. 18, No. 1, 2007, pp. 50-60.
[39] Vandenbroucke, R.E., et al., "Cellular entry pathway and gene transfer capacity of TAT-modified lipoplexes," *Biochim Biophys Acta*, Vol. 1768, No. 3, 2007, pp. 571-9.
[40] Fischer, R., et al., "A targeted protease substrate for a quantitative determination of protease activities in the endolysosomal pathway," *Chembiochem*, Vol. 7, No. 9, 2006, pp. 1428-34.
[41] Rinne, J., et al., "Internalization of novel non-viral vector TAT-streptavidin into human cells," *BMC Biotechnol*, Vol. 7, No. 2007, pp. 1.
[42] Hyndman, L., et al., "HIV-1 Tat protein transduction domain peptide facilitates gene transfer in combination with cationic liposomes," *J Control Release*, Vol. 99, No. 3, 2004, pp. 435-44.
[43] Khalil, I.A., et al., "Octaarginine-modified multifunctional envelope-type nanoparticles for gene delivery," *Gene Ther*, Vol. 14, No. 8, 2007, pp. 682-9.
[44] Yamada, Y., et al., "MITO-Porter: A liposome-based carrier system for delivery of macromolecules into mitochondria via membrane fusion," *Biochim Biophys Acta*, Vol. 1778, No. 2, 2008, pp. 423-32.
[45] El-Andaloussi, S., et al., "Induction of splice correction by cell-penetrating peptide nucleic acids," *J Gene Med*, Vol. 8, No. 10, 2006, pp. 1262-73.
[46] Plank, C., et al., "The influence of endosome-disruptive peptides on gene transfer using synthetic virus-like gene transfer systems," *J Biol Chem*, Vol. 269, No. 17, 1994, pp. 12918-24.
[47] Sugita, T., et al., "Improved cytosolic translocation and tumor-killing activity of Tat-shepherdin conjugates mediated by co-treatment with Tat-fused endosome-disruptive HA2 peptide," *Biochem Biophys Res Commun*, Vol. 363, No. 4, 2007, pp. 1027-32.
[48] Sirsi, S.R., et al., "Functionalized PEG-PEI copolymers complexed to exon-skipping oligonucleotides improve dystrophin expression in mdx mice," *Hum Gene Ther*, Vol. 19, No. 8, 2008, pp. 795-806.
[49] Suk, J.S., et al., "Gene delivery to differentiated neurotypic cells with RGD and HIV Tat peptide functionalized polymeric nanoparticles," *Biomaterials*, Vol. 27, No. 29, 2006, pp. 5143-50.

[50] Shiraishi, T., Pankratova, S., and Nielsen, P.E., "Calcium ions effectively enhance the effect of antisense peptide nucleic acids conjugated to cationic tat and oligoarginine peptides," *Chem Biol*, Vol. 12, No. 8, 2005, pp. 923-9.
[51] Shiraishi, T., and Nielsen, P.E., "Enhanced delivery of cell-penetrating peptide-peptide nucleic acid conjugates by endosomal disruption," *Nat Protoc*, Vol. 1, No. 2, 2006, pp. 633-6.
[52] Christiaens, B., et al., "Membrane interaction and cellular internalization of penetratin peptides," *Eur J Biochem*, Vol. 271, No. 6, 2004, pp. 1187-97.
[53] Zatsepin, T.S., et al., "Conjugates of oligonucleotides and analogues with cell penetrating peptides as gene silencing agents," *Curr Pharm Des*, Vol. 11, No. 28, 2005, pp. 3639-54.
[54] Schwarze, S.R., et al., "In vivo protein transduction: delivery of a biologically active protein into the mouse," *Science*, Vol. 285, No. 5433, 1999, pp. 1569-72.
[55] Lewin, M., et al., "Tat peptide-derivatized magnetic nanoparticles allow in vivo tracking and recovery of progenitor cells," *Nat Biotechnol*, Vol. 18, No. 4, 2000, pp. 410-4.
[56] Juliano, R., et al., "Mechanisms and strategies for effective delivery of antisense and siRNA oligonucleotides," *Nucleic Acids Res*, Vol. 36, No. 12, 2008, pp. 4158-71.
[57] Kim, W.J., et al., "Cholesteryl oligoarginine delivering vascular endothelial growth factor siRNA effectively inhibits tumor growth in colon adenocarcinoma," *Mol Ther*, Vol. 14, No. 3, 2006, pp. 343-50.
[58] Morris, M.C., et al., "Cell-penetrating peptides: from molecular mechanisms to therapeutics," *Biol Cell*, Vol. 100, No. 4, 2008, pp. 201-17.
[59] Meade, B.R., and Dowdy, S.F., "Exogenous siRNA delivery using peptide transduction domains/cell penetrating peptides," *Adv Drug Deliv Rev*, Vol. 59, No. 2-3, 2007, pp. 134-40.
[60] Morris, M.C., et al., "A peptide carrier for the delivery of biologically active proteins into mammalian cells," *Nat Biotechnol*, Vol. 19, No. 12, 2001, pp. 1173-6.
[61] Kumar, P., et al., "Transvascular delivery of small interfering RNA to the central nervous system," *Nature*, Vol. 448, No. 7149, 2007, pp. 39-43.
[62] Lundberg, P., et al., "Delivery of short interfering RNA using endosomolytic cell-penetrating peptides," *Faseb J*, Vol. 21, No. 11, 2007, pp. 2664-71.
[63] Fawell, S., et al., "Tat-mediated delivery of heterologous proteins into cells," *Proc Natl Acad Sci U S A*, Vol. 91, No. 2, 1994, pp. 664-8.
[64] Gros, E., et al., "A non-covalent peptide-based strategy for protein and peptide nucleic acid transduction," *Biochim Biophys Acta*, Vol. 1758, No. 3, 2006, pp. 384-93.
[65] El-Andaloussi, S., Holm, T., and Langel, U., "Cell-penetrating peptides: mechanisms and applications," *Curr Pharm Des*, Vol. 11, No. 28, 2005, pp. 3597-611.
[66] Gupta, B., Levchenko, T.S., and Torchilin, V.P., "Intracellular delivery of large molecules and small particles by cell-penetrating proteins and peptides," *Adv Drug Deliv Rev*, Vol. 57, No. 4, 2005, pp. 637-51.
[67] Mae, M., and Langel, U., "Cell-penetrating peptides as vectors for peptide, protein and oligonucleotide delivery," *Curr Opin Pharmacol*, Vol. 6, No. 5, 2006, pp. 509-14.
[68] Dietz, G.P., and Bahr, M., "Delivery of bioactive molecules into the cell: the Trojan horse approach," *Mol Cell Neurosci*, Vol. 27, No. 2, 2004, pp. 85-131.
[69] Snyder, E.L., and Dowdy, S.F., "Recent advances in the use of protein transduction domains for the delivery of peptides, proteins and nucleic acids in vivo," *Expert Opin Drug Deliv*, Vol. 2, No. 1, 2005, pp. 43-51.
[70] Snyder, E.L., et al., "Treatment of terminal peritoneal carcinomatosis by a transducible p53-activating peptide," *PLoS Biol*, Vol. 2, No. 2, 2004, pp. E36.
[71] Knight, J.S., et al., "A peptide-based inhibitor for prevention of B cell hyperproliferation induced by Epstein-Barr virus," *Virology*, Vol. 354, No. 1, 2006, pp. 207-14.

[72] Kwon, Y.M., et al., "PTD-modified ATTEMPTS system for enhanced asparaginase therapy: a proof-of-concept investigation," *J Control Release*, Vol. 130, No. 3, 2008, pp. 252-8.
[73] Kwon, Y.M., et al., "The ATTEMPTS delivery systems for macromolecular drugs," *Expert Opin Drug Deliv*, Vol. 5, No. 11, 2008, pp. 1255-66.
[74] Massodi, I., et al., "Inhibition of ovarian cancer cell metastasis by a fusion polypeptide Tat-ELP," *Clin Exp Metastasis*, Vol. 26, No. 3, 2009, pp. 251-60.
[75] Moy, P., et al., "Tat-mediated protein delivery can facilitate MHC class I presentation of antigens," *Mol Biotechnol*, Vol. 6, No. 2, 1996, pp. 105-13.
[76] Shibagaki, N., and Udey, M.C., "Dendritic cells transduced with protein antigens induce cytotoxic lymphocytes and elicit antitumor immunity," *J Immunol*, Vol. 168, No. 5, 2002, pp. 2393-401.
[77] Wang, H.Y., et al., "Induction of CD4(+) T cell-dependent antitumor immunity by TAT-mediated tumor antigen delivery into dendritic cells," *J Clin Invest*, Vol 109, No. 11, 2002, pp. 1463-70.
[78] Kabouridis, P.S., et al., "Inhibition of NF-kappa B activity by a membrane-transducing mutant of I kappa B alpha," *J Immunol*, Vol. 169, No. 5, 2002, pp. 2587-93.
[79] Cao, G., et al., "In Vivo Delivery of a Bcl-xL Fusion Protein Containing the TAT Protein Transduction Domain Protects against Ischemic Brain Injury and Neuronal Apoptosis," *J Neurosci*, Vol. 22, No. 13, 2002, pp. 5423-31.
[80] Khafagy el, S., et al., "Effect of cell-penetrating peptides on the nasal absorption of insulin," *J Control Release*, Vol. 133, No. 2, 2009, pp. 103-8.
[81] Wheeler, D.S., Dunsmore, K.E., and Wong, H.R., "Intracellular delivery of HSP70 using HIV-1 Tat protein transduction domain," *Biochem Biophys Res Commun*, Vol. 301, No. 1, 2003, pp. 54-9.
[82] Eum, W.S., et al., "In vivo protein transduction: biologically active intact pep-1-superoxide dismutase fusion protein efficiently protects against ischemic insult," *Free Radic Biol Med*, Vol. 37, No. 10, 2004, pp. 1656-69.
[83] Gallo, G., "Making proteins into drugs: assisted delivery of proteins and peptides into living neurons," *Methods Cell Biol*, Vol. 71, No. 2003, pp. 325-38.
[84] Cornelissen, B., et al., "Cellular penetration and nuclear importation properties of 111In-labeled and 123I-labeled HIV-1 tat peptide immunoconjugates in BT-474 human breast cancer cells," *Nucl Med Biol*, Vol. 34, No. 1, 2007, pp. 37-46.
[85] Josephson, L., et al., "High-efficiency intracellular magnetic labeling with novel superparamagnetic-Tat peptide conjugates," *Bioconjug Chem*, Vol. 10, No. 2, 1999, pp. 186-91.
[86] Dodd, C.H., et al., "Normal T-cell response and in vivo magnetic resonance imaging of T cells loaded with HIV transactivator-peptide-derived superparamagnetic nanoparticles," *J Immunol Methods*, Vol. 256, No. 1-2, 2001, pp. 89-105.
[87] Kaufman, C.L., et al., "Superparamagnetic iron oxide particles transactivator protein-fluorescein isothiocyanate particle labeling for in vivo magnetic resonance imaging detection of cell migration: uptake and durability," *Transplantation*, Vol. 76, No. 7, 2003, pp. 1043-6.
[88] Tkachenko, A.G., et al., "Cellular trajectories of peptide-modified gold particle complexes: comparison of nuclear localization signals and peptide transduction domains," *Bioconjug Chem*, Vol. 15, No. 3, 2004, pp. 482-90.
[89] Zhao, M., et al., "Differential conjugation of tat peptide to superparamagnetic nanoparticles and its effect on cellular uptake," *Bioconjug Chem*, Vol. 13, No. 4, 2002, pp. 840-4.
[90] Pittet, M.J., et al., "Labeling of immune cells for in vivo imaging using magnetofluorescent nanoparticles," *Nat Protoc*, Vol. 1, No. 1, 2006, pp. 73-9.

[91] Cryan, S.A., et al., "Increased intracellular targeting to airway cells using octaarginine-coated liposomes: in vitro assessment of their suitability for inhalation," *Mol Pharm*, Vol. 3, No. 2, 2006, pp. 104-12.
[92] Liu, J., et al., "Nanostructured materials designed for cell binding and transduction," *Biomacromolecules*, Vol. 2, No. 2, 2001, pp. 362-8.
[93] Becker, M.L., et al., "Peptide-derivatized shell-cross-linked nanoparticles. 1. Synthesis and characterization," *Bioconjug Chem*, Vol. 15, No. 4, 2004, pp. 699-709.
[94] Becker, M.L., Bailey, L.O., and Wooley, K.L., "Peptide-derivatized shell-cross-linked nanoparticles. 2. Biocompatibility evaluation," *Bioconjug Chem*, Vol. 15, No. 4, 2004, pp. 710-7.
[95] Santra, S., et al., "TAT conjugated, FITC doped silica nanoparticles for bioimaging applications," *Chem Commun (Camb)*, Vol. 24, 2004, pp. 2810-1.
[96] de la Fuente, J.M., and Berry, C.C., "Tat peptide as an efficient molecule to translocate gold nanoparticles into the cell nucleus," *Bioconjug Chem*, Vol. 16, No. 5, 2005, pp. 1176-80.
[97] Nativo, P., Prior, I.A., and Brust, M., "Uptake and intracellular fate of surface-modified gold nanoparticles," *ACS Nano*, Vol. 2, No. 8, 2008, pp. 1639-44.
[98] Zhang, K., et al., "Shape effects of nanoparticles conjugated with cell-penetrating peptides (HIV Tat PTD) on CHO cell uptake," *Bioconjug Chem*, Vol. 19, No. 9, 2008, pp. 1880-7.
[99] Medintz, I.L., et al., "Quantum dot bioconjugates for imaging, labelling and sensing," *Nat Mater*, Vol. 4, No. 6, 2005, pp. 435-46.
[100] Santra, S., et al., "Rapid and effective labeling of brain tissue using TAT-conjugated CdS:Mn/ZnS quantum dots," *Chem Commun (Camb)*, Vol. 25, 2005, pp. 3144-6.
[101] Chen, B., et al., "Transmembrane delivery of the cell-penetrating peptide conjugated semiconductor quantum dots," *Langmuir*, Vol. 24, No. 20, 2008, pp. 11866-71.
[102] Ballou, B., et al., "Noninvasive imaging of quantum dots in mice," *Bioconjug Chem*, Vol. 15, No. 1, 2004, pp. 79-86.
[103] Silver, J., and Ou, W., "Photoactivation of quantum dot fluorescence following endocytosis," *Nano Lett*, Vol. 5, No. 7, 2005, pp. 1445-9.
[104] Delehanty, J.B., et al., "Self-assembled quantum dot-peptide bioconjugates for selective intracellular delivery," *Bioconjug Chem*, Vol. 17, No. 4, 2006, pp. 920-7.
[105] Rozenzhak, S.M., et al., "Cellular internalization and targeting of semiconductor quantum dots," *Chem Commun (Camb)*, Vol. 17, 2005, pp. 2217-9.
[106] Lasic, D.D., *Liposomes: From Physics to Applications*, Amersterdam: Elsevier, 1993.
[107] Torchilin, V.P., "Recent advances with liposomes as pharmaceutical carriers," *Nat Rev Drug Discov*, Vol. 4, No. 2, 2005, pp. 145-60.
[108] Lasic, D.D., and Martin, F.J., *Stealth Liposomes*, Boca Raton: CRC Press, 1995.
[109] Torchilin, V.P., et al., "Poly(ethylene glycol)-coated anti-cardiac myosin immunoliposomes: factors influencing targeted accumulation in the infarcted myocardium," *Biochim Biophys Acta*, Vol. 1279, No. 1, 1996, pp. 75-83.
[110] Torchilin, V.P., et al., "p-Nitrophenylcarbonyl-PEG-PE-liposomes: fast and simple attachment of specific ligands, including monoclonal antibodies, to distal ends of PEG chains via p-nitrophenylcarbonyl groups," *Biochim Biophys Acta*, Vol. 1511, No. 2, 2001, pp. 397-411.
[111] Torchilin, V.P., "Structure and design of polymeric surfactant-based drug delivery systems," *J Control Release*, Vol. 73, No. 2-3, 2001, pp. 137-72.
[112] Torchilin, V.P., "Micellar nanocarriers: pharmaceutical perspectives," *Pharm Res*, Vol. 24, No. 1, 2007, pp. 1-16.
[113] Maeda, H., et al., "Tumor vascular permeability and the EPR effect in macromolecular therapeutics: a review," *J Control Release*, Vol. 65, No. 1-2, 2000, pp. 271-84.

[114] Maeda, H., Bharate, G.Y., and Daruwalla, J., "Polymeric drugs for efficient tumor-targeted drug delivery based on EPR-effect," *Eur J Pharm Biopharm*, Vol.71, No.3, 2009, pp. 409-19.
[115] Lukyanov, A.N., and Torchilin, V.P., "Micelles from lipid derivatives of water-soluble polymers as delivery systems for poorly soluble drugs," *Adv Drug Deliv Rev*, Vol. 56, No. 9, 2004, pp. 1273-89.
[116] Lukyanov, A.N., et al., "Polyethylene glycol-diacyllipid micelles demonstrate increased accumulation in subcutaneous tumors in mice," *Pharm Res*, Vol. 19, No. 10, 2002, pp. 1424-9.
[117] Torchilin, V.P., et al., "TAT peptide on the surface of liposomes affords their efficient intracellular delivery even at low temperature and in the presence of metabolic inhibitors," *Proc Natl Acad Sci U S A*, Vol. 98, No. 15, 2001, pp. 8786-91.
[118] Torchilin, V.P., et al., "Cell transfection in vitro and in vivo with nontoxic TAT peptide-liposome-DNA complexes," *Proc Natl Acad Sci U S A*, Vol. 100, No. 4, 2003, pp. 1972-7.
[119] Tseng, Y.L., Liu, J.J., and Hong, R.L., "Translocation of liposomes into cancer cells by cell-penetrating peptides penetratin and tat: a kinetic and efficacy study," *Mol Pharmacol*, Vol. 62, No. 4, 2002, pp. 864-72.
[120] Fretz, M.M., et al., "OVCAR-3 cells internalize TAT-peptide modified liposomes by endocytosis," *Biochim Biophys Acta*, Vol. 1665, No. 1-2, 2004, pp. 48-56.
[121] Marty, C., et al., "Enhanced heparan sulfate proteoglycan-mediated uptake of cell-penetrating peptide-modified liposomes," *Cell Mol Life Sci*, Vol. 61, No. 14, 2004, pp. 1785-94.
[122] Sawant, R.R., et al., "The architecture of ligand attachment to nanocarriers controls their specific interaction with target cells," *J Drug Target*, Vol. 16, No. 7, 2008, pp. 596-600.
[123] Ignatovich, I.A., et al., "Complexes of plasmid DNA with basic domain 47-57 of the HIV-1 Tat protein are transferred to mammalian cells by endocytosis-mediated pathways," *J Biol Chem*, Vol. 278, No. 43, 2003, pp. 42625-36.
[124] Rudolph, C., et al., "Application of novel solid lipid nanoparticle (SLN)-gene vector formulations based on a dimeric HIV-1 TAT-peptide in vitro and in vivo," *Pharm Res*, Vol. 21, No. 9, 2004, pp. 1662-9.
[125] Huang, Z., et al., "Thiocholesterol-based lipids for ordered assembly of bioresponsive gene carriers," *Mol Ther*, Vol. 11, No. 3, 2005, pp. 409-17.
[126] Gupta, B., Levchenko, T.S., and Torchilin, V.P., "TAT peptide-modified liposomes provide enhanced gene delivery to intracranial human brain tumor xenografts in nude mice," *Oncol Res*, Vol. 16, No. 8, 2007, pp. 351-9.
[127] Pappalardo, J.S., et al., "Improved transfection of spleen-derived antigen-presenting cells in culture using TATp-liposomes," *J Control Release*, Vol. 134, No. 1, 2009, pp. 41-6.
[128] Ko, Y.T., et al., "Gene delivery into ischemic myocardium by double-targeted lipoplexes with anti-myosin antibody and TAT peptide," *Gene Ther*, Vol. 16, No. 1, 2009, pp. 52-9.
[129] Kogure, K., et al., "Development of a non-viral multifunctional envelope-type nano device by a novel lipid film hydration method," *J Control Release*, Vol. 98, No. 2, 2004, pp. 317-23.
[130] Kleemann, E., et al., "Nano-carriers for DNA delivery to the lung based upon a TAT-derived peptide covalently coupled to PEG-PEI," *J Control Release*, Vol. 109, No. 1-3, 2005, pp. 299-316.
[131] Nguyen, J., et al., "Effects of cell-penetrating peptides and pegylation on transfection efficiency of polyethylenimine in mouse lungs," *J Gene Med*, Vol. 10, No. 11, 2008, pp. 1236-46.
[132] Juliano, R.L., "Intracellular delivery of oligonucleotide conjugates and dendrimer complexes," *Ann N Y Acad Sci*, Vol. 1082, No. 2006, pp. 18-26.

[133] Coles, D.J., et al., "The characterization of a novel dendritic system for gene delivery by isothermal titration calorimetry," *Biopolymers*, Vol. 90, No. 5, 2008, pp. 651-4.
[134] Kim, T.I., et al., "Synthesis and characterization of a novel arginine-grafted dendritic block copolymer for gene delivery and study of its cellular uptake pathway leading to transfection," *Bioconjug Chem*, Vol. 18, No. 2, 2007, pp. 309-17.
[135] Meade, B.R., and Dowdy, S.F., "Enhancing the cellular uptake of siRNA duplexes following noncovalent packaging with protein transduction domain peptides," *Adv Drug Deliv Rev*, Vol. 60, No. 4-5, 2008, pp. 530-6.
[136] Simeoni, F., et al., "Insight into the mechanism of the peptide-based gene delivery system MPG: implications for delivery of siRNA into mammalian cells," *Nucleic Acids Res*, Vol. 31, No. 11, 2003, pp. 2717-24.
[137] Davidson, T.J., et al., "Highly efficient small interfering RNA delivery to primary mammalian neurons induces MicroRNA-like effects before mRNA degradation," *J Neurosci*, Vol. 24, No. 45, 2004, pp. 10040-6.
[138] Zhang, C., et al., "siRNA-containing liposomes modified with polyarginine effectively silence the targeted gene," *J Control Release*, Vol. 112, No. 2, 2006, pp. 229-39.
[139] Law, M., Jafari, M., and Chen, P., "Physicochemical characterization of siRNA-peptide complexes," *Biotechnol Prog*, Vol. 24, No. 4, 2008, pp. 957-63.
[140] Muratovska, A., and Eccles, M.R., "Conjugate for efficient delivery of short interfering RNA (siRNA) into mammalian cells," *FEBS Lett*, Vol. 558, No. 1-3, 2004, pp. 63-8.
[141] Nakamura, Y., et al., "Octaarginine-modified multifunctional envelope-type nano device for siRNA," *J Control Release*, Vol. 119, No. 3, 2007, pp. 360-7.
[142] Moschos, S.A., et al., "Lung delivery studies using siRNA conjugated to TAT(48-60) and penetratin reveal peptide induced reduction in gene expression and induction of innate immunity," *Bioconjug Chem*, Vol. 18, No. 5, 2007, pp. 1450-9.
[143] Moschos, S.A., Williams, A.E., and Lindsay, M.A., "Cell-penetrating-peptide-mediated siRNA lung delivery," *Biochem Soc Trans*, Vol. 35, No. Pt 4, 2007, pp. 807-10.
[144] Torchilin, V.P., "Targeted polymeric micelles for delivery of poorly soluble drugs," *Cell Mol Life Sci*, Vol. 61, No. 19-20, 2004, pp. 2549-59.
[145] Jaracz, S., et al., "Recent advances in tumor-targeting anticancer drug conjugates," *Bioorg Med Chem*, Vol. 13, No. 17, 2005, pp. 5043-54.
[146] Gabizon, A., et al., "Tumor cell targeting of liposome-entrapped drugs with phospholipid-anchored folic acid-PEG conjugates," *Adv Drug Deliv Rev*, Vol. 56, No. 8, 2004, pp. 1177-92.
[147] Widera, A., Norouziyan, F., and Shen, W.C., "Mechanisms of TfR-mediated transcytosis and sorting in epithelial cells and applications toward drug delivery," *Adv Drug Deliv Rev*, Vol. 55, No. 11, 2003, pp. 1439-66.
[148] Sawant, R.M., et al., " "SMART" drug delivery systems: double-targeted pH-responsive pharmaceutical nanocarriers," *Bioconjug Chem*, Vol. 17, No. 4, 2006, pp. 943-9.
[149] Kale, A.A., and Torchilin, V.P., "Design, synthesis, and characterization of pH-sensitive PEG-PE conjugates for stimuli-sensitive pharmaceutical nanocarriers: the effect of substitutes at the hydrazone linkage on the ph stability of PEG-PE conjugates," *Bioconjug Chem*, Vol. 18, No. 2, 2007, pp. 363-70.
[150] Kale, A.A., and Torchilin, V.P., "Enhanced transfection of tumor cells in vivo using "Smart" pH-sensitive TAT-modified pegylated liposomes," *J Drug Target*, Vol. 15, No. 7-8, 2007, pp. 538-45.
[151] Sethuraman, V.A., and Bae, Y.H., "TAT peptide-based micelle system for potential active targeting of anti-cancer agents to acidic solid tumors," *J Control Release*, Vol. 118, No. 2, 2007, pp. 216-24.

[152] Futaki, S., "Oligoarginine vectors for intracellular delivery: design and cellular-uptake mechanisms," *Biopolymers*, Vol. 84, No. 3, 2006, pp. 241-9.
[153] Fuchs, S.M., and Raines, R.T., "Pathway for polyarginine entry into mammalian cells," *Biochemistry*, Vol. 43, No. 9, 2004, pp. 2438-44.
[154] Potocky, T.B., Menon, A.K., and Gellman, S.H., "Cytoplasmic and nuclear delivery of a TAT-derived peptide and a beta-peptide after endocytic uptake into HeLa cells," *J Biol Chem*, Vol. 278, No. 50, 2003, pp. 50188-94.
[155] Fischer, R., et al., "A stepwise dissection of the intracellular fate of cationic cell-penetrating peptides,"*J Biol Chem*, Vol. 279, No. 13, 2004, pp. 12625-35.
[156] Hitz, T., et al., "Interaction of alpha-and beta-oligoarginine-acids and amides with anionic lipid vesicles: a mechanistic and thermodynamic study," *Biochemistry*, Vol. 45, No. 18, 2006, pp. 5817-29.
[157] Hafez, I.M., and Cullis, P.R., "Roles of lipid polymorphism in intracellular delivery," *Adv Drug Deliv Rev*, Vol. 47, No. 2-3, 2001, pp. 139-48.
[158] Zhou, X., and Huang, L., "DNA transfection mediated by cationic liposomes containing lipopolylysine: characterization and mechanism of action," *Biochim Biophys Acta*, Vol. 1189, No. 2, 1994, pp. 195-203.
[159] Kogure, K., Akita, H., and Harashima, H., "Multifunctional envelope-type nano device for non-viral gene delivery: concept and application of Programmed Packaging," *J Control Release*, Vol. 122, No. 3, 2007, pp. 246-51.
[160] Kogure, K., et al., "Multifunctional envelope-type nano device (MEND) as a non-viral gene delivery system," *Adv Drug Deliv Rev*, Vol. 60, No. 4-5, 2008, pp. 559-71.
[161] Nakamura, Y., et al., "Significant and prolonged antisense effect of a multifunctional envelope-type nano device encapsulating antisense oligodeoxynucleotide," *J Pharm Pharmacol*, Vol. 58, No. 4, 2006, pp. 431-7.
[162] Suzuki, R., Yamada, Y., and Harashima, H., "Efficient cytoplasmic protein delivery by means of a multifunctional envelope-type nano device," *Biol Pharm Bull*, Vol. 30, No. 4, 2007, pp. 758-62.
[163] Nakamura, T., et al., "Efficient MHC class I presentation by controlled intracellular trafficking of antigens in octaarginine-modified liposomes," *Mol Ther*, Vol. 16, No. 8, 2008, pp. 1507-14.
[164] Kaplan, I.M., Wadia, J.S., and Dowdy, S.F., "Cationic TAT peptide transduction domain enters cells by macropinocytosis," *J Control Release*, Vol. 102, No. 1, 2005, pp. 247-53.
[165] Lo, S.L., and Wang, S., "An endosomolytic Tat peptide produced by incorporation of histidine and cysteine residues as a nonviral vector for DNA transfection," *Biomaterials*, Vol. 29, No. 15, 2008, pp. 2408-14.
[166] Midoux, P., and Monsigny, M., "Efficient gene transfer by histidylated polylysine/pDNA complexes," *Bioconjug Chem*, Vol. 10, No. 3, 1999, pp. 406-11.
[167] Boussif, O., et al., "A versatile vector for gene and oligonucleotide transfer into cells in culture and in vivo: polyethylenimine," *Proc Natl Acad Sci U S A*, Vol. 92, No. 16, 1995, pp. 7297-301.
[168] Huang, R.Q., Pei, Y.Y., and Jiang, C., "Enhanced gene transfer into brain capillary endothelial cells using Antp-modified DNA-loaded nanoparticles," *J Biomed Sci*, Vol. 14, No. 5, 2007, pp. 595-605.

Section 3

Cell Responsive Biomaterials in Tissue Engineering

CHAPTER 10

BIOMIMETIC MATRICES FOR INTEGRIN-MEDIATED CELL ADHESION

Keshia M. Ashe, Duron A. Lee, Kevin W.-H. Lo, Lakshmi S. Nair and Cato T. Laurencin*

Department of Orthopaedic Surgery, University of Connecticut, Farmington, CT 06030, USA
**E-mail: Laurencin@uchc.edu*

1. Introduction

Tissue engineering is a relatively new field, involving "the application of biological, chemical, and engineering principles towards the repair, restoration, or regeneration of living tissues using biomaterials, cells, and factors, alone or in combination" [1]. The use of synthetic biomaterials as implants has been a central theme due to limited availability of autologous tissue, relative ease of material attainment or fabrication, and favorable biocompatibility characteristics inherently present in many of these biomaterials [2]. However, in order for these implants to successfully enhance tissue regeneration, cells must be able to use transmembrane surface adhesion receptors, or integrins, to effectively adhere to material surfaces via adsorbed or immobilized proteins. This adhesion promotes normal cellular behaviors such as proliferation, migration, and differentiation [3]. Without proper osteoblast integrin-mediated adhesion, poor cell-substrate interactions can lead to problems such as *in vivo* fibrosis and implant encapsulation, foreign body reaction, inflammation, aseptic loosening and local bone resorption [2]. In order to circumvent these problems, researchers have looked to biological mimicry (or biomimetics) in an attempt to fabricate materials with certain chemical, biological and morphological surface properties that are capable of eliciting or modulating specific cellular responses, and ultimately enhance new tissue formation *in situ* [4]. By modeling biological properties or processes that naturally occur in the body, biologically inert materials can be enhanced with functional biomolecules derived from the biological microenvironment and incorporated directly onto or within a biomaterial. As such, biomaterials have been created with the incorporation of specific biomolecules for several tissue engineering applications, among which the addition of molecular ligands for engagement with cell-surface receptors has received much attention [5]. Further, materials with intrinsic bioactive characteristics, such as hydroxyapatite, have been explored extensively for orthopaedic applications due to their unique bone forming abilities.

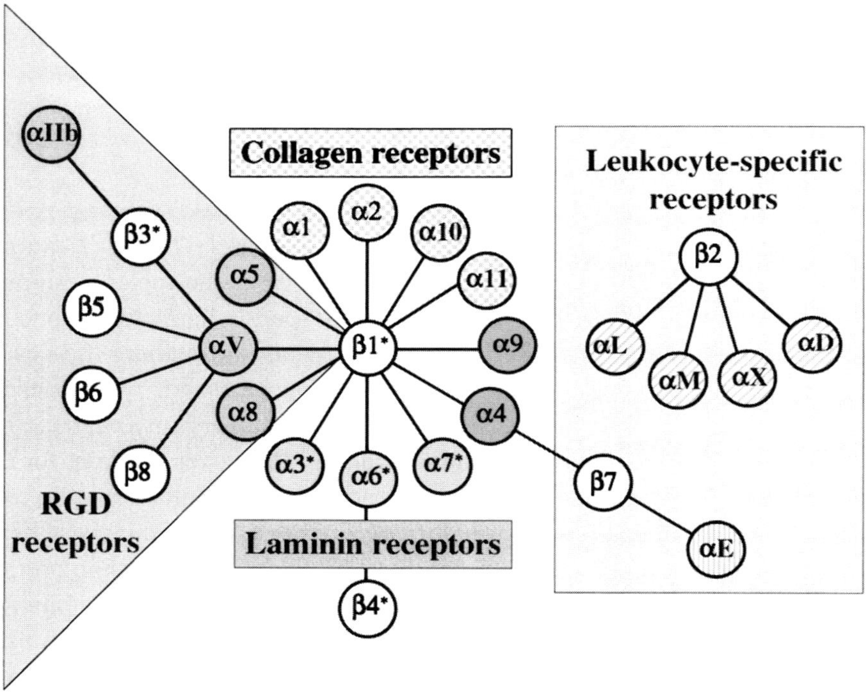

Fig. 1. Diagram of the integrin superfamily (Reprinted from [13], with permission from publisher).

In the present review, we will explore how the integrin-mediated interactions of cells with proteins of the extracellular matrix (ECM), a fibrous network connecting cells together in tissues, can serve as a model system for developing biomimetic materials for tissue engineering applications. We will focus on two main strategies used to modify biomaterials with ECM-derived biomolecules for tissue regeneration: 1) the alteration of surface physicochemical properties to modulate ECM protein adsorption and subsequent cell interactions and 2) the immobilization ECM-derived biomolecules to the surface of biomaterials. As such, we will look at various physical and chemical immobilization schemes used to modify biomaterial surfaces with biologically active ECM-derived molecules for directed cell and tissue responses. In addition, we will discuss how bioactive ceramics have been shown to enhance favorable cell responses, such as bone mineralization, in tissue engineered biomimetic implants.

2. Integrin-mediated Cell Adhesion

Integrins, a family of glycoprotein heterodimers, are transmembrane cell surface adhesion receptors that represent a major pathway used by virtually all cell types to interact with different extracellular matrix components [6]. Integrins play a central role in the development, organization, maintenance and repair of various tissues by providing anchorage and triggering signals that direct cell survival, migration, cell cycle progression, and expression of differentiated phenotypes [7]. Integrins also play a crucial role in immune and inflammatory responses [8-10]. Each integrin is comprised of a large α-subunit containing several cation-binding sites and a smaller β-subunit. There are over 18 α- and 8 β-subunits, which non-covalently assemble together in the presence of extracellular calcium to form at least 24 distinct integrin units [11] [Figure 1]. Broadly defined by their β-subunit, the composition of the αβ heterodimer determines the specificity of the integrin towards various ECM protein ligands. Some of the heterodimer combinations are highly specific, while others demonstrate promiscuity toward multiple ECM ligands. Accordingly, many ECM proteins serve as ligands for several integrin molecules [12]. Thus, the binding of integrins to their ligand is not one-to-one and varies within cell type, local environment and material substrate. This interaction is also affected by the conformation (section 4.1), concentration, and spatial distribution (section 5.2) of the ligand to which the integrin binds.

3. Cellular Adhesion to Implanted Biomaterials

In native tissues, the ECM serves many functions, including providing physical support for cell anchorage and regulating cellular behavior. The ECM is a complex structural entity composed of structural fibrillar proteins (collagen, elastin); amorphous, high-molecular weight interfibrillar proteoglycans; and specialized proteins (fibronectin, laminin, growth factors). The type, amount, and composition of the ECM is diverse in nature, varies by tissue type, and gives tissues their unique physical, structural and biological properties [25,26]. Resident cells interact with their surrounding ECM through a process of biological recognition, which involves the specific binding of integrins with their corresponding ligands present in the ECM. Such ligands can exist within structural adhesion proteins of the ECM or as cellular growth factors sequestered within the ECM. Upon receptor-ligand binding, specific cell responses, including attachment, proliferation and differentiation, regulate the behavior of anchorage-dependent cells and ultimately direct tissue formation [7]. Thus, the ECM serves a dual function: as a substratum for physical support and cell anchorage, as well as a key regulator of cell behavior by providing molecular signals to resident cell populations. Moreover, the specific interaction between cells and the ECM ligands through biorecognition is crucial for the maintenance of normal tissue structure and function [20,25-28].

A similar process of biorecognition occurs when host cells interact with implanted biomaterials [29]. Once biomaterials are introduced into the biological environment, non-specific adsorption of soluble ECM proteins occurs spontaneously on the biomaterial surface [30,31]. These long chain proteins range in various orientations, 3-dimensional conformations, size and binding

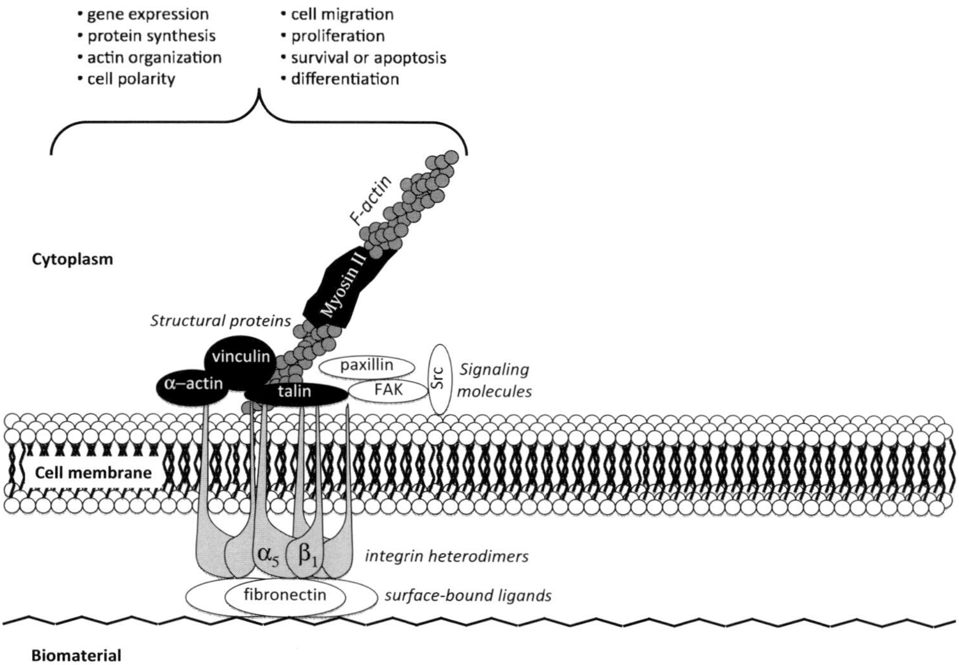

Fig. 2. Diagram Representation of the cell proteins involved in integrin-mediated cell adhesion to biomaterials.

affinity. The exact concentration, composition and conformational state of the adsorbed proteins depend highly on the surface properties of the implanted biomaterial, and how these surfaces bind various biomolecules [31]. Cells interact with the implanted biomaterial through this intervening adsorbed protein layer via membrane-associated proteins and integrin receptors [5] [Figure 2]. The specificity of the cell-surface interaction, in part, is derived from the composition and organization of the protein layer [32]. Thus, the adsorbed protein layer is essential in regulating subsequent cellular behavior at the interface of these implanted biomaterials.

4. Biomimetic Materials for Tissue Engineering using ECM Proteins

Within the last 30 years, in an effort to mimic the integrin-mediated signaling phenomenon detailed in section 2, researchers have developed surface modification techniques to endow otherwise biologically inert biomaterials with ECM proteins [3,33-36]. These materials include polymeric films and scaffolds [37], metallic implants [38], and bioceramics [39]. Surface modifications are

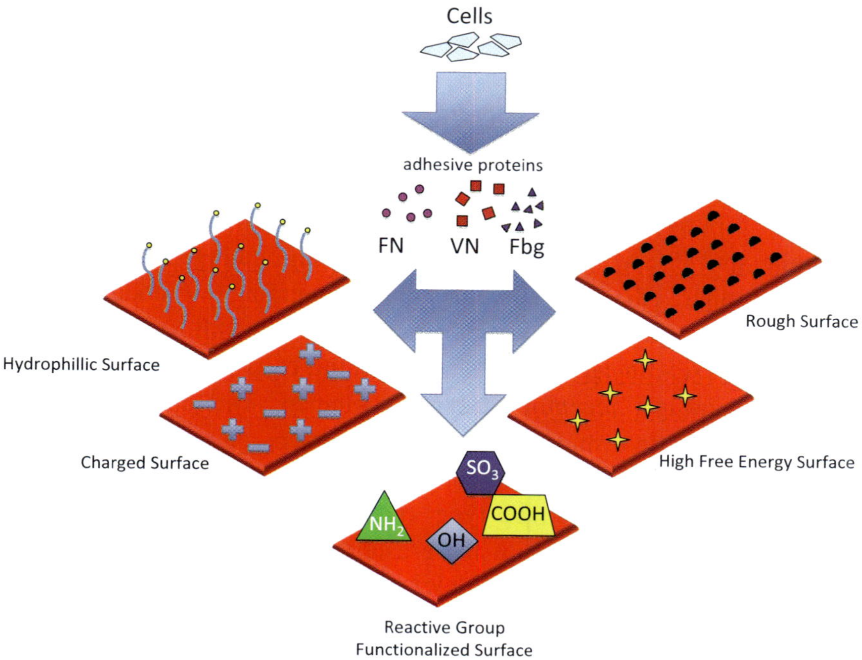

Fig. 3. Integrin interactions with adhesive proteins such as fibronectin (FN), vitronectin (VN) and fibrinogen (Fbg) to adhere to modified biomaterials surfaces.

advantageous because they allow for the modulation of material surface properties within the first few outermost molecular layers of a solid surface, while retaining the beneficial properties of the bulk material such as biocompatibility, degradability, and mechanical integrity [40]. Methods to accomplish these modifications range from simple non-specific protein adsorption [36] to more complex techniques that change the surface properties of a material, such as hydrophilicity, charge, topology, and chemical makeup, to enhance protein adsorption from serum or plasma [40] [Figure 3]. As reviewed below, each technique has unique advantages and disadvantages, and varies highly depending on the biomaterial, target protein, technique used, physiological environment, and cell type of interest.

4.1. *Physical adsorption of ECM proteins to biomaterials*

Physical adsorption of ECM proteins is the oldest, easiest, and most widely used technique to enhance the bioactivity of any material. When a foreign material such as a polymeric film or metallic substrate is introduced into a physiological environment, proteins such as fibronectin (FN) and vitronectin (VN) are non-specifically and spontaneously adsorbed on the surface of the material [36,41]. As demonstrated by García et al. [42], the increasing density of a FN adsorbed layer results in a linear increase in density of $\alpha_5\beta_1$ integrin-FN bonds, as predicted by simple receptor-ligand equilibrium. However, as Nikolovski et al. [43] demonstrated, the amount of non-specific protein absorbed from serum-containing solutions differs with material used. Results revealed that in solutions with equal protein concentrations, VN adsorbs favorably over FN onto polyglycolic acid (PGA), polylactic acid (PLA), and collagen 2D films and 3D scaffolds. Further, the proteins adsorbed specifically modulate integrin expression. The adhesion of smooth muscle cells (SMCs) is mediated by adhesion of the $\alpha_v\beta_5$ integrin receptor to VN, the $\alpha_5\beta_1$ integrin receptor to FN, and the $\alpha_2\beta_1$ integrin receptor to type-I collagen. This integrin expression, however, is tunable. In a study conducted by Stephansson et al. [44], the binding and clustering of MC3T3-E1 osteoblast-like cell $\alpha_5\beta_1$ integrins into focal adhesions varied with substrate type (untreated, tissue culture, and type-I collagen-coated polystyrene), with the greatest binding and clustering observed on the biomimetic surface. This resulting integrin expression has been shown in countless studies to modulate cell behavior. For instance, Chastain and colleagues [45] showed that mesenchymal stem cell (MSC) osteogenic differentiation was particularly enhanced with collagen-I mediated adhesion to thin films of poly(lactic-co-glycolic acid) (PLAGA), as opposed to VN mediated adhesion to thin films of poly-ε-caprolactone (PCL). Similarly, El-Amin and colleagues [46] found that human osteoblasts expressed higher levels of the osteoblast marker protein, osteocalcin, and adhered to PLAGA at a rate significantly higher than on PLA polymers at 3, 6 and 12 h. This adhesion was confirmed by higher expression levels of the integrin subunits α_1, α_2, α_3, α_4, α_5, α_6, and β_1, with $\alpha_2\beta_1$ and β_5 showing the greatest difference in levels between the two surfaces. Studies carried out on metallic implants, such as Titanium (Ti), show increased osteoblast collagen synthesis, but decreased bone formation, or alkaline phosphatase (ALP) activity and calcium deposition, on type-III collagen Ti coatings as compared to non-coated substrates. [47]. These studies are representative of the myriad of studies conducted on protein adsorption, integrin expression, and subsequent cell behavior, and indicate the inherent complexity of mimicking interactions.

The most important aspect of surface bioactivation is preservation of the protein biological activity after attachment to the bio-inert surface. Upon adsorption, proteins frequently undergo conformational changes from protein native structures to denatured states [41]. This event changes the available binding sequences for cell adhesive integrins and thus affects cell adherence ability to biomaterials. Protein denaturing can be prompted by solution related factors such as concentration. For instance, MacDonald et al. [48] demonstrated that at low concentrations protein conformation of human plasma FN coated on commercially pure Ti scaffolds had a small globular structure (similar to that in solution), while at higher concentrations it appeared as a thin cross-linked monolayer. Rico et al. confirmed this phenomenon on polymer surfaces as well [49]. Also, protein denaturation can occur because of specific surface properties such as hydrophobicity, electric charge, topography, and chemistry. As demonstrated by García et al. [50], different substrates change FN conformations, which alter the quantity of bound C2C12 myoblast integrin α_5- and β_1-subunits and affects myoblast proliferation and differentiation. Martínez et al. [51] elucidated the effects of crystallinity, showing how FN tended to expand its arms and form a protein network on smooth poly-L-lactide (PLLA) substrates, unlike the maintenance of its globular structure on semicrystalline PLLA. Thus, investigating the effects of these surface physiochemical properties on the conformation, density, and spatial distribution of the intervening adsorbed protein layer and ensuing integrin binding is critical in understanding how various cell types will adhere, proliferate, and differentiate on an implanted material [29,52].

4.1.1. *Influencing ECM protein adsorption*

The surface properties and structure of a biomaterial play an essential role in protein adsorption. As such, changes in the surface physicochemical properties and micro/nano-structure of biomaterials may in turn alter their bioactivity.

Hydrophilicity/Hydrophilicity: Many studies have investigated hydrophilicity and hydrophobicity as it relates to protein adsorption and subsequent cell adhesion. Highly hydrophobic surfaces (water contact angle > 30°) favor the adsorption of proteins from aqueous solutions thermodynamically, but these tight bonds may result in denatured protein structures and overall decrease in bioactivity [51]. On the other hand, highly hydrophilic surfaces (water contact angle < 150°) may expel proteins molecules and inhibit adsorption [52]. Therefore neither highly hydrophobic nor hydrophilic surfaces are preferred for protein adsorption. This has lead to the widely accepted concept that proteins and cells attach well to surfaces with moderate wettability so proteins are adsorbed while also maintaining their native conformations [52].

Table 1. Effects of plasma treatments on hydrophilicity of PDLLA and collagen-coated surfaces. Adapted from [40].

Modification Method	Contact Angle (°)	
	θH_2O	θCH_2I_2
None	78.0	37.0
NH_3 plasma	21.5	40.0
N_2 plasma	25.5	33.5
O_2 plasma	45.0	26.5
(O_2 + NH_3 plasma)*	17.0	32.0
Collagen coating	61.9	38.3
(Collagen anchorage)**	54.3	42.8

* 60 s for O_2 and then 60 s for NH_3
**NH_3 plasma pre-treated

There are several methods used to increase hydrophilicity, notably plasma treatments [Table 1] and polymer grafting. For plasma treatments, low-pressure gases such as argon [53], ammonia [54] or oxygen [55] are ionized into free radicals, ions, protons, electrons, gas atoms, and molecules of different energies. These high-energy species are driven onto the material surface to result in chemical and physical changes ranging in depths of several hundred angstroms to 10 microns [36]. Introducing hydroxyl, carboxyl, amino, and sulfate groups on substrate surfaces, not only increases hydrophilicity, but also prepares these surfaces for the covalent immobilization of ECM-derived proteins (section 5.1). The other common method to increase hydrophilicity on polymer surfaces is to graft hydrophilic polymers such as poly(acrylamide) (PAM) or poly(hydroxylethyl methacrylate) (PHEMA) onto hydrophobic polymers such as PCL [56] and PLA [57]. The introduction of initiators can be achieved by argon plasma treatment, ozone oxidation, γ-ray, electron irradiation, and laser treatment [58-60]

Numerous studies have explored the role of hydrophilicity on protein adsorption, integrin expression, focal adhesion formations, and whole cell adhesion. Alves et al. [61] recently showed that oxygen radio frequency glow discharge on poly (D, L, lactide) (PDLLA) affects protein adsorption and bone cell behavior. Plasma treated films showed an increase in hydrophilicity and surface energy, which lead to higher percentages of FN deposition and increased MG63 osteoblast-like cell and fetal rat calvarial cell adhesion as compared to untreated films. To explore the effects of hydrophobicity on integrin expression, Liu et al. [62] compared α_2, α_3, α_4, α_5, α_v, β_1, and β_3 integrin subunit expression by human fetal osteoblastic (hFOB) cells cultured on hydrophilic and hydrophobic surfaces for 3 and 6 days. They found that hFOB cells cultured on hydrophillic surfaces initially expressed significantly higher levels of α_v and β_3 subunits than on hydrophobic surfaces, but this difference decreased with time in culture. In another study, researchers quantified downstream signaling events associated with successful integrin-mediated adhesion of human alveolar osteoblasts (AOBs) to Ti surfaces. They observed that within 3 hours, the attachment rates of AOBs cultured on chemically modified hydrophilic SLA (modSLA) surfaces were significantly higher than that on hydrophobic sandblasted and acid-etched surfaces (SLA). Further, after 6 hours the AOBs developed more defined actin stress fibers and expressed FAK at higher levels on modSLA [63]. Cell proliferation is enhanced on plasma-treated surfaces as well, as demonstrated by the two-fold increase in mouse 3T3 fibroblast cell number on PDLLA plasma-modified surfaces as compared to untreated PLA surfaces [54].

This general hydrophilicity rule varies with specific polymer surfaces and cell types, as well as method used. For instance, Zhu et al. [56] demonstrated that the best water contact angle for endothelial cell attachment and proliferation on

UV-induced PCL-g-poly(methyl acrylate) (PMA) is 70°, while Ma et al. [57] found that for chondrocytes on PLLA-g-poly(methyl methal acrylate) (PMAA) it is 76°. Even further, when Fe^{2+} was used to initiate grafting polymerization, the chrondrocytes on PLLA-g-PMMA favored the surface with a water contact angle of 52° [57]. These results show there is no clear rule of thumb when it comes to polymer surface hydrophilicity, protein adsorption, and subsequent integrin-mediated cell adhesion.

Surface Charge: Modulating surface charge is yet another way to influence proteins adsorption and cell adhesion and spreading. Electrostatically driven protein adsorption is mainly directed by global charges on proteins and surfaces [41]. Since proteins are generally positively charged to attract negatively charged cell membranes, negatively charging biomaterial surfaces have been shown to enhance protein adsorption [41]. There are also instances when negatively charged proteins are attracted to negatively charged surfaces. This takes place when positively charged patches on the protein are exposed and oriented towards the negatively charged surface, resulting in electrostatic attraction and protein adsorption. Negative charges can be introduced to biomaterial surfaces in a number of ways, including but not limited to grafting, hydrolysis, and electrical stimulation [64-66]. Mayingi and colleagues [64] functionalized oxidized titanium (Ti) surfaces by the covalent grafting of sodium styrene sulfonate NaSS. The anionic groups of polyNaSS enhanced osteoblast-like cell adhesion to the surface modified metallic substrate, showing a 19% increase in mineralization as compared to unmodified surfaces. Similarly, Bisson et al. [65] induced an electrostatic attraction between poly(acrylic acid) (PAA) grafted poly(ethylene terephthalate) (PET) to spur the interaction between the negatively charged surface and positively charged collagen proteins to coat the PET surface. Human bladder SMCs cultured on this surface exhibited 100% confluence within one week. Lastly, Kotwal and Schmidt [66] found that the electrical stimulation of polymer polypyrrole (PP) increases FN adsorption from purified FN and serum-containing solutions, resulting in longer neurite expression from PC-12 cells.

Surface Topography: The effect of surface topology on cell behavior such as morphology, migration, protein synthesis and gene expression has long been recognized in the literature [67]. Whether texture is inherently incorporated in a biomaterial's topology, unconsciously introduced during material processing, or intentionally fabricated into scaffold materials (physically and chemically patterned surfaces), it is generally perceived to have a tunable effect on cell adhesion, proliferation, and differentiation. The scale of these modifications is important to consider because they are believed to influence cell behavior in different ways. Micro-modifications have been reported to mainly influence cell positioning behaviors, namely migration activity via "contact guidance" [68]. However, researchers have recently reported that micro-modified surfaces can also enhance protein adsorption, integrin expression, and resulting cell behaviors. Chen et al. [69] showed that on chemically homogenous poly(dimethylsiloxane) (PDMS) surfaces with microtopology introduced by soft lithography, protein adsorption was increased by 46% as compared to flat surfaces. Researchers have also reported the roles of integrins in cell adhesion to micro-modified surfaces. As shown by Keselowsky et al. [70], Ti substrates with increasing micro-scale rough topographies enhance FAK activation and $\alpha_5\beta_1$ integrin binding of MG63 human osteoblast-like cells. Surface roughness impacts protein adsorption and cell adhesion on metallic substrates as well. It has been demonstrated that roughened Ti surfaces exhibited better early cell attachment than smooth surfaces in the presence of serum, though cells attached to roughened Ti were less spread than those attached to machined Ti [71]. Protivínský et al. [72] showed that as compared to a machined surface or sodium hydroxide treated acid etched Ti, acid etched Ti surfaces exhibit a greater affinity for FN adsorption, which enhanced cell adhesion, ALP activity, and osteocalcin and osteopontion expression of human embryonic palatal MCs. Furthermore, Kramer et al. [73] found that on Ti substrates with a range of micro-modifications, suppressing integrin expression with anti-β_1 antibodies and blocking molecules significantly decreased cellular attachment. Silencing the α_2-subunit integrin also blocked increases in β_1, osteocalcin, and ALP activity typical of MG63 osteoblast-like cells cultured on SLA and modSLA surfaces, thus indicating the importance of the $\alpha_2\beta_1$ heterodimer in osteoblast differentiation caused by Ti microstructure [74]. These recent studies indicate that further investigations into the effects of microtopology on protein adsorption, integrin expression, and cell adhesion are warranted.

On the other hand, it is well known that nanoscale surface features within the range of 1-100 nm tend to affect the adsorption and conformation of integrin-binding proteins, changing the availability of binding sites and modifying integrin signaling [75,76]. Moreover, since the native cellular milieu is in the nanoscale, many cell types are naturally adept to functioning within a complex nanotopographical environment [77-79]. For this reason, much focus has been placed on nano-modifications for the enhancement of cell adhesion. As evidenced in numerous studies where random nanoroughness or isotropic nanopatterns were introduced to polymeric, metallic, and bioceramic surfaces, results tend to show the enhancement of cell adhesion.

It is relatively easy to endow nano-features on polymeric surfaces because of inherent material flexibility, as reviewed by many papers [78-81]. In particular, Biggs et al. [82] used electron beam lithography to create nanoscale pits and grooves on PMMA. They observed that the nanopit arrays disrupted the focal adhesion formation and cellular spreading of human osteoblasts (HOBs) and the FAK mediated activation of the ERK/MAPK signaling pathway (osteospecific differentiation) in mesenchymal populations. However, HOBs cultured on 100 mm wide groove arrays increased integrin mediated adhesion formation and cellular spreading, likely through $\alpha_5\beta_1$ integrin binding. In another study Heydarkhan-Hagvall et al. [83] investigated the effects of human fibroblast adhesion behavior on silicon surfaces with nano-post and nano-grate structure modifications. While the integrin subunits $\alpha_5\beta_1$ and β_3 were all detected, β_3 exhibited stronger signals on nano-grates. Furthermore, paxillin and phosphorylated FAK (pFAK) were observed as elongated and aligned on nano-grates, as opposed to the small dot-like patterns at the cell-periphery exhibited on nano-posts. This indicates that nano-grates may be more effective in inducing human fibroblast adhesion and downstream signaling. In addition to influencing protein adsorption through nanotopology, proteins can also be arranged in clusters to modulate cell adhesion. Nanopatterning of FN with controlled size and pitch against nonadhesive polyethylene glycol (PEG) surfaces led to the controlled number of FN proteins within each adhesion site and cell adherance to these nanopatterns with even distributions as compared to that on a glass control [84].

Researchers and clinicians have also investigated the effects of nanoroughness on metallic substrates. There are several ways to introduce surface nanoroughness, including but not limited to plasma-spraying, grit blasting, acid-etching, anodization or calcium phosphate coatings. For instance, researchers have shown how Fbg [85] and FN [86] adsorption increased with increasing nanoroughness of tantalum films. The positive effect of nanostructures on protein adsorption [87] and osteoblast adhesion [88] was also confirmed on the most commonly used bone implant, Ti. In contrast, Cai et al. [89] reported that there were no significant differences between Fbg adsorption on smooth and nano-modified Ti substrates. Thus, further investigation into the effects of nano-modifications on protein adsorption and integrin-mediated cell adhesion is warranted.

Surface Chemistry: Surface chemistry is yet another property that can be modified to enhance protein adsorption from serum solutions. Keselowsky et al. [90] studied how self-assembled monolayers (SAMs) presenting different terminal functionalities (CH_3, OH, COOH, and NH_2) affected integrin-mediated cell adhesion to equal densities of adsorbed FN. The binding of $\alpha_5\beta_1$ integrin to adsorbed FN was controlled by SAM surface chemistry (OH > COOH = NH_2 > CH_3), and cell adhesion strength followed this trend. On the other hand, the binding of $\alpha_V\beta_3$ integrin displayed the relationship COOH>NH_2>>OH=CH_3 [91]. Surface chemistry has been further shown to modulate focal adhesion composition [91] and osteoblastic differentiation and matrix mineralization [92]. In all three studies, OH- and NH_2- terminated surfaces proved to be the best surfaces to enhance cell adhesion, focal adhesion formation, and up-regulate osteoblast-specific gene expression, ALP activity, and matrix mineralization. On the other hand, blocking the β_3 integrin increased mineralization on the COOH substrate. The differences in integrin binding, cell adhesion strength, and subsequent cell behaviors were attributed to conformational changes that FN undergoes on different terminal-presenting surfaces.

While protein adsorption has historically been the most common approach to developing biomimetic materials, as discussed above, adsorption behavior strongly depends on the surface properties of the biomaterial and quantity and conformations of adsorbed ECM proteins [36]. It has been shown that nonspecifically adsorbed layers frequently result in uneven and unstable protein distributions, or in some cases, no protein layer at all [52,61]. Even when the long chained proteins are adsorbed, cell adhesion capabilities are diminished if they loose their structural conformation [36], exhibit improper orientation with the surface and sterically hinder receptor domain binding [93], or desorb entirely [41]. Protein adsorption can be time-consuming, expensive, and may induce competitive adsorption of other factors from the environment, which could lead to a change in the composition and configuration of the adsorbed molecules [40]. Further, this method is not ideal when working with 3D scaffolds, where its complex structure prevents high yields of protein immobilization due to inaccessible reactive sites on the ligand molecules. This leads to lower cell-receptor interactions and thus lower integrin-mediated cell adhesion [36]. Thus, the discovery of certain short amino acid sequences that bind to integrins on cell surfaces to mediate cell adhesion has made a great impact on bioactivation research. These signaling domains are taken from the receptor-binding domains of long chain ECM proteins. The most popular peptide, RGD (Arg-Gly-Asp) is found in the cell-binding domain of FN, VN, and collagen. These short peptide fragments have been used for surface modification in numerous studies [5].

5. Biomimetic Materials for Tissue Engineering using ECM Peptides

Upon the discovery of ECM peptides, the development of biomimetic materials shifted focus from the adsorption of whole ECM proteins to the immobilization of peptides sequences. These fragments are functional signaling domains from ECM proteins that are composed of a short stretch of amino acid sequences that primarily interact with integrin receptors. The use of short peptide sequence for surface modification is advantageous over the use of native or recombinant ECM proteins because the short peptide sequence is generally more stable and resistant to denaturizing insults during the modification process [94]. As such, nearly all adsorbed peptides are available for interacting with the cell surface's receptors [5]. Furthermore, peptide sequences can be used to target specific cellular interactions, while eliminating possible undesired responses of an intact protein. Moreover, short peptide sequences can be produced economically and synthetically in a laboratory, allowing precise control over their chemical composition and avoiding issues related to concerns on proteins from animal sources.

To date, the most commonly used peptide for surface modification is Arg-Gly-Asp (RGD), which represents the signaling domain derived from fibronectin (FN) and vitronectin (VN). RGD peptides have been shown to enhance adhesion, proliferation, differentiation, and mineralization when attached to the surface of various biodegradable materials [95]. Additionally, other non RGD-containing short peptide sequences derived from ECM protein such as Tyr-Ile-Gly-Ser-Arg

Table 2. Selective synthetic peptide sequences of ECM proteins used in tissue engineering applications.

Sequences	Orgin	Function	Application	Reference
RGD	Fibronectin, Vitronectin	Osteoblast adhesion	bone	[98,99]
REDV	Fibronectin	Endothelial cell adhesion	vascular	[97]
YIGSR	Laminin B1	Neurite adhesion	nerve	[96]
KRSR	Heparin binding protein	Osteoblast adhesion	bone	[100]
KHIFSDDSSE	Neural cell adhesion molecules	Astrocyte adhesion	nerve	[101]

(YIGSR), and Ile-Lys-Val-Ala-Val (IKVAV) have been used to enhance cell adhesion on various surfaces [96,97]. Commonly used peptide sequences used in tissue engineering applications are summarized in Table 2.

5.1. *Covalent immobilzation of ECM-derived peptides to biomaterials*

Peptide immobilization on a material is generally accomplished by formation of covalent bonds between a material surface and introduced components, or rarely by non-covalent interactions [102]. Non-covalent adsorption of small peptides onto biomaterial surfaces however, will usually lead to poor immobilization and in turn, poor cellular attachment. In order to create biomimetic materials that can withstand long-term survival, stable immobilization of these small peptides to the biomaterial surface is crucial. The most extensively investigated approach to immobilize small, bioactive oligopeptide sequences is through covalent coupling directly to the biomaterial surface. Covalent immobilization via chemical methods is often times hampered by the lack of chemical reactivity at the material surface. In order to provide stable covalent linkages between the peptide and biomaterial, surface reactive groups need to be available on the biomaterial surface, which is not always the case with certain materials (e.g. polypyrole, poly(a-hydroxy acids)).

In order to accomplish the covalent immobilization of small peptides onto chemically inert biomaterials, surface reactive groups must first be introduced or exposed to serve as coupling sites for the peptide molecules. A number of methods have been utilized to introduce reactive groups, including graft polymerization, plasma treatment, hydrolysis, aminolysis, oxidation/reduction and combinations of the above methods [Table 3]. For example, hydroxyl groups can be introduced to surfaces via alkaline hydrolysis, while aminolysis can be produced by reacting surfaces with diamines (e.g. hydrazine hydrate, ethylenediamine and hexanediamine) resulting in amino-functionalized surfaces [103]. Once reactive groups are available, various chemical immobilization schemes can be utilized to create stable covalent linkages usually the N-terminus amine group of the peptide molecule and the activated surface functional groups of the biomaterial. Peptides have been immobilized by reacting the N-terminus amine groups with surface carboxyl, hydroxyl, epoxide and aldehyde groups.

Biomaterials with carboxyl (-COOH) surface functionality can be on activated using peptide-coupling agents, such as carbodiimides. Water-soluble carbodiimides, like 1-ethyl-3-(3-dimethylaminopropyl)-carbodiimide (EDC) and the organic-soluble derivative, N,N'-dicyclohexyl-carbodiimide (DCC), serve as heterobifunctional cross-linkers that mediate the formation of amide bonds between surface carboxyl (or phosphate) groups and N-terminus amines, via the formation of an amine-reactive intermediate [95]. What results is a stable, covalent bond between the introduced peptide molecule and the activated biomaterial surface. Other bi-functional cross-linkers with long spacer arm lengths have also been used for peptide immobilization. The advantage of using cross-linkers with long spacer arm lengths is that they negate steric hinderence of bulky peptide molecules and enable them to move flexibly in the biological environment [104]. N-hydroxysuccinimide (NHS) is often used to assist carbodiimide-mediated peptide coupling by forming an active ester intermediate via condensation of the surface carboxyl group and NHS. The NHS-reactive ester intermediate is susceptible to nucleophilic attack by primary amines and results in the formation of stable amide bonds between the biomaterial surface and the N-terminus of the peptide. Poly(glycolide) sutures have been immobilized with bioactive molecules using carbodiimide chemistry [105], while poly(L-lactide) microspheres were used to immobilize RGD peptides to their surfaces for use as chondrocyte microcarriers in dynamic culture conditions [106].

Biomaterial surfaces containing aminated groups can be activated with homobifunctional linkers, such as glutaraldehyde (GL), disuccinimidyl glutarate (DSG) or phenylene diisothiocyanate [107-109], and used for peptide molecule immobilization through reaction with the N-terminus amine of the peptide. Surface amine groups can also be converted into other reactive molecular species, such as carboxyl and thiol. Surface amine groups can be converted into carboxyl-containing surfaces by reacting with succinic anhydride, bis-activated moieties (disuccinimidyl tartrate, ethylene glycol-bis(succinimidyl succinate) and N,N'–disuccinimidyl carbonate [110,111]. Carlisle et al. [112] used bistresyl-PEG in this manner as a linker molecule to immobilize RGD peptides to amine-functionalized surfaces for improved hepatocyte adhesion. Aminated surfaces have beeen converted into thiol-reactive surfaces and used for covalent attachment of bioactive molecules. Matsuya et al. [113] fabricated nanospheres with PEG tethered chains on the surface bearing primary amino groups at the distal ends. The amino terminal groups were converted into thiol-reactive moieties by reacting the nanospheres with N-succinimidyl-4-(N-maleimidomethyl)cyclohexane-1-carboxylate (SMCC) to produce maleimide-functional surfaces. Thiol-containing biomolecules, such as anti-human a-fetoprotein Fab' fragment and cysteine-rich peptides, were then covalently conjugated to the nanosphere surfaces via reaction with the surface maleimide groups [113].

Biomaterial surfaces with hydroxyl groups present can be used for peptide immobilization through the use of highly reactive sulfonyl chlorides, such as

Table 3. Summary of common surface functionalization and activation techniques.

Functionalization techniques	Reactive Moiety	Activating agent	References
Hydrolysis	Carboxyl	Carbodiimides (EDC, DCC); long spacer arm (NHS)	[106,129]
Aminolysis	Amino	GL, DSG, phenylene diisothiocyanate	[109-111]
Alkaline hydrolysis	Hydroxyl	Highly reactive sulfonyl chlorides (tres chloride); DSC; p-NPC	[114,126-128]

2,2,2-trifluoroethanesulfonyl chloride (tresyl chloride) [114]. Surfaces can be pre-activated with tresyl chloride [115-118] to yield sulfonated surfaces that are susceptible to nucleophilic attack by primary amines, thiols and imidazole groups [119-121]. Further, tresyl chloride can activate hydroxyl-containing biomaterials, such as silica and agarose, to form tresylated hydroxyl groups and couple enzymes and peptides by direct reaction with their primary amine groups or sulfhydryl side-groups [11,119]. FN cell-adhesive proteins and Polymyxin B peptide antibiotic have been successfully immobilized on Ti surfaces [122-124], and ethyl acrylate and 2-hydroxyethyl methacrylate copolymers [125], respectively, via tresyl chloride reactions. Alternatively, surface hydroxyl groups can also be activated with N,N'-disuccinimidyl carbonate (DSC) or p-nitrophenyl chlorocarbonate (p-NPC) and coupled with peptides under aqueous conditions [110,126-128].

Chemoselective ligation is a more recent approach to chemically modify biomaterial surfaces. This process immobilizes peptide molecules to biomaterial surfaces via stable covalent bonds by selectively coupling unique and mutually reactive functional groups under mild conditions without the need of activating agents or interfering with other functional groups [130]. These reactions are highly chemoselective and behave like molecular "velcro" [131]. Oxime ligation is a chemoselective reaction between aldehyde groups and hydroxyl amino groups and serves as a site-specific method to link unprotected aminooxy-functionalized peptides to material substrates. Researchers have used aminooxy-aldehyde coupling reactions to attach proteins and aminooxy-terminated RGD cyclopeptides to various substrate surfaces [132,133]. Hydrazone ligation has been used to immobilize synthetic hydrazine-like peptides onto aldehyde- or α-oxoaldehyde-functionalized surfaces. Synthetic peptidoliposomes have been prepared by chemoselectively creating α-oxohydrazone bonds between lysosomal-associated membrane protein (LAMP)-derived peptides and lipidic anchors [134]. Other chemoseletive strategies have been used to modify thiol-functionalized surfaces with bromoacetyl-containing RGD cyclopeptides [135] and maleimide-functionalized surfaces with thiol-containing RGD peptides [136-138].

5.2. *Effects of immobilized peptide concentration and distribution*

Biomimetic scaffolds for tissue engineering can be fabricated by chemically immobilizing small peptides to the surfaces of various biomaterials. The cellular responses to these modified biomaterials are dictated not only by the type of biomimetic peptide molecule immobilized to the biomaterial surface, but also by the ECM ligand concentration, spatial distribution, orientation and receptor-ligand affinity [5].

Early studies that investigated the cellular response to various concentrations of adsorbed cell adhesive ECM proteins demonstrated that a minimum surface concentration of FN and VN was needed for sufficient cell spreading, ranging from approximately 100 fmol/cm^2 to 1300 fmol/cm^2 [139-141]. For surfaces immobilized with RGD peptides, cellular attachment and spreading appeared to demonstrate a sigmoidal increase as a function of increasing RGD surface concentration [142-146]. Thus, a minimum surface density is needed to elicit certain cellular responses. Massia et al. [99] performed quantitative studies to examine the cellular response to GRGDY immobilized onto polymer-modified glass substrates via the N-terminal glycine residue. A minimal amount of RGD peptide (1 fmol/cm^2) was found to be sufficient for fibroblast cell spreading, while at least 10 fmol/cm^2 was needed for $\alpha_V\beta_3$ integrin binding, focal contact formation and cytoskeletal organization of F-actin stress fibers. At this surface concentration, approximately 60 RGD ligands/mm2 were available for binding to cell-surface integrins, demonstrating the biological potency of these synthetic, EMC-derived oligopeptides for use in biomimetic scaffold fabrication [29]. Drumheller et al. [146,147] also examined the cellular response to RGD- and YIGSR-containing peptides grafted at various concentrations within cross-linked poly(acrylic acid) hydrogels via a PEG linker molecule. Fibroblast cells required a peptide concentration of 12 pmol/cm^2 for cell spreading and 66 pmol/cm^2 for focal contact formation on these interpenetrating networks. While higher RGD surface densities are generally associated with enhanced cell adhesion and spreading, there is a point at which greater peptide immobilization may impede cellular responsiveness. Neff et al. [148] demonstrated that maximum fibroblast proliferation occurred on polystyrene surfaces immobilized RGD peptides at an intermediate surface concentration of approximately 1.33 pmol/cm^2. Similarly, smooth muscle cell attachment and spreading was enhanced at intermediate peptide concentrations without limiting cell migration, proliferation and matrix production [149]. Cell migration has also been shown to demonstrate a bi-phasic response to ligand density *in vitro* [150].

Cellular responsiveness to surface modified biomaterials can also be influenced by the nanoscale spatial distribution of biomimetic peptides on the material surface. By distributing peptide ligands in a manner that can facilitate cell adhesion receptor aggregation, specific cellular responses may be enhanced [151]. A synthetic polymer-linking method was employed that allowed for variation of both the average surface density and the local spatial distribution of surface immobilized peptides [152]. YGRGD peptides were attached to PEG hydrogel-modified coverslips using star PEO tethers, composed of many PEO arms emanating from a central core. Peptide-polymer hybrid molecules were synthesized containing 1, 5, and 9 peptide ligands per star molecule and immobilized at a range of average ligand densities (1,000-200,000 ligands/mm^2) for cell culture. Maheshwari et al. observed that a significantly greater fraction of cells resisted higher shear stresses on clustered surfaces following centrifugation. Cell adhesion and migration on YGRGD-modified surfaces increased with average surface density and local cluster size. Cells also demonstrated well-formed stress fibers and focal contacts when peptide ligands were presented in clustered forms.

While nanoscale RGD clustering allows for the enhancement of specific cellular responses, the distance from which peptides are oriented from the substrate surface can also influence cell behavior. Cells may require RGD peptides to be immobilized with a minimum spacing between them and the anchoring substrate surface [97,153,154] such that they are flexible and experience minimal steric hindrance [5]. Short bionert polymer and amino acid chains (e.g. PEG, Gly-Gly-Gly-Gly, Pro-Val-Glu-Leu-Pro) have been used as spacers for peptide immobilization [98,142,155,156]. Hern et al. [142] observed that surfaces modified with RGD peptides containing PEG spacers at a low surface density of 0.01 pmol/cm^2, promoted and enhanced cell adhesion, while surfaces modified with RGDs without PEG spacers exhibited limited cell adhesion even at higher surface densities. Platelet binding to poly(acrylonitrile) beads was shown to be enhanced by coupling up to 13 glycine residues to the N-terminus of a RGDF peptide [154]. Beer et al. [154] suggested that the majority of RGD bonding sites could be reached by peptides that extend 11-32Å from the substrate surface and most cell receptors could be reached with a spacer length of 46Å. Craig et al. [153] discovered that 12 amino acid residues were optimal for spacer length in novel oligopeptide coatings. There are examples where no spacer molecule is needed for adequate cell adhesion as well as where reduced cell adhesion when the spacer molecule is too long [157-161]. Nevertheless, the use of spacers in peptide immobilization may serve to: allow RGD peptides to access the integrin binding site located within the globular head of the molecule; facilitate the arrangement of peptides into spatial micro-domains on substrate surfaces for enhanced cellular attachment; or compensate for substrate surface micro-scale roughness [95].

Receptor-ligand affinity and cell selectivity contributes to successful cell attachment and the modulation of cellular behavior on peptide-modified surfaces. Since each cell type has its own typical pattern of integrin expression, RGD peptides can be used to promote selective cell adhesion with high receptor affinity on modified surfaces [162]. Hirano et al. [163] cultured 5 different cell lines on surfaces modified with RGD, RGDS and RGDT peptides. The tetrapeptides derived from FN and collagen elicited greater cellular attachment compared to the tripeptide sequences due to greater integrin affinity towards the tetrapeptides molecules. Employing more affine RGD cyclopeptides in surface modification schemes can further enhance cellular attachment. Groups have observed increased cell attachment on surfaces modified with cyclic peptides compared to their respective linear conformations [164,165]. Some *in vitro* studies have demonstrated the feasibility of incorporating integrin specificity onto RGD-modified surfaces for selective cell adhesion [157]. Cyclo(RGDfV) peptides have demonstrated similar affinity towards $\alpha_5\beta_1$ and $\alpha_{IIb}\beta_3$ integrins, however they have significantly higher affinity towards $\alpha_5\beta_3$ integrins [166]. Cyclic peptides G*PenGRGDSPC*A [167] and cyclo(RGDf(NMe)V) [168] can mediated selective $\alpha_v\beta_3$ integrin interactions, while linear RGD-derived peptides promote $\alpha_5\beta_1$ integrin-mediated cell adhesion [167,169,170]. These same linear RGD peptides, with lipophilic amino acid residues introduced next to aspartic acid (e.g. GRGDF, GRGDY, GRGDVY, GRGDYPC), demonstrated higher affinity towards $\alpha_v\beta_3$ and $\alpha_{IIb}\beta_3$ integrins and selective cell attachment via these receptors [142,154,171,172]. Platelet agglutination can selectively proceed on GRGDF surfaces via $\alpha_{IIb}\beta_3$ integrins [173], while endothelial cells selectively adhere to GRGDVY surfaces via $\alpha_V\beta_3$ integrins [142,172]. RGDSPASSKP tethered surfaces demonstrated preferential adhesion to fibroblasts rather than endothelial cells via $\alpha_5\beta_1$ integrin selectivity [11]. Similarly, the more $\alpha_v\beta_3$ integrin-selective cyclo(RGDfK) surfaces promoted the adhesion of bone related cells and chondrocytes, while $\alpha_5\beta_1$ selective GRGDSP peptide functionalized surfaces enhanced fibroblast attachment and the $\alpha_5\beta_3$ selective cyclic

G*PenGRGDSPC*A surfaces supported higher smooth muscle cell and endothelial cell densities [174].

Whole protein and peptide immobilization techniques have been used widely in tissue engineering research due to their ability to bioactive other bio-inert materials. However, other materials inherently exhibit bioactive qualities without physical or chemical conjugations with adhesive proteins. These bioactive ceramics have been used extensively in the bone tissue engineering applications.

6. Bioactive Ceramics for Bone Tissue Engineering

Bioactive materials generally possess native characteristics that, without an intervening protein layer, can evoke specific behaviors when in contact with constituents from a biological environment. Moreover, when extracellular matrix (ECM) proteins such as collagen and fibronectin (FN) are adsorbed or immobilized on these surfaces, cell-material interactions are enhanced due to integrin-mediated adhesion. In the realm of bone tissue engineering, such bioactive materials promote the precipitation of calcium and phosphate ions from physiological environments to enhance the bone formation, or osseointegration, on materials designed for orthopedic applications. A major class of these materials is bioceramics, which are specially designed and fabricated ceramics for the repair and reconstruction of diseased, damaged, or "worn out" parts of the skeletal framework. The use of bioceramics as bone graft substitutes has a long history [2,175,176] due to inherent material properties, such as biocompatibility, bio-resorbability, and structural similarities to bone [177]. However, for loading-bearing functions, research has more heavily focused on applying bioceramics as coatings for metallic implants. Such coatings have been shown to enhance the overall osseointegration rate of foreign implants, reducing aseptic loosening, encapsulation fibrosis, and extending the lifetime of orthopedic devices. Since bone tissue itself is 30 mass% organic proteins and 70 mass% inorganic calcium phosphate (CaP) in the forms of crystallized hydroxyapatite (HA) and amorphous CaP, CaP compounds have gained much attention due to many physical and chemical similarities to bone.

6.1. *Surface coatings*

Modifying surfaces of biomaterials with inorganic layers of calcium phosphate serves two main purposes: 1) coatings of CaP can induce the precipitation of CaP, or biological apatite, in physiological environments improving implant osteointegration with surrounding tissues [178]; and 2) CaP can alter the topographical properties of a biomaterial by inducing various levels of surface roughness or porosity, which has been shown to directly influence protein adsorption and cellular behavior. These surfaces can be further modified by the covalent attachment of adhesion proteins and peptides. Hydroxyapatite ($Ca_{10}(PO_4)_6(OH)_2$) has been successfully used as coating on metallic hips and dental implants for a number of years [179]. These metallic implant coatings encourage ingrowth of bone to implant device, enhance fixation of the implants, and improve the lifetime of the prostheses [180]. Commercially pure titanium (cpTi) or titanium alloy compounds (ie: Ti6Al4V) are frequently used as the metal of choice for HA coatings due to their high mechanical properties and corrosion resistance [181].

Technically, several procedures have been developed to coat metallic substrates, such as high temperature plasma-spraying, magnetron sputtering, electrospraying, pulsed laser deposition, and hot isostatic pressing [94,182]. Coatings carried out at high temperatures usually receive post-immersion in SBF to induce the formation of an amorphous CaP layer [178]. The pre-treatment of Ti substrates also is important in the resulting properties of the HA coating. Researchers have shown how Ti substrates modified prior to the electrochemical deposition of HA result in inorganic layers with different surface textures and contact angles [183]. Furthermore, as discussed in greater detail in later sections, pre- and post-treatments also affected the precipitation of CaP from aqueous solutions.

6.1.1. *Biological apatite*

The formation of a CaP, or biological apatite, layer at the bone-bioceramic interface is critical to the biomimetic nature of HA coated metallic implants. During bone remodeling old bone is resorbed by the local acidification of bone mineral prompted by integrin-mediated adhesion of osteoclasts. New bone is formed by CaP precipitation from aqueous solution, protein adsorption, and osteoblast adherence, maturation into osteocytes, and mineralization. Biomimetic CaP compounds similarly sustain dissolution-reprecipitation cascades in physiological solution due to the surface hydration of calcium and phosphate ions present in the biomaterial, along with ionic transfers from surrounding fluids onto the CaP substrate. Such exchanges at the solid-liquid interface lead to the formation of biological apatite on the material surface [180]. As reviewed by Kokubo [184], there is a correlation between apatite formation on surfaces pre-implantation and *in vivo* bone bioactivity: "a material able to have apatite form on its surface in SBF can bond to living bone through the apatite layer formed on its surface in the living body, as long as the material does not contain any substance that induces toxic or antibody reactions". Moreover, proteins and cells can also be incorporated into this newly mineralized bone. Since overall success of an implant largely depends on proper osseointegration at the biomaterial interface [185], the ion exchange phenomena that occurs with CaP compounds validates its use as coatings on biologically inert materials, such as a metallic hip implants, insuring the cohesion between the foreign implant and native bone tissue.

As mentioned, pre- and post- treatments of the Ti-coated substrate can affect the resulting apatite layer. Eliaz et al. [186] showed despite the increased wettability by the H_2O_2 pre-treatment, bone-forming cells adhered more to HA precipitated (HAp) surfaces of NaOH-treated Ti surfaces because of the associated increase in surface area. Post-treatments aimed at modifying the roughness of CaP coatings also have an effect on HAp. Paital et al. [187] found that when CaP-coated Ti6Al6V substrates were increasingly laser-textured, the HAp in SBF was decreased. Both of these examples verify the importance of pre- and post-treatments on HA precipitation and resulting cell adhesion.

6.1.2. *Surface bound ECM-derived proteins and peptides*

Despite the favorable bone-bonding outcomes of HA coated Ti implants, the addition of adhesive proteins such as collagen, fibronectin (FN), vitronectin (VN), and fibrinogen (Fbg) have been explored in order to truly mimic native bone. Proteins are necessary for integrin-mediated cell adhesion and subsequent related cell behaviors [Table 4]. The specific role of integrins has been investigated in several integrin-blocking studies. Kramer et al. [188] used antibodies and peptides to block the integrin-mediated attachment of periodontal ligament fibroblasts to HA-coated Ti surfaces. They found significant reduction of fibroblast attachment, indicating that these receptors are necessary in periodontal ligament attachment to HA-coated Ti surfaces. Similarly, Siebers et al. [189] discovered that blocking integrin subunit–β_1 and –β_3 negatively affected osteoblast-like cell adhesion to CaP-coated Ti. The properties of the underlying substrate also affect integrin expression. By varying the thickness of the HA coat on anodized Ti, human osteoblast-like cells integrin expression has been shown to be up-regulated [190]. These aforementioned studies only touch on the breadth of research currently being carried out on integrin-mediated cell adhesion studies related to bioceramic coatings and metal implants.

As Wilson et al. explained: "the ability of materials to adsorb such proteins (in an active state) from serum determines their ability to support cell adhesion

Table 4. α- and β-subunits involved in ECM protein integrin-mediated musculoskeletal cell adhesion (Adapted from [191]).

Cells	Ligands	β-	α-
Bone cells, cultured osteoblastic cells, smooth muscle cells	collagen-I, collagen-IV, laminin	β_1	α_1
Bone cells, cultured osteoblastic cells, fibroblasts	Collagens-I to –IV, laminin and possibly fibronectin		α_2
Cultured osteoblastic cells	fibronectin, collagen-I, laminin		α_3
Cultured osteoblastic cells	fibronectin		α_4
Bone cells, cultured osteoblastic cells, fibroblasts, smooth muscle cells	fibronectin		α_5
	laminin-1, -2, -4, and -5 (only *in vitro*)		α_6
Skeletal and cardiac muscle cells are specific stages during muscle development	laminin-1		α_7
	fibronectin		α_8
Adult skeletal muscle and visceral smooth muscle	osteopontin		α_9
Cultured osteoblastic cells	fibronectin, vitronectin		α_V
Smooth muscle cells	collagen		α_2
Bone cells and cultured osteoblastic cells	fibrinogen, fibronectin, vitronectin, osteopontin	β_3	α_V
fibroblasts	laminin-1	β_4	α_6
Cultured osteoblastic cells, fibroblasts, smooth muscle cells	vitronectin	β_5	α_V
	fibronectin	β_6	α_V
	fibronectin	β_7	α_4

and spreading and, hence, is an important aspect of their biocompatibility" [41]. After protein adsorption, cells such as osteoprogenitor, pre-osteoblasts (human bone marrow stromal cells), and primary osteoblasts use integrins to strongly adhere to CaP surfaces in order to proliferate, migrate, and start their differentiation phase [180]. As with the polymeric and metallic materials already discussed (section 4.1) adhesion proteins are spontaneously adsorbed onto bioceramic surfaces after only a few minutes of contact with fetal bovine serum (FBS) [41,192-194] and endogenous plasma [195]. Several studies have independently investigated the adsorption of FN [196-198], VN [193,199], and Fbg [200]. Research indicates that adsorbed proteins FN and VN are present on the HA surface in conformations appropriate for the binding of purified integrin receptors $\alpha_5\beta_1$ and $\alpha_v\beta_3$ and cells such as MSCs and pre-osteoblasts [193,194]. Also, in reference to the previous section (section 6.1.1), the presence of Fbg has been shown to stimulate CaP formation on HA-coated titanium surfaces from SBF [201]. While FN and Fbg are not necessary for cell adhesion to HA, as Zreiqat et al. demonstrated, the serum protein VN is necessary for human bone derived (HBD) cell adherence [202]. Another protein that is critical to osteoblast survival is extracellular collagen. Collagen is an organic compound that makes up 95% of the 30 mass% organic component of bone [203]. It has been incorporated [204,205] or coated on the HA scaffolds [206,207], with *in vitro* and *in vivo* studies indicating excellent outcomes with improved initial osteoblast attachment [206,208], reportedly mediated by the α_2 integrin subunit [209].

In specific relation to metallic coatings, several studies demonstrate how type 1 collagen has also been augmented to HA surfaces to more accurately mimic the unique nano-composite structure of bone tissue. [94] When Park and colleagues [210] examined the effects of adhesive proteins on HA-coated Ti disks, results showed that interactions between $\alpha_2\beta_1$ integrin and type I collagen facilitated the adhesion and spreading of fibroblasts and osteoblast-like cells on these coated disks. Furthermore, Schliephake and colleagues [211] found that over a period of 1 to 3 months, composite coatings of HA and collagen of dental screw-type implant surfaces significantly enhanced bone-implant contact and peri-implant bone formation, as compared to surfaces with either coating alone. On the other hand, studies have shown that uniform, homogenous biomimetic collagen-CaP coatings did not improve early bone ingrowth in implanted constructs as compared to CaP only coatings [212]. Nevertheless, collagen-CaP composites exhibit superior behavior mechanically [213]. Other non-collagenous proteins, such as osteocalcin, osteonectin, osteopontin, bone sialoprotein have also been reviewed for their adhesion capabilities and differentiation influences on bone cells [214,215].

Furthermore, as detailed in section 5.2, motifs derived from larger ECM proteins can be immobilized onto bioceramic surfaces. The presence of such peptides increases integrin expression, which in turn activates osteoblast signaling pathways that direct cell survival, cell-cycle progression, gene expression, and matrix mineralization. Researchers first sought to further enhance bioceramic cell adhesive properties by functionalizing HA with RGD (Arg-Gly-Asp), which is widely believed to promote cell/biomaterial interactions. However, it was discovered that in comparison with unfunctionalized disks, these peptides actually inhibit MSC adhesion and survival in vitro and new bone formation in vivo [192,195]. This inhibition is likely due to competition with adsorbed proteins such as FN, VN, and Fbg for binding to cell surface integrins, including $\alpha_5\beta_1$, $\alpha_v\beta_3$, and $\alpha_{II}\beta_3$, respectively. As an alternative, Hennessy et al. investigated the effects of functionalizing HA disks with the collagen-mimic peptides DGEA, P15, and GFOGER because they bind with RGD-independent integrins receptors [216]. They found that *in vitro* HA disks coated with DGEA and P15 equally supported greater cell adhesion as compared with uncoated HA. *In vivo* the modified disks did not enhance cell adhesion, but did improve bone formation on tibial implants, likely due to the activation of the collagen-selective integrin, $\alpha_2\beta_1$, which induces osteoblastic differentiation [217-219]. Other peptides have also been investigated for their integrin-dependent signaling pathways in MC3T3-E1 osteoblasts [220].

The material reviewed in this section specifically focuses on HA coatings on Ti implants. In addition to observing osteoblastic cell adhesion markers on HA discs of varying porosity [221], other CaP compounds such as tricalcium phosphate (TCP) [203,222] and biphasic ceramics (BPC) [223] have also been investigated for their bone forming properties. Additionally, CaP coatings are used with other substrates, such as on Ti foams [224,225] and meshes [226], as well as polymeric scaffolds [40,227-231]. CaP compounds and polymers have also been used as composites [232,233].

7. Conclusion

In recent years, biomimetic materials have emerged as the premier construct for tissue engineering applications. Thus, several techniques have been developed to endow the surfaces of normally bio-inert materials with functional biomolecules such as physically adsorbed adhesive proteins, covalently bound ECM-protein derived peptides, and coatings of hydroxyapatite. Numerous accounts have shown how cells can then interact with a variety of materials, ranging from biodegradable polymers to metallic implants, through integrin-mediated adhesion to proliferate, differentiate, and exhibit other behaviors ultimately aimed towards the formation of new tissue. These strategies combined open up further options towards enhanced cell and tissue regeneration through biological cues incorporated directly on tissue engineered constructs.

References

1. Laurencin CT, Ambrosio AMA, Borden MD, Cooper JA. Tissue Engineering: Orthopedic Applications. Annu Rev Biomed Eng 1999;1:19-46.
2. Khan Y, Yaszemski MJ, Mikos AG, Laurencin CT. Tissue Engineering of Bone: Material and Matrix Considerations. J Bone Joint Surg Am 2008;90:36-42.
3. García AJ, Keselowsky BG. Biomimetic surfaces for control of cell adhesion to facilitate bone formation. Crit Rev Eukaryot Gene Expr 2002;12:151-62.
4. Hench LL, Polak JM. Third-Generation Biomedical Materials. Science 2002;295:1014-7.
5. Shin H, Jo S, Mikos AG. Biomimetic materials for tissue engineering. Biomaterials 2003;24:4353-64.
6. Yamada KM, Pankov R, Cukierman E. Dimensions and dynamics in integrin function. Brazilian Journal of Medical and Biological Research 2003;36:959-66.
7. Danen EH, Sonnenberg A. Erratum: Integrins in regulation of tissue development and function. *J Pathol*; 200: 471-480. J Pathol 2003;201:632-41.
8. Ruoslahti E, Pierschbacher M. New perspectives in cell adhesion: RGD and integrins. Science 1987;238:491-7.
9. Albelda S, Buck C. Integrins and other cell adhesion molecules. FASEB J 1990;4:2868-80.
10. Travis J. Biotech gets a grip on cell adhesion. Science 1993;260:906-8.
11. van der Flier A, Sonnenberg A. Function and interactions of integrins. Cell Tissue Res 2001;305:285-98.
12. Plow EF, Haas TA, Zhang L, Loftus J, Smith JW. Ligand Binding to Integrins. J Biol Chem 2000;275:21785-8.
13. Hynes RO. Integrins: Bidirectional, Allosteric Signaling Machines. Cell 2002;110:673-87.
14. Gottschalk KE, Adams PD, Brunger AT, Kessler H. Transmembrane signal transduction of the alpha$_{IIb}$beta$_3$ integrin. Protein Science 2002;11:1800-12.
15. LeBaron RG, Athanasiou KA. Extracellular Matrix Cell Adhesion Peptides: Functional Applications in Orthopedic Materials. Tissue Eng 2000;6:85-103.
16. Zamir E, Geiger B. Molecular complexity and dynamics of cell-matrix adhesions. J Cell Sci 2001;114:3583-90.
17. Geiger B, Bershadsky A. Assembly and mechanosensory function of focal contacts. Curr Opin Cell Biol 2001;13:584-92.
18. Pande G. The role of membrane lipids in regulation of integrin functions. Curr Opin Cell Biol 2000;12:569-74.
19. Ziegler WH, Gingras AR, Critchley DR, Emsley J. Integrin connections to the cytoskeleton through talin and vinculin. Biochem Soc Trans 2008;36:235-9.
20. Berrier AL, Yamada KM. Cell-matrix adhesion. J Cell Physiol 2007;213:565-73.
21. Boudreau NJ, Jones PL. Extracellular matrix and integrin signalling: the shape of things to come. Biochem J 1999;339:481-8.
22. Schwartz MA. Integrin signaling revisited. Trends Cell Biol 2001;11:466-70.
23. Critchley DR, Holt MR, Barry ST, Priddle H, Hemmings L, Norman J. Integrin-mediated cell adhesion: the cytoskeletal connection. Biochem Soc Symp 1999;65:77-9.
24. Bilezikian JP, Raisz LG, Rodan GA. Principles of Bone Biology. 1996;:1398.
25. Culav EM, Clark CH, Merrilees MJ. Connective Tissues: Matrix Composition and Its Relevance to Physical Therapy. Phys Ther 1999;79:308-19.
26. Hamilton DW. Functional role of periostin in development and wound repair: implications for connective tissue disease. J Cell Commun Signal 2008;2:9-17.
27. Lukashev ME, Werb Z. ECM signalling: orchestrating cell behaviour and misbehaviour. Trends Cell Biol 1998;8:437-41.

28. Stamenkovic I. Extracellular matrix remodelling: the role of matrix metalloproteinases. J Pathol 2003;200:448-64.
29. Elbert DL, Hubbell JA. Surface Treatments of Polymers for Biocompatibility. Annual Review of Materials Science 1996;26:365-294.
30. Anderson JM. Biological Responses to Materials. Annu Rev Mater Res 2001;31:81-110.
31. Ratner BD, Bryant SJ. Biomaterials: Where We Have Been and Where We are Going. Annu Rev Biomed Eng 2004;6:41-75.
32. Brash JL. Composition of the protein layers adsorbed from blood or plasma to solid surfaces: A perspective. Die Makromolekulare Chemie 1985;9:69-80.
33. Langer R, Cima LG, Tamada JA, Wintermantel E. Future directions in biomaterials. Biomaterials 1990;11:738-45.
34. Hubbell JA. Bioactive biomaterials. Curr Opin Biotechnol 1999;10:123-9.
35. Tessmar J, Kellner K, Schulz MB, Blunk T, Göpferich A. Towards the development of biomimetic polymers by protein immobilization: PEGylation of insulin as a model reaction. Tissue Eng 2004;10:441-53.
36. Vasita R, Shanmugam IK, Katt DS. Improved Biomaterials for Tissue Engineering Applications: Surface Modification of Polymers. Curr Top Med Chem 2008;8:341-53.
37. Nair LS, Laurencin CT. Polymers as Biomaterials for Tissue Engineering and Controlled Drug Delivery. Adv Biochem Engin/Biotechnol 2006;102:47-90.
38. Medeiros WSd, Oliveira MVd, Pereira LC, Andrade MCd. Bioactive Porous Titanium: An Alternative to Surgical Implants. Artif Organs 2008;32:277-82.
39. Guda T, Appleford M, Oh S, Ong JL. A Cellular Perspective to Bioceramic Scaffolds for Bone Tissue Engineering: the State of the Art. Curr Top Med Chem 2008;8:290-9.
40. Wang S, Cui W, Bei J. Bulk and surface modifications of polylactide. Anal Bioanal Chem 2005;381:547-56.
41. Wilson CJ, Clegg RE, Leavesley DI, and Pearcy MJ. Mediation of Biomaterial–Cell Interactions by Adsorbed Proteins: A Review. Tissue Eng 2005;11:1-18.
42. García AJ, Boettiger D. Integrin–fibronectin interactions at the cell-material interface: initial integrin binding and signaling. Biomaterials 1999;20:2427-33.
43. Nikolovski J, Mooney DJ. Smooth muscle cell adhesion to tissue engineering scaffolds. Biomaterials 2000;21:2025-32.
44. Stephansson SN, Byers BA, García AJ. Enhanced expression of the osteoblastic phenotype on substrates that modulate fibronectin conformation and integrin receptor binding. Biomaterials 2002;23:2527-34.
45. Chastain SR, Kundu AK, Dhar S, Calvert JW, Putnam AJ. Adhesion of mesenchymal stem cells to polymer scaffolds occurs via distinct ECM ligands and controls their osteogenic differentiation. Journal of Biomedical Materials Research Part A 2006;78A:73-85.
46. El-Amin SF, Attawia M, Lu HH, et al. Integrin expression by human osteoblasts cultured on degradable polymeric materials applicable for tissue engineered bone. Journal of Orthopaedic Research 2002;20:20-8.
47. Bierbaum S, Hempel U, Geissler U, et al. Modification of Ti6AL4V surfaces using collagen I, III, and fibronectin. II. Influence on osteoblast responses. J Biomed Mater Res A 2003;67:431-8.
48. MacDonald DE, Markovic B, Allen M, Somasundaran P, Boskey AL. Surface analysis of human plasma fibronectin adsorbed to commercially pure titanium materials. J Biomed Mater Res 1998;41:120-30.
49. Rico P, Rodriguez Hernandez JC, Moratal D, Altankov G, Monleon Pradas M, Salmeron M. Substrate-induced assembly of fibronectin into networks. Influence of surface chemistry and effect on osteoblast adhesion. Tissue Eng Part A 2009;15:[ePub ahead of print].

50. García AJ, Vega MD, Boettiger D. Modulation of Cell Proliferation and Differentiation through Substrate-dependent Changes in Fibronectin Conformation. Mol Biol Cell 1999;10:785-98.
51. Martínez CE, Rodríguez Hernández JC, Machado M, et al. Human chondrocyte morphology, its dedifferentiation, and fibronectin conformation on different PLLA microtopographies. Tissue Eng Part A 2009;14:1751-62.
52. Ma PX. Biomimetic materials for tissue engineering. Adv Drug Deliv Rev 2008;60:184-98.
53. Lee SG, An Ey, Lee JB, Park JC, Shin JW, Kim JK. Enhanced cell affinity of poly(D,L-lactic-co-glycolic acid) (50/50) by plasma treatment with β-(1 →3) (1→ 6)-glucan. Surface Coat Technol 2007;201:5128-31.
54. Yang J, Bei J, Wang S. Improving cell affinity of poly(d,l-lactide) film modified by anhydrous ammonia plasma treatment. Polym Adv Technol 2002;13:220-6.
55. Yamaguchi M, Shinbo T, Kanamori T, et al. Surface modification of poly(l-lactic acid) affects initial cell attachment, cell morphology, and cell growth. Artif Organs 2004;7:187-93.
56. Zhu Y, Gao C, Shen J. Surface modification of polycaprolactone with poly(methacrylic acid) and gelatin covalent immobilization for promoting its cytocompatibility. Biomaterials 2002;23:4889-95.
57. Ma Z, Gao C, Gong Y, Shen J. Chondrocyte behaviors on poly--lactic acid (PLLA) membranes containing hydroxyl, amide or carboxyl groups. Biomaterials 2003;24:3725-30.
58. Steffens GCM, Nothdurft L, Buse G, Thissen H, Hocker H, Klee D. High density binding of proteins and peptides to poly(d,l-lactide) grafted with polyacrylic acid. Biomaterials 2002;23:3523-31.
59. Abbasi F, Mirzadeh H, Katbab AA. Bulk and surface modification of silicone rubber for biomedical applications, Polym Int 2002;51:882-8.
60. Shim JK, Na HS, Lee YM, Huh H, Nho YC. Surface modification of polypropylene membranes by gamma-ray induced graft copolymerization and their solute permeation characteristics. J Membr Sci 2001;190:215-26.
61. Alves CM, Yang Y, Marton D, et al. Plasma surface modification of poly(D,L-lactic acid) as a tool to enhance protein adsorption and the attachment of different cell types. Journal of Biomedical Materials Research Part B: Applied Biomaterials 2008;87B:59-66.
62. Liu X, Lim JY, Donahue HJ, Dhurjati R, Mastro AM, Vogler EA. Influence of substratum surface chemistry/energy and topography on the human fetal osteoblastic cell line hFOB 1.19: Phenotypic and genotypic responses observed in vitro. Biomaterials 2007;28:4535-50.
63. Lai H, Zhuang L, Liu X, Wieland M, Zhang Z, Zhang Z. The influence of surface energy on early adherent events of osteoblast on titanium substrates. Journal of Biomedical Materials Research Part A 2009;9999:NA.
64. Mayingi J, Hélary G, Noirclere F, Bacroix B, Migonney V. Synthèse et greffage de polymères bioactifs sur des surfaces en titane pour favoriser l'ostéointégration. IRBM 2008;29:1-6.
65. Bisson I, Kosinski M, Ruault S, et al. Acrylic acid grafting and collagen immobilization on poly(ethylene terephthalate) surfaces for adherence and growth of human bladder smooth muscle cells. Biomaterials 2002;23:3149-58.
66. Kotwal A, Schmidt CE. Electrical stimulation alters protein adsorption and nerve cell interactions with electrically conducting biomaterials. Biomaterials 2001;22:1055-64.
67. Martínez E, Engel E, Planell JA, Samitier J. Effects of artificial micro- and nano-structured surfaces on cell behaviour. Annals of Anatomy - Anatomischer Anzeiger 2009;191:126-35.
68. Li J, McNally H, Shi R. Enhanced neurite alignment on micro-patterned poly-L-lactic acid films. Journal of Biomedical Materials Research Part A 2008;87A:392-404.

69. Chen H, Song W, Zhou F, et al. The effect of surface microtopography of poly(dimethylsiloxane) on protein adsorption, platelet and cell adhesion. Colloids and Surfaces B: Biointerfaces 2009;71:275-81.
70. Keselowsky BG, Wang L, Schwartz Z, Garcia AJ, Boyan BD. Integrin alpha$_5$ controls osteoblastic proliferation and differentiation responses to titanium substrates presenting different roughness characteristics in a roughness independent manner. Journal of Biomedical Materials Research Part A 2007;80A:700-10.
71. Nishimoto SK, Nishimoto M, Park SW, et al. The effect of titanium surface roughening on protein absorption, cell attachment, and cell spreading. Int J Oral Maxillofac Implants 2008;23:675-80.
72. Protivínský J, Appleford M, Strnad J, Helebrant A, Ong JL. Effect of chemically modified titanium surfaces on protein adsorption and osteoblast precursor cell behavior. The International journal of oral & maxillofacial implants 2007;22:542-50.
73. Kramer PR, JanikKeith A, Cai Z, Ma S, Watanabe I. Integrin mediated attachment of periodontal ligament to titanium surfaces. Dental Materials 2009;25:877-83.
74. Olivares-Navarrete R, Raz P, Zhao G, et al. Integrin $\alpha 2\beta 1$ plays a critical role in osteoblast response to micron-scale surface structure and surface energy of titanium substrates. Proceedings of the National Academy of Sciences 2008;105:15767-72.
75. Nair LS, Laurencin CT. Nanofibers and Nanoparticles for Orthopaedic Surgery Applications. J Bone Joint Surg Am 2008;90:128-31.
76. Webster TJ, Schadler LS, Siegel RW, Bizios R. Mechanisms of enhanced osteoblast adhesion on nanophase alumina involve vitronectin. Tissue Eng 2001;7:291-301.
77. Variola F, Vetrone F, Richert L, et al. Improving Biocompatibility of Implantable Metals by Nanoscale Modification of Surfaces: An Overview of Strategies, Fabrication Methods, and Challenges. Small 2009;5:996-1006.
78. Yim EKF, Leong KW. Significance of synthetic nanostructures in dictating cellular response. Nanomedicine: Nanotechnology, Biology and Medicine 2005;1:10-21.
79. Flemming RG, Murphy CJ, Abrams GA, Goodman SL, Nealey PF. Effects of synthetic micro- and nano-structured surfaces on cell behavior. Biomaterials 1999;20:573-88.
80. Lim JY, Donahue HJ. Cell Sensing and Response to Micro- and Nanostructured Surfaces Produced by Chemical and Topographic Patterning. Tissue Eng 2007;13:1879-91.
81. Ma Z, Mao Z, Gao C. Surface modification and property analysis of biomedical polymers used for tissue engineering. Colloids and Surfaces B: Biointerfaces 2007;60:137-57.
82. Biggs MJP, Richards RG, Gadegaard N, Wilkinson CDW, Oreffo ROC, Dalby MJ. The use of nanoscale topography to modulate the dynamics of adhesion formation in primary osteoblasts and ERK/MAPK signalling in STRO-1+ enriched skeletal stem cells. BiomaterialsIn Press, Corrected Proof.
83. Heydarkhan-Hagvall S, Choi C, Dunn J, et al. Influence of Systematically Varied Nano-Scale Topography on Cell Morphology and Adhesion. Cell Communication & Adhesion 2007;14:181.
84. Slater JH, Frey W. Nanopatterning of fibronectin and the influence of integrin clustering on endothelial cell spreading and proliferation. Journal of Biomedical Materials Research Part A 2008;87A:176-95.
85. Rechendorff K, Hovgaard MB, Foss M, Zhdanov VP, Besenbacher F. Enhancement of Protein Adsorption Induced by Surface Roughness. Langmuir 2006;22:10885-10888.
86. Hovgaard MB, Rechendorff K, Chevallier J, Foss M, Besenbacher F. Fibronectin Adsorption on Tantalum: The Influence of Nanoroughness. J Phys Chem B 2008;112:8241-8249.
87. Galli C, Collaud Coen M, Hauert R, et al. Protein adsorption on topographically nanostructured titanium. Surf Sci 2001;474:L180-4.

88. Divya RVV, Manzoor K, Menon D, Selvamurugan N, Nair SV. The design of novel nanostructures on titanium by solution chemistry for an improved osteoblast response. Nanotechnology 2009;20:195101.
89. Cai K, Bossert J, Jandt KD. Does the nanometre scale topography of titanium influence protein adsorption and cell proliferation? Colloids and Surfaces B: Biointerfaces 2006;49:136-44.
90. Keselowsky BG, Collard DM, García AJ. Surface chemistry modulates fibronectin conformation and directs integrin binding and specificity to control cell adhesion. Journal of Biomedical Materials Research Part A 2003;66A:247-59.
91. Keselowsky BG, Collard DM, García AJAJ. Surface chemistry modulates focal adhesion composition and signaling through changes in integrin binding. Biomaterials 2004;25:5947-54.
92. Keselowsky BG, Collard DM, García AJ. Integrin binding specificity regulates biomaterial surface chemistry effects on cell differentiation. Proceedings of the National Academy of Sciences of the United States of America 2005;102:5953-7.
93. Trzaskowski B, Leonarski F, Leś A, Adamowicz L. Altering the Orientation of Proteins on Self-Assembled Monolayers: A Computational Study. Biomacromolecules 2008;9:3239-3245.
94. de Jonge LT, Leeuwenburgh SC, Wolke JG, Jansen JA. Organic–Inorganic Surface Modifications for Titanium Implant Surfaces. Pharm Res 2008;25:2357-2369.
95. Hersel U, Dahmen C, Kessler H. RGD modified polymers: biomaterials for stimulated cell adhesion and beyond. Biomaterials 2003;24:4385-415.
96. Ranieri JP, Bellamkonda R, Bekos EJ, Vargo TG, Gardella JA, Aebischer P. Neuronal cell attachment to fluorinated ethylene propylene films with covalently immobilized laminin oligopeptides YIGSR and IKVAV. II. J Biomed Mater Res 1995;29:779-85.
97. Hubbell JA, Massia SP, Desai NP, Drumheller PD. Endothelial cell-selective materials for tissue engineering in the vascular graft via a new receptor. Biotechnology (N Y) 1991;9:568-72.
98. Shin H, Jo S, Mikos AG. Modulation of marrow stromal osteoblast adhesion on biomimetic oligo(poly(ethylene glycol) fumarate) hydrogels modified with Arg-Gly-Asp peptides and a poly(ethylene glycol) spacer. J Biomed Mater Res 2002;61:169-79.
99. Massia S, Hubbell J. An RGD spacing of 440 nm is sufficient for integrin alpha V beta 3-mediated fibroblast spreading and 140 nm for focal contact and stress fiber formation. J Cell Biol 1991;114:1089-100.
100. Dee KC, Andersen TT, Bizios R. Design and function of novel osteoblast-adhesive peptides for chemical modification of biomaterials. J Biomed Mater Res 1998;40:371-7.
101. Kam L, Shain W, Turner JN, Bizios R. Selective adhesion of astrocytes to surfaces modified with immobilized peptides. Biomaterials 2002;23:511-5.
102. Yamada KM, Kennedy DW. Amino acid sequence specificities of an adhesive recognition signal. J Cell Biochem 1985;28:99-104.
103. Massia S, Hubbell J. Immobilized amines and basic amino acids as mimetic heparin-binding domains for cell surface proteoglycan-mediated adhesion. J Biol Chem 1992;267:10133-41.
104. Rezania A, Healy KE. Biomimetic Peptide Surfaces That Regulate Adhesion, Spreading, Cytoskeletal Organization, and Mineralization of the Matrix Deposited by Osteoblast-like Cells. Biotechnol Prog 1999;15:19-32.
105. Lee K, Yoon KR, Woo SI, Choi IS. Surface modification of poly(glycolic acid) (PGA) for biomedical applications. J Pharm Sci 2003;92:933-7.

106. Chen R, Curran SJ, Curran JM, Hunt JA. The use of poly(l-lactide) and RGD modified microspheres as cell carriers in a flow intermittency bioreactor for tissue engineering cartilage. Biomaterials 2006;27:4453-60.
107. Benters R, Niemeyer CM, Wöhrle D. Dendrimer-Activated Solid Supports for Nucleic Acid and Protein Microarrays. ChemBioChem 2001;2:686-94.
108. Yang M, Kong RYC, Kazmi N, Leung AKC. Covalent immobilization of oligonucleotides on modified glass/ silicon surfaces for solid-phase DNA hybridization and amplification. Chem Lett 1994;27:257-8.
109. Pack SP, Kamisetty NK, Nonogawa M, et al. Direct immobilization of DNA oligomers onto the amine-functionalized glass surface for DNA microarray fabrication through the activation-free reaction of oxanine. Nucleic Acids Research 2007;35:e110.
110. Morpurgo M, Bayer EA, Wilchek M. N-hydroxysuccinimide carbonates and carbamates are useful reactive reagents for coupling ligands to lysines on proteins. J Biochem Biophys Methods 1999;38:17-28.
111. Kondoh A, Makino K, Matsuda T. 2-Dimensional artificial extracellular-matrix-bioadhesive peptide-immobilized surface design. J Appl Polym Sci 1993;47:1983-8.
112. Carlisle ES, Mariappan MR, Nelson KD, et al. Enhancing hepatocyte adhesion by pulsed plasma deposition and poly-ethylene glycol coupling. Tissue Eng 2000;6:45-52.
113. Matsuya T, Tashiro S, Hoshino N, Shibata N, Nagasaki Y, Kataoka K. A core-shell-type fluorescent nanosphere possessing reactive poly(ethylene glycol) tethered chains on the surface for zeptomole detection of protein in time-resolved fluorometric immunoassay. Anal Chem 2003;75:6124-32.
114. Jennissen HP. Cyanogen bromide and tresyl chloride chemistry revisited: the special reactivity of agarose as a chromatographic and biomaterial support for immobilizing novel chemical groups. Journal of Molecular Recognition 1995;8:116-24.
115. Banerjee P, Irvine DJ, Mayes AM, Griffith LG. Polymer latexes for cell-resistant and cell-interactive surfaces. J Biomed Mater Res 2000;50:331-9.
116. Tong YW, Shoichet MS. Peptide surface modification of poly(tetrafluoroethylene-*co*-hexafluoropropylene) enhances its interaction with central nervous system neurons. J Biomed Mater Res 1998;42:85-95.
117. Massia SP, Hubbell JA. Human endothelial cell interactions with surface-coupled adhesion peptides on a nonadhesive glass substrate and two polymeric biomaterials. J Biomed Mater Res 1991;25:223-42.
118. Massia SP, Hubbell JA. Covalently Attached GRGD on Polymer Surfaces Promotes Biospecific Adhesion of Mammalian Cells[a]. Ann N Y Acad Sci 1990;589:261-70.
119. Nilsson K, Mosbach K. Immobilization of enzymes and affinity ligands to various hydroxyl group carrying supports using highly reactive sulfonyl chlorides. Biochem Biophys Res Commun 1981;102:449-57.
120. Nilsson K, Mosbach K. Tresyl chloride-activated supports for enzyme immobilization. Methods Enzymol 1987;135:65-78.
121. Nilsson KM, K. Immobilization of ligands with organic sulfonyl chlorides. Meth Enzymol 1984;104:56-69.
122. Hayakawa T, Yoshinari M, Nagai M, Yamamoto M, Nemoto K. X-ray photoelectron spectroscopic studies of the reactivity of basic terminal OH of titanium towards tresyl chloride and fibronectin. Biomed Res 2003;24:223-30.
123. Hayakawa T, Yoshinari M, Nemoto K. Direct attachment of fibronectin to tresyl chloride-activated titanium. Journal of Biomedical Materials Research Part A 2003;67A:684-8.

124. Hayakawa T, Yoshinari M, Nemoto K. Quartz-crystal microbalance-dissipation technique for the study of initial adsorption of fibronectin onto tresyl chloride-activated titanium. Journal of Biomedical Materials Research Part B: Applied Biomaterials 2005;73B:271-6.
125. Tzorisa A, Hall EAH, Besselinkb GAJ, Bergveld P. Testing the Durability of Polymyxin B Immobilization on a Polymer Showing Antimicrobial Activity: A Novel Approach with the Ion-Step Method. Analytical Letters 2003;36:1781-803.
126. Jo S, Shin H, Mikos AG. Modification of Oligo(poly(ethylene glycol) fumarate) Macromer with a GRGD Peptide for the Preparation of Functionalized Polymer Networks. Biomacromolecules 2001;2:255-261.
127. Li JT, Carlsson J, Lin JN, Caldwell KD. Chemical modification of surface active poly(ethylene oxide)-poly(propylene oxide) triblock copolymers. Bioconjug Chem 1996;7:592-9.
128. Woerly S, Laroche G, Marchand R, Pato J, Subr V, Ulbrich K. Intracerebral implantation of hydrogel-coupled adhesion peptides: tissue reaction. J Neural Transplant Plast 1995;5:245-55.
129. Lee K, Yoon KR, Woo SI, Choi IS. Surface modification of poly(glycolic acid) (PGA) for biomedical applications. J Pharm Sci 2003;92:933-7.
130. Tam JP, Yu Q, Miao Z. Orthogonal ligation strategies for peptide and protein. Peptide Science 1999;51:311-32.
131. Camarero JA, Kwon Y, Coleman MA. Chemoselective attachment of biologically active proteins to surfaces by expressed protein ligation and its application for "protein chip" fabrication. J Am Chem Soc 2004;126:14730-1.
132. Thumshirn G, Hersel U, Goodman SL, Kessler H. Multimeric Cyclic RGD Peptides as Potential Tools for Tumor Targeting: Solid-Phase Peptide Synthesis and Chemoselective Oxime Ligation. Chemistry - A European Journal 2003;9:2717-25.
133. Scheibler L, Dumy P, Boncheva M, et al. Functional molecular thin films: topological templates for the chemoselective ligation of antigenic peptides to self-assembled monolayers. Angewandte {C}hemie, {I}nternational {E}dition 1999;38:696-9.
134. Bourel-Bonnet L, Pécheur EI, Grandjean C, et al. Anchorage of Synthetic Peptides onto Liposomes via Hydrazone and r-Oxo Hydrazone Bonds. Preliminary Functional Investigations. Bioconjugate Chem 2005;16:450-7.
135. Ivanov B, Grzesik W, Robey FA. Synthesis and use of a new bromoacetyl-derivatized heterotrifunctional amino acid for conjugation of cyclic RGD-containing peptides derived from human bone sialoprotein. Bioconjug Chem 1995;:3-269.
136. Fields GB, Lauer JL, Dori Y, Forns P, Yu Y, Tirrell M. Proteinlike molecular architecture: Biomaterial applications for inducing cellular receptor binding and signal transduction. Peptide Science 1998;47:143-51.
137. Houseman BT, Gawalt ES, Mrksich M. Maleimide functionalized self-assembled monolayers for the preparation of peptide and carbohydrate biochips. Langmuir 2003;19:1522-31.
138. Lateef SS, Boateng S, Hartman TJ, Crot CA, Russell B, Hanley L. GRGDSP peptide-bound silicone membranes withstand mechanical flexing in vivo and display enhanced fibroblast adhesio. Biomaterials 2002;23:3159-68.
139. Hubbell JA, Massia SP, Drumheller PD. Surface-grafted Cell-binding Peptides in Tissue Engineering of the Vascular Graft. Ann N Y Acad Sci 1992;665:253-8.
140. Humphries M, Akiyama S, Komoriya A, Olden K, Yamada K. Identification of an alternatively spliced site in human plasma fibronectin that mediates cell type-specific adhesion. J Cell Biol 1986;103:2637-47.
141. Underwood P, Bennett F. A comparison of the biological activities of the cell-adhesive proteins vitronectin and fibronectin. J Cell Sci 1989;93:641-9.

142. Hern DL, Hubbell JA. Incorporation of adhesion peptides into nonadhesive hydrogels useful for tissue resurfacing. J Biomed Mater Res 1998;39:266-76.
143. Kantlehner M, Schaffner P, Finsinger D, et al. Surface Coating with Cyclic RGD Peptides Stimulates Osteoblast Adhesion and Proliferation as well as Bone Formation. ChemBioChem 2000;1:107-14.
144. Jeschke B, Meyer J, Jonczyk A, et al. RGD-peptides for tissue engineering of articular cartilage. Biomaterials 2002;23:3455-63.
145. Danilov YN, Juliano RL. (Arg-Gly-Asp)n-Albumin conjugates as a model substratum for integrin-mediated cell adhesion. Exp Cell Res 1989;182:186-96.
146. Drumheller PD, Hubbell JA. Polymer Networks with Grafted Cell Adhesion Peptides for Highly Biospecific Cell Adhesive Substrates. Anal Biochem 1994;222:380-8.
147. Drumheller PD, Elbert DL, Hubbell JA. Multifunctional poly(ethylene glycol) semi-interpenetrating polymer networks as highly selective adhesive substrates for bioadhesive peptide grafting. Biotechnol Bioeng 1994;43:772-80.
148. Neff JA, Tresco PA, Caldwell KD. Surface modification for controlled studies of cell–ligand interactions. Biomaterials 1999;20:2377-93.
149. Mann BK, West JL. Cell adhesion peptides alter smooth muscle cell adhesion, proliferation, migration, and matrix protein synthesis on modified surfaces and in polymer scaffolds. J Biomed Mater Res 2002;60:86-93.
150. Palecek SP, Loftus JC, Ginsberg MH, Luffenburger DA, Horwitz AF. Integrin-ligand binding properties govern cell migration speed through cell-substratrum adhesiveness. Nature 1997;385:537-40.
151. Irvine DJ, Hue K, Mayes AM, Griffith LG. Simulations of Cell-Surface Integrin Binding to Nanoscale-Clustered Adhesion Ligands. Biophys J 2002;82:120-32.
152. Maheshwari G, Brown G, Lauffenburger D, Wells A, Griffith L. Cell adhesion and motility depend on nanoscale RGD clustering. J Cell Sci 2000;113:1677-86.
153. Craig WS, Cheng S, Mullen DG, Blevitt J, Pierschbacher MD. Concept and progress in the development of RGD-containing peptide pharmaceuticals. Biopolymers 1995;37:157-75.
154. Beer J, Springer K, Coller B. Immobilized Arg-Gly-Asp (RGD) peptides of varying lengths as structural probes of the platelet glycoprotein IIb/IIIa receptor. Blood 1992;79:117-28.
155. Loebsack A, Greene K, Wyatt S, et al. *In vivo* characterization of a porous hydrogel material for use as a tissue bulking agent. J Biomed Mater Res 2001;57:575-81.
156. Sakiyama-Elbert SE, Panitch A, Hubbell JA. Development of growth factor fusion proteins for cell-triggered drug delivery. FASEB J 2001;.
157. Elbert DL, Hubbell JA. Conjugate addition reactions combined with free-radical cross-linking for the design of materials for tissue engineering. Biomacromolecules 200;2:430-1.
158. Pelham RJ,Jr, Wang YL. Cell Locomotion and Focal Adhesions Are Regulated by the Mechanical Properties of the Substrate. Biol Bull 1998;194:348-50.
159. Mammen M, Choi S, Whitesides GM. Polyvalent Interactions in Biological Systems: Implications for Design and Use of Multivalent Ligands and Inhibitors. Angewandte Chemie International Edition 1998;37:2754-94.
160. Wong JY, Kuhl TL, Israelachvili JN, Mullah N, Zalipsky S. Direct Measurement of a Tethered Ligand-Receptor Interaction Potential. Science 1997;275:820-2.
161. Lo C, Wang H, Dembo M, Wang Y. Cell Movement Is Guided by the Rigidity of the Substrate. Biophys J 2000;79:144-52.
162. Ruoslahti E. The RGD story: a personal account. Matrix Biology 2003;22:459-65.
163. Hirano Y, Okuno M, Hayashi T, Goto K, Nakajima A. Cell-attachment activities of surface immobilized oligopeptides RGD, RGDS, RGDV, RGDT, and YIGSR toward five cell lines. J Biomater Sci Polym Ed 1993;4:235-43.

164. Delforge D, Gillon B, Art M, Dewelle J, Raes M, Remacle J. Design of a synthetic adhesion protein by grafting RGD tailed cyclic peptides on bovine serum albumin. Lett Pept Sci 1998;5:87-91.
165. van der Pluijm G, Vloedgraven HJM, Ivanov B, et al. Bone Sialoprotein Peptides Are Potent Inhibitors of Breast Cancer Cell Adhesion to Bone. Cancer Res 1996;56:1948-55.
166. Pfaff M, Tangemann K, Muller B, et al. Selective recognition of cyclic RGD peptides of NMR defined conformation by αIIbβ3, αvβ3, and α5β1 integrins. J Biol Chem 1994;269:20233-8.
167. Pierschbacher M, Ruoslahti E. Influence of stereochemistry of the sequence Arg-Gly-Asp-Xaa on binding specificity in cell adhesion. J Biol Chem 1987;262:17294-8.
168. Dechantsreiter MA, Planker E, Mathä B, et al. N-methylated cyclic RGD peptides as highly active and selective αvβ3 integrin antagonists. J Med Chem 1999;42:3033-40.
169. Kao WJ, Hubbell JA. Murine macrophage behavior on peptide-grafted polyethyleneglycol-containing networks. Biotechnol Bioeng 1998;59:2-9.
170. Kao WJ, Hubbell JA, Anderson JM. Protein-mediated macrophage adhesion and activation on biomaterials: a model for modulating cell behavior. J Mater Sci Mater Med 1999;10:601-5.
171. Lin HB, Sun W, Mosher DF, et al. Synthesis, surface, and cell adhesion properties of polyurethanes containing covalently grafted RGD-peptides. J Biomed Mater Res 1994;28:329-42.
172. Lin HB, Garciaecheverria C, Asakura S, Sun W, Mosher DF, Cooper SL. Endothelial-cell adhesion on polyurethanes containing covalently attached RGD-peptides. Biomaterials 1992;13:905-14.
173. Rezania A, Healy KE. Integrin subunits responsible for adhesion of human osteoblast-like cells to biomimetic peptide surfaces. Journal of Orthopaedic Research 1999;17:615-23.
174. Massia SP, Stark J. Immobilized RGD peptides on surface grafted dextran promotes biospecific cell attachment. J Biomed Mater Res 2001;56:390-9.
175. Albee FH, Morrison HF. Studies in bone growth: triple calcium phosphate as stimulus to osteogenesis. Ann Surg 1920;71:32-9.
176. Ray RD, Degge J, Gloyd P, Mooney G. Bone regeneration; an experimental study of bone-grafting materials. J Bone Joint Surg 1952;34A:638-47.
177. Giannoudis PV, Dinopoulos H, Tsiridis E. Bone substitutes: An update. Injury 2005;36:S20-7.
178. Xin R, Leng Y, Chen J, Zhang Q. A comparative study of calcium phosphate formation on bioceramics in vitro and in vivo. Biomaterials 2005;26:6477-86.
179. Epinette J, Manley MT. Fifteen Years of Clinical Experience with Hydroxyapatite Coatings in Joint Arthroplasty. Springer, 2009.
180. Barrère F, van Blitterswijk CA, de Groot K. Bone regeneration: molecular and cellular interactions with calcium phosphate ceramics. Int J Nanomedicine 2006;1:317-32.
181. Balazic M, Kopac J, Jackson MJ, Ahmed W. Review: titanium and titanium alloy applications in medicine. International Journal of Nano and Biomaterials 2007;1:3-34.
182. Narayanan R, Seshadri SK, Kwon TY, Kim KH. Calcium phosphate-based coatings on titanium and its alloys. Journal of Biomedical Materials Research Part B: Applied Biomaterials 2008;85B:279-99.
183. Hu K, Yang X, Cai Y, Cui Z, Wei Q. Comparison of physical characteristics and cell culture test of hydroxyapatite/collagen composite coating on NiTi SMA: electrochemical deposition and chemically biomimetic growth. Frontiers Of Materials Science In China 2007;1:229-36.
184. Kokubo T, Kim H, Kawashita M. Novel bioactive materials with different mechanical properties. Biomaterials 2003;24:2161-75.

185. Ramaswamy Y, Wu C, Dunstan CR, et al. Sphene ceramics for orthopedic coating applications: An in vitro and in vivo study. Acta BiomaterialiaIn Press, Corrected Proof.
186. Eliaz N, Shmueli S, Shur I, Benayahu D, Aronov D, Rosenman G. The effect of surface treatment on the surface texture and contact angle of electrochemically deposited hydroxyapatite coating and on its interaction with bone-forming cells. Acta BiomaterialiaIn Press, Corrected Proof.
187. Paital SR, Dahotre NB. Wettability and kinetics of hydroxyapatite precipitation on a laser-textured Ca–P bioceramic coating. Acta BiomaterialiaIn Press, Corrected Proof.
188. Kramer PR, JanikKeith A, Cai Z, Ma S, Watanabe I. Integrin mediated attachment of periodontal ligament to titanium surfaces. Dental Materials 2009;25:877-83.
189. Siebers MC, Walboomers XF, van den Dolder J, Leeuwenburgh SC, Wolke JG, Jansen JA. The behavior of osteoblast-like cells on various substrates with functional blocking of integrin-beta1 and integrin-beta3. J Mater Sci Mater Med 2008;19:861-8.
190. Sohn SH, Jun HK, Kim CS, et al. Biological responses in osteoblast-like cell line according to thin layer hydroxyapatite coatings on anodized titanium. J Oral Rehabil 2006;33:898-911.
191. Anselme K. Osteoblast adhesion on biomaterials. Biomaterials 2000;21:667-81.
192. Sawyer AA, Hennessy KM, Bellis SL. Regulation of mesenchymal stem cell attachment and spreading on hydroxyapatite by RGD peptides and adsorbed serum proteins. Biomaterials 2005;26:1467-75.
193. Kilpadi KL, Chang P, Bellis SL. Hydroxylapatite binds more serum proteins, purified integrins, and osteoblast precursor cells than titanium or steel. J Biomed Mater Res 2001;57:258-67.
194. Matsuura T, Hosokawa R, Okamoto K, Kimoto T, Akagawa Y. Diverse mechanisms of osteoblast spreading on hydroxyapatite and titanium. Biomaterials 2000;21:1121-7.
195. Hennessy KM, Clem WC, Phipps MC, Sawyer AA, Shaikh FM, Bellis SL. The effect of RGD peptides on osseointegration of hydroxyapatite biomaterials. Biomaterials 2008;29:3075-83.
196. Deligianni D, Korovessis P, Porte-Derrieu MC, Amedee J. Fibronectin preadsorbed on hydroxyapatite together with rough surface structure increases osteoblasts' adhesion "in vitro": the theoretical usefulness of fibronectin preadsorption on hydroxyapatite to increase permanent stability and longevity in spine implants. J Spinal Disord Tech 2005;18:257-62.
197. Pecheva E, Pramatarova L, Altankov G. Hydroxyapatite grown on a native extracellular matrix: initial interactions with human fibroblasts. Langmuir 2007;23:9386-92.
198. Schonmeyr BH, Wong AK, Li S, Gewalli F, Cordiero PG, Mehrara BJ. Treatment of hydroxyapatite scaffolds with fibronectin and fetal calf serum increases osteoblast adhesion and proliferation in vitro. Plast Reconstr Surg 2008;121:751-62.
199. Preissner KT. Structure and biological role of vitronectin. Annu Rev Cell Biol 1991;7:275-310.
200. Phang MY, Ng MH, Tan KK, Aminuddin BS, Ruszymah BH, Fauziah O. Evaluation of suitable biodegradable scaffolds for engineered bone tissue. Med J Malaysia 2004;59:198-9.
201. Arvidsson A, Currie F, Kjellin P, Sul YT, Stenport V. Nucleation and growth of calcium phosphates in the presence of fibrinogen on titanium implants with four potentially bioactive surface preparations. An in vitro study. J Mater Sci Mater Med 2009;[E pub ahead of print].
202. Zreiqat H, Standard OC, Gengenbach T, Steele JG, Howlett CR. The role of surface characteristics in the initial adhesion of human bone-derived cells on ceramics. Cell Mater 1996;6:45-56.

203. Kamitakahara M, Ohtsuki C, Miyazaki T. Review paper: Behavior of Ceramic Biomaterials Derived from Tricalcium Phosphate in Physiological Condition. J Biomater Appl 2008;23:197-212.
204. Yamauchi K, Goda T, Takeuchi N, Einaga H, Tanabe T. Preparation of collagen/calcium phosphate multilayer sheet using enzymatic mineralization. Biomaterials 2004;25:5481-9.
205. John A, Hong L, Ikada Y, Tabata Y. A trial to prepare biodegradable collagen-hydroxyapatite composites for bone repair. J Biomater Sci Polym Ed 2001;12:689-705.
206. Brodie JC, Goldie E, Connel G, Merry J, Grant MH. Osteoblast interactions with calcium phosphate ceramics modified by coating with type I collagen. J Biomed Mater Res A 2005;73:409-21.
207. Rodrigues CVM, Serricella P, Linhares ABR, et al. Characterization of a bovine collagen–hydroxyapatite composite scaffold for bone tissue engineering. Biomaterials 2003;24:4987-97.
208. Dawson JI, Wahl DA, Lanham SA, Kanczler JM, Czernuszka JT, Oreffo ROC. Development of specific collagen scaffolds to support the osteogenic and chondrogenic differentiation of human bone marrow stromal cells. Biomaterials 2008;29:3105-16.
209. Vohra S, Hennessy KM, Sawyer AA, Zhuo Y, Bellis SL. Comparison of mesenchymal stem cell and osteosarcoma cell adhesion to hydroxyapatite. J Mater Sci Mater Med 2008;19:3567-74.
210. Park BS, Heo SJ, Kim CS, et al. Effects of adhesion molecules on the behavior of osteoblast-like cells and normal human fibroblasts on different titanium surfaces. J Biomed Mater Res A 2005;74:640-51.
211. Schliephake H, Scharnweber D, Roesseler S, Dard M, Sewing A, Aref A. Biomimetic calcium phosphate composite coating of dental implants. Int J Oral Maxillofac Implants 2006;21:738-46.
212. Schliephake H, Scharnweber D, Dard M, Röbetaler S, Sewing A, Hüttmann C. Biological performance of biomimetic calcium phosphate coating of titanium implants in the dog mandible. J Biomed Mater Res 2003;64A:225-34.
213. Wahl DA, Czernuszka JT. Collagen-hydroxyapatite composites for hard tissue repair. Eur Cell Mater 2006;11:43-56.
214. Bernards MT, Qin C, Jiang S. MC3T3-E1 cell adhesion to hydroxyapatite with adsorbed bone sialoprotein, bone osteopontin, and bovine serum albumin. Colloids Surf B Biointerfaces 2008;62:236-47.
215. Roach HI. Why does bone matrix contain non-collagenous proteins? The role of osteocalcon, osteonectin, osteopontin and bone sialoprotein in bone mineralization and resoprtion. Cell Biol Int 1994;18:617-26.
216. Hennessy KM, Pollot BE, Clem WC, et al. The effect of collagen I mimetic peptides on mesenchymal stem cell adhesion and differentiation, and on bone formation at hydroxyapatite surfaces. Biomaterials 2009;30:1898-909.
217. Mizuno M, Fujisawa R, Kuboki Y. Type I collagen-induced osteoblastic differentiation of bone-marrow cells mediated by collagen-alpha2beta1 integrin interaction. J Cell Physiol 2000;184:207-13.
218. Salasznyk RM, Williams WA, Boskey A, Batorsky A, Plopper GE. Adhesion to vitronectin and collagen I promotes osteogenic differentiation of human mesenchymal stem cells. J Biomed Biotechnol 2004;2004:24-34.
219. Carvalho RS, Kostenuik PJ, Salih E, Bumann A, Gerstenfeld LC. Selective adhesion of osteoblastic cells to different integrin ligands induces osteopontin gene expression. Matrix Biology 2003;22:241-9.

220. Gilbert M, Giachelli CM, Stayton PS. Biomimetic peptides that engage specific integrin-dependent signaling pathways and bind to calcium phosphate surfaces. J Biomed Mater Res A 2003;67:69-77.
221. Rouahi M, Champion E, Hardouin P, Anselme K. Quantitative kinetic analysis of gene expression during human osteoblastic adhesion on orthopaedic materials. Biomaterials 2006;27:2829-44.
222. dos Santos EA, Farina M, Soares GA, Anselme K. Chemical and topographical influence of hydroxyapatite and beta-tricalcium phosphate surfaces on human osteoblastic cell behavior. Journal of Biomedical Materials Research Part A 2009;89A:510-20.
223. Zhao BH, Bai W, Feng HL, Cui FZ. Effects of TCP/HA-coating titanium on the adhesion behavior of human gingival fibroblasts. Zhonghua Kou Qiang Yi Xue Za Zhi 2004;39:501-4.
224. Jalota S, Bhaduri SB, Tas AC. Osteoblast proliferation on neat and apatite-like calcium phosphate-coated titanium foam scaffolds. Materials Science and Engineering: C 2007;27:432-40.
225. Spoerke ED, Murray NG, Li H, Brinson LC, Dunand DC, Stupp SI. A bioactive titanium foam scaffold for bone repair. Acta Biomaterialia 2005;1:523-33.
226. Vehof JW, Mahmood J, Takita H, et al. Ectopic bone formation in titanium mesh loaded with bone morphogenetic protein and coated with calcium phosphate. Plast Reconstr Surg 2001;108:434-43.
227. Woo KM, Seo J, Zhang R, Ma PX. Suppression of apoptosis by enhanced protein adsorption on polymer/hydroxyapatite composite scaffolds. Biomaterials 2007;28:2622-30.
228. Ring A, Steinstraesser L, Muhr G, Steinau HU, Hauser J, Langer S. Improved Neovascularization of PEGT/PBT Copolymer Matrices in Response to Surface Modification by Biomimetic Coating. Eur Surg Res 2007;39:75-81.
229. Zhang R, Ma PX. Biomimetic Polymer/Apatite Composite Scaffolds for Mineralized Tissue Engineering. Macromolecular Bioscience 2004;4:100-11.
230. Wei G, Ma PX. Macroporous and nanofibrous polymer scaffolds and polymer/bone-like apatite composite scaffolds generated by sugar spheres. Journal of Biomedical Materials Research Part A 2006;78A:306-15.
231. Chesnutt BM, Yuan Y, Brahmandam N, et al. Characterization of biomimetic calcium phosphate on phosphorylated chitosan films. Journal of Biomedical Materials Research Part A 2007;82A:343-53.
232. Khan YM, Cushnie EK, Kelleher JK, Laurencin CT. In situ synthesized ceramic–polymer composites for bone tissue engineering: bioactivity and degradation studies. J Mater Sci 2007;42:4183-90.
233. Laurencin CT, Khan Y. Polymer/Calcium Phosphate Scaffolds for Bone tissue Engineering. In Scaffolding in Tissue Engineering. In: Ma PX, Elisseeff J, ed. Scaffolding in Tissue Engineering. Boca Raton, FL, US: Taylor and Francis Group, 2005:253-263.

CHAPTER 11

ENGINEERING ARTIFICIAL STEM CELL NICHES

Matthias P. Lutolf*
Laboratory of Stem Cell Bioengineering and Institute of Bioengineering, Ecole Polytechnique Fédérale de Lausanne (EPFL), Lausanne, Switzerland
**E-mail: matthias.lutolf@epfl.ch*

1. Introduction

Owing to their unique dual function to renew themselves ('self-renewal') and to specialize ('differentiation'), stem cells are responsible for maintaining and regenerating tissues. Consequently, stem cells possess an intriguing potential to be utilized clinically for the treatment of numerous genetic diseases or trauma. At least two recent breakthroughs in stem cell biology have propelled the field to the forefront of the Life Sciences: First, the discovery and characterization of adult stem cells in virtually every tissue promises new clinical strategies to augment tissue regeneration via recruitment and manipulation of these endogenous stem cells. Second, already specialized tissue cells can be forced to change their identity to a stem cell state ('reprogramming') when exposed to a defined set of so far at least two transcription factors,[1] proteins that control the transfer of genetic information from DNA to RNA within the cell. The resulting stem cells, induced pluripotent stem (iPS) cells, promise the generation of any patient-specific cell type for cell-based therapy, or other emerging applications such as disease models for drug discovery, without the use of embryonic material.

These advances are extremely encouraging. Nonetheless, they should not prompt us to expect that a broad therapeutic usage of stem cells, beyond blood and skin stem cells, is within reach. Many stumbling blocks remain to be overcome to tap the true potential of stem cells in human medicine.[2] Apart from major technical and logistic challenges in producing 'clinical grade' stem cells, many challenges root in our limited understanding of adult stem cell biology, likely a consequence of the extraordinary complexity of adult stem cell systems and a lack of simplified models to study them. For example, we lack a good understanding of the cellular and molecular factors and mechanisms that are responsible for stem cell self-renewal and specialization, or the reversion of somatic cells to an iPS state. As a result, we do not know how to grow stem cells in culture once they are removed from their niche: most adult stem cell types rapidly specialize upon extraction from their tissue, and it is still very cumbersome to specialize in a well-controlled, directed manner pluripotent embryonic stem or iPS cells into the many differentiated cell types of the body.

To shed light on the mechanisms that regulate stem cells, technologies that allow us to study the function of an isolated component of the complex in vivo regulatory system are crucial. Biomaterials are one such emerging area that is poised to assist stem cell biology and move it one step closer to the clinic. The prime driving force for the application of biomaterials in stem cell biology is the possibility to fabricate matrices that recapitulate, nearly down to the molecular details, the microenvironment, or niche, in which stem cells reside naturally. Biomaterials could then, for example, be exploited as modular toolboxes to construct *de novo* niches with diverse biochemical and biophysical properties, enabling quantitative analyses of stem cell behavior in a manner previously not possible. Furthermore, an integration of biomaterials technologies with microfabrication platforms such as biomolecule micropatterning or microfluidics could open up new avenues for identifying stem cell regulators and investigating stem cell behavior at the single cell level and in high-throughput. Equally exciting, knowledge gleaned from such studies could feed into efforts that aim to reconstruct tissue-like multicellular constructs with applications in many areas of Life Science. This chapter highlights, by way of selected examples, biomaterials approaches to probe and manipulate stem cells, changing their fate in a predictable manner.

1.1. *Adult stem cells are regulated by niches*

Adult stem cells are harbored in anatomically well-defined locations termed niches.[3,4,5,6,7,8] Niches are composed of countless biomolecular signals that, in concert with cell-intrinsic regulatory networks, regulate stem cell function. The presence of the niche is crucial, as its absence often leads to the loss of stem cell function, which in turn can have dramatic consequences for tissue function and can completely impair regeneration. The niche concept was postulated first on hematopoietic (blood) stem cells more than two decades ago by Schofield,[9] but concrete proof of the existence and function of niches was only provided ca. one decade ago in seminal studies of stem cells in fruit flies (e.g.: [10,11,12,13]). More recently, niches have been identified and characterized in nearly all tissues of mammals, including the skin (in the bulge region of the hair follicle), intestine (in the epithelium), brain (in the subventricular zone of the hippocampus), bone marrow (on the endosteal surface and near blood vessels) and muscle (beneath the muscle fiber basal lamina).[5,7,8,14] Interestingly, the characteristic niche structure and biochemical composition of stem cell niches appears to be conserved from fruit flies to mammals.

The signals that control stem cells function in the niche in a spatially and temporally well-controlled manner can be grouped into three main categories **(Fig. 1)**: *(i)* direct physical contact with *support cells* via cell-cell interactions providing short-range signals, *(ii)* contact with a surrounding protein- and sugar-rich extracellular matrix (ECM), and *(iii)* exposure to soluble signals such as growth factors, cytokines, chemokines or metabolic cues such as Calcium ions or reactive oxygen species. Notably, blood vessels are often found near niches (or are perhaps niches themselves),[15,16,17,18] presumably to transport long-range signals and serve as a conduit for recruitment of circulating cells into the niche. In addition, stem cells in niches can respond to inputs from the nervous system, as demonstrated in the hematopoietic stem cell (HSC) niche.[19]

1.2. *Cell-cell interactions in the niche*

Support cells provide transmembrane signals such as Cadherin proteins that anchor the stem cells to their niches for example via so-called adherens junctions **(Fig. 1a and b)**. The extracellular domain of Cadherins on support cells can interact either with stem cell-derived Cadherins of the same kind (*i.e.* homophilic binding) or with different Cadherins (*i.e.* heterophilic binding).[20] In studies on fruit flies it has been shown that loss of Cadherin in stem cell niches leads to stem cell loss as well,[21] underscoring the importance of adhesive cell-cell interactions in the niche. In as much the Cadherin-mediated cell-cell interactions are involved in regulating stem cell self-renewal is not well understood.

Cell-cell communication via transmembrane receptors in the stem cell niche can also regulate functions beyond cell adhesion. For example, the family of Notch receptors and their ligands Jagged and Delta have been associated with an important role in stem cell regulation in diverse tissues.[22,23,24,25] Lack of Notch signaling can for example result in a reduction of neural stem/progenitor cell numbers, suggesting a role for this pathway in stem cell maintenance.[22]

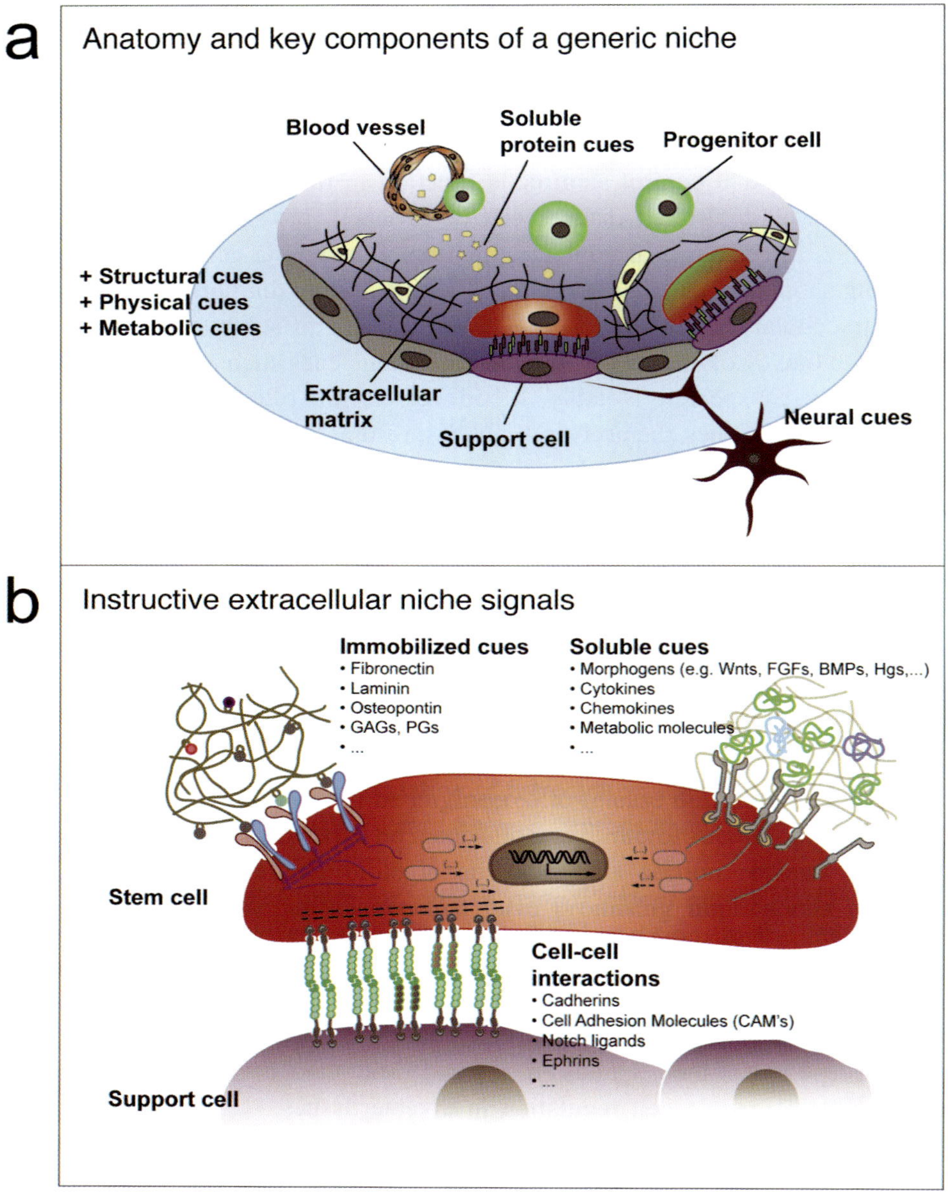

Fig. 1. Architecture and composition of a stem cell niche: Adult stem cells are located within instructive microenvironments comprised of complex mixtures of extracellular cues delivered by support cells in close proximity (a). The main components of a niche are support cells and their secreted transmembrane cell-cell adhesion proteins, soluble factors and the surrounding extracellular matrix (b). Reproduced with permission from[100]. Copyright 2009 Wiley InterScience.

1.3. *Stem cell-ECM interactions in the niche*

Stem cells in the niche also interact via specific receptors such as integrins with their surrounding ECM **(Fig. 1a and 1b)** The ECM can be either a 2-dimensional (2D) or a 3-dimensional (3D) crosslinked network of proteins and sugars. For example, epithelial stem cells[26] or satellite cells, the canonical muscle stem cells,[27] are exposed to a 2D basal lamina, while HSC in the bone marrow appear to be embedded in a 3D matrix.[16,28] The ECM provides cell adhesion and controls cell shape, cell motility, such as during homing of stem cells back to the niche,[29,30,31] but also stem cell maintenance[32,33]. The list of ECM components that has been associated with adult stem cell regulation is extensive. Important examples include osteopontin[34,35], fibronectin[36] or the glycosaminoglycan hyaluronic acid[37] which all have been described to play a role in HSC regulation. Apart from adhesive functions, integrins can also control the cell cycle, and are involved in signal transduction to regulate stem cell maintenance or differentiation.[32,33]

1.4. *Stem cell interaction with soluble niche signals*

Many soluble signals such as growth factors have been described to play a role in regulating adult stem cells. One class of molecules, the developmental morphogen proteins, have been identified to play a role in many niches across different species. For example, HSC maintenance seems to be controlled by several of these proteins including Wnt-3a[38,39], Sonic hedgehog (Shh)[40,41], c-kit ligand[42], or FGF-1[43]. However, many proteins that are often studied in vitro in a soluble form may not actually be soluble in vivo, but rather bound to the ECM via intermolecular interactions such as electrostatic interactions. Heparin, a heparan sulfate proteoglycan, can bind many morphogens with high affinitiy, localizing their response to the niche and possibly protecting them from rapid proteolytic inactivation.[44]

1.5. *Stem cell functions controlled by the niche*

An understanding of the dynamic behavior of individual stem cells and their responsiveness to niche signals may be the key to the understanding of processes that occur at the tissue level. Excluding death, we can distinguish between four main single cell fate changes **(Fig. 2)**: *(i)* a stem cell never divides (quiescence; **Fig. 2a)**, *(ii)* a stem cell undergoes self-renewal divisions that result in one daughter stem cell and one differentiated cell (termed *asymmetric* divisions -

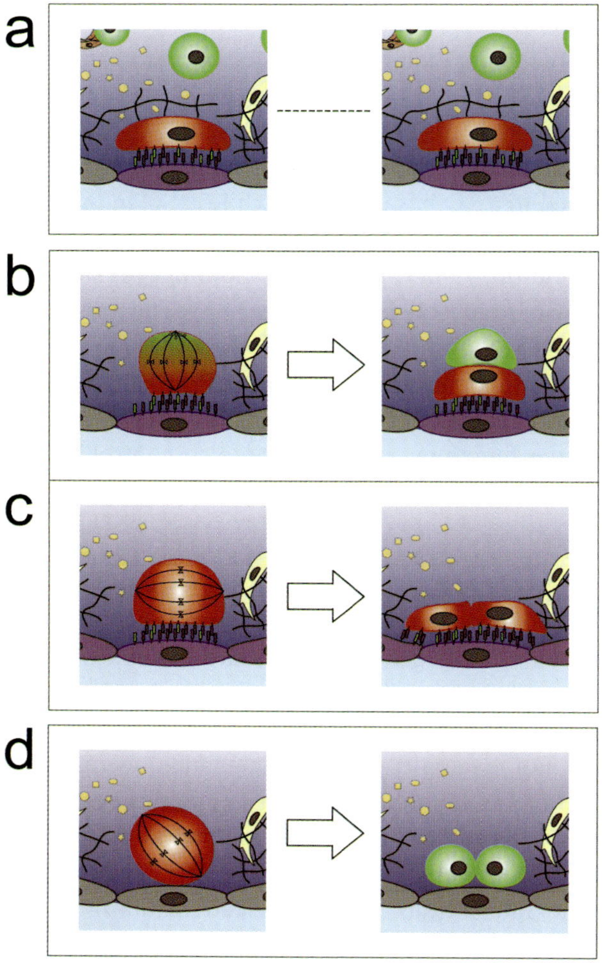

Fig. 2. Schematic stem cell fates in the niche: Stem cells are red, progenitor cells are green. Adult stem cells are generally considered to be quiescent in their niches (a) unless they are activated to proliferate in response to the demands of a tissue (e.g. stress or trauma). Quiescence is actively regulated by niche proteins such as cell-cell adhesion proteins. During homeostatic conditions, self-renewal divisions are asymmetric, generating one daughter cell retaining stem cell identity and another one being already partially differentiated (b). Asymmetric divisions can be controlled inside the cell via localization of cell fate determinants segregated to the cytoplasm of just one daughter cell. A hallmark of this type of division is the regulated orientation of the mitotic spindle that retains only one daughter in the niche. During development and/or stress the stem cell pool needs to expand via symmetric self-renewal divisions (c). Both daughter cells are exposed to the same niche environment and therefore keep their stem cell identity. A fourth possible fate is that of (symmetric) differentiation division, whereby both daughter cells lose stem cell function (d). This fate can be observed in many cases during in vitro culture of adult stem cells as well. Reproduced with permission from [100]. Copyright 2009 Wiley InterScience.

asymmetric with regard to the identity of the two daughter cells; **Fig. 2b**), *(iii)* a stem cell undergoes self-renewal divisions that result in two daughter stem cells (termed *symmetric* divisions; **Fig. 2c**), *(iv)* a stem cell undergoes divisions that result in two differentiated progeny, which could occur, for example, due to an absence of the niche or important niche cues **(Fig. 2d)**. All of these fates must be actively regulated and coordinated by the niche in order to ensure an appropriate size of the stem cell pool during homeostasis and regeneration, and over the course of the lifetime of an organism **(Fig. 3)**.

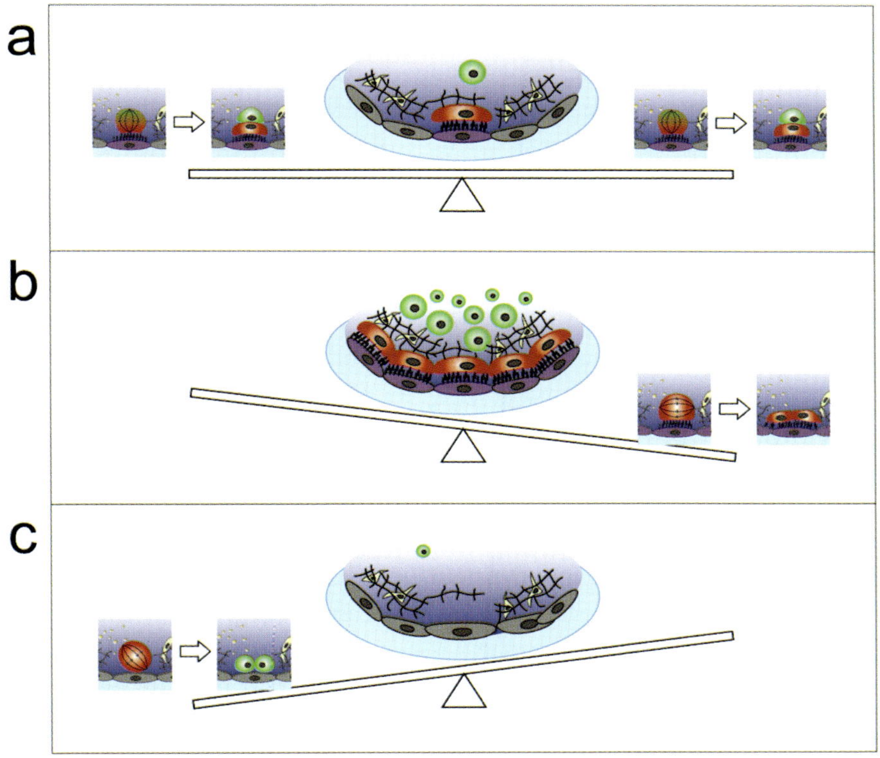

Fig. 3. Control of the stem cell pool size: The ensemble of single cell fates (Fig. 2) determines the size of the stem cell pool in response to the demands of the tissue. Cell numbers in the niche need to be tightly controlled as an imbalance could have dramatic consequences for tissue function. Under homeostatic conditions, niche signals keep the number of stem cells in the niche constant (a). During stress or in pathological situations such as cancer, the demand is higher and symmetric self-renewal divisions dominate, allowing the stem cell pool to expand (b). Predominant symmetric differentiation divisions could lead to a depletion of the stem cell pool in the niche which would compromise regeneration (c). Reproduced with permission from [100]. Copyright 2009 Wiley InterScience.

The mechanisms that regulate the above fates, in particular the delicate balance between cell divisions that lead to self-renewal and/or differentiation, are still under intense investigation.[45,46,47,48] The decision of a stem cell to undergo an asymmetric division may be controlled by cell-intrinsic and/or cell-extrinsic mechanisms. In the first scenario, intracellular segregation of certain intracellular protein components may drive asymmetry.[46] On the other hand, the asymmetric positioning of daughter cells relative to external niche components may also induce asymmetric divisions.[48] In this case, both daughter cells may initially be equivalent, but their different microenvironments may impose two disparate identities. During development or when experiencing stress, adult stem cells in the niche must increase in numbers which can only occur via symmetric self-renewal divisions giving rise to two daughter stem cells **(Fig. 2c)**. A symmetric division could, for example, be controlled by cell-extrinsic mechanisms, if both daughter cells encounter the same niche environment after division and remain in the niche as stem cells. Notably, the same stem cell populations appear to switch from symmetric divisions during embryonic development or regeneration in the adult to asymmetric cell divisions during late fetal development and homeostasis.[49,50]

The interplay between stem cells and their niches therefore creates a dynamic and reciprocal system that balances stem cell numbers in response to the physiological demands of the tissue **(Fig. 3)**. Consequently, the size of the stem cell pool has been shown to correlate with the size of the niche.[7] For example, when a change in numbers of support osteoblasts in the bone marrow niche was induced[51,52], accompanying changes in the HSC pool size were observed. Specific signals keep the number of stem cells in the niche constant during homeostasis **(Fig. 3a)** and allow the stem cell pool to expand under physiological stress and in pathological situations such as cancer **(Fig. 3b)** where the tightly orchestrated regulation of cell numbers is misregulated.

Finally, it is conceivable that multiple types of niches exist for each stem cell type. Although still debated, HSCs are believed to transit from an endosteal niche, wherein they adhere to osteoblasts and remain quiescent, to a vascular niche, wherein they become activated due to interaction with endothelial cells on blood vessel walls. Thus, the nature of the two niches may dictate the state of activity of the stem cell[18,53,54,55]. As well, it is likely that niches can be formed or destroyed in response to physiological needs. In the absence of functional niches, symmetric differentiation divisions **(Fig. 2d)** could lead to a rapid depletion of the stem cell pool **(Fig. 3c)**, therefore impairing further production and leading to loss of tissue function. This may explain why to date many adult stem cell populations cannot be maintained in culture. Indeed, when plated on a conventional cell culture substrate such as tissue culture plastic these cells often undergo differentiation divisions due to the lack of instructive components from the niche.

2. Engineering *in vitro* Surrogate Models of Stem Cell Niches

An emerging route towards overcoming the translational hurdles that stem cell biology faces today involves the combination of stem cell biology with biomolecular materials engineering and microfabrication technologies in order to generate novel cell culture platforms that mimic crucial biochemical or structural aspects of complex in vivo niches. Several lines of research towards such 'artificial niches' appear particularly promising and are briefly discussed below.

2.1. *Engineering biomaterials with niche-like physicochemical characteristics*

Stem cell niches are soft and highly hydrated structures, rich in proteins and sugars. Synthetic approaches that mimic these characteristics may be crucial in controlling adult stem cell fate outside the niche.[56,57] A striking example of the influence of matrix stiffness on stem cell fate was demonstrated by Engler and colleagues.[58] Mesenchymal stem/progenitor cells were shown to alter their gene expression patterns in response to the elasticity of a substrate, lending credence to the notion that non-physiological rigid plastic surfaces could induce the commitment of stem cells to undesired lineages. Modular hydrogel networks[59] formed from synthetic building blocks, should be a promising route to mimic the physicochemical niche characteristics. Gel substrates are typically composed of 95-99% water and as a consequence are rather soft, with elastic moduli on the order of hundreds of Pa to a few kPa. Moreover, many polymer hydrogels are resistant to protein adsorption and cell adhesion. Biomolecular functionalization can thus be conducted on an inert background, re-constructing complexity from the 'bottom-up'.

Since many signaling cues in stem cell niches are presented in an immobilized fashion, chemical schemes that permit the recapitulation of the natural presentation mode of niche proteins have received increasing attention. The well-controlled tethering of desired protein signals to a synthetic polymer is not an easy obstacle to overcome, as non-specific crosslinking may compromise the protein's bioactivity. Alberti and colleagues have presented interesting approaches towards artificial niches with tethered protein cues whereby signaling ligands can be immobilized to maleic anhydride copolymer thin-film coatings.[60] Tethered leukemia inhibitory factor (LIF), a signal that controls ESC self-renewal in feeder-free cultures, led to retention of pluripotency for at least 2 weeks in the absence of soluble LIF in the culture medium.

Thus, the choice of a substrate that *(i)* mimics the physicochemical niche properties, *(ii)* can be selectively functionalized with regulatory cues, and *(iii)* can be molecularly tuned in its key properties within a wide range, may be important in controlling stem cell behavior outside of their natural microenvironment.

2.2. *Microwell arrays for high-throughput single stem cell studies*

As discussed above, an understanding of the mechanisms that control *individual* stem cells in their niche may be crucial in moving the stem cell field forward. Unfortunately, conventional cell culture platforms are not readily amenable to investigating stem cells at the single cell level. For example, standard multiwell plates such as 96-well plate would require large amounts of expensive culture media components and do not offer enough throughput. This problem has been solved by the introduction of microwell arrays for cell biology.[61,62,63,64,65,66,67,68]

These platforms permit the analysis of a large number of individual, spatially confined cells. They have recently been successfully applied to stem cell biology, on both embryonic and adult stem cells.[65,66,67,68,69,70,71,72] For example, Dykstra and colleagues tracked the dynamic behavior of single mouse hematopoietic stem cells on PDMS microwell arrays and were able to correlate proliferative behavior in vitro with in vivo function, that is, the multilineage reconstitution of the blood.[70] As a result of the achieved single cell resolution, these authors detected new hallmarks of proliferating HSCs that are, to some extent, predictive of self-renewal divisions. Cordey *et al.* reported the application of a novel hydrogel microwell array platform based on poly(ethylene glycol) (PEG) to explore the development of single neural stem cells (NSC) into multicellular spheroids ('neurospheres').[71] Compared to conventional neurosphere culture methods on flat plastic dishes, single NSC viability on soft hydrogels more than doubled. Effective confinement of single proliferating cells to microwells led to neurosphere formation of vastly different sizes, a high percentage of which maintained stem cell phenotypes after one week in culture.

In an effort to also recapitulate the signaling characteristics of niches on such (otherwise biochemically 'passive') microwell array platforms, topographical hydrogel patterning was recently combined with microcontact printing (**Fig. 4**).[72]

Protein tethering was achieved by attaching a heterofunctional PEG linker to a protein of interest and then crosslinking this conjugate into the forming gel network. To ensure site-selectivity in protein immobilization, engineered Fc-chimeric proteins were linked on the gel surface via binding to an intermediate auxiliary protein, ProteinA, that contains four high-affinity binding sites ($K_a = 10^8$ per mole) for the Fc-region of human, mouse and rabbit immunoglobulins (**Fig. 4a**). To specifically functionalize gels and immobilize proteins only at the bottom of microwells, rather than homogeneously distributing proteins across the entire array (bulk modification), the commonly used micromolding process was augmented by adding a protein microcontact printing step (**Fig. 4b**): PEG-functionalized ProteinA was adsorbed onto the posts of the PDMS stamp (step 1,2) and the hydrogel polymerized onto the ProteinA/PDMS (step 3,4), transferring both the topographic pattern and protein pattern onto the gel surface. Immunofluorescence microscopy revealed that microcontact printed proteins, such as a BSA-FITC model protein were localized at the bottom of the microwells (**Fig. 4c**). When ProteinA was used, Fc-chimeric proteins such as N-Cadherin (N-Cad) were shown via immunostaining to be effectively tethered (**Fig. 4d**). Indeed, selective modification of microwells with adhesion proteins such as fibronectin or Fc-chimeric Vascular Cell Adhesion Molecule-1 (VCAM-1) ensured efficient confinement and tracking of HSCs over long culture periods, whereas the cells escaped from the microwells within a few hours when the bulk of the surface was modified. Using this platform, individual HSCs were exposed to selected putative protein components and their growth tracked by time-lapse microscopy. It was demonstrated that single HSCs can undergo self-renewal divisions in vitro in response to selected immobilized proteins in these artificial niches. Notably, a reduction in proliferation kinetics or an increase in asynchronous division of single HSCs in microwells in response to the protein Wnt3a or N-Cadherin correlated well with subsequent serial long-term blood reconstitution in mice in vivo. These results validate the protein-tethered hydrogel microwell platform as a broadly applicable paradigm for dissecting the regulatory role of specific signals within a complex stem cell niche.

Ochsner and colleagues recently demonstrated that it is possible to form microwells having dimensions comparable to that of single cells in order to achieve complete cell confinement in protein-functionalized microwells.[73] If it were possible to pattern the microwell surfaces with different types of proteins (or protein mixtures) on these arrays, a true mimicry of a single stem cell niche with spatially well-defined polarization of protein cues could become possible.

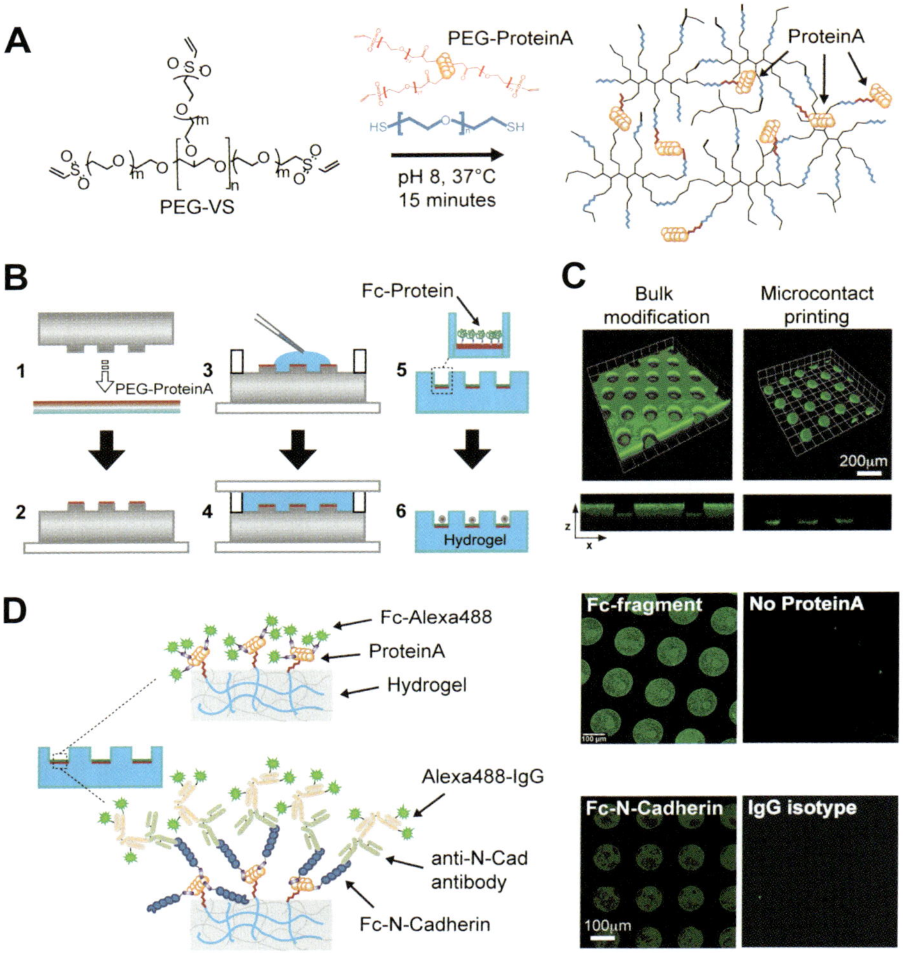

Fig. 4. Microcontact printing to generate artificial niches via site-selective attachment of niche proteins: A heterofunctional PEG linker is used to covalently attach ProteinA to PEG hydrogel networks (a). Subsequently, ProteinA site-selectively anchors Fc-chimeric proteins on hydrogel microwell arrays. Overview of multistep process to locally immobilize Fc-chimeric proteins to the bottom of hydrogel microwells (b). Proof-of-principle experiments demonstrating the spatial control of protein (here: FITC-labeled BSA) immobilization afforded by the hydrogel microcontact printing process (c). Scale bar = 200 μm. Anchoring on the bottom of individual microwells (right panel) rather than on the entire surface of the microwell array (left panel) can be achieved. 3D confocal micrographs of projection of 84 stacks acquired at a constant slice thickness of 1.8 m. Immobilization of Fc-chimeric proteins via selective binding to ProteinA. Alexa-conjugated Fc-fragment and Fc–N-Cadherin were tethered and detected via fluorescence microscopy according to the schemes (d, left & middle panels). Scale bar = 100 μm. As negative controls (right panels), microwell arrays are shown that are not tethered with ProteinA or treated with isotype control primary antibody. Reproduced with permission from [72]. Copyright 2008 Royal Society of Chemistry.

2.3. *Niche protein microarrays*

An outstanding challenge in stem cell biology is to unravel the complexity of biomolecular signaling that controls stem cell behavior. Conventional experimental paradigms, *i.e.* the testing of one signal at a time, fail to deal with this complexity. Several groups have started to address this challenge by screening the effects of combinations of multiple putative microenvironmental signals on stem cell fate.[74,75,76,77] Mixtures of protein signaling cues such as ECM components, morphogens, and other signaling proteins were microarrayed on flat glass substrates using robotic spotting technology. Stem cells can be exposed to such multicomponent artificial niches, and their response quantified at the single cell level via multi-parameter analyses involving, for example, immunocytochemistry-based read-outs (i.e. staining of cell surface markers). These high-throughput analyses of signaling networks have begun to characterize the effects of combinations of stem cell regulatory proteins on self-renewal and differentiation. In one seminal study by Soen et *al.*,[75] primary human neural precursor cells were cultured on printed protein arrays to explore the extent and direction of differentiation into neurons and glias (**Fig. 5**). Co-stimulation with two specific developmental morphogens (Wnt and Notch ligands) maintained stem cells in an undifferentiated-like state suggesting that this combination of signals may be found in the native niche, in contrast to bone morphogenetic protein-4, which led to the expression of differentiation markers. In another study by LaBarge, Bissell and co-authors, protein microarrays were utilized to dissect the instructive function of the microenvironment in human mammary progenitor cell regulation.[77] In combination with organotypic 3D culture models and micropatterned substrates, previously unrecognized combinatorial microenvironments of cell-extrinsic mammary gland proteins (including the Notch ligand Jagged-1, P- and E-Cadherin) as well as ECM molecules (including Laminin-1) were identified. Bhatia and colleagues, who pioneered this approach, recently expanded the breadth of these platforms by compartmentalizing protein arrays using gaskets to produce a multi-well plate. This advance allowed them to simultaneously probe the interactions of ECM components and soluble growth factors on stem cell fate.[78] The application of robotic spotting technologies to hydrogels, and also to microwell arrays in order to probe nonadherent stem cell populations, should allow the effects of combinatorial signaling to be studied in stem cells grown under physicochemical conditions, more closely resembling niches.

While the above studies have resulted in important discoveries with regards to extrinsic stem cell regulation, they have invariably been conducted on flat

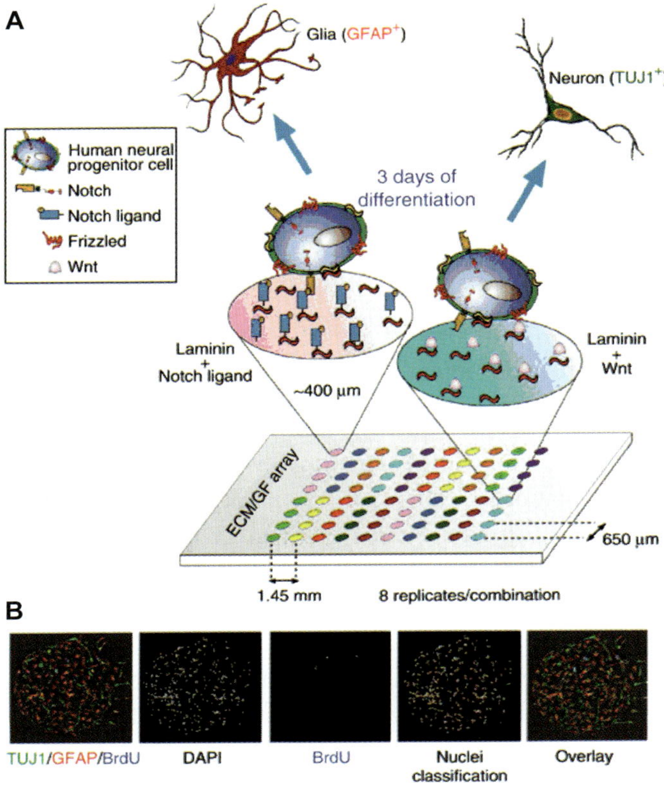

Fig. 5. Design and application of a niche protein microarray. Schematics of a molecular microenvironment array experiment (a). Arrays of pre-mixed combinations of signaling molecules were printed using a non-contact, piezoelectric arrayer. Each spot typically included a combination of Laminin (Ln) and one or more recombinant proteins that were previously implicated in cell fate decision processes. Each combination was printed in two separate groups of four replicates. Bi-potent human neural precursors were captured onto the printed spots by adherence to the Ln. Thereafter, the cells were cultured on the array under defined, differentiation-promoting conditions for about 3 days. Differentiation and proliferation responses to each microenvironment were analyzed by immunostaining with TUJ1, GFAP, and BrdU. A basic feature extraction example (b). Arrays were imaged with four wavelengths using automated fluorescent microscopy. Cell- and image-based information were extracted from each image using an analysis script that measured multiple phenotypes from each cell and computed ensemble average phenotypes. All the nuclei within a spot were detected using the DAPI channel and each nucleus was defined as an object representing a cell. Subsequent measurements were performed with respect to each nucleus and were associated with the corresponding cell. Perinuclear cytoplasmic region was defined by expanding a narrow ring of specified width (0.55 mum) around each nucleus. Cell fate and extent of differentiation were evaluated by measuring TUJ1 and GFAP intensities within the perinuclear ring. Proliferating cells were identified based on intranuclear BrdU threshold crossing. Green and orange circles indicate non-proliferating neuron-like and glial-like cells, respectively (right panel). Blue and white circles correspond, respectively, to proliferating neuron-like and glial-like cells. Reproduced with permission from [75]. Copyright 2006 Nature Publishing Group.

substrates and not in a near-physiological 3D setting. Since a stem cell in 3D is exposed to an environment with a wide range of matrix porosities, stiffnesses, proteolytic sensitivities, cell adhesion and cell signalling components, using conventional experimental approaches, it would possibly take years to achieve a comprehensive understanding of how the niche controls stem cell fate, just on one stem cell type. Therefore, novel approaches aiming at high-throughput screening of 3D microenvironmental conditions are urgently needed. In order to achieve high-throughput micro-arraying of 3D matrices,[79] robotic liquid dispensing and printing approaches could be combined with mild biomaterials crosslinking chemistries. Combinatorial mixtures of liquid precursors of hydrogel networks could for example be deposited in tiny volumes and high density onto solid substrates. Murphy et al. fabricated 3D PEG hydrogel arrays to screen for the individual and combinatorial effects of gel degradability, cell adhesion ligand type, and cell adhesion ligand density on human MSC viability.[80] PEG network degradability and the presence of cell adhesion ligands were shown to increase MSC viability in a dose-dependent manner. In future studies it will be important to increase the throughput of such technologies, and to expand the read-outs to relevant stem cell functions such as self-renewal or differentiation.

2.4. *Dissecting cell-cell interactions in the niche in 3D*

It is still poorly understood how cell membrane-bound signals emanating from support cells in the niche control stem cell function. In order to study such cell-cell signalling interactions in near-physiological 3D environments, novel model systems based on 3D cell patterning technologies need to be devised. Bhatia et al. have presented an interesting approach based on electropatterning of mammalian cells within hydrogels.[81,82] Electropatterning allows localizing live cells within hydrogels, such as photopolymerized PEG gels, using dielectrophoretic forces. Parallel formation of large numbers of living multicellular cell clusters of precise size and shape were formed in 3D. By modulating the size of 3D clusters, this microscale tissue organization was for example shown to influence bovine articular chondrocyte biosynthesis. This platform should be interesting to apply to the study of the crosstalk of stem cells with support cells in 3D. Another promising approach to investigate 3D cell-cell interactions was demonstrated by Kamm and colleagues who combined gel patterning with microfluidic technology to analyze angiogenesis in 3D co-cultures.[83] Primary liver and vascular cells were cultured on each sidewall of a collagen gel between two microfluidic channels. Morphogenesis of 3D hepatocyte cultures was found to depend on diffusion and convection across the nascent tissues. Remarkably, vascular cells formed 3D capillary-like structures that extended across an intervening gel to the hepatocyte tissues. Since microvascular networks are considered to be important components of stem cell niches, this approach of 3D engineered tissues in vitro in a microfluidic environment should have interesting applications to address fundamental questions in stem cell biology.

2.5. *3D biomolecule gradients as model niches*

A question of paramount importance in developmental and stem cell biology is how protein morphogen gradients regulate cell fate and tissue or organ development. Biomolecule gradients are indeed crucial regulatory components of dynamic tissue processes, not only during development, but also homeostasis and regeneration. Therefore, biomolecule gradients should become an important element of the emerging 3D biomaterials toolbox for stem cell biology. Protein gradients can be exploited in two ways: First, as a means of high-throughput screening for the optimal dose of stem cell signaling molecules. In this case, a large number of individual stem cells can be exposed to a relatively large-scale gradient, each cell being exposed to different protein concentration. Second, steeper gradients can serve as a means to probe the effect of a gradient on the fate of one single stem cell. Thereby, the individual cell could sense two different biomolecule concentrations across its length, possibly influencing directional stem cell migration in chemotaxis, such as in stem cell homing, or the symmetry of stem cell division (symmetric vs. asymmetric division). Arguably the most precise and robust way of generating biomolecule gradient is using microfluidic technology.[84] Microfluidic gradient platforms have already been applied to stem cell biology, albeit in 2D, (e.g. [85]). However, 3D gradient systems are rapidly emerging.[86,87] Choi and colleagues have for example presented a microfluidics-based approach whereby cells within alginate gels could be exposed to desirable soluble gradients in 3D microenvironments.[86] Applied to adult stem cell culture, such intricate control over the biochemical microenvironment in 3D constitutes an important step towards the in vitro recapitulation of more complex stem cell microenvironments. The advantages of combining biomaterials engineering with microfluidics for such applications are clearly apparent, since apart from affording excellent spatiotemporal control in biomolecule presentation, microfluidic technology also allows to array cell culture chambers that are individually addressable.[88] Since many protein morphogens are bound to the

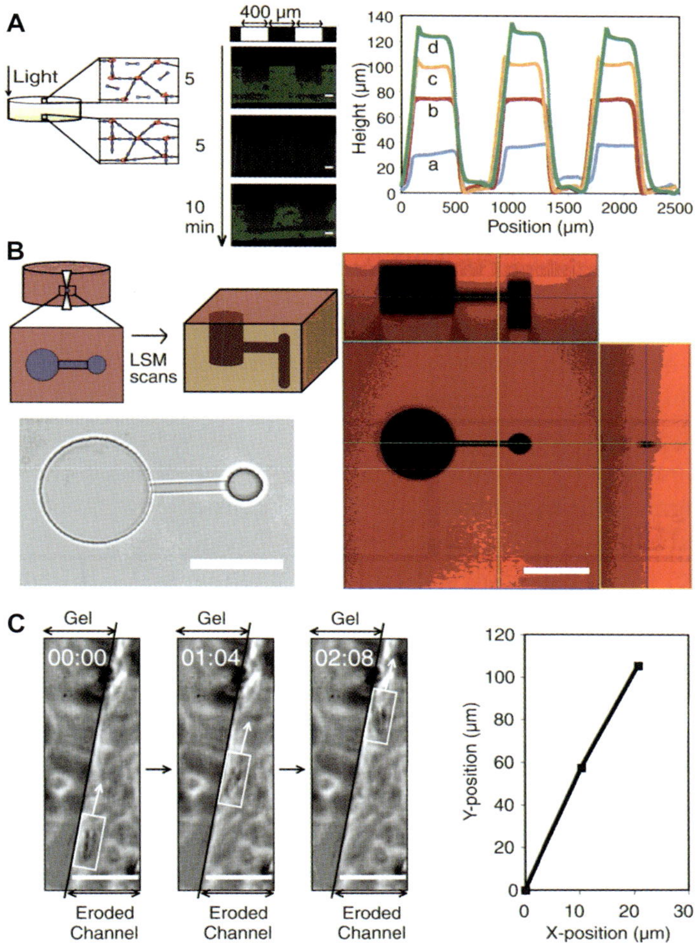

Fig. 6. 2D and 3D patterning of photodegradable hydrogels. (A) Thick gels demonstrate surface erosion upon irradiation (left). A gel covalently labeled with fluorescein was eroded spatially through masked flood irradiation (320 to 500 nm at 40 mW/cm2, 400 μm line periodic photomask). Channel depth increased linearly with irradiation, and no changes in hydrogel dimensions due to increased swelling were observed (middle). Feature dimensions were quantified with profilometry: (a) 2.5, (b) 5, (c) 7.5, and (d) 10 min irradiation (right). Scale bar, 100 μm. (B) Interconnected 3D channels were fabricated within a photodegradable gel, covalently labeled with rhodamine B, using a two-photon laser scanning microscopy (LSM). A thin horizontal channel connected two offset vertical channels of different diameter, which was visualized in brightfield (bottom left) and with confocal LSM (right, intact gel is red and the created feature is black; corresponding cross sections are noted by blue, green, and orange lines). Scale bar, 100 μm. (C) Channels were eroded within a hydrogel encapsulating fibrosarcoma cells, releasing cells into the degraded channel and enabling migration. Migration of a cell along the edge of a channel is shown in time-lapsed brightfield images (left) and its corresponding position trace (right). Scale bar, 50 μm. Reproduced with permission from [91]. Copyright 2009 The American Association for the Advancement of Science.

extracellular matrix with relatively high affinity, one open challenge in this area will be to tether 3D gradients to hydrogel networks.

2.6. *Mimicking the spatial 3D niche heterogeneity*

How do stem cells sense and respond to spatially heterogeneous 3D microenvironments? As described previously, many in vivo stem cell microenvironments are 'polarized' structures, exposing individual stem cells to differential niche components. A case in point is the niche of the muscle (satellite) stem cell, which is located between the muscle fiber membrane and the surrounding basal lamina. An ideal 3D in vitro model of a stem cell niche would allow recapitulating such complex architectures and manipulate it at a desired time during an experiment, for example to address the question whether microenvironmental polarity dictates the symmetry of stem cell division. Clever hydrogel engineering tricks based on photochemistry now promise to do that, with impressive precision and control over the dynamics as well (Figure 6).[89,90,91] For example, using photopolymerized PEG hydrogels, Anseth and colleagues have synthesized photo-labile building blocks that can be cleaved by a controlled light beam to locally modulate biophysical and biochemical gel properties at a given time point. MSCs were shown to respond to locally induced network changes in stiffness and cell adhesion properties: in a densely crosslinked gel, the decrease in crosslinking density obtained via cleavage of the photolabile chain backbone induced a significant morphological change in the encapsulated stem cells. Moreover, the controlled manipulation of cell-adhesive peptide ligand concentration in the PEG gel led to inducible changes in chondrocytic differentiation. These new methods of locally manipulating the 3D microenvironment using light will surely be powerful to explore a wealth of question in stem cell biology.

2.7. *From artificial niches to 3D in vitro 'tissues'*

Knowing how stem cell fate is controlled by niche signals should be a cornerstone in starting to build tissues outside of an organism. The 3D approaches discussed above serve as powerful model systems to elucidate extrinsic stem cell regulation, but they would not be appropriate to start re-constructing large-scale tissue models using stem cells and biomaterials as building blocks. 'Bioprinting' could perhaps be the technology of choice to facilitate such difficult endeavors. Indeed, bioprinting technologies are increasingly being scrutinized to try to recreate the 3D spatial organization of tissues (e.g. [92,93,94]) In bioprinting, custom-designed inkjet printers are applied to deposit, in a controlled layer-by-layer fashion, cells and biomaterials in nearly picoliter-sized droplets at a rate of tens of thousands per second. Upon deposition on a substrate, these droplets can be polymerized to form a solid gel that could encapsulate stem cells or contain biomolecules with locally modular composition. Although the bioprinting field has arguably had little impact on stem cell biology so far, the already obtained results look promising. Lee and colleagues for example have presented an approach to pattern in 3D viable constructs of neurons and astrocytes in multilayered collagen. Clearly, if bioprinting were to become more robust and a suitable 'bioink' available (which is arguably not the case), it would represent a tremendous step forward in realizing the long-standing dream of tissue-engineers, that is, the formation of functional tissues outside the human body.

3. Conclusions and Outlook

The merger of concepts and know-how from biomaterials science, microfabrication technology and stem cell biology has already resulted in novel experimental tools that begin to impact stem cell biology. A simplification of the niche complexity, combined with advanced imaging approaches on live stem cells, allows the investigation of the role of specific niche components and the 3D niche architecture in regulating fundamental behaviors such as mechanisms of cell division, self-renewal and differentiation. Applied in vitro, this may well lead to the generation of adequate numbers of stem cells and the ability to precisely control their differentiation in order to maximize their clinical utility as cell-based therapeutics for tissue regeneration.

However, it can be expected that many in vitro findings will result in new approaches to manipulate stem cells in vivo as well. For example, biomaterials concepts could be devised to locally and specifically deliver bioactive niche components or inhibitory/stimulatory molecules or drugs to a particular stem cell niche, to increase stem cell numbers for example. This could be realized either from the 'bulk' (solid) phase **(Fig. 7a)**, by forming a drug/biomolecule-releasing scaffold in close proximity to a stem cell niche, or via targeted delivery of soluble micro- or nanoparticles **(Fig. 7b)**.[95] Biofunctional polymer particles can now be engineered to render them efficient for such applications, as they can be functionalized to confer molecular targeting, environmental responsiveness, controlled drug release or designed cell uptake as demonstrated by Hubbell and

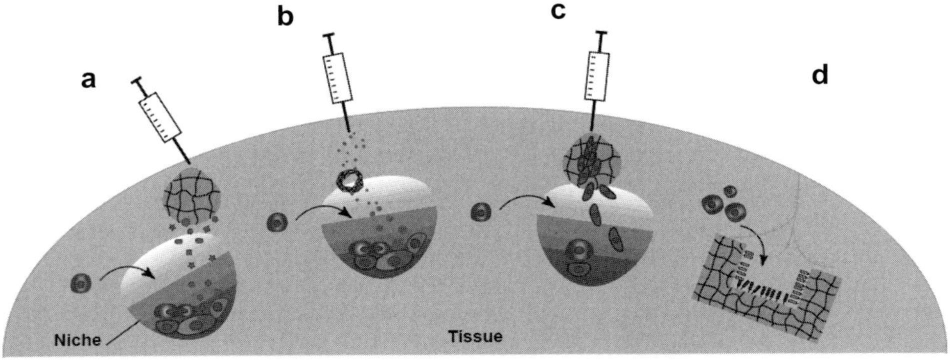

Fig. 7. Therapeutic manipulation of the natural niche using biomaterials-based approaches. Local delivery of bioactive niche components or inhibitory/stimulatory molecules from a solid (injectable) biomaterial scaffold (a). Targeting the niche via micro- or nanoparticles that carry and delivery bioactive molecules to manipulate the niche (b). Local delivery of support cells to augment or manipulate stem cell fates in vivo (c). Cell delivery could be facilitated using (injectable) biomaterials carriers that likely improve the survival and engraftment of the transplanted cells. Implanted, multicomponent artificial niche that could possibly attract stem cells to populate it (d). Reproduced with permission Reproduced with permission from [100]. Copyright 2009 Wiley InterScience.

colleagues and others.[96,97,98] Secondly, biomaterials concepts could be harnessed to locally deliver cellular components of stem cell niches **(Fig. 7c)**. 'Smart' cell delivery systems which have been shown to improve the survival, engraftment, and fate of transplanted cells are now available, as has been reviewed elsewhere.[99] Finally and maybe most excitingly, it is conceivable that multicomponent, potentially injectable materials could be designed to act as *de novo* niches in vivo **(Fig. 7d)**. If appropriate 'homing' signals were present to attract endogenous stem cells to these artificial niches and localize the stem cells via known cell-cell or cell-matrix adhesive interactions, and signals were present, which could control stem cell function, such efforts have an important impact in the near future.

References

1 Takahashi, K. & Yamanaka, S. Induction of pluripotent stem cells from mouse embryonic and adult fibroblast cultures by defined factors. *Cell* **126**, 663-676 (2006).

2 Daley, G. Q. & Scadden, D. T. Prospects for stem cell-based therapy. *Cell* **132**, 544-548, doi:Doi 10.1016/J.Cell.2008.02.009 (2008).

3 Watt, F. M. & Hogan, B. L. Out of Eden: stem cells and their niches. *Science* **287**, 1427-1430 (2000).

4 Spradling, A., Drummond-Barbosa, D. & Kai, T. Stem cells find their niche. *Nature* **414**, 98-104 (2001).

5 Fuchs, E., Tumbar, T. & Guasch, G. Socializing with the neighbors: stem cells and their niche. *Cell* **116**, 769-778 (2004).

6 Yamashita, Y. M., Fuller, M. T. & Jones, D. L. Signaling in stem cell niches: lessons from the Drosophila germline. *Journal of Cell Science* **118**, 665-672 (2005).

7 Scadden, D. T. The stem-cell niche as an entity of action. *Nature* **441**, 1075-1079 (2006).

8 Moore, K. A. & Lemischka, I. R. Stem cells and their niches. *Science* **311**, 1880-1885 (2006).

9 Schofield, R. Relationship between Spleen Colony-Forming Cell and Hematopoietic Stem-Cell - Hypothesis. *Blood Cells* **4**, 7-25 (1978).

10 Xie, T. & Spradling, A. C. A niche maintaining germ line stem cells in the Drosophila ovary. *Science* **290**, 328-330 (2000).

11 Tran, J., Brenner, T. J. & DiNardo, S. Somatic control over the germline stem cell lineage during Drosophila spermatogenesis. *Nature* **407**, 754-757 (2000).

12 Kiger, A. A., White-Cooper, H. & Fuller, M. T. Somatic support cells restrict germline stem cell self-renewal and promote differentiation. *Nature* **407**, 750-754 (2000).

13 Kiger, A. A., Jones, D. L., Schulz, C., Rogers, M. B. & Fuller, M. T. Stem cell self-renewal specified by JAK-STAT activation in response to a support cell cue. *Science* **294**, 2542-2545 (2001).

14 Li, L. & Xie, T. Stem cell niche: structure and function. *Annu Rev Cell Dev Biol* **21**, 605-631 (2005).

15 Palmer, T. D., Willhoite, A. R. & Gage, F. H. Vascular niche for adult hippocampal neurogenesis. *J Comp Neurol* **425**, 479-494 (2000).

16 Heissig, B. *et al.* Recruitment of stem and progenitor cells from the bone marrow niche requires MMP-9 mediated release of kit-ligand. *Cell* **109**, 625-637 (2002).

17 Avecilla, S. T. *et al.* Chemokine-mediated interaction of hematopoietic progenitors with the bone marrow vascular niche is required for thrombopoiesis. *Nat Med* **10**, 64-71 (2004).

18 Kiel, M. J. & Morrison, S. J. Maintaining hematopoietic stem cells in the vascular niche. *Immunity* **25**, 862-864 (2006).

19 Katayama, Y. *et al.* Signals from the sympathetic nervous system regulate hematopoietic stem cell egress from bone marrow. *Cell* **124**, 407-421 (2006).

20 Halbleib, J. M. & Nelson, W. J. Cadherins in development: cell adhesion, sorting, and tissue morphogenesis. *Genes & Development* **20**, 3199-3214 (2006).

21 Song, X., Zhu, C. H., Doan, C. & Xie, T. Germline stem cells anchored by adherens junctions in the Drosophila ovary niches. *Science* **296**, 1855-1857 (2002).

22 Yoon, K. & Gaiano, N. Notch signaling in the mammalian central nervous system: insights from mouse mutants. *Nature Neuroscience* **8**, 709-715 (2005).

23 Ohlstein, B. & Spradling, A. Multipotent Drosophila intestinal stem cells specify daughter cell fates by differential Notch signaling. *Science* **315**, 988-992 (2007).

24 Conboy, I. M. *et al.* Rejuvenation of aged progenitor cells by exposure to a young systemic environment. *Nature* **433**, 760-764 (2005).

25 Adams, G. B. *et al.* Osteoblasts participate in the stem cell niche regulating stem cell numbers by Jagged1 activation of notch. *Blood* **102**, 18A-18A (2003).

26 Tumbar, T. *et al.* Defining the epithelial stem cell niche in skin. *Science* **303**, 359-363 (2004).

27 Sacco, A., Doyonnas, R., Kraft, P., Vitorovic, S. & Blau, H. M. Self-renewal and expansion of single transplanted muscle stem cells. *Nature* **456**, 502-506 (2008).

28 Wilson, A. & Trumpp, A. Bone-marrow haematopoietic-stem-cell niches. *Nature Reviews Immunology* **6**, 93-106 (2006).

29 Scott, L. M., Priestley, G. V. & Papayannopoulou, T. Deletion of alpha4 integrins from adult hematopoietic cells reveals roles in homeostasis, regeneration, and homing. *Mol Cell Biol* **23**, 9349-9360 (2003).

30 Whetton, A. D. & Graham, G. J. Homing and mobilization in the stem cell niche. *Trends Cell Biol* **9**, 233-238 (1999).

31 Prosper, F. & Verfaillie, C. M. Regulation of hematopoiesis through adhesion receptors. *J Leukoc Biol* **69**, 307-316 (2001).

32 Zhu, A. J., Haase, I. & Watt, F. M. Signaling via beta 1 integrins and mitogen-activated protein kinase determines human epidermal stem cell fate in vitro. *Proceedings of the National Academy of Sciences of the United States of America* **96**, 6728-6733 (1999).

33 Campos, L. S. *et al.* beta 1 integrins activate a MAPK signalling pathway in neural stem cells that contributes to their maintenance. *Development* **131**, 3433-3444 (2004).

34 Nilsson, S. K. *et al.* Osteopontin, a key component of the hematopoietic stem cell niche and regulator of primitive hematopoietic progenitor cells. *Blood* **106**, 1232-1239 (2005).

35 Stier, S. *et al.* Osteopontin is a hematopoietic stem cell niche component that negatively regulates stem cell pool size. *Journal of Experimental Medicine* **201**, 1781-1791 (2005).

36 Simmons, P. J., Levesque, J. P. & Zannettino, A. C. Adhesion molecules in haemopoiesis. *Baillieres Clin Haematol* **10**, 485-505 (1997).

37 Nilsson, S. K. *et al.* Hyaluronan is synthesized by primitive hemopoietic cells, participates in their lodgment at the endosteum following transplantation, and is involved in the regulation of their proliferation and differentiation in vitro. *Blood* **101**, 856-862 (2003).

38 Reya, T. *et al.* A role for Wnt signalling in self-renewal of haematopoietic stem cells. *Nature* **423**, 409-414 (2003).

39 Willert, K. *et al.* Wnt proteins are lipid-modified and can act as stem cell growth factors. *Nature* **423**, 448-452 (2003).

40 Bhardwaj, G. *et al.* Sonic hedgehog induces the proliferation of primitive human hematopoietic cells via BMP regulation. *Nat Immunol* **2**, 172-180 (2001).

41 Trowbridge, J. J., Scott, M. P. & Bhatia, M. Hedgehog modulates cell cycle regulators in stem cells to control hematopoietic regeneration. *Proceedings of the National Academy of Sciences of the United States of America* **103**, 14134-14139 (2006).

42 Bowie, M. B., Kent, D. G., Copley, M. R. & Eaves, C. J. Steel factor responsiveness regulates the high self-renewal phenotype of fetal hematopoietic stem cells. *Blood* **109**, 5043-5048 (2007).

43 de Haan, G. *et al.* In vitro generation of long-term repopulating hematopoietic stem cells by fibroblast growth factor-1. *Dev Cell* **4**, 241-251 (2003).

44 Ramirez, F. & Rifkin, D. B. Cell signaling events: a view from the matrix. *Matrix Biol* **22**, 101-107 (2003).

45 Doe, C. Q. & Bowerman, B. Asymmetric cell division: fly neuroblast meets worm zygote. *Current Opinion in Cell Biology* **13**, 68-75 (2001).

46 Betschinger, J. & Knoblich, J. A. Dare to be different: Asymmetric cell division in Drosophila, C-elegans and vertebrates. *Current Biology* **14**, R674-R685 (2004).

47 Yamashita, Y. M. & Fuller, M. T. Asymmetric stem cell division and function of the niche in the Drosophila male germ line. *International Journal of Hematology* **82**, 377-380 (2005).

48 Morrison, S. J. & Kimble, J. Asymmetric and symmetric stem-cell divisions in development and cancer. *Nature* **441**, 1068-1074 (2006).

49 Chenn, A. & Mcconnell, S. K. Cleavage Orientation and the Asymmetric Inheritance of Notch1 Immunoreactivity in Mammalian Neurogenesis. *Cell* **82**, 631-641 (1995).

50 Noctor, S. C., Martinez-Cerdeno, V., Ivic, L. & Kriegstein, A. R. Cortical neurons arise in symmetric and asymmetric division zones and migrate through specific phases. *Nature Neuroscience* **7**, 136-144 (2004).

51 Calvi, L. M. *et al.* Osteoblastic cells regulate the haematopoietic stem cell niche. *Nature* **425**, 841-846 (2003).

52 Zhang, J. *et al.* Identification of the haematopoietic stem cell niche and control of the niche size. *Nature* **425**, 836-841 (2003).

53 Bryder, D., Rossi, D. J. & Weissman, I. L. Hematopoietic stem cells - The paradigmatic tissue-specific stem cell. *American Journal of Pathology* **169**, 338-346 (2006).

54 Wilson, A. *et al.* Dormant and self-renewing hematopoietic stem cells and their niches. *Ann N Y Acad Sci.* **1106**, 64-75 (2007).

55 Kaplan, R. N., Psaila, B. & Lyden, D. Niche-to-niche migration of bone-marrow-derived cells. *Trends in Molecular Medicine* **13**, 72-81 (2007).

56 Langer, R. & Tirrell, D. A. Designing materials for biology and medicine. *Nature* **428**, 487-492 (2004).

57 Lutolf, M. P. & Hubbell, J. A. Synthetic biomaterials as instructive extracellular microenvironments for morphogenesis in tissue engineering. *Nat Biotechnol* **23**, 47-55 (2005).

58 Engler, A. J., Sen, S., Sweeney, H. L. & Discher, D. E. Matrix elasticity directs stem cell lineage specification. *Cell* **126**, 677-689 (2006).

59 Kopecek, J. & Yang, J. Y. Hydrogels as smart biomaterials. *Polymer International* **56**, 1078-1098 (2007).

60 Alberti, K. *et al.* Functional immobilization of signaling proteins enables control of stem cell fate. *Nature Methods* **5**, 645-650 (2008).

61 Revzin, A. *et al.* Fabrication of poly(ethylene glycol) hydrogel microstructures using photolithography. *Langmuir* **17**, 5440-5447 (2001).

62 Koh, W. G. & Pishko, M. Photoreaction injection molding of biomaterial microstructures. *Langmuir* **19**, 10310-10316 (2003).

63 Dusseiller, M. R., Schlaepfer, D., Koch, M., Kroschewski, R. & Textor, M. An inverted microcontact printing method on topographically structured polystyrene chips for arrayed micro-3-D culturing of single cells. *Biomaterials* **26**, 5917-5925 (2005).

64 Chin, V. I. *et al.* Microfabricated platform for studying stem cell fates. *Biotechnology and Bioengineering* **88**, 399-415 (2004).

65 Mohr, J. C., de Pablo, J. J. & Palecek, S. P. 3-D microwell culture of human embryonic stem cells. *Biomaterials* **27**, 6032-6042 (2006).

66 Khademhosseini, A. *et al.* Co-culture of human embryonic stem cells with murine embryonic fibroblasts on microwell-patterned substrates. *Biomaterials* **27**, 5968-5977 (2006).

67 Karp, J. M. *et al.* Controlling size, shape and homogeneity of embryoid bodies using poly(ethylene glycol) microwells. *Lab on a Chip* **7**, 786-794 (2007).

68 Moeller, H. C., Mian, M. K., Shrivastava, S., Chung, B. G. & Khademhosseini, A. A microwell array system for stem cell culture. *Biomaterials* **29**, 752-763 (2008).

69 Ungrin, M. D., Joshi, C., Nica, A., Bauwens, C. & Zandstra, P. W. Reproducible, ultra high-throughput formation of multicellular organization from single cell suspension-derived human embryonic stem cell aggregates. *PLoS ONE* **3**, 1565 (2008).

70 Dykstra, B. *et al.* High-resolution video monitoring of hematopoietic stem cells cultured in single-cell arrays identifies new features of self-renewal. *Proceedings of the National Academy of Sciences of the United States of America* **103**, 8185-8190 (2006).
71 Cordey, M., Limacher, M., Kobel, S., Taylor, V. & Lutolf, M. P. Enhancing the Reliability and Throughput of Neurosphere Culture on Hydrogel Microwell Arrays. *Stem Cells* **26**, 2586-2594 (2008).
72 Lutolf, M. P., Doyonnas, R., Havenstrite, K., Koleckar, K. & Blau, H. M. Perturbation of Single Hematopoietic Stem Cell Fates in Artificial Niches. *Integr. Biol.* **DOI:10.1039/B815718A** (2009).
73 Ochsner, M. *et al.* Micro-well arrays for 3D shape control and high resolution analysis of single cells. *Lab on a Chip* **7**, 1074-1077 (2007).
74 Flaim, C. J., Chien, S. & Bhatia, S. N. An extracellular matrix microarray for probing cellular differentiation. *Nature Methods* **2**, 119-125 (2005).
75 Soen, Y., Mori, A., Palmer, T. D. & Brown, P. O. Exploring the regulation of human neural precursor cell differentiation using arrays of signaling microenvironments. *Molecular Systems Biology*, - (2006).
76 Derda, R. *et al.* Defined substrates for human embryonic stem cell growth identified from surface arrays. *Acs Chemical Biology* **2**, 347-355 (2007).
77 LaBarge, M. A. *et al.* Human mammary progenitor cell fate decisions are products of interactions with combinatorial microenvironments. *Integr. Biol.* **DOI: 10.1039/b816472j** (2009).
78 Flaim, C. J., Teng, D., Chien, S. & Bhatia, S. N. Combinatorial signaling microenvironments for studying stem cell fate. *Stem Cells and Development* **17**, 29-39 (2008).
79 Lee, M. Y. *et al.* Three-dimensional cellular microarray for high-throughput toxicology assays. *Proceedings of the National Academy of Sciences of the United States of America* **105**, 59-63, doi:Doi 10.1073/Pnas.0708756105 (2008).
80 Jongpaiboonkit, L., King, W. J. & Murphy, W. L. Screening for 3D Environments That Support Human Mesenchymal Stem Cell Viability Using Hydrogel Arrays. *Tissue Engineering Part A* **15**, 343-353, doi:Doi 10.1089/Ten.Tea.2008.0096 (2009).
81 Albrecht, D. R., Underhill, G. H., Wassermann, T. B., Sah, R. L. & Bhatia, S. N. Probing the role of multicellular organization in three-dimensional microenvironments. *Nature Methods* **3**, 369-375 (2006).
82 Albrecht, D. R., Underhill, G. H., Mendelson, A. & Bhatia, S. N. Multiphase electropatterning of cells and biomaterials. *Lab on a Chip* **7**, 702-709 (2007).
83 Sudo, R. *et al.* Transport-mediated angiogenesis in 3D epithelial coculture. *FASEB* **Mar 6. [Epub ahead of print]** (2009).
84 Whitesides, G. M. The origins and the future of microfluidics. *Nature* **442**, 368-373 (2006).
85 Chung, B. G. *et al.* Human neural stem cell growth and differentiation in a gradient-generating microfluidic device. *Lab on a Chip* **5**, 401-406 (2005).
86 Choi, N. W. *et al.* Microfluidic scaffolds for tissue engineering. *Nature Materials* **6**, 908-915 (2007).
87 Peret, B. J. & Murphy, W. L. Controllable Soluble Protein Concentration Gradients in Hydrogel Networks. *Advanced Functional Materials* **18**, 3410-3417, doi:Doi 10.1002/Adfm.200800218 (2008).
88 Lii, J. *et al.* Real-time microfluidic system for studying mammalian cells in 3D microenvironments. *Analytical Chemistry* **80**, 3640-3647 (2008).

89 Hahn, M. S., Miller, J. S. & West, J. L. Three-dimensional biochemical and biomechanical patterning of hydrogels for guiding cell behavior. *Advanced Materials* **18**, 2679- (2006).
90 Wosnick, J. H. & Shoichet, M. S. Three-dimensinal chemical patterning of transparent hydrogels. *Chem. Mater.* **20**, 55-60 (2008).
91 Kloxin, A. M., Kasko, A. M., Salinas, C. N. & Anseth, K. S. Photodegradable Hydrogels for Dynamic Tuning of Physical and Chemical Properties. *Science* **324**, 59-63 (2009).
92 Mironov, V., Boland, T., Trusk, T., Forgacs, G. & Markwald, R. R. Organ printing: computer-aided jet-based 3D tissue engineering. *Trends Biotechnol* **21**, 157-161 (2003).
93 Campbell, P. G. & Weiss, L. E. Tissue engineering with the aid of inkjet printers. *Expert Opinion on Biological Therapy* **7**, 1123-1127 (2007).
94 Mironov, V., Kasyanov, V., Drake, C. & Markwald, R. R. Organ printing: promises and challenges. *Regenerative Medicine* **3**, 93-103 (2008).
95 Zhang, L. *et al.* Nanoparticles in medicine: Therapeutic applications and developments. *Clinical Pharmacology & Therapeutics* **83**, 761-769 (2008).
96 Rehor, A., Schmoekel, H., Tirelli, N. & Hubbell, J. A. Functionalization of polysulfide nanoparticles and their performance as circulating carriers. *Biomaterials* **29**, 1958-1966 (2008).
97 Rothenfluh, D. A., Bermudez, H., O'Neil, C. P. & Hubbell, J. A. Biofunctional polymer nanoparticles for intra-articular targeting and retention in cartilage. *Nature Materials* **7**, 248-254 (2008).
98 Gu, F. *et al.* Precise engineering of targeted nanoparticles by using self-assembled biointegrated block copolymers. *Proceedings of the National Academy of Sciences of the United States of America* **105**, 2586-2591 (2008).
99 Mooney, D. J. & Vandenburgh, H. Cell delivery mechanisms for tissue repair. *Cell Stem Cell* **2**, 205-213 (2008).
100 Lutolf, M. P. & Blau, H. M. Artificial stem cell niches. *Advanced Materials* DOI: 10.1002/adma.200802582 (2009) (2009).

CHAPTER 12

ENGINEERING PEPTIDES IN HYDROGELS FOR CARTILAGE TISSUE REGENERATION

Zhaoyang Ye and Jennifer Elisseeff*

Department of Biomedical Engineering, Johns Hopkins University, Baltimore, MD 21218, USA

**E-mail: jhe@bme.jhu.edu*

1. Introduction

It is estimated that severe cartilage degeneration due to osteoarthritis (OA) afflicts 26.9 million of Americans with joint pain and life-long debilitation in some cases [1]. Articular cartilage covers the subchondral bone and serves to reduce joint stress and surface friction in normal diarthrodial joint. Trauma and diseases of the synovial joint can result in structural damages to the articular cartilage layer. Articular cartilage in adults is a comparatively avascular, alymphatic, and aneural tissue with cellular volume averaging only approximately 2% of the total cartilage volume. Chondrocytes are the principle resident cells, which are responsible for the secretion of extracellular matrix (ECM), even though mesenchymal progenitor cells (MPCs) might exist as well [2]. Chondrocytes receive oxygen and nutrients only through diffusion through tissue fluid or synovium in cartilage. When damaged, there is only limited spontaneous repair [3]. Clinically, to induce cartilage tissue repair, mechanical penetration of the subchondral bone to stimulate marrow infusion (e.g., microfracture), cartilage/osteochondral, periosteum and perichondrium grafts or autologous chondrocyte implantation (ACI) have been exploited with some success. However, these procedures are effective only for chondral defects of limited sizes and generally, the long-term biomechanical and biochemical properties of the resulting tissue fail to match that of native cartilage [4]. Functional restoration of degenerated articular cartilage still remains unobtainable.

Tissue engineering is a field of exploiting cells and biomaterials to regenerate or substitute damaged tissues and organs [5]. Articular cartilage is typically composed of 75-80% water and a solid matrix, that is 50-73% collagen II and 15-30% proteoglycan macromolecules [6]. While insoluble collagen fibrils withstand tension, proteoglycans such as aggrecan are resistant to compression, due to their extremely hydrophilicity. Engineering cartilage tissue *ex vivo* for implantation or directly inducing cartilage regeneration *in vivo* represents an exciting strategy to recapitulate the biochemical and biomechanical properties of hyaline cartilage through the appropriate combination of cells (e.g., chondrocytes and stem cells), scaffolds and biofactors (e.g., transforming growth factor β, TFG-β and bone morphogenetic proteins, BMPs) [7, 8]. The three-dimensional (3D) scaffolds not only fill tissue defects and provide the shape, but also is to mimic the native microenvironment of cells, which is very critical in maintaining the phenotype of chondrocytes and conducting lineage-specific differentiation of stem cells [9, 10]. In general, scaffolds should have appropriate porosity for accommodating cells and permeable to nutrients, waste and gas (O_2, CO_2) and bearing appropriate biological cues, while with adequate, initial biomechanical strength, which is especially important for cartilage tissue engineering. Balanced biodegradable properties that coordinate the rates of neotissue formation are also desirable, which also facilitate the integration of neo-tissue with host tissue.

Scaffolds in a variety of physical forms (i.e., fibers, sponges, meshes and hydrogels) have been exploited for cartilage tissue engineering [11]. Hydrogels due to their high water content, which mimics the native ECM, have been most attractive by offering many advantages over other scaffold [12-14]. For example, hydrogels enable homogenous cell seeding. Biofactors and other molecules can diffuse freely throughout hydrogels. *In situ* gelation allows hydrogels to accurately and completely fill irregularly shaped defects [15]. Hydrogel formation can be initiated via chemical crosslinking (e.g., initiated by redox reaction or UV radiation), self-assembling (e.g., initiated by temperature and pH change) and ionic interactions of both natural and synthetic materials. Natural materials including polysaccharides (e.g., alginate) and proteins (e.g., collagens) are advantageous because of their inherent properties of biological recognition. However, the lack of control over the gelation process, the relative weak mechanical strength and the complexities associated with purification, immunogenicity and pathogen transmission limit their applications. Synthetic materials such as poly(ethylene glycol) (PEG) can be easily subjected to chemical modifications to modulate the composition and structures of hydrogels [12]. PEG-based hydrogels are particularly exciting, which can be prepared by photopolymerization of PEG-diacrylate (PEGDA) and have been extensively used in cartilage tissue engineering [16-18]. Recently, nanofibrillar hydrogels by self-assembly of small peptides, which resembles the structural organization of native collagen fibrils, may present another attractive material for cartilage tissue engineering [19].

Optimal hydrogels for cartilage tissue engineering should be chondroconductive and chondroinductive to facilitate long-term *in vivo* phenotypic stability of chondrocytes. To achieve this goal, the interaction between biomaterials and cells are greatly appreciated [20, 21]. It is recognized that the most important step is to provide cells (chondrocytes and stem cells) with an appropriate environment for their growth and differentiation. It is well known that isolated chondrocytes will lose their differentiated phenotype (so-called dedifferenation) in two-dimensional (2D) culture [22]. It has been established that dedifferentiated chondrocytes can recover their differentiated phenotype when they are relocated into a 3D environment [23-25]. ECM is a highly hydrated network consisted of fibrillar proteins such as collagens, noncollagenous glycoproteins such as fibronectin, elastin or laminin and hydrophilic proteoglycans such as aggrecan and is also a reservoir of soluble macromolecules such as growth factors, chemokines and cytokines. ECM sequesters, modulates and potentiates secreted factors such as binding of BMP2 to GAGs [26] and enhancing the bFGF activities by heparin sulfate proteoglycans [27, 28]. The adhesion, migration, proliferation and differentiation of cells are regulated by the molecular interactions with these ECM components [20]. Biophysical and biochemical signals, transmitted from the ECM via various cell surface receptors and integrated by intracellular signaling pathways, converge to regulate gene expression and ultimately establish cell phenotype. Adhesion to fibronectin has been shown to be necessary for pre-cartilage condensation of chick limb bud cells [29]. In a recent study, MSCs were seeded onto a scaffold derived by decellularizing porcine cartilage [30]. The chondrogenesis of MSCs could be induced without any exogenous growth factors. Therefore, to mimic native extracellular microenvironment for cells is the most promising strategy for both *ex vivo* tissue engineering and *in vivo* tissue regeneration.

Peptides are the most important signaling transducers and constitute the recognition domains of proteins and therefore the functionalization of biomaterials with peptides represents the most important step in preparing biomimetic scaffolds. It is well known that synthetic polymers are normally bio-inert to cells. For example, PEG hydrogels lack adhesiveness, which largely limited their capability in promoting the cell survival and controlling differentiation for stem cells [31]. Therefore, ligands (in most cases, peptides) with motifs that mimic the natural ECM- and cell-cell interactions (e.g., cell adhesion peptides and ECM binding peptides) are engineered in hydrogel matrices with the aim to improve cell performance and achieve functional cartilage tissue regeneration [32-35]. Peptide-conjugated hydrogels represent a very promising strategy in creating biomimetic scaffolds for cartilage tissue engineering. The use of peptides and their mimics in tissue engineering is attractive for several reasons. Peptides can be produced synthetically, allowing precise control of their chemical composition and permitting immobilization on an inert surface and more resistant to denaturing insults compared to high-molecular-weight proteins. Different chemistries have been exploited to establish both efficient and controllable methodologies for introducing peptides into hydrogels. However, functionalization of peptides for their attachment, crosslinking or simply self-assembling into hydrogel systems should not compromise the biological activity of peptides. Research efforts on understanding the cell-ECM interactions further can provide insights in developing novel peptides that are promising in tissue engineering. The utilization of powerful molecular approaches such as phage display technology [36] facilitates identifying specific amino acid sequences involved in protein-protein interactions and sequences that are preferentially recognized by chondrocytes as well as stem cells. Furthermore, the development of recombinant DNA technology enables delicate design and synthesis of multi-functional peptides [37]. Recent progress in utilizing systematic, combinatorial and parallel approaches might help to expedite the identification of optimized bio-mimetic synthetic stem cell niches [38-41].

In this chapter, we first briefly summarize different hydrogel systems and cells for cartilage tissue engineering. The discussion of rational selection of peptides and the conjugation chemistry applied to introduce peptides into hydrogels will be followed. The biological influence of the modified hydrogel systems for cartilage regeneration will be thoroughly reviewed. Specifically, conjugation of peptides into hydrogels to improve cell survival, proliferation, and differentiation will be discussed in details. Excellent examples of cartilage regeneration and tissue engineering using peptide-conjugate hydrogels are presented in order to highlight the current knowledge and limitations in this area. In the end, the authors conclude with perspectives for future direction.

2. Hydrogel Systems for Cartilage Tissue Engineering

2.1. *Synthetic polymer-based hydrogels*

PEG-based hydrogels have been applied as biomaterials for both medical use and drug delivery extensively [12]. PEG molecules are highly hydrophilic. The structures of PEG molecules can be linear, branched, or star-shaped. The end hydroxyl groups on PEG are easily modified with a variety of functionalities to prepare macromers for polymerization, many of which are commercially available. PEG is normally reacted with acryloyl chloride or methacryloyl chloride in the presence of triethylamine for introducing photoreactive vinyl groups [42, 43]. PEG hydrogels can be created with a range of properties (i.e., mechanical properties and porosity) by adjusting molecular weights and the amount of PEG as well as using PEG with different topologies. Especially, PEG-based hydrogels by photopolymerization of PEGDA and or with other macromers are the most extensively exploited in cartilage tissue engineering [16, 17, 44-48]. Optimal conditions for cell encapsulation as well as *in situ* gel formation by photocrosslinking PEGDA with Irgacure ® 2959 as photoinitiator have been carefully studied for ensuring high cell viability and biocompatibility [18, 49]. A 10% of PEGDA (Mw=3400Da) is normally selected for cell encapsulation with optimized crosslinking density, i.e., porosity of the hydrogels and appropriate mechanical strength. However, pure PEG hydrogels are normally non-degradable. Therefore, oligomers of α-hydroxy acids such as lactic acid are introduced between the PEG and photoreactive groups to produce degradable macromers, such as PEG-*b*-poly(lactic acid) (PEG-*b*-PLA) [50]. Anesth and colleagues have thoroughly explored hydrogels of PEG-*b*-PLA for cartilage regeneration and showed more favorable results than PEG hydrogels [51-54]. However, the disadvantage is acidic by-products generated by the degradation of PLA. Therefore, it is thus critical to modify synthetic materials with biological or favorable chemical entities such as cyclic acetals [55, 56], which are more biocompatible to cells.

Poly(propylene fumarate)s (PPFs) are linear polyesters consisting of repeat units with multiple ester groups and unsaturated carbon-carbon double bonds available for crosslinking. Hydrogels are formed with crosslinkers (usually, PEGDA) via thermal- or photoinitiators [57, 58]. The advantage of PPFs in preparing hydrogels is their degradability. In addition, depending on the molecular weight of the PEG block, PPF-based hydrogels exhibit adjustable bulk properties (tensile and swelling properties) [59]. Specifically, hydrogels prepared with PPFs with PEGDA (3400Da) showed very good biocompatibility [57, 60] and have been successfully applied in cartilage tissue engineering [61-67].

Poly(vinyl alcohol) (PVA) has been used to prepare hydrogels for cartilage tissue engineering, too. The most attractive feature of using PVA is the abundance of pendant hydroxyl groups along the backbone which allow for various chemical modifications such as the introduction of methacrylate groups or biological molecules like fibronectin [68-71]. PVA can be modified with acrylic acid [72], methacrylic acid, glycidyl acrylate, methacrylamidoacetaldehyde dimethyl acetal [73] and 2-isocyanatoethyl methacrylate [71]. Copolymers of PVA and PEG [70] as well as PVA and chondroitin sulfate (CS) [71] have been created and used to encapsulate chondrocytes for cartilage tissue engineering applications. Thermoreversible hydrogels, like poly(N-isopropylacrylamide-co-acrylic acid) (PNiPAAm-co-AAc), have also been used to expand chondrocytes without loss of phenotype *in vitro* [74]. PNiPAAm-co-AAc is able to gel at 37°C (lower critical solution temperature, LCST) or above, and becoming liquid at lower temperatures, which allows for easy cell recovery.

2.2. *Polysaccharide-based hydrogels*

Alginate derived from brown sea algae is the most extensively studied native polysaccharide for cartilage tissue engineering. It is a polymer of (1, 4)-linked β-D mannuronic and α-L guluronic acid repeating units. The alginate forms hydrogels through very simple ionic interactions between the guluronic acid groups and divalent calcium cations (usually calcium chloride solution) [75]. Due to very high hydrophilicity, it is also non-adhesive to cells like PEG hydrogels. Studies have demonstrated that articular chondrocytes do not dedifferentiate within the alginate *in vitro* [76-78] and *in vivo* [79-81]. Short-term study in rabbits also showed positive repair of cartilage defects by chondrocytes in alginate beads [82]. Clinical Studies using chondrocytes cultured in alginate to treat full-thickness cartilage or osteochondral lesions showed some improvement after 12 months with the defects filled with both hyaline-like cartilage and fibrocartilage [83]. By culturing MSCs in alginate beads and pre-differentiated with TGF-β, the transdifferentiation of MSCs was inhibited [84] and the stable chondrogenic phenotype could be achieved [85].

Agarose is a linear polysaccharide derived from Asian seaweeds that solidifies when cooled and is known to improve the differentiation of chondrocytes [86]. Agarose gels have been used to encapsulate chondrocytes due to its non-adhesive nature and to investigate factors that affect chondrocyte metabolism including various growth factors, cell morphology, synthesis of cartilaginous ECM, cell phenotype and the efficacy to promote repair of articular cartilage defects in animal models [87-91]. A recent 2-year clinical trial suggested that autologous chondrocyte implantation within an alginate-agarose hydrogel might support hyaline cartilage-like repair tissue [92]. The chondrogenic differentiation of MSCs has also been established in agarose-based hydrogels [93-95]. Hydrogels made of hydroxypropyl methylcellulose (HPMC) grafted with silanol groups also showed to be appropriate for encapsulation of human nasal chondrocytes and support their differentiation *in vitro* [96, 97] and induce repairing articular cartilage defects *in vivo* [98].

Hyaluronic acid (HA) is an unmodified glycosaminoglycan (GAG) in ECM in all connective tissues playing major biological functions, such as cell motility, tissue organization, wound healing and angiogenesis [99]. It is a linear copolymer of D-glucuronic acid and N-acetyl-D-glucosamine with molecular weight up to 1-2 million Da. In articular cartilage, HA has the ability to bear compressive loads in joints, and provides lubrication to articulating surfaces. Akmal et al. [100] examined the effect of varying concentrations of HA on bovine chondrocytes encapsulated in alginate beads and demonstrated that low concentrations of HA significantly increased DNA, GAG and collagen synthesis of the chondrocytes. However, it is evidenced that the biological activity of HA differs depending on the molecular weight [99]. While low molecular weight HA (below 3.5×10^4 Da) can induce inflammatory response and angiogenesis, high molecular weight HA (above 2×10^5 Da) inhibits cell proliferation. HA can be degraded by hyaluronidase, which is secreted by chondrocytes. Therefore, hydrogels made of HA can facilitate migration of chondrocytes. HA can be functionalized with mono and polyfunctional hydrazides [101, 102], amino or aldehyde functional groups [103] and methacrylate groups [104, 105]. Hydrogels prepared from HA modified with methacrylic anhydride have been used to encapsulate porcine chondrocytes [106] and the chondrocytes maintained viability and were able to produce neocartilage tissue. It has also been shown that MSCs encapsulated in HA hydrogels, had improved chondrogenic differentiation over those in PEG hydrogels [107]. HA can been copolymerized with other macromers to prepare hybrid hydrogels. N-succinyl-chitosan and aldehyde modified HA formed hydrogels via Schiff-base reaction between amino and aldehyde functionalities [108]. The hydrogels were demonstrated to support the growth and differentiation of encapsulated bovine chondrocytes.

Chondroitin sulfate (CS), like HA, is one of the major components of native cartilage tissue aggrecans, capable of absorbing large quantities of water, and responsible for the compressive strength of the tissue. It is also an enzymatically degradable proteoglycan composed of repeating units of glucuronic acid and Nacetylgalactosamine with a sulfate and carboxyl group located on each disaccharide unit. CS has been modified for photocrosslinking by reaction with glycidyl methacrylate [105, 109]. Hydrogels created by copolymerization between CS and PEG have been shown to improved chondrocyte metabolism [110] and chondrogenic differentiation of MSCs [111], while hydrogels prepared by pure CS did not support chondrogenesis [110, 111].

2.3. *Protein-based hydrogels*

Collagens, specifically type II collagen, are the most abundant components in ECM of articular cartilage. However, gels made from type I collagen are extensively exploited due to its high availability. Although *ex vivo* type I collagen gels do not to support the synthesis of a cartilaginous ECM by chondrocytes, they increase chondrocyte proliferation [112]. It has been reported that the collagen-chondrocyte composite implants enhanced the cartilage repair processes *in vivo*, even though the resulting graft did not form normal morphological zones and subchondral bony plate was not produced [113-115]. Studies comparing chondrogenic differentiation of MSCs in alginate, type I and II collagen gels showed that type II collagen gels provided most favorable condition for the expression of chondrogenic phenotype [116]. Type II collagen and its analogs have been shown to support the migration of chondrocytes [117, 118], which is very important in cartilage tissue repair. Clinically, collagen gels have been applied in delivery of chondrocytes for cartilage tissue regeneration [119]. However, repair tissue comparable to native cartilage tissue is not obtainable.

Fibrin is a biopolymer of fibrinogen in blood clotting. Fibrin can be applied as hydrogels or fibrin glue depending on the preparation methods [120]. However, fibrin is a relatively weak gel and easily degraded, leading to the shrinkage of the gel. Additional crosslinking, for example, via Genipin can be used to stabilize fibrin hydrogels [120]. Fibrin hydrogels containing chondrocytes have been applied to treat chondral detects [121]. Other types of cells including MSCs have also been exploited for chondrogenic differentiation in fibrin [122-124]. Fibrin has also been applied in combination with other polymers such as collagen [125], alginate [126] and HA [127] to maintain chondrogenic phenotype of chondrocytes. Recently, fibrin glue mixed with particles made of a tri-copolymer of gelatin, HA, and CS was shown to enhance its mechanical strength and may be promising for cartilage tissue engineering [128].

Recombinant proteins due to possible artificial manipulation with rational design present another attractive source of biomaterials. These large molecular weight polymers normally consist of repeating blocks of peptides with precise composition, sequence and length and generally are biocompatible [129]. Elastin-like polypeptides (ELPs) consisting of oligomeric repeats of the pentapeptide sequence Val-Pro-Gly-Xaa-Gly (Xaa is any amino acid except proline) are one example, which can form hydrogels above the inverse phase transition temperature (T_t) and have been applied for cartilage tissue engineering [130]. The chondrogenic phenotype of chondrocytes could be maintained when encapsulated in ELP-hydrogels [131]. The chondrogenic differentiation of MSCs could be induced in these hydrogels even without the additional chondrogenic supplements such as TGF-β1 and dexamethasone [132]. Further modifications to make them more bio-recognizable will be possible via genetic design to obtain optimal scaffolds [133]. Another similar polypeptide is the silk-elastin-like protein copolymer SELP-47 K, composed of four silk-like blocks, seven elastin-like blocks, and one modified elastin block containing a lysine (K) substitution [134]. SELP-47 K can also gel at physiological temperature and has been proved to support the chondrogenic differentiation of hMSCs [134]. By recombinant technology, polypeptides consisted of repeating sequences of a specific domain of type II collagen responsible for chondrocyte migration were also constructed and shown to support chondrogenesis [118].

2.4. *Self-assembling peptide-based hydrogels*

Hydrogels prepared by self-assembling of peptides present another promising class of scaffolds for cartilage tissue engineering [19, 135, 136]. Synthetic peptides with designed peptide sequences of alternating ionic hydrophobic and uncharged hydrophilic side groups (e.g., RAD-, ELK-, ELD- and EAK-based peptides) form stable β-sheets of interwoven nanofibers at physiological conditions [137], which resemble the intricate fibrillar architecture of natural ECM. RAD16-I, a AcN-$(RADA)_4$-$CONH_2$ peptide has been commercially available for tissue culture [138]. These hydrogels have been shown to accommodate the differentiation of chondrocytes and MSCs, are highly biocompatible and can be constructed to bear cell-recognizable peptide sequences [136]. Another class of self-assembling peptides, so called peptide amphiphiles are peptides coupled with short fatty acid chains thereby amphiphile, which are also able to self-assemble into nanofibrous structures and then form gels by trapping water macroscopically [139-141]. In this case, the self-assembling process is driven by formation of a hydrophobic core composed of closely packed alkyl tails, whereby fibrous strands can build because of hydrogen bond formation between the amino acids. In cell culture media or other physiological fluids, cells can be encapsulated during gelation process. Hydrogels prepared by self-assembling of peptides have been shown to support proliferation and differentiation of cells [142-144].

3. Cell Sources for Cartilage Tissue Regeneration Chondrocytes

3.1. *Chondrocytes*

Chondrocytes are the resident cells of cartilage and are responsible for maintaining homeostasis of the cartilage ECM and, hence, functional properties. Therefore, autologous chondrocytes represent the logical choice for cell-based therapies in cartilage tissue regeneration. They have been extensively used in cartilage repair clinically [119]. Chondrocytes are easily isolated from mature articular cartilage by enzymatic digestion (e.g., collagenase and trypsin) of the cartilage tissue. Chondrocytes from nasal cartilage may also be a promising cell source [145]. Carticel®, the only FDA-approved cell-based cartilage repair product in USA, involves the harvesting and dissociation of cartilage from a less weight-bearing site, followed by *in vitro* expansion of the isolated chondrocytes, and their implantation into the damaged site [146, 147]. Implantation of cells in conjunction with scaffolds has been shown to improve cartilage repair, but in most cases the defects had been filled with a mix of fibrous and cartilaginous tissues, suggesting that dedifferentiation of the chondrogenic cells to fibroblast-like cells had taken place over time [148]. The needs to *ex vivo* expand isolated chondrocytes to obtain sufficient number of cells for tissue engineering and the concomitant dedifferentiation present a big obstacle for the application of chondrocytes. When chondrocytes undergo dedifferentiation, they decrease in production of type II collagen and proteoglycans, and acquire a fibroblastic morphology and produce type I collagen [149, 150].

3.2. *Mesenchymal stem cells*

MSCs are a very promising cellular source for cartilage tissue regeneration due to their non-limiting capability in self-proliferation and differentiation into plural lineages including chondrocytes [151-153]. The known resistance to low-oxygen conditions of MSCs makes them attractive in cartilage tissue engineering

[154-156] since cartilage is an avascular tissue. MSCs can be isolated from bone marrow, adipose tissue and many other adult tissues [157]. Normally, MSCs are characterized by their capacity to adhere to plastic, their phenotype ($CD73^+$, $CD90^+$, $CD105^+$, $CD14^-$ or $CD11b^-$, $CD19^-$ or $CD79a^-$, $CD45^-$ and HLA^-DR^-; with CD34 being expressed solely by adipose-derived MSCs) and their potential to differentiate into adipocytes, chondrocytes and osteoblasts [158] even though comprehensive protocols to confirm their identities are not available yet. It is still not clear whether MSCs from different tissues are the same population of cells [152]. Both bone-marrow-derived and adipose-derived MSCs have been mostly studied due to their ease in isolation [11, 159]. However, tissue source, donor age, and disease stage can directly affect MSC yield, rate of proliferation and multipotency. In a comparative study of MSCs isolated from 5 different tissue sources, synovium-derived stem cells were shown to have the greatest chondrogenic potential [160]. One exciting finding is that the zonal organization of chondrocytes in articular cartilage tissue might be able to be recapitulated by MSCs [161, 162]. Recently, MSCs have also been described as immunoregulatory cells and thus hold great potential for allogeneic use in treating arthritic diseases as well [163]. Murphy et al found that MSCs could delay cartilage destruction in a traumatic injury model by a direct intra-articular injection of MSCs [164]. This suggests different mechanisms of cartilage tissue engineering between *ex vivo* engineering and direct *in vivo* delivery. Therefore, MSCs are clearly not just considered as a cell source of chondrocytes, but also as a vehicle of many biofactors for inducing tissue regeneration.

It has been established that biofactors TGF-β superfamily members including TGF-β1, TGF-β2, TGF-β3 and BMPs, as well as insulin-like growth factors, Wnt proteins and fibroblast growth factors (FGFs) are essential for *in vitro* chondrogenic differentiation of MSCs [163]. Extensive studies [163] have been performed for *in vitro* chondrogenic differentiation of MSCs with the optimization of biomaterials, biofactors, mechanical stimulations (fluid flow, shear stress, intermittent hydrostatic pressure, and dynamic deformation loading). At current stage, most of *in vivo* studies for cartilage repair using MSCs have combined the delivery of biofactors via either directly encapsulated in scaffolds or incorporated into microspheres for better controlled release [165-167]. Studies [91, 95] comparing the biochemical and mechanical properties of tissue constructs engineered by MSCs and chondrocytes clearly suggested that further optimization is needed before MSCs exclusively can be used for functional cartilage tissue engineering. In a clinical trial on human OA patients, autologous bone-marrow MSCs embedded in collagen gel were transplanted into the articular defects showed improvement in their arthroscopic and histologic score while the clinical improvement did not show statistical significance [168].

3.3. *Embryonic stem cells*

Embryonic stem cells (ESCs) [7] as well as embryonic germ cells [169, 170] have been exploited in cartilage tissue engineering. ESCs, derived from the inner cell mass of the blastocyst, represent another promising cell source for tissue regeneration because of their unlimited self-renewal and ability to differentiate into all somatic cell lineages [171]. Kramer et al [172, 173] were the first to demonstrate cartilage differentiation of mouse ESCs through formation of embryoid bodies (EBs) at the presence of BMPs. Studies showed that different mouse ESCs lines exhibited varying degrees of spontaneous chondrogenic differentiation [174] and the size of EBs also influenced the chondrogenesis [175]. Both mouse [176] and human [177] ESCs have been shown to undergo complete chondrogenesis from chondrogenic induction to hypertrophic maturation. However, mouse ESC-derived chondrocytes exhibited certain differentiation plasticity into osteogenic and adipogenic lineages [178]. Current efforts are still focusing on establishing protocols for chondrogenic differentiation of ESCs [179, 180]. Hydrogels have been exploited in improving chondrogenesis of ESCs [181]. When mouse EBs were encapsulated in PEG hydrogels with the stimulation of TGF-β1, chondrogenesis with upregulation of cartilage specific markers and basophilic ECM deposition characteristic of neocartilage were observed [47]. Recently, human mesenchymal cells derived from EB out-growth were also established and encapsulated in PEG-based hydrogels, and the chondrogenic differentiation was significantly improved [182]. *In vivo* application of these ESC-derived cells showed the establishment of normal cartilage architecture in rat osteochondral defects [183]. Co-culture of human ESCs with primary chondrocytes, which enabled a feeder-free culture of ESCs and without undergoing EB formation, was shown to improve chondrogenesis, and cells derived as such when seeded in 3D scaffolds and implanted *in vivo* produced cartilaginous tissue [184, 185]. However, the potential to form teratomas and the associated legal, ethical and political issues have hampered the development of ESCs in tissue engineering. Recently developed induced pluripotent stem (iPS) cells may provide other source of chondrocytes with the advantages of avoiding legal, ethical and political issues [186, 187].

4. Rational Selection of Peptides for Cartilage Tissue Engineering

4.1. *Cell adhesion*

Cell adhesion is very critical for the survival and growth of anchorage-dependent cells (e.g., MSCs) [188]. Cells retain the round morphology when encapsulated in hydrogels consisted of alginate, agarose or PEG. Fibronectin and vitronectin are the primary glycoproteins that promote adhesion of various cell types to otherwise-inert support scaffolds [189]. Therefore, the deposition of these glycoproteins onto the surfaces of scaffolds is necessary for the interaction with integrins and subsequent cell adhesion. Integrins are principle cell adhesion receptors that mediate cell survival, proliferation, and migration in response to cues from ECM [190]. The integrins, composed of an association of one α-subunit and one β-subunit, are a large family of transmembrane, heterodimeric, cell-surface molecules and transmit information from ECM molecules across the cell membrane [191]. Chondrocytes express a variety of integrin subunits including α_1, α_2, α_3, α_4, α_5, α_6, α_{10}, α_v, and β_1, β_3, β_4, β_5 depending on their differentiated status [192, 193]. Integrin-mediated interactions of chondrocytes to ECM were implicated to be critical in various physiological cell functions such as their survival, proliferation and differentiation *in vivo* [194, 195]. For example, $\alpha_5\beta_1$ integrin is involved in chondrocyte adhesion, spreading, proliferation on fibronectin [195], and acts as a mechanoreceptor as well [196, 197]. Blocking the expression of focal adhesion kinase in integrin signaling pathway could inhibit redifferentiation of chondrocytes cultured in alginate with collagen II [198].

Peptides containing an RGD motif, which is naturally occurring in several extracellular matrix proteins (e.g., fibronectin, vitronectin, fibrinogen, etc), have been identified as the ligands for most of integrins [199]. By covalent modification of RGD peptides, attachment and spreading of cells like fibroblasts and endothelial cells on various coated substrates were stimulated suggesting their high potential in tissue engineering [200-202]. Different peptide sequences (e.g., RGD with different flanking amino acids) have different binding affinities and may bind preferentially to different integrins. Research has recently shown that cyclo(Arg-Gly-Asp-D-Phe-Lys) [c(RGDfK)] and cyclo(Arg-Gly-Asp-D-Phe-Glu) [c(RGDfE)] more efficiently compete with fibronectin for specific binding to integrin $\alpha_v\beta_3$, compared with the linear GRGDSP peptide [203]. Furthermore, the optimal density and the contextual presentation of RGD peptides for cell adhesion are required for their favorable effects [204, 205]. Intermediate adhesion is required for enabling cell migration [206]. Caution should be taken since steric hindrance introduced by adding additional sequences to an active peptide or by immobilizing a peptide to a material may result in a reduction in peptide activity.

4.2. *Interaction with ECM components*

Reconstruction of ECM for encapsulated cells in 3D scaffolds involves the organization of ECM components by cells. Organized ECM is recognizable to cells. In a recent study, when MSCs were seeded onto a scaffold derived from porcine cartilage tissue, the chondrogenesis could be induced without any exogenous growth factors [30]. However, physically entrapping ECM components such as collagen, HA and CS into hydrogels results in the unknown distorted structures. Therefore, peptides that can bind to ECM components including collagens, proteoglycans and soluble growth factors provide an alternative way to retain these molecules to maintain cell favorable niches while minimally affecting the physical-chemical properties of hydrogels. Collagens are the major components in ECM of cells and can maintain the growth and differentiation of both chondrocytes and stem cells. Retaining collagens secreted by resident cells should improve the efficiency in tissue engineering by facilitating the organization of ECM produced by resident cells. A collagen mimetic peptide (CMP, -(Pro-Hyp-Gly)$_{(x)}$-, where Hyp = hydroxyproline) was developed and found to be able to binds to type I collagen molecules through a process involving both strand invasion and triple-helix assembly [207, 208]. When PEG hydrogel is conjugated with CMP, diffusional loss of type I collagen that was added to the hydrogel was limited [209]. Decorin is a small leucine-rich proteoglycan (SLRP) and interacts with ECM components such as type II collagen and growth factors, such as fibronectin and TGF-β [210]. Therefore, decorin plays very important roles in matrix organization of cartilage [211, 212]. Specifically, type II collagen is stabilized by binding to decorin at two major sites, RELH and KLER [213, 214] against collagenase degradation [215]. Therefore, peptides derived from decorin hold potential application in cartilage tissue engineering by facilitating retaining type II collagen. Heparin binds a wide variety of growth factors, which are selected to provide suitable inductive cues, including acidic and basic fibroblast growth factor (aFGF, bFGF) and TGF-β. Park et al. [216] entrapped low molecular weight heparin (4500Da)-bound TGF-β3 in p(NiPAAm-co-AAc) hydrogels for chondrogensis of MSCs. On the other hand, the heparin-binding domains have been derived from anti-thrombin III (K(bA)FAKLAARLYRKA), modified anti-thrombin III (R(bA)FARLAARLYRRA), neural cell adhesion molecule (KHKGRDVILKKDVR), or platelet factor-4 (YKKIIKKL) [217, 218]. Therefore, introducing heparin binding sequences into hydrogels will result in enrichment of heparin, which is then available to bind a wide variety of heparin-binding growth factors and enables sequestered growth factors to be slowly released by a cell-mediated degradation of the scaffolds by heparinase and plasmin enzyme activities. A heparin-binding domain has been functionalized with a transglutaminase substrate sequence for subsequent crosslinking to fibrin [217].

4.3. *ECM remodeling*

Remodeling of ECM is required for cell migration and organization [219]. Therefore, designing peptides that can be specifically degraded by proteinases such as studies collagenase, plasmin, or MMPs secreted by resident cells will definitely offer attractive properties to hydrogels for tissue engineering. Many proteinases including MMPs are suggested to be very critical in the differentiation of chondrocytes and cartilage tissue repair. Studies show that the upregulation of MMP-13, also known as collagenase-3, occurs within 7-12 days of hMSC chondrogenesis [220]. Further, the upregulation of this enzyme coincides with the cell's down-regulation of fibronectin as seen in vivo [221]. MMP-13 is a highly active enzyme often seen in patients suffering from osteoarthritis, which is known to degrade collagen, decorin, biglycan, aggrecan and various components of the cartilage ECM [222-224]. A major MMP-13 cleavage site found on aggrecan, a cartilage ECM component, is PENFF (proline-glutamic acid-asparagine-phenylalanine-phenylalanine) [225, 226]. Acrylated hyaluronic acids with low molecular weights (MW 50,000 Da and 10,000 Da) were crosslinked with MMP-sensitive peptides (GCRDGPQGIWGQDRCG) [227]. The hydrogels prepared could be degraded by both hyaluronidase and collagenase.

5. Strategies for Bioconjugation of Peptides with Hydrogels

5.1. *Pendant attachment of peptides*

Attachment of peptides to polymers via covalent linkage formation is the straight forward way to present biological cues into hydrogels. Natural and synthetic polymers normally bear diverse functionalities, e.g., hydroxyl, carboxylate and amine, which are available for chemical conjugations while peptides normally bear amine, carboxylate, thiol groups. Modification of RGD peptides with polymerizable vinyl function is the most extensively exploited strategy to introduce them into hydrogels. For example, YRGDS has been conjugated with acryloyl-PEG-N-hydroxysuccinimide (Acryl-PEG-NHS, Mw=3400Da) in very mild conditions (in 50mM Tris buffer (pH=8.2) for 2 h at room temperature) [182, 228-231]. Acryloyl-PEG-NHS is commercially available with high purity. Acrylated peptide was also prepared through aminolysis of the N-hydroxysuccinimide (NHS) ester of acrylic acid [228]. However, the incorporation efficiency was lower compared to that with PEG spacer, which can normally reach above 80%. In addition, the PEG spacer is also able to inhibit non-specific adhesion of cells. Possible side reactions of the peptide YRGDS attributed to reaction of the Tyr or Ser hydroxyl with the NHS ester could be inhibited by selecting appropriate reaction conditions (e.g., NHS ester: peptides = 10 and a reaction time of 2 h) [228]. Similar methodologies were also applied for preparing RGD modified OPF hydrogels [232, 233]. However, the extent of incorporation of RGD-modified PEG monoacrylate into PEGDA hydrogels is limited because increasing incorporation of monoacrylated monomers affects the mechanical properties and the swelling ratio of the resultant hydrogels.

Rowley et al [234] incorporated the peptide GRGDY into alginate gels. The carbodiimide chemistry with 1-ethyl-(dimethylaminopropyl) carbodiimide (EDC)/N-hydroxysulfosuccinimide (sulfo-NHS) was used to form amide linkages between amine containing molecules (RGD peptides) and the carboxylate moieties on alginate back bone. The reaction conditions were optimized to achieve high incorporation efficiency with minimized O-acylurea rearrangement side reaction to N-acylurea, which can stably modify alginate therefore affecting ionic gelling capacity. Agarose gel can also be modified with peptides. A heterobifunctional sulfo-SANPAH cross-linker was used to functionalize peptides at the primary amines [235, 236]. The functionalized peptides are then attached to agarose by exposing to 365 nm UV light for 3 min to activate the photoreactive groups of the sulfo-SANPAH and conjugate the peptide to free CH-groups in the agarose.

Peptides can also be pendantly attached onto PNiPAAm-co-AAc hydrogels [237]. PNiPAAm-co-AAc was synthesized with certain amount of AAc to obtain LCST of 37°C. PEG-diamine was first conjugated onto the carboxylate groups of AAc as a spacer. The other amine group of PEG-diamine was then activated with sulfosuccinimidyl 4-(*N*-maleimidomethyl) cyclohexane-1-carboxlyate (Sulfo-SMCC), where the peptides (RGD peptide: Ac-CGGNGEPRGDTYRAY-NH_2 and a heparin binding peptide: Ac-CGGFHRRIKA-NH_2) was conjugated via the thiol addition to maleimide group. Aminopropyl methacrylate can also be copolymerized with PNiPAAm to have hydrogels with additional amine groups for conjugation [238]. In this study, a maleimide group was introduced by EDC coupling of ε-maleimidocaproic acid to the primary amines. Peptides with cysteine (i.e., a thiol group) are then attached to the maleimide.

Attaching peptides to fibrin hydrogels can be carried out by native enzymes, such as transglutaminase factor XIIIa, which can recognize NQEQVSP peptide sequence as its substrate [239]. Peptide sequences such as IKVAV, YIGSR or RNIAEIIKDI derived from laminin, DGEA derived from collagen and RGD have all been coupled with a transglutaminase substrate sequence to generate a biofunctional peptide for subsequent incorporation into other proteins (e.g., fibrin gel) [239, 240]. This methodology is very attractive without using chemicals and subsequent tedious purifications.

5.2. *Crosslinking via peptides*

Peptides can be functionalized with two functionalities, which enable them to be used as crosslinkers. The hydrogels prepared via peptide crosslinkers can be biologically degradable. Cell responsive remodeling of the scaffolds is also becoming possible, which makes hydrogels more attractive in tissue engineering. Vinylsulfone-functionalized PEG macromers have been cross-linked via a Michael-type addition reaction between the vinylsulfone end groups and thiol-bearing peptides [241]. These reactions can be conducted under physiological conditions and allow for the preparation of hydrogels in the presence of cells or *in vivo* [242]. Acrylated hyaluronic acids with low molecular weights (Mw=50,000 Da and 10,000 Da) were also crosslinked with MMP-sensitive peptides (GCRDGPQGIWGQDRCG) [227]. The hydrogels prepared could be degraded by both hyaluronidase and collagenase. On the other hand, photoinititated reaction between thiol-methacrylate [243] can result in networks with step-wise growth (thiol-methacrylate reaction) and chain polymerization (methacrylate homopolymerization). Therefore, when RGD peptides containing cysteines at both termini (CCRGDSCC) were reacted with PEG dimethylacrylate with the presence of Irgacure® 2959 as a photoinitiator under 365-nm UV light [244], hydrogels with RGD peptides in the backbone of the polymer or as crosslinker can be created.

Zhu et al [245] developed a new method to create peptide-modified PEG hydrogels. A cyclic RGD peptide functionalized with two lysine moieties with three continuous serine as a spacer (cyclo[RGDfE(SSSKK-NH_2)]) was synthesized. Two molecules of Acryl-PEG-NHS were attached to one molecule of the peptide to make macromers. The extent of incorporation of peptides can easily be controlled with minimal influence on the physical properties of hydrogels. The degradable peptide sequences with two primary amines in the sequences such as GGLGPAGGK (collagenase-sensitive) and AAAAAAAAK (elastase-sensitive) were reacted with Acryl-PEG-NHS to generate block copolymer, which are then crosslinked as PEGDA [229, 246].

Combination of different chemistries can be exploited to construct more exquisite biological cues into hydrogels. Lutolf et al [247] attached a RGD peptide (RGDSP) to vinylsulfone-functionalized PEGs and cross-linked the macromers with MMP-sensitive peptide sequences. RGD peptide enhances the cell adhesion, while MMP-sensitive peptide attributes the cell-responsive degradation to hydrogels. In addition, using recombinant DNA technology, a laminin-derived peptide (PPFLMLLKGSTR, which has a strong affinity for $\alpha_3\beta_1$ integrin) was able to be fused with a collagen-binding polypeptide domain at either one terminus or both termini [37]. Therefore, multi-functional peptides can be synthesized for conjugation into hydrogels.

5.3. *Direct designing self-assembling peptides*

New developments in peptide chemistry (e.g., self-assembling peptides) have greatly enhanced its application in biomaterials [248]. As mentioned before, by appropriate designing of peptide sequences or including a hydrophobic chain, peptides can be afforded capability of self-assembling into macroscopic hydrogels in cell-favorable conditions. Furthermore, different bioactive motifs can be constructed into self-assembling structures thereby self-assembling of peptides presents another way of incorporating peptides into hydrogels. The hydrogels prepared by self-assembling of peptides without any bioactive motifs has been shown to support the chondrogenic phenotype of encapsulated chondrocytes [19]. Introducing bioactive sequences into the self-assembling peptides will improve the efficiency of cartilage tissue engineering. For example, a laminin derived peptide, IKVAVPA, could be designed into a peptide amphiphile to promote neurite sprouting and to direct neurite growth [249]. In another study, a peptide amphiphile was designed to be consisted of different domains [250]. The peptide sequence contained an MMP-2-cleavable site composed of GTAGLIGQ; a glutamic acid to assist in calcium binding for self-assembling; and a cell-adhesion sequence, RGDS. Even though few reports could be found in literatures about the application of self-assembling peptides in cartilage tissue engineering, these hydrogels definitely present a very promising way for cell delivery.

5.4. *Controlled presentation of peptides*

Temporal and spatially controlled presentation (i.e., micro/nanopatterning) of peptides in hydrogels is desirable such as to develop a scaffold with anisotropic adhesion characteristics or other bioactive cues so that cells can be directed to respond differentially within hydrogels, which may allow for engineering of complex tissue constructs. Studies have shown that cells are more responsive to the nanoscale spatial organization of RGD peptides (such as clustered rather than random) [251, 252]. The layered organization of chondrocytes within cartilage implicates the importance to engineer a stratified structure. Microfabrication methods are developed to create patterned structures for 3D hydrogels, for example, photolithographic patterning [253] and 3D printing [254]. Guided cell growth along the patterns can be achieved by patterned adhesive peptides [253, 255]. Shoichet and colleagues developed bioactive channels (bioactive cues at confined regions) within hydrogels by using a focused laser [256-258], which provides a practical way of spatially controlling the presentation of peptides. First, an agarose hydrogel was modified with a cysteine derivative containing a photosensitive sulphydryl protecting group (S-2-nitrobenzyl-cysteine) via ester bond formation at the presence of 1,1′-carbonyldiimidazole (CDI) [256]. Then, upon exposure to the laser, which can be focused to defined regions, patterned channels with free sulphydryl groups could be created. The adhesive peptide, GRGDS with a maleimide terminus could therefore be conjugated onto agarose only within those channels. The guidance effects of GRGDS oligopeptide-modified channels on the 3D cell migration and neurite outgrowth was observed *in vitro*. Similarly, West and colleagues applied two-photon laser scanning (TPLS) photolithographic technique to create an RGD micropatterning within degradable PEG hydrogels for guided cell migration [259, 260]. In these studies, acrylate-PEG–(GGGLGPAGGK–PEG)$_n$–acrylate, n≥3, was pre-crosslinked with the presence of cells in fibrin gel. The gel was then soaked in RGDSK–PEG–acrylate solution and exposed to TPLS across an x-y plane within the hydrogel according to the pre-defined regions. Very complicated patterns could be created [260]. Migration of cells along RGD patterned pathways within degradable PEG hydrogels was observed [259]. By exploiting Huigsen [3+2] cycloaddition reaction for gelation and thiol-ene photocoupling for peptide patterning, the independently tuning the materials physical and biochemical properties can be achieved [261]. In a very recent publication, Kloxin et al. [262] conceptualized a real-time manipulation for the presentation of RGD peptides in hydrogels. In their studies, the RGD peptide was functionalized with nitrobenzyl ether moiety, which is photolabile and bearing an acrylic group for polymerization with PEGDA. By irradiation with laser, the releasing of RGD peptides can be realized with controlled patterns and at demanded time. This provides a promising strategy in controlling microenvironments on demand.

6. Peptide Conjugated Hydrogels for Cartilage Tissue Engineering

6.1. *Promoting survival, proliferation and chondrogenesis of cells via RGD conjugation*

Anchorage-dependent cells, when encapsulated in 3D scaffolds, i.e., hydrogels, have to initiate integrin-mediated attachment for their survival [263]. However, most scaffolds prepared from synthetic polymers, such as PEG, are bio-inert to cells. When MSCs are immobilized in hydrogels, they take a spherical morphology [18, 264]. Nuttelman et al [31] examined the viability of hMSCs when encapsulated in PEG hydrogels (10% PEGDA, 3400Da) and found hMSC viability drops to 15% after 1 week cultured in MSC medium (DMEM plus 10% FBS). However, when the PEG hydrogels were modified with RGD (Acryl-PEG-RGD, 2.8mM in pre-gel solution), around 75% of cells survived after 1 week in culture. This was obviously due to the improvement of cell attachment and spreading in hydrogels containing RGD peptides. Salinas et al. [244] prepared PEG hydrogel modified with an RGD peptide (CCRGDSCC) via a photoinitiated reaction between thiol and acrylate groups. Molar concentrations of RGD peptides were found to be important in maintaining viability of hMSCs. While hydrogels with 5 mM RGD peptides were found to maintain 77% of cell viability after 2 weeks in MSC medium, only 50% of cell viability was maintained in hydrogels with 0 mM RGD peptides and hydrogels with 15 mM of RGD peptides did not support cell growth at all. The chondrogenic differentiation was also significantly enhanced with 5 mM RGD peptides. Nathaniel et al. developed hESC-derived cells [182] as well as feeder-free cultured hESCs (**Figure 1** and **2**), which were chondrogenically committed by co-culturing with chondrocytes and also showed superior chondrogenesis when encapsulated them in RGD-modified PEG hydrogels compared to PEG hydrogels. However, cell adhesion may not be necessary for chondrocytes. A RGD-peptide coated surface was found to accelerate the dedifferentiation of chondrocytes [193]. Disruption of the

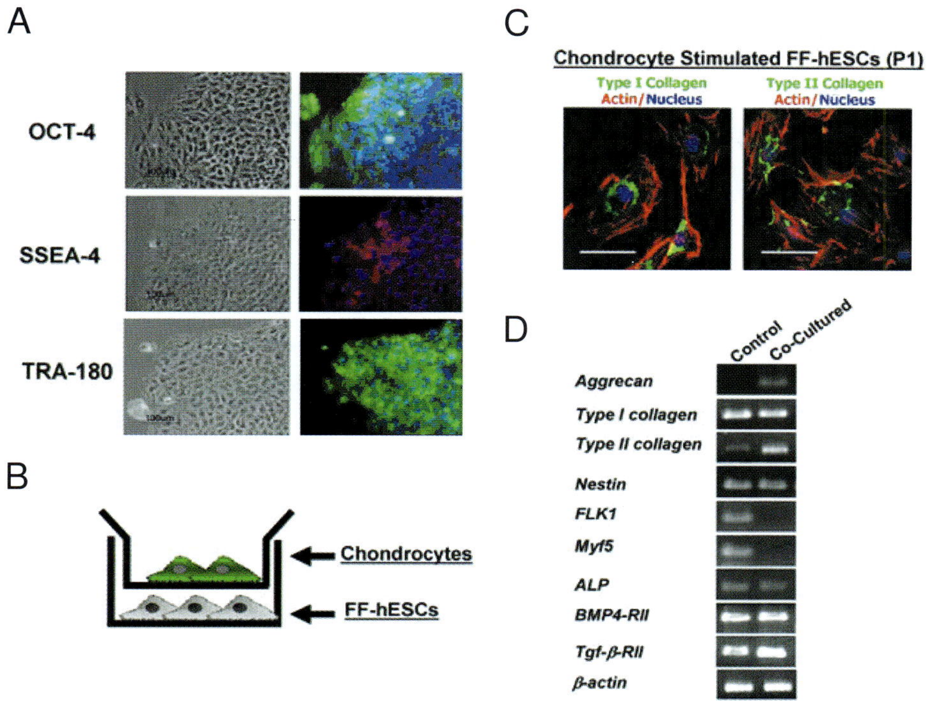

Fig. 1. Derivation of chondrogenically-committed cells from feeder-free hESCs. (Reprinted with permission from Hwang NS, Varghese S, Elisseeff J (2008) PLoS ONE 3(6): e2498).

F-actin cytoskeleton with cytochalasin D inhibits this dedifferentiation process [265], while culturing chondrocytes within three-dimensional hydrogels preserves their rounded morphology and chondrocytic phenotype [266]. Chondrocytes, which are anchorage-independent, remained highly viable in PEG hydrogels even after 2 weeks in culture [44], even though Alsberg et al. [267] demonstrated that incorporating RGD peptides into alginate gel was advantageous to promote the differentiation of chondrocytes after subcutaneous implantation in mice, which resulted in growing cartilage tissue.

The contextual presentation of RGD peptide motifs within the hydrogels may have very important roles in cartilage tissue engineering with peptide-conjugated hydrogels. Studies have shown that cell attachment and migration can be regulated by spatial presentation of RGD peptides at the nanoscale level [251]. Minimum distance required for ligands extending out from scaffold surfaces was also determined to be 3.0-3.5 nm [268]. Naturally, RGD peptide is presented to the cell via a loop-like conformation within the fibronectin molecule [269, 270].

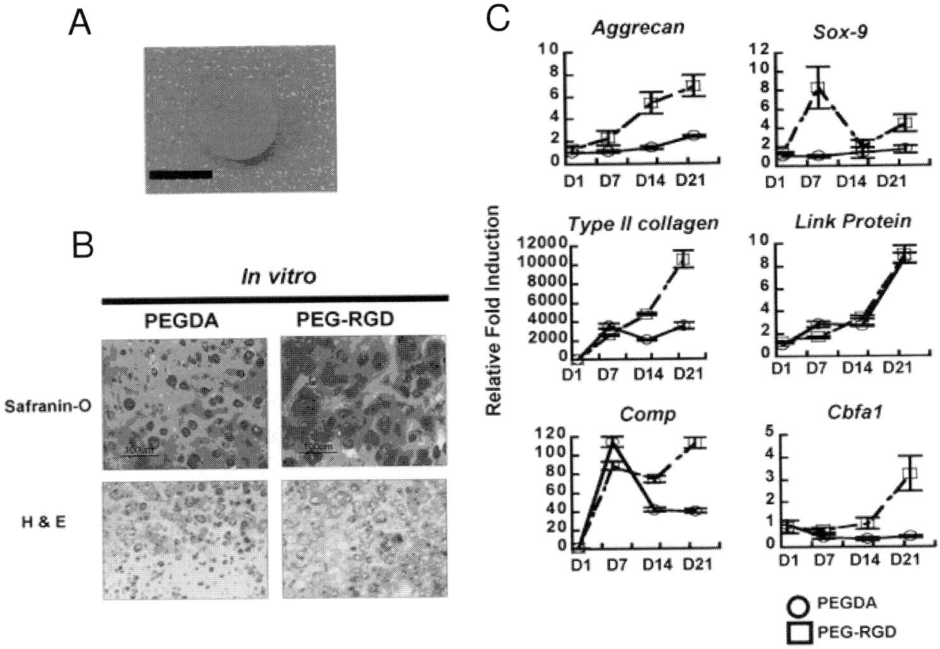

Fig. 2. *In vitro* chondrogenic differentiation of chondrogenic-committed cells derived from hESCs in PEG-based hydrogels. (Reprinted with permission from Hwang NS, Varghese S, Elisseeff J (2008) PLoS ONE 3(6): e2498).

In a study by Salinas et al. [244, 271] the RGD peptides were incorporated into PEG hydrogels either as pendant attachments or dually attached as crosslinker or embedded in the backbone of the polymer. In addition, a RGD peptide with an eight-glycine spacer ($C(G)_8RGDSG$) was also used to modify hydrogels. The viability of hMSCs in hydrogels after 2 weeks of culturing in MSC medium was found to be 79%, 84% and 61% for pendantly attached without a spacer, pendantly attached with the spacer and dully attached, respectively. Therefore, the spacer and pendant attachment of RGD peptide sequences for cell adhesion are favorable. Furthermore, integrin receptors for $\alpha_v\beta_3$ correlated to the trends in hMSC survival [244].

Now, it becomes clear that the integrin-mediated adhesion is only necessary at the onset of differentiation down the chondrogenic path for MSCs [221]. Down-regulation of fibronectin is correlated with maturation of chondrocytes [221, 272]. Therefore, the presence of RGD peptides in hydrogels is favorable for early stages of chondrogenesis, while limiting complete differentiation of MSCs. In one study, the chondrogenesis of MSCs in RGD-modified alginate was

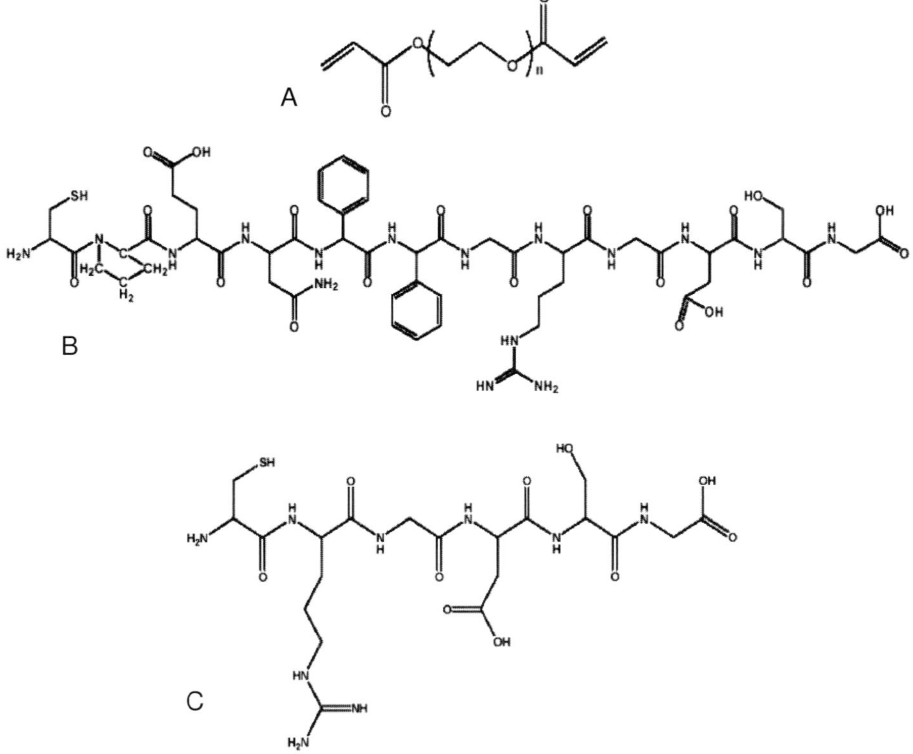

Fig. 3. Chemical structures for PEGDA (A), a bifunctional peptide containing RGD and MMP-sensitive motifs, CPENFFGRGDSG (B) and a RGD peptide, CRGDSG (C). (Reprinted with permission from Salinas CN, Anseth KS (2008) Biomaterials 29(15): 2370 and with permission from Elsevier Ltd, Copyright © 2008).

found to be lower than that in RGE (a non-adhesion peptide)-modified alginate, even though increased proliferation in RGD-modified alginate was observed [264]. The introduction of MMP-13 cleavage motif (PENFF) to the RGD peptide sequence could enable cellular responsive release of RGD peptides from the hydrogels along with the differentiation process of MSCs [273]. In this study, the bifunctional peptide (CPENFFGGRGDSG) was incorporated in PEG hydrogels via photoinitiated mixed-mode thiol-acrylate addition with PEG dimethacrylate (**Figure 3**). Therefore, the peptide was only pendantly attached since only one cysteine in the sequence. hMSCs encapsulated in hydrogels with cleavable RGD peptides produced 10 times as much GAG as those in hydrogels with uncleavable RGD peptides by day 21 of culture. However, the cell viability was observed to be decreasing dramatically after day 11 culture in chondrogenic medium probably due to the detachment of cells from the scaffolds. Further optimization for enhanced cell survival will be needed for the application of this concept in cartilage tissue engineering. A photodegradable PEG hydrogel was constructed with real-time manipulation of the physical and chemical properties by Kloxin et al. [262]. The RGD peptide was functionalized with nitrobenzyl ether moiety, which is photolabile and bearing an acrylic group for polymerization with PEGDA. By inducing the releasing RGD peptides via photo-irradiation at day 10 in chondrogenic medium, the production of both GAG and type II collagen was significantly increased compared to hydrogels with persistent RGD peptides by day 21. The viability in these hydrogels was maintained during the culture time.

Therefore, it suggests that while RGD peptide modification improves the overall viability and proliferation of cells in otherwise non-adhesive hydrogels, the integrin mediated interactions with scaffolds may also have direct effects on the differentiation of cells [264, 274]. There is possibility that the adhesion to specific matrix molecules might influence TGF-β and other growth factor signals in regulating the chondrogenic differentiation process [275]. Care should be taken when modifying biomaterials with peptides, such as RGD peptides. Connelly et al found that when bone-marrow derived MSCs were encapsulated in RGD modified alginate gels, the stimulating effect of TGF-β on chondrogenic differentiation was inhibited [264]. Even though the inhibition mechanism is not clear yet, modulating cytoskeletal organization by integrin mediated adhesion might be attributed to this [236]. Studies [274, 276] have also demonstrated that specific receptors, such as $\alpha_v\beta_3$, can play distinct roles in adhesion and spreading while other integrins, such as $\alpha_5\beta_1$, are more important for differentiation. Integrin can act as a mechanoreceptor in regulating chondrocyte activity when encapsulated in hydrogels [277]. RGD conjugation can inhibit collagen production (at low RGD concentrations) when hydrogels subjected to dynamic compressive strains, but stimulate GAG synthesis (at higher RGD concentrations).

6.2. *Enhanced chondrogenesis with ECM-binding peptides*

Lee et al. [209] conjugated the collagen mimetic peptide (CMP, -(Pro-Hyp-Gly)$_7$-) to PEGDA hydrogels by functionalizing the peptide with Acryl-PEG-NHS. When chondrocytes were encapsulated, the ECM production was significantly improved compared to cells in PEG hydrogels. In another study [278], bone marrow-derived MSCs were encapsulated in the CMP-conjugated PEG hydrogels and the chondrogenic differentiation was investigated *in vitro*. More than 2-fold increase in the production of both GAG and collagen was achieved compared to those by MSCs encapsulated PEG hydrogels. In addition, by incorporation of CMP peptides, the hypertrophic differentiation was inhibited, which was evidenced by down-regulation of both type X collagen and *cbfa*-1, an essential transcriptional factor for osteoblast differentiation. Improved retention of MSC-secreted collagen was believed to contribute to enhanced chondrogenic differentiation of MSCs. Salinas and Anseth [279] derived a peptide (CKLERG) containing KLER, one of the two major decorin binding sites for type II collagen and pendantly conjugated the peptide into PEG hydrogels via a photoinitiated thiol-acrylate polymerization with PEGDA. A RGD peptide CRGDSG was also incorporated into the gels for promoting cell survival. hMSCs were encapsulated in the hydrogels with 1 mM of CRGDSG and 5 mM of CKLERG. During a 6-week period of culture in chondrogenic medium, the production of both GAG and type II collagen was much higher compared to all controls including hydrogels with RGD peptides only. The expression of chondrogenic gene markers such as *aggrecan* and type II collagen was also increased in hydrogels conjugated with decorin peptides. These improvements in chondrogenesis were suggested to the better ECM organization by decorin moieties.

6.3. *Remodeling for neo-cartilage tissue formation and integration of engineered tissue*

Hydrogels with degradable property or even more sophisticated cell-responsive degradation is highly desirable for cartilage tissue engineering [52]. Scaffolds provide temporal physical support for cells in tissue engineering. However, following neo-tissue formation, it will be very important for the scaffolds to be remodeled passively or actively by cells to accommodate cellular residents and newly deposited ECM. This will result in organizing cellular contents in engineering tissue constructs and inducing desirable tissue regeneration as well as integration of neo-tissue. As discussed above, MMPs, especially MMP-13, play very important roles in the chondrogenesis [220]. Their expression is coincident with the process of chondrogenic differentiation. Based on these, MMP-degradable scaffolds have been exploited in cartilage tissue engineering. Hubbell and colleagues [247, 280] pioneered the application of MMP-sensitive hydrogels in tissue engineering and showed that degradation of the hydrogels by cell-secreted MMPs facilitated cell invasion [280]. Park et al. [281] applied the same MMP-degradable PEG hydrogels for chondrocytes. MMP-sensitive peptides (GCRDGPQGIWGQDRCG) were designed to bear thiol functionalities for crosslinking with four- and eight-armed PEG-VS macromers. Primary bovine calf chondrocytes were encapsulated for 1 month in culture with more than 90% viability in all gels. The chondrogenic gene markers of chondrocytes in these degradable gels were increased comparing to those in non-degradable gels prepared from PEG-VS and PEG-dithiol, while the expression of MMP-13 was decreased. In addition, more diffused collagen fibrils and much larger cell clusters were observed in degradable hydrogels, even though cell numbers were not increased. In addition, eight-armed PEG hydrogels were not favorable for chondrogenesis due to much higher crosslinking density.

6.4. *In vivo cartilage tissue regeneration*

Alsberg et al. [267] demonstrated that incorporating RGD peptides into alginate gel was required for the proliferation of encapsulated chondrocytes after implantation, while minimal growth of the implanted constructs was observed. By co-transplantation of osteoblasts with chondrocytes in RGD-modified alginate, organization of chondrocytes into the grow-plate-like tissue could be obtained. This also suggests that the patterned presentation of adhesive peptides may lead to engineered complex tissues with organized cell contents.

Recently, chondrogenic commitment of feeder-free cultured hESC by co-culturing them with chondrocytes on Transwell™ inserts was established [185]. These chondrogenic committed cells could be expanded while maintaining the expression of chondrogenic gene markers and applied for cartilage tissue engineering. The expanded cells (Passage 8) were encapsulated in PEG-based hydrogels and subcutaneously transplanted into athymic nude mice for up to 24 weeks. The stability of chondrogenic phenotype of the derived cells was well maintained. Greater amounts of GAG and collagen were observed in PEG-RGD hydrogels compared to PEGDA hydrogels at 12 weeks. However, after 24 weeks, more GAG accumulated in PEGDA hydrogels, with comparable amounts of collagen detected in both hydrogels [185].

7. Conclusions and Perspectives

At current stage, the engineered cartilage tissue is still not comparable to native cartilage tissue. Not only the biochemical content and tensile properties of the *ex vivo* engineering tissue in hydrogels by stem cells are not matching those by chondrocyte-loaded hydrogels [91], but also tissue constructs by both cell types are still inferior to native ones [282]. Different hydrogels demonstrated distinct properties in supporting chondrogenesis for stem cells and chondrocytes [91], especially *in vivo* [283]. Long-term stable cartilage-like transplants *in vivo* have still not obtainable by tissue engineering. Even though peptide-conjugated hydrogels have been extensively studied for chondrogenesis *in vitro*, there are only very few reports on the *in vivo* performance of either implanted *ex vivo* engineered tissue constructs or direct *in situ* formed composites. In addition, integration of repaired tissue with surrounding tissue is very important in assessing the cartilage tissue repair. Implanting undifferentiated cells in scaffolds is believed to able to achieve better integration between neotissue and host tissue [284]. A partially developed cartilaginous material (defined as an intermediate) would facilitate integration of the implant with host tissue [285]. The hydrogels with cell-remodeling properties may facilitate the neo-tissue integration due to the possible cell invasion and cell migration. All these potential advantages warrant intensive studies on the *in vivo* cartilage tissue engineering using peptide-conjugated hydrogel systems

References

[1] R.C. Lawrence, D.T. Felson, C.G. Helmick, L.M. Arnold, H. Choi, R.A. Deyo, S. Gabriel, R. Hirsch, M.C. Hochberg, G.G. Hunder, J.M. Jordan, J.N. Katz, H.M. Kremers and F. Wolfe, Arthritis Rheum, 58 (2008) 26.

[2] S. Alsalameh, R. Amin, T. Gemba and M. Lotz, Arthritis Rheum, 50 (2004) 1522.

[3] E.B. Hunziker, Osteoarthritis Cartilage, 7 (1999) 15.

[4] M.W. Kessler, G. Ackerman, J.S. Dines and D. Grande, Sports Med Arthrosc, 16 (2008) 246.

[5] L.G. Griffith and G. Naughton, Science, 295 (2002) 1009.

[6] R.G. LeBaron and K.A. Athanasiou, Biomaterials, 21 (2000) 2575.

[7] M.J. Stoddart, S. Grad, D. Eglin and M. Alini, Regen Med, 4 (2009) 81.

[8] C. Vinatier, D. Mrugala, C. Jorgensen, J. Guicheux and D. Noel, Trends Biotechnol, 27 (2009) 307.

[9] N.S. Hwang, S. Varghese and J. Elisseeff, Adv Drug Deliv Rev, 60 (2008) 199.

[10] P.X. Ma, Adv Drug Deliv Rev, 60 (2008) 184.

[11] C. Chung and J.A. Burdick, Adv Drug Deliv Rev, 60 (2008) 243.

[12] A.S. Hoffman, Ann N Y Acad Sci, 944 (2001) 62.

[13] J.L. Drury and D.J. Mooney, Biomaterials, 24 (2003) 4337.

[14] F. Brandl, F. Sommer and A. Goepferich, Biomaterials, 28 (2007) 134.

[15] J. Elisseeff, Expert Opin Biol Ther, 4 (2004) 1849.

[16] J. Elisseeff, K. Anseth, D. Sims, W. McIntosh, M. Randolph, M. Yaremchuk and R. Langer, Plast Reconstr Surg, 104 (1999) 1014.

[17] J. Elisseeff, W. McIntosh, K. Anseth, S. Riley, P. Ragan and R. Langer, J Biomed Mater Res, 51 (2000) 164.

[18] C.G. Williams, T.K. Kim, A. Taboas, A. Malik, P. Manson and J. Elisseeff, Tissue Eng, 9 (2003) 679.

[19] J. Kisiday, M. Jin, B. Kurz, H. Hung, C. Semino, S. Zhang and A.J. Grodzinsky, Proc Natl Acad Sci U S A, 99 (2002) 9996.

[20] H.K. Kleinman, D. Philp and M.P. Hoffman, Curr Opin Biotechnol, 14 (2003) 526.

[21] K. Saha, J.F. Pollock, D.V. Schaffer and K.E. Healy, Curr Opin Chem Biol, 11 (2007) 381.

[22] E.M. Darling and K.A. Athanasiou, J Orthop Res, 23 (2005) 425.

[23] J. Bonaventure, N. Kadhom, L. Cohen-Solal, K.H. Ng, J. Bourguignon, C. Lasselin and P. Freisinger, Exp Cell Res, 212 (1994) 97.
[24] C. Domm, M. Schunke, K. Christesen and B. Kurz, Osteoarthritis Cartilage, 10 (2002) 13.
[25] J. Malda, C.A. van Blitterswijk, M. Grojec, D.E. Martens, J. Tramper and J. Riesle, Tissue Eng, 9 (2003) 939.
[26] M. Grunert, C. Dombrowski, M. Sadasivam, K. Manton, S.M. Cool and V. Nurcombe, J Mol Histol, 38 (2007) 393.
[27] M. Fannon, K.E. Forsten and M.A. Nugent, Biochemistry, 39 (2000) 1434.
[28] D.A. Rider, C. Dombrowski, A.A. Sawyer, G.H. Ng, D. Leong, D.W. Hutmacher, V. Nurcombe and S.M. Cool, Stem Cells, 26 (2008) 1598.
[29] O.S. Bang, E.J. Kim, J.G. Chung, S.R. Lee, T.K. Park and S.S. Kang, Biochem Biophys Res Commun, 278 (2000) 522.
[30] N.C. Cheng, B.T. Estes, H.A. Awad and F. Guilak, Tissue Engineering Part A., 15 (2009) 231.
[31] C.R. Nuttelman, M.C. Tripodi and K.S. Anseth, Matrix Biol, 24 (2005) 208.
[32] M.P. Lutolf and J.A. Hubbell, Nat Biotechnol, 23 (2005) 47.
[33] R. Stoop, Injury, 39 Suppl 1 (2008) S77.
[34] C.C. Lin and K.S. Anseth, Pharm Res, 26 (2009) 631.
[35] G.D. Nicodemus and S.J. Bryant, Tissue Eng Part B Rev, 14 (2008) 149.
[36] J.K. Scott and G.P. Smith, Science, 249 (1990) 386.
[37] M. Hiraoka, K. Kato, T. Nakaji-Hirabayashi and H. Iwata, Bioconjug Chem, (2009).
[38] D.G. Anderson, S. Levenberg and R. Langer, Nat Biotechnol, 22 (2004) 863.
[39] S. Neuss, C. Apel, P. Buttler, B. Denecke, A. Dhanasingh, X. Ding, D. Grafahrend, A. Groger, K. Hemmrich, A. Herr, W. Jahnen-Dechent, S. Mastitskaya, A. Perez-Bouza, S. Rosewick, J. Salber, M. Woltje and M. Zenke, Biomaterials, 29 (2008) 302.
[40] L. Jongpaiboonkit, W.J. King, G.E. Lyons, A.L. Paguirigan, J.W. Warrick, D.J. Beebe and W.L. Murphy, Biomaterials, 29 (2008) 3346.
[41] L. Jongpaiboonkit, W.J. King and W.L. Murphy, Tissue Eng Part A, (2008).
[42] G.M. Cruise, D.S. Scharp and J.A. Hubbell, Biomaterials, 19 (1998) 1287.
[43] D.K. Han and J.A. Hubbell, Macromolecules, 30 (1997) 6077.
[44] S.J. Bryant and K.S. Anseth, Biomaterials, 22 (2001) 619.
[45] J. Elisseeff, K. Anseth, D. Sims, W. McIntosh, M. Randolph and R. Langer, Proc Natl Acad Sci U S A, 96 (1999) 3104.
[46] J. Elisseeff, W. McIntosh, K. Fu, B.T. Blunk and R. Langer, J Orthop Res, 19 (2001) 1098.
[47] N.S. Hwang, M.S. Kim, S. Sampattavanich, J.H. Baek, Z. Zhang and J. Elisseeff, Stem Cells, 24 (2006) 284.
[48] N.S. Hwang, S. Varghese, P. Theprungsirikul, A. Canver and J. Elisseeff, Biomaterials, 27 (2006) 6015.
[49] C.G. Williams, A.N. Malik, T.K. Kim, P.N. Manson and J.H. Elisseeff, Biomaterials, 26 (2005) 1211.
[50] A.S. Sawhney, C.P. Pathak and J.A. Hubbell, Macromolecules, 26 (1993) 581.
[51] S.J. Bryant and K.S. Anseth, J Biomed Mater Res, 59 (2002) 63.
[52] S.J. Bryant and K.S. Anseth, J Biomed Mater Res A, 64 (2003) 70.
[53] S.J. Bryant, K.L. Durand and K.S. Anseth, J Biomed Mater Res A, 67 (2003) 1430.
[54] M.A. Rice and K.S. Anseth, J Biomed Mater Res A, 70 (2004) 560.
[55] S. Kaihara, S. Matsumura and J.P. Fisher, Eur J Pharm Biopharm, 68 (2008) 67.
[56] M.W. Betz, P.C. Modi, J.F. Caccamese, D.P. Coletti, J.J. Sauk and J.P. Fisher, J Biomed Mater Res A, 86 (2008) 662.
[57] H. Shin, P. Quinten Ruhe, A.G. Mikos and J.A. Jansen, Biomaterials, 24 (2003) 3201.
[58] J.S. Temenoff, H. Park, E. Jabbari, D.E. Conway, T.L. Sheffield, C.G. Ambrose and A.G. Mikos, Biomacromolecules, 5 (2004) 5.

[59] J.S. Temenoff, K.A. Athanasiou, R.G. LeBaron and A.G. Mikos, J Biomed Mater Res, 59 (2002) 429.
[60] H. Shin, J.S. Temenoff and A.G. Mikos, Biomacromolecules, 4 (2003) 552.
[61] T.A. Holland, Y. Tabata and A.G. Mikos, J Control Release, 101 (2005) 111.
[62] T.A. Holland, E.W. Bodde, L.S. Baggett, Y. Tabata, A.G. Mikos and J.A. Jansen, J Biomed Mater Res A, 75 (2005) 156.
[63] H. Park, J.S. Temenoff, T.A. Holland, Y. Tabata and A.G. Mikos, Biomaterials, 26 (2005) 7095.
[64] M. Dadsetan, J.P. Szatkowski, M.J. Yaszemski and L. Lu, Biomacromolecules, 8 (2007) 1702.
[65] H. Park, J.S. Temenoff, Y. Tabata, A.I. Caplan and A.G. Mikos, Biomaterials, 28 (2007) 3217.
[66] H. Park, J.S. Temenoff, Y. Tabata, A.I. Caplan, R.M. Raphael, J.A. Jansen and A.G. Mikos, J Biomed Mater Res A, 88 (2009) 889.
[67] H. Park, X. Guo, J.S. Temenoff, Y. Tabata, A.I. Caplan, F.K. Kasper and A.G. Mikos, Biomacromolecules, (2009).
[68] C.R. Nuttelman, D.J. Mortisen, S.M. Henry and K.S. Anseth, J Biomed Mater Res, 57 (2001) 217.
[69] C.R. Nuttelman, S.M. Henry and K.S. Anseth, Biomaterials, 23 (2002) 3617.
[70] P.J. Martens, S.J. Bryant and K.S. Anseth, Biomacromolecules, 4 (2003) 283.
[71] S.J. Bryant, K.A. Davis-Arehart, N. Luo, R.K. Shoemaker, J.A. Arthur and K.S. Anseth, Macromolecules, 37 (2004) 6726.
[72] A. Muhlebach, B. Muller, C. Pharisa, M. Hofmann, B. Seiferling and D. Guerry, Journal of Polymer Science: Part A: Polymer Chemistry, 35 (1997) 3603.
[73] R.H. Schmedlen, K.S. Masters and J.L. West, Biomaterials, 23 (2002) 4325.
[74] Y.H. An, D. Webb, A. Gutowska, V.A. Mironov and R.J. Friedman, Anat Rec, 263 (2001) 336.
[75] K. Smetana, Jr., Biomaterials, 14 (1993) 1046.
[76] H.J. Hauselmann, R.J. Fernandes, S.S. Mok, T.M. Schmid, J.A. Block, M.B. Aydelotte, K.E. Kuettner and E.J. Thonar, J Cell Sci, 107 (Pt 1) (1994) 17.
[77] J.L. van Susante, P. Buma, G.J. van Osch, D. Versleyen, P.M. van der Kraan, W.B. van der Berg and G.N. Homminga, Acta Orthop Scand, 66 (1995) 549.
[78] D.A. Lee, T. Reisler and D.L. Bader, Acta Orthop Scand, 74 (2003) 6.
[79] D.J. Park, J.P. Bong, S.Y. Park and K.S. Hong, Ann Otol Rhinol Laryngol, 109 (2000) 1157.
[80] W.J. Marijnissen, G.J. van Osch, J. Aigner, H.L. Verwoerd-Verhoef and J.A. Verhaar, Biomaterials, 21 (2000) 571.
[81] W.J. Marijnissen, G.J. van Osch, J. Aigner, S.W. van der Veen, A.P. Hollander, H.L. Verwoerd-Verhoef and J.A. Verhaar, Biomaterials, 23 (2002) 1511.
[82] E. Fragonas, M. Valente, M. Pozzi-Mucelli, R. Toffanin, R. Rizzo, F. Silvestri and F. Vittur, Biomaterials, 21 (2000) 795.
[83] C.M. Hettrich, D. Crawford and S.A. Rodeo, Sports Med Arthrosc, 16 (2008) 230.
[84] L. Song and R.S. Tuan, FASEB J, 18 (2004) 980.
[85] A.T. Mehlhorn, H. Schmal, S. Kaiser, G. Lepski, G. Finkenzeller, G.B. Stark and N.P. Sudkamp, Tissue Eng, 12 (2006) 1393.
[86] P.D. Benya and J.D. Shaffer, Cell, 30 (1982) 215.
[87] B. Rahfoth, J. Weisser, F. Sternkopf, T. Aigner, K. von der Mark and R. Brauer, Osteoarthritis Cartilage, 6 (1998) 50.
[88] R.L. Mauck, M.A. Soltz, C.C. Wang, D.D. Wong, P.H. Chao, W.B. Valhmu, C.T. Hung and G.A. Ateshian, J Biomech Eng, 122 (2000) 252.
[89] X. Xu, J.P. Urban, U. Tirlapur, M.H. Wu and Z. Cui, Biotechnol Bioeng, 93 (2006) 1103.

[90] M.A. Dimicco, J.D. Kisiday, H. Gong and A.J. Grodzinsky, Osteoarthritis Cartilage, 15 (2007) 1207.
[91] I.E. Erickson, A.H. Huang, C. Chung, R.T. Li, J.A. Burdick and R.L. Mauck, Tissue Eng Part A, 15 (2009) 1041.
[92] T.A. Selmi, P. Verdonk, P. Chambat, F. Dubrana, J.F. Potel, L. Barnouin and P. Neyret, J Bone Joint Surg Br, 90 (2008) 597.
[93] H.A. Awad, M.Q. Wickham, H.A. Leddy, J.M. Gimble and F. Guilak, Biomaterials, 25 (2004) 3211.
[94] C.Y. Huang, P.M. Reuben, G. D'Ippolito, P.C. Schiller and H.S. Cheung, Anat Rec A Discov Mol Cell Evol Biol, 278 (2004) 428.
[95] R.L. Mauck, X. Yuan and R.S. Tuan, Osteoarthritis Cartilage, 14 (2006) 179.
[96] C. Vinatier, D. Magne, P. Weiss, C. Trojani, N. Rochet, G.F. Carle, C. Vignes-Colombeix, C. Chadjichristos, P. Galera, G. Daculsi and J. Guicheux, Biomaterials, 26 (2005) 6643.
[97] C. Vinatier, D. Magne, A. Moreau, O. Gauthier, O. Malard, C. Vignes-Colombeix, G. Daculsi, P. Weiss and J. Guicheux, J Biomed Mater Res A, 80 (2007) 66.
[98] C. Vinatier, O. Gauthier, A. Fatimi, C. Merceron, M. Masson, A. Moreau, F. Moreau, B. Fellah, P. Weiss and J. Guicheux, Biotechnol Bioeng, 102 (2009) 1259.
[99] D.D. Allison and K.J. Grande-Allen, Tissue Eng, 12 (2006) 2131.
[100] M. Akmal, A. Singh, A. Anand, A. Kesani, N. Aslam, A. Goodship and G. Bentley, J Bone Joint Surg Br, 87 (2005) 1143.
[101] K.P. Vercruysse, D.M. Marecak, J.F. Marecek and G.D. Prestwich, Bioconjug Chem, 8 (1997) 686.
[102] G.D. Prestwich, D.M. Marecak, J.F. Marecek, K.P. Vercruysse and M.R. Ziebell, J Control Release, 53 (1998) 93.
[103] P. Bulpitt and D. Aeschlimann, J Biomed Mater Res, 47 (1999) 152.
[104] J. Baier Leach, K.A. Bivens, C.W. Patrick, Jr. and C.E. Schmidt, Biotechnol Bioeng, 82 (2003) 578.
[105] Y.D. Park, N. Tirelli and J.A. Hubbell, Biomaterials, 24 (2003) 893.
[106] J.A. Burdick, C. Chung, X. Jia, M.A. Randolph and R. Langer, Biomacromolecules, 6 (2005) 386.
[107] C. Chung and J.A. Burdick, Tissue Eng Part A, 15 (2009) 243.
[108] H. Tan, C.R. Chu, K.A. Payne and K.G. Marra, Biomaterials, 30 (2009) 2499.
[109] Q. Li, C.G. Williams, D.D. Sun, J. Wang, K. Leong and J.H. Elisseeff, J Biomed Mater Res A, 68 (2004) 28.
[110] S.J. Bryant, J.A. Arthur and K.S. Anseth, Acta Biomater, 1 (2005) 243.
[111] S. Varghese, N.S. Hwang, A.C. Canver, P. Theprungsirikul, D.W. Lin and J. Elisseeff, Matrix Biol, 27 (2008) 12.
[112] L. Schuman, P. Buma, D. Versleyen, B. de Man, P.M. van der Kraan, W.B. van den Berg and G.N. Homminga, Biomaterials, 16 (1995) 809.
[113] A.E. Sams and A.J. Nixon, Osteoarthritis Cartilage, 3 (1995) 47.
[114] S.R. Frenkel, B. Toolan, D. Menche, M.I. Pitman and J.M. Pachence, J Bone Joint Surg Br, 79 (1997) 831.
[115] S. Wakitani, T. Goto, R.G. Young, J.M. Mansour, V.M. Goldberg and A.I. Caplan, Tissue Eng, 4 (1998) 429.
[116] D. Bosnakovski, M. Mizuno, G. Kim, S. Takagi, M. Okumura and T. Fujinaga, Biotechnol Bioeng, 93 (2006) 1152.
[117] A. Fertala, W.B. Han and F.K. Ko, J Biomed Mater Res, 57 (2001) 48.
[118] H. Ito, A. Steplewski, T. Alabyeva and A. Fertala, J Biomed Mater Res A, 76 (2006) 551.
[119] E. Kon, M. Delcogliano, G. Filardo, C. Montaperto and M. Marcacci, Sports Med Arthrosc, 16 (2008) 221.
[120] T.A. Ahmed, E.V. Dare and M. Hincke, Tissue Eng Part B Rev, (2008).

[121] D. Eyrich, F. Brandl, B. Appel, H. Wiese, G. Maier, M. Wenzel, R. Staudenmaier, A. Goepferich and T. Blunk, Biomaterials, 28 (2007) 55.
[122] X.L. Xu, J. Lou, T. Tang, K.W. Ng, J. Zhang, C. Yu and K. Dai, J Biomed Mater Res B Appl Biomater, 75 (2005) 289.
[123] G.I. Im, Y.W. Shin and K.B. Lee, Osteoarthritis Cartilage, 13 (2005) 845.
[124] F. Chang, T. Ishii, T. Yanai, H. Mishima, H. Akaogi, T. Ogawa and N. Ochiai, J Orthop Res, 26 (2008) 18.
[125] C. Perka, O. Schultz, K. Lindenhayn, R.S. Spitzer, M. Muschik, M. Sittinger and G.R. Burmester, Clin Exp Rheumatol, 18 (2000) 13.
[126] K.F. Almqvist, L. Wang, J. Wang, D. Baeten, M. Cornelissen, R. Verdonk, E.M. Veys and G. Verbruggen, Ann Rheum Dis, 60 (2001) 781.
[127] C. Perka, R.S. Spitzer, K. Lindenhayn, M. Sittinger and O. Schultz, J Biomed Mater Res, 49 (2000) 305.
[128] C.H. Chou, W.T. Cheng, T.F. Kuo, J.S. Sun, F.H. Lin and J.C. Tsai, J Biomed Mater Res A, 82 (2007) 757.
[129] Z. Megeed, J. Cappello and H. Ghandehari, Adv Drug Deliv Rev, 54 (2002) 1075.
[130] D.E. Meyer and A. Chilkoti, Biomacromolecules, 3 (2002) 357.
[131] H. Betre, L.A. Setton, D.E. Meyer and A. Chilkoti, Biomacromolecules, 3 (2002) 910.
[132] H. Betre, S.R. Ong, F. Guilak, A. Chilkoti, B. Fermor and L.A. Setton, Biomaterials, 27 (2006) 91.
[133] E.R. Welsh and D.A. Tirrell, Biomacromolecules, 1 (2000) 23.
[134] M. Haider, J. Cappello, H. Ghandehari and K.W. Leong, Pharm Res, 25 (2008) 692.
[135] J.D. Kisiday, M. Jin, M.A. DiMicco, B. Kurz and A.J. Grodzinsky, J Biomech, 37 (2004) 595.
[136] J.D. Kisiday, P.W. Kopesky, C.H. Evans, A.J. Grodzinsky, C.W. McIlwraith and D.D. Frisbie, J Orthop Res, 26 (2008) 322.
[137] T.C. Holmes, Trends Biotechnol, 20 (2002) 16.
[138] S. Zhang, T.C. Holmes, C.M. DiPersio, R.O. Hynes, X. Su and A. Rich, Biomaterials, 16 (1995) 1385.
[139] J.D. Hartgerink, E. Beniash and S.I. Stupp, Science, 294 (2001) 1684.
[140] J.D. Hartgerink, E. Beniash and S.I. Stupp, Proc Natl Acad Sci U S A, 99 (2002) 5133.
[141] E. Beniash, J.D. Hartgerink, H. Storrie, J.C. Stendahl and S.I. Stupp, Acta Biomater, 1 (2005) 387.
[142] D.A. Harrington, E.Y. Cheng, M.O. Guler, L.K. Lee, J.L. Donovan, R.C. Claussen and S.I. Stupp, J Biomed Mater Res A, 78 (2006) 157.
[143] K. Rajangam, H.A. Behanna, M.J. Hui, X. Han, J.F. Hulvat, J.W. Lomasney and S.I. Stupp, Nano Lett, 6 (2006) 2086.
[144] H. Hosseinkhani, M. Hosseinkhani, F. Tian, H. Kobayashi and Y. Tabata, Biomaterials, 27 (2006) 4079.
[145] W. Kafienah, M. Jakob, O. Demarteau, A. Frazer, M.D. Barker, I. Martin and A.P. Hollander, Tissue Eng, 8 (2002) 817.
[146] L. Peterson, T. Minas, M. Brittberg, A. Nilsson, E. Sjogren-Jansson and A. Lindahl, Clin Orthop Relat Res, (2000) 212.
[147] G. Knutsen, L. Engebretsen, T.C. Ludvigsen, J.O. Drogset, T. Grontvedt, E. Solheim, T. Strand, S. Roberts, V. Isaksen and O. Johansen, J Bone Joint Surg Am, 86-A (2004) 455.
[148] K. Gelse, C. Muhle, O. Franke, J. Park, M. Jehle, K. Durst, M. Goken, F. Hennig, K. von der Mark and H. Schneider, Arthritis Rheum, 58 (2008) 475.
[149] M. Schnabel, S. Marlovits, G. Eckhoff, I. Fichtel, L. Gotzen, V. Vecsei and J. Schlegel, Osteoarthritis Cartilage, 10 (2002) 62.
[150] S. Thirion and F. Berenbaum, Methods Mol Med, 100 (2004) 1.

[151] D. Magne, C. Vinatier, M. Julien, P. Weiss and J. Guicheux, Trends Mol Med, 11 (2005) 519.
[152] F.H. Chen, K.T. Rousche and R.S. Tuan, Nat Clin Pract Rheumatol, 2 (2006) 373.
[153] N.S. Hwang and J. Elisseeff, J Knee Surg, 22 (2009) 60.
[154] D.P. Lennon, J.M. Edmison and A.I. Caplan, J Cell Physiol, 187 (2001) 345.
[155] D.W. Wang, B. Fermor, J.M. Gimble, H.A. Awad and F. Guilak, J Cell Physiol, 204 (2005) 184.
[156] K. Scherer, M. Schunke, R. Sellckau, J. Hassenpflug and B. Kurz, Biorheology, 41 (2004) 323.
[157] R.S. Tuan, G. Boland and R. Tuli, Arthritis Res Ther, 5 (2003) 32.
[158] M. Dominici, K. Le Blanc, I. Mueller, I. Slaper-Cortenbach, F. Marini, D. Krause, R. Deans, A. Keating, D. Prockop and E. Horwitz, Cytotherapy, 8 (2006) 315.
[159] C. Merceron, C. Vinatier, J. Clouet, S. Colliec-Jouault, P. Weiss and J. Guicheux, Joint Bone Spine, 75 (2008) 672.
[160] Y. Sakaguchi, I. Sekiya, K. Yagishita and T. Muneta, Arthritis Rheum, 52 (2005) 2521.
[161] S. Wakitani, T. Goto, S.J. Pineda, R.G. Young, J.M. Mansour, A.I. Caplan and V.M. Goldberg, J Bone Joint Surg Am, 76 (1994) 579.
[162] W.J. Li, R. Tuli, C. Okafor, A. Derfoul, K.G. Danielson, D.J. Hall and R.S. Tuan, Biomaterials, 26 (2005) 599.
[163] F.H. Chen and R.S. Tuan, Arthritis Res Ther, 10 (2008) 223.
[164] J.M. Murphy, D.J. Fink, E.B. Hunziker and F.P. Barry, Arthritis Rheum, 48 (2003) 3464.
[165] B. Sharma, C.G. Williams, M. Khan, P. Manson and J.H. Elisseeff, Plast Reconstr Surg, 119 (2007) 112.
[166] H. Fan, Y. Hu, L. Qin, X. Li, H. Wu and R. Lv, J Biomed Mater Res A, 77 (2006) 785.
[167] T.A. Holland, E.W. Bodde, V.M. Cuijpers, L.S. Baggett, Y. Tabata, A.G. Mikos and J.A. Jansen, Osteoarthritis Cartilage, 15 (2007) 187.
[168] S. Wakitani, K. Imoto, T. Yamamoto, M. Saito, N. Murata and M. Yoneda, Osteoarthritis Cartilage, 10 (2002) 199.
[169] M.S. Kim, N.S. Hwang, J. Lee, T.K. Kim, K. Leong, M.J. Shamblott, J. Gearhart and J. Elisseeff, Stem Cells, 23 (2005) 113.
[170] S. Varghese, P. Theprungsirikul, A. Ferran, N. Hwang, A. Canver and J. Elisseeff, Conf Proc IEEE Eng Med Biol Soc, 1 (2006) 2643.
[171] J.A. Thomson, J. Itskovitz-Eldor, S.S. Shapiro, M.A. Waknitz, J.J. Swiergiel, V.S. Marshall and J.M. Jones, Science, 282 (1998) 1145.
[172] J. Kramer, C. Hegert, K. Guan, A.M. Wobus, P.K. Muller and J. Rohwedel, Mech Dev, 92 (2000) 193.
[173] J. Kramer, C. Hegert and J. Rohwedel, Methods Enzymol, 365 (2003) 251.
[174] J. Kramer, C. Hegert, G. Hargus and J. Rohwedel, Cell Biol Int, 29 (2005) 139.
[175] J.M. Messana, N.S. Hwang, J. Coburn, J.H. Elisseeff and Z. Zhang, J Tissue Eng Regen Med, 2 (2008) 499.
[176] J. Kramer, C. Hegert, G. Hargus and J. Rohwedel, Cytotechnology, 41 (2003) 177.
[177] W.S. Toh, Z. Yang, H. Liu, B.C. Heng, E.H. Lee and T. Cao, Stem Cells, 25 (2007) 950.
[178] C. Hegert, J. Kramer, G. Hargus, J. Muller, K. Guan, A.M. Wobus, P.K. Muller and J. Rohwedel, J Cell Sci, 115 (2002) 4617.
[179] J.S. Khillan, Methods Mol Biol, 330 (2006) 161.
[180] J.M. Jukes, L. Moroni, C.A. van Blitterswijk and J. de Boer, Tissue Eng Part A, 14 (2008) 135.
[181] N.S. Hwang, S. Varghese and J. Elisseeff, Methods Mol Biol, 407 (2007) 351.
[182] N.S. Hwang, S. Varghese, Z. Zhang and J. Elisseeff, Tissue Eng, 12 (2006) 2695.
[183] N.S. Hwang, S. Varghese, H.J. Lee, Z. Zhang, Z. Ye, J. Bae, L. Cheng and J. Elisseeff, Proc Natl Acad Sci U S A, 105 (2008) 20641.

[184] A. Vats, R.C. Bielby, N. Tolley, S.C. Dickinson, A.R. Boccaccini, A.P. Hollander, A.E. Bishop and J.M. Polak, Tissue Eng, 12 (2006) 1687.
[185] N.S. Hwang, S. Varghese and J. Elisseeff, PLoS ONE, 3 (2008) e2498.
[186] J. Yu, M.A. Vodyanik, K. Smuga-Otto, J. Antosiewicz-Bourget, J.L. Frane, S. Tian, J. Nie, G.A. Jonsdottir, V. Ruotti, R. Stewart, Slukvin, II and J.A. Thomson, Science, 318 (2007) 1917.
[187] K. Takahashi, K. Tanabe, M. Ohnuki, M. Narita, T. Ichisaka, K. Tomoda and S. Yamanaka, Cell, 131 (2007) 861.
[188] D.G. Stupack, X.S. Puente, S. Boutsaboualoy, C.M. Storgard and D.A. Cheresh, J Cell Biol, 155 (2001) 459.
[189] C.R. Howlett, M.D. Evans, W.R. Walsh, G. Johnson and J.G. Steele, Biomaterials, 15 (1994) 213.
[190] F.G. Giancotti and E. Ruoslahti, Science, 285 (1999) 1028.
[191] A. Howe, A.E. Aplin, S.K. Alahari and R.L. Juliano, Curr Opin Cell Biol, 10 (1998) 220.
[192] R.G. LeBaron and K.A. Athanasiou, Tissue Eng, 6 (2000) 85.
[193] B. Jeschke, J. Meyer, A. Jonczyk, H. Kessler, P. Adamietz, N.M. Meenen, M. Kantlehner, C. Goepfert and B. Nies, Biomaterials, 23 (2002) 3455.
[194] M.S. Hirsch, L.E. Lunsford, V. Trinkaus-Randall and K.K. Svoboda, Dev Dyn, 210 (1997) 249.
[195] M. Enomoto-Iwamoto, M. Iwamoto, K. Nakashima, Y. Mukudai, D. Boettiger, M. Pacifici, K. Kurisu and F. Suzuki, J Bone Miner Res, 12 (1997) 1124.
[196] M.O. Wright, K. Nishida, C. Bavington, J.L. Godolphin, E. Dunne, S. Walmsley, P. Jobanputra, G. Nuki and D.M. Salter, J Orthop Res, 15 (1997) 742.
[197] S.J. Millward-Sadler, M.O. Wright, H. Lee, H. Caldwell, G. Nuki and D.M. Salter, Osteoarthritis Cartilage, 8 (2000) 272.
[198] Y.H. Kim and J.W. Lee, J Cell Physiol, 218 (2009) 623.
[199] E. Ruoslahti, Annu Rev Cell Dev Biol, 12 (1996) 697.
[200] S.P. Massia and J.A. Hubbell, Anal Biochem, 187 (1990) 292.
[201] K.C. Olbrich, T.T. Andersen, F.A. Blumenstock and R. Bizios, Biomaterials, 17 (1996) 759.
[202] A.D. Cook, J.S. Hrkach, N.N. Gao, I.M. Johnson, U.B. Pajvani, S.M. Cannizzaro and R. Langer, J Biomed Mater Res, 35 (1997) 513.
[203] C. Tang, F. Kligman, C.C. Larsen, K. Kottke-Marchant and R.E. Marchant, J Biomed Mater Res A, 88 (2009) 348.
[204] S.P. Massia and J.A. Hubbell, J Cell Biol, 114 (1991) 1089.
[205] P. Schaffner, J. Meyer, M. Dard, R. Wenz, B. Nies, S. Verrier, H. Kessler and M. Kantlehner, J Mater Sci Mater Med, 10 (1999) 837.
[206] S.P. Palecek, J.C. Loftus, M.H. Ginsberg, D.A. Lauffenburger and A.F. Horwitz, Nature, 385 (1997) 537.
[207] X. Mo, Y. An, C. Yun and S.M. Yu, Angew Chem Int Ed, 118 (2006) 2325.
[208] A.Y. Wang, X. Mo, C.S. Chen and S.M. Yu, J. Am. Chem. Soc, 127 (2005) 4130.
[209] H.J. Lee, J.S. Lee, T. Chansakul, C. Yu, J.H. Elisseeff and S.M. Yu, Biomaterials, 27 (2006) 5268.
[210] R.V. Iozzo, J Biol Chem, 274 (1999) 18843.
[211] G. Zhang, Y. Ezura, I. Chervoneva, P.S. Robinson, D.P. Beason, E.T. Carine, L.J. Soslowsky, R.V. Iozzo and D.E. Birk, J Cell Biochem, 98 (2006) 1436.
[212] T.A. Dugan, V.W. Yang, D.J. McQuillan and M. Hook, J Biol Chem, 281 (2006) 38208.
[213] J.E. Scott, Biochemistry, 35 (1996) 8795.
[214] I.T. Weber, R.W. Harrison and R.V. Iozzo, J Biol Chem, 271 (1996) 31767.
[215] Y. Geng, D. McQuillan and P.J. Roughley, Matrix Biol, 25 (2006) 484.
[216] J.S. Park, D.G. Woo, H.N. Yang, H.J. Lim, H.M. Chung and K.H. Park, Transplantation, 85 (2008) 589.

[217] S.E. Sakiyama-Elbert and J.A. Hubbell, J Control Release, 65 (2000) 389.
[218] A.C. Lee, V.M. Yu, J.B. Lowe, 3rd, M.J. Brenner, D.A. Hunter, S.E. Mackinnon and S.E. Sakiyama-Elbert, Exp Neurol, 184 (2003) 295.
[219] M.D. Sternlicht and Z. Werb, Annu Rev Cell Dev Biol, 17 (2001) 463.
[220] I. Sekiya, J.T. Vuoristo, B.L. Larson and D.J. Prockop, Proc Natl Acad Sci U S A, 99 (2002) 4397.
[221] S. Tavella, G. Bellese, P. Castagnola, I. Martin, D. Piccini, R. Doliana, A. Colombatti, R. Cancedda and C. Tacchetti, J Cell Sci, 110 (Pt 18) (1997) 2261.
[222] J. Monfort, G. Tardif, P. Reboul, F. Mineau, P. Roughley, J.P. Pelletier and J. Martel-Pelletier, Arthritis Res Ther, 8 (2006) R26.
[223] P. Reboul, J.P. Pelletier, G. Tardif, J.M. Cloutier and J. Martel-Pelletier, J Clin Invest, 97 (1996) 2011.
[224] G. Tardif, P. Reboul, J.P. Pelletier and J. Martel-Pelletier, Mod Rheumatol, 14 (2004) 197.
[225] S.J. Deng, D.M. Bickett, J.L. Mitchell, M.H. Lambert, R.K. Blackburn, H.L. Carter, 3rd, J. Neugebauer, G. Pahel, M.P. Weiner and M.L. Moss, J Biol Chem, 275 (2000) 31422.
[226] A.J. Fosang, K. Last, V. Knauper, G. Murphy and P.J. Neame, FEBS Lett, 380 (1996) 17.
[227] J. Kim, Y. Park, G. Tae, K.B. Lee, S.J. Hwang, I.S. Kim, I. Noh and K. Sun, J Mater Sci Mater Med, 19 (2008) 3311.
[228] D.L. Hern and J.A. Hubbell, J Biomed Mater Res, 39 (1998) 266.
[229] B.K. Mann, A.S. Gobin, A.T. Tsai, R.H. Schmedlen and J.L. West, Biomaterials, 22 (2001) 3045.
[230] J.A. Burdick and K.S. Anseth, Biomaterials, 23 (2002) 4315.
[231] F. Yang, C.G. Williams, D.A. Wang, H. Lee, P.N. Manson and J. Elisseeff, Biomaterials, 26 (2005) 5991.
[232] H. Shin, S. Jo and A.G. Mikos, J Biomed Mater Res, 61 (2002) 169.
[233] H. Shin, J.S. Temenoff, G.C. Bowden, K. Zygourakis, M.C. Farach-Carson, M.J. Yaszemski and A.G. Mikos, Biomaterials, 26 (2005) 3645.
[234] J.A. Rowley, G. Madlambayan and D.J. Mooney, Biomaterials, 20 (1999) 45.
[235] M.C. Dodla and R.V. Bellamkonda, J Biomed Mater Res A, 78 (2006) 213.
[236] J.T. Connelly, A.J. Garcia and M.E. Levenston, J Cell Physiol, 217 (2008) 145.
[237] R.A. Stile and K.E. Healy, Biomacromolecules, 2 (2001) 185.
[238] W.H. Blackburn, E.B. Dickerson, M.H. Smith, J.F. McDonald and L.A. Lyon, Bioconjug Chem, (2009).
[239] J.C. Schense and J.A. Hubbell, Bioconjug Chem, 10 (1999) 75.
[240] J.C. Schense, J. Bloch, P. Aebischer and J.A. Hubbell, Nat Biotechnol, 18 (2000) 415.
[241] M.P. Lutolf and J.A. Hubbell, Biomacromolecules, 4 (2003) 713.
[242] D.L. Elbert, A.B. Pratt, M.P. Lutolf, S. Halstenberg and J.A. Hubbell, J Control Release, 76 (2001) 11.
[243] L. Lecamp, F. Houllier, B. Youssef and C. Bunel, Polymer, 42 (2001) 2727.
[244] C.N. Salinas, B.B. Cole, A.M. Kasko and K.S. Anseth, Tissue Eng, 13 (2007) 1025.
[245] J. Zhu, C. Tang, K. Kottke-Marchant and R.E. Marchant, Bioconjug Chem, 20 (2009) 333.
[246] J.L. West and J.A. Hubbell, Macromolecules, 32 (1999) 241.
[247] M.P. Lutolf, J.L. Lauer-Fields, H.G. Schmoekel, A.T. Metters, F.E. Weber, G.B. Fields and J.A. Hubbell, Proc Natl Acad Sci U S A, 100 (2003) 5413.
[248] L. Gentilucci, A. Tolomelli and F. Squassabia, Curr Med Chem, 13 (2006) 2449.
[249] G.A. Silva, C. Czeisler, K.L. Niece, E. Beniash, D.A. Harrington, J.A. Kessler and S.I. Stupp, Science, 303 (2004) 1352.
[250] K.M. Galler, A. Cavender, V. Yuwono, H. Dong, S. Shi, G. Schmalz, J.D. Hartgerink and R.N. D'Souza, Tissue Eng Part A, 14 (2008) 2051.
[251] G. Maheshwari, G. Brown, D.A. Lauffenburger, A. Wells and L.G. Griffith, J Cell Sci, 113 (Pt 10) (2000) 1677.

[252] D.J. Irvine, A.M. Mayes and L.G. Griffith, Biomacromolecules, 2 (2001) 85.
[253] M.S. Hahn, L.J. Taite, J.J. Moon, M.C. Rowland, K.A. Ruffino and J.L. West, Biomaterials, 27 (2006) 2519.
[254] V. Mironov, T. Boland, T. Trusk, G. Forgacs and R.R. Markwald, Trends Biotechnol, 21 (2003) 157.
[255] J.P. Ranieri, R. Bellamkonda, E.J. Bekos, J.A. Gardella, Jr., H.J. Mathieu, L. Ruiz and P. Aebischer, Int J Dev Neurosci, 12 (1994) 725.
[256] Y. Luo and M.S. Shoichet, Nat Mater, 3 (2004) 249.
[257] Y. Luo and M.S. Shoichet, Biomacromolecules, 5 (2004) 2315.
[258] P. Musoke-Zawedde and M.S. Shoichet, Biomed Mater, 1 (2006) 162.
[259] S.H. Lee, J.J. Moon and J.L. West, Biomaterials, 29 (2008) 2962.
[260] M.S. Hahn, J.S. Miller and J.L. West, Advanced Materials, 18 (2006) 2679.
[261] B.D. Polizzotti, B.D. Fairbanks and K.S. Anseth, Biomacromolecules, 9 (2008) 1084.
[262] A.M. Kloxin, A.M. Kasko, C.N. Salinas and K.S. Anseth, Science, 324 (2009) 59.
[263] E. Ruoslahti and J.C. Reed, Cell, 77 (1994) 477.
[264] J.T. Connelly, A.J. Garcia and M.E. Levenston, Biomaterials, 28 (2007) 1071.
[265] P. Newman and F.M. Watt, Exp Cell Res, 178 (1988) 199.
[266] E. Kolettas, L. Buluwela, M.T. Bayliss and H.I. Muir, J Cell Sci, 108 (Pt 5) (1995) 1991.
[267] E. Alsberg, K.W. Anderson, A. Albeiruti, J.A. Rowley and D.J. Mooney, Proc Natl Acad Sci U S A, 99 (2002) 12025.
[268] M. Kantlehner, D. Finsinger, J. Meyer, P. Schaffner, A. Jonczyk, B. Diefenbach, B. Nies and H. Kessler, Angew Chem Int Ed 38 (1999) 560.
[269] M.D. Pierschbacher and E. Ruoslahti, Nature, 309 (1984) 30.
[270] S. Johansson, G. Svineng, K. Wennerberg, A. Armulik and L. Lohikangas, Front Biosci, 2 (1997) d126.
[271] C.N. Salinas and K.S. Anseth, J Tissue Eng Regen Med, 2 (2008) 296.
[272] D.A. Frenz, N.S. Jaikaria and S.A. Newman, Dev Biol, 136 (1989) 97.
[273] C.N. Salinas and K.S. Anseth, Biomaterials, 29 (2008) 2370.
[274] B.G. Keselowsky, D.M. Collard and A.J. Garcia, Proc Natl Acad Sci U S A, 102 (2005) 5953.
[275] M.M. Schneiderbauer, C.M. Dutton and S.P. Scully, Cell Signal, 16 (2004) 1133.
[276] T.A. Petrie, J.R. Capadona, C.D. Reyes and A.J. Garcia, Biomaterials, 27 (2006) 5459.
[277] S.J. Bryant, G.D. Nicodemus and I. Villanueva, Pharm Res, 25 (2008) 2379.
[278] H.J. Lee, C. Yu, T. Chansakul, N.S. Hwang, S. Varghese, S.M. Yu and J.H. Elisseeff, Tissue Eng Part A, 14 (2008) 1843.
[279] C.N. Salinas and K.S. Anseth, J Biomed Mater Res A, (2008).
[280] M.P. Lutolf, F.E. Weber, H.G. Schmoekel, J.C. Schense, T. Kohler, R. Muller and J.A. Hubbell, Nat Biotechnol, 21 (2003) 513.
[281] Y. Park, M.P. Lutolf, J.A. Hubbell, E.B. Hunziker and M. Wong, Tissue Eng, 10 (2004) 515.
[282] A.H. Huang, M. Yeger-McKeever, A. Stein and R.L. Mauck, Osteoarthritis Cartilage, 16 (2008) 1074.
[283] A. Dickhut, E. Gottwald, E. Steck, C. Heisel and W. Richter, Front Biosci, 13 (2008) 4517.
[284] S. Wakitani, M. Nawata, K. Tensho, T. Okabe, H. Machida and H. Ohgushi, J Tissue Eng Regen Med, 1 (2007) 74.
[285] D.A. Grande, A.S. Breitbart, J. Mason, C. Paulino, J. Laser and R.E. Schwartz, Clin Orthop Relat Res, (1999) S176.

CHAPTER 13

BIOMIMETIC MATERIALS FOR ENGINEERING OF NEURAL TISSUES: CONTROL OF CELL ADHESION AND GUIDING NEURAL CELL OUTGROWTH WITH PEPTIDE-CONJUGATED POLYMER STRUCTURES

Jianming Li[1] and Riyi Shi[1,2*]

[1]*Weldon School of Biomedical Engineering*
[2]*Department of Basic Medical Sciences, School of Veterinary Medicine*
Purdue University, West Lafayette, IN 47907, USA
[*]*E-mail: riyi@purdue.edu*

1. Introduction

The extracellular matrix (ECM) is a marvel of complexity and highlights multiple biologic structure-function relationships. The ECM provides essential physical and biochemical elements required for homeostasis, while improper interactions between cells and the ECM can alter gene expression and govern cell fate. In disease or injury, the cellular and matrix components are compromised and the challenge in tissue engineering is to recreate a surrogate environment that encourages natural wound healing and regeneration. Whether using a cellular therapy or acellularized constructs aimed to recruit endogenous cell remodeling, appropriate host integration is dependent upon the implant's ability to modulate cell attachment, migration and growth. Within the nervous system, the challenge is even greater, given the microenvironment after injury is either non-permissive or non-instructional to regeneration. In this chapter, we discuss the dichotomy between the central and peripheral nervous system biology and how the chain of biochemical and cellular events following damage play a role in dictating the design and implementation of ECM analogs. Strategies essential for facilitating cell adhesion, neurite extension and functional reconnection are further discussed.

2. The Cellular and Architectural Landscape of the Nervous System

Neurons are unique cells from a functional and morphological perspective. Neurons are electrically excitable and single cells can span several feet in length or have as many as 200,000 synaptic contacts. The multiple neuronal phenotypes observed within the body highlight the range of functional specialization. Complex, multi-dendritic neurons perform signal integration and processing while the long axons of many PNS neurons act as conduits for impulse transmission. However, neurons are only part of the nervous system landscape. In the brain, neurons are outnumbered by glia on a scale of 2:1 [1]. In the CNS, glia serve many pertinent roles including nutritional support of neurons, maintenance of local homeostasis, axon myelination and facilitating synaptic transmission. Glia also have vital functions in early development where they act as guidepost cells in directing neuronal projections [2]. In the PNS, Schwann cells are responsible for myelination, but after injury they are key players in the regenerative process.

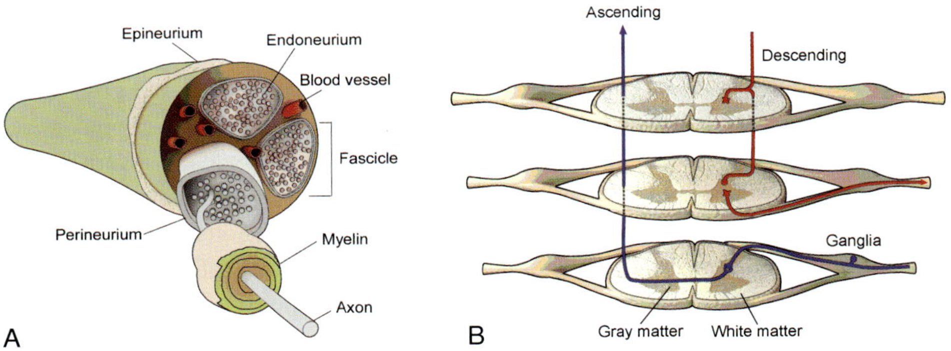

Fig. 1. (A) Hierarchal arrangement of peripheral nerve. Conducting axons are surrounded by a layer of basement membrane, which aggregate into bundles (fascicles). Around each fascicle is a collagen sheath called the perineurium. Multiple fascicles group together to comprise the nerve trunk. (B) Representation of select ascending and descending pathways in the spinal cord. Also shown are gray and white matter regions and sensory ganglia.

The asymmetry between the CNS and PNS is not just limited to cellular components. Indeed, the connective tissue composition and architecture differ noticeably. For example, the anatomical framework of peripheral nerve is comparable to other hierarchal structures such as ligaments, tendons and skeletal muscle (Figure 1). Peripheral nerves contain 25-50% connective tissue and the collagen fibrils are longitudinally oriented to resist physiologic tensile forces [3].

Yet in spinal cord, the vertebral column withstands cyclical mechanical loads and the amount of collagenous material within the cord is comparatively low. In brain, the local tissue arrangement can be extremely complex, but a global organization is lacking. The cellular vs. connective tissue proportion further influences observed mechanical properties. Not surprisingly, CNS tissue has a different set of biomechanical characteristics compared to peripheral nerve.

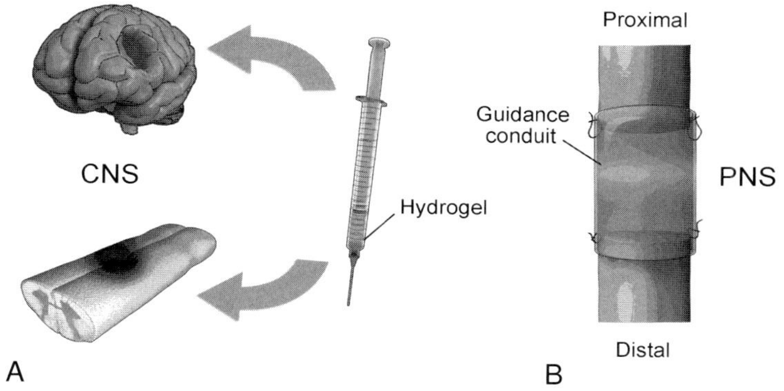

Fig. 2. (A) Hydrogel based therapy is well suited for CNS repair. In this schematic, solubilized polymer (with or without cells) is injected into the lesion and cross-linked *in situ*. The polymerized polymer conforms to the defect and directly interfaces with surrounding tissue. (B) For PNS gap defects, nerve guidance conduits (NGCs) are used to bridge the proximal and distal segments. The NGC is designed to enclose the injury site and provide the necessary guidance cues to accelerate and direct regeneration through the lesion.

While the diversity of neuronal networks underpins functional adaptations, certain challenges also arise in terms of repair. For example, disparities between the CNS and PNS anatomy predispose particular injuries. Localized crush injuries are prevalent in the spinal cord, while in the PNS, stretch and lacerations occur with higher frequency. Within brain, traumatic brain injury (TBI) or disease states may cause patterns of damage that are either focal or diffuse. These dissimilar injury modalities, coupled with the structural variations (and mechanical properties) within the nervous system can define intra-operative decision making and the therapeutic regime. Severe damage to the spinal cord or brain resulting in significant tissue loss may warrant *in situ* polymerization with hydrogels (Figure 2). In contrast, transection of peripheral nerve is generally repaired via pre-fabricated implants that bridge the proximal and distal segments. Thus, medical therapies intended for the CNS or PNS will need to consider the native mechanical, structural and cellular characteristics.

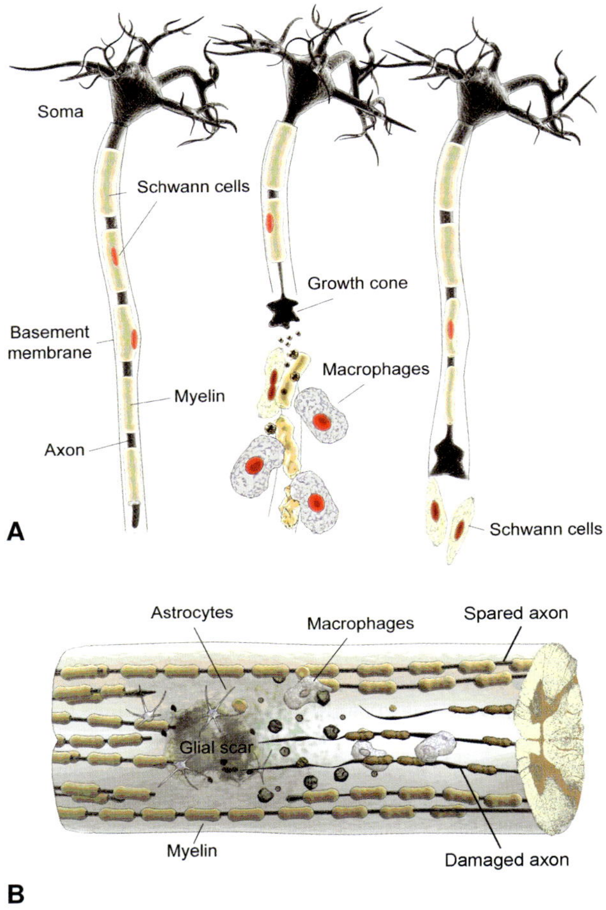

Fig. 3. (A) Sequence of cellular events following PNS injury. Left: Undamaged myelinated axon and its corresponding basement membrane sheath. Center: After trauma, the proximal segment first retracts, but later sprouts new processes. The axon tip (growth cone) surveys the local microenvironment for directional and growth cues. Meanwhile, the distal axonal segment undergoes Wallerian degeneration, a process marked by axon disintegration, macrophage infiltration and Schwann cell migration/proliferation. Right: Regenerating axons that cross the lesion follow the residual basement membrane tubes and paths outlined by Schwann cells. (B) The damaged spinal cord (as well as brain) presents a series of biochemical and physical obstacles for regeneration. Secondary injury induces a feedback mechanism that causes more cell death. Hypertrophic astrocytes create a glial scar that blocks axon growth. Spontaneous regeneration is absent in the degenerated CNS.

2.1. *Pathophysiology*

In both the CNS and PNS, tissue damage induces a cascade of regulated cellular, physical and biochemical events that are time and severity dependent. In a damaged axon, the proximal nerve segment first swells and retracts in a process known as dieback (retrograde degeneration). Within hours, the distal nerve undergoes Wallerian degeneration, events characterized by disruption of microfilaments, axonal swelling, myelin breakdown and eventual disintegration of the distal segment (Figure 3). If the initial trauma does not incur cell death, the proximal axon sprouts multiple new projections.

In the PNS, new axonal branches are stimulated and guided by a host of biochemical, cellular and physical factors [4]. Many of these cues are presented by proliferating Schwann cells that have migrated into and distal to the injury zone. However, even in the presence of Schwann cells, axons projecting into the lesion are often "confused" due to insufficient guidance mechanisms. Moreover, intrafascicular fibrosis is common as myofibroblasts invading the area can synthesize scar tissue. The lack of directional stimulation and the accumulation of scar can lead to aberrant regeneration, a condition signified by abnormal axonal projection, misdirection and improper reinnervation [5]. Axons that traverse the lesion eventually follow paths outlined by endoneurial tube remnants. However, the rate of axonal regeneration is slow, on the order of 1mm/day. At these regeneration speeds, other problems arise, including motor endplate degradation, intramuscular fibrosis and muscle atrophy [6].

In the adult CNS, the landscape is markedly different. The dogma that CNS neurons cannot regenerate after injury has been recanted [7]. Indeed adult CNS neurons have an intrinsic ability for regeneration and this observation was known as early as 1911 [8]. However, the poor regenerative outcomes clinically observed are predominately determined by a growth inhibiting microenvironment. Endogenous molecules such as myelin-associated glycoprotein, Nogo-A, oligodendrocyte-myelin glycoprotein and chondroitin sulfate proteoglycans contribute to non-permissive milieu that causes abortive regeneration [9]. Hypertrophic astrocytes also form a barrier to regeneration, either through induction of a stop signal [10] or via formation of a physical scar. Moreover, primary CNS damage often leads to secondary injury, which is a progressive malady that incurs additional cell death. Secondary injury is initiated by initial damage to cell membranes, which permits the influx of extracellular ions, including Ca^{+2}. Calcium dependent processes are then set into motion, causing depolymerization of cytoskeleton, membrane damage and eventual cell death. Dying neurons in turn, emit toxins, which spread to neighboring cells.

This vicious cycle can result in significant neuronal loss in the CNS and is extremely devastating given the non-proliferative status of neurons.

2.2. *Design challenges and biomaterials for neural engineering*

A consensus within the field of neural tissue engineering supports a multi-faceted approach that addresses the numerous biologic events following injury to the CNS or PNS. In the CNS, the challenges are substantial: containment of secondary injury and recapitulation of development. In contrast, the PNS is already primed for regeneration but the quality of regeneration is poor. Therapeutic objectives should strive to accelerate the regenerative process and minimize aberrant reinnervation. In either scenario, instructional biomaterials can address some of these issues and provide a platform for cell or drug delivery. In addition to manufacturing ease and scalability, neural biomaterials should in general, satisfy the following criteria:

i) *Integrate with host tissue and encourage cell-specific attachment, migration and growth:* Host integration is key in minimizing the foreign body response and for promoting cell-specific interactions *in vivo*. In the PNS, proper neuron-biomaterial as well as Schwann cell –substrate interactions are critical in dictating biomaterial success. Ideal substrates should encourage Schwann cell attachment, migration and also facilitate axon pathfinding. Additionally, discouraging fibroblast adhesion will reduce intrafascicular scarring. In the CNS, minimization of astrocyte attachment and proliferation is vital to diminishing glial scars, whereas neurons should readily adhere and elongate along the biomaterial.
ii) *Provide directional cues for guided axonal extension:* Controlled axonal targeting is key to successful functional reconnection. In the PNS, axonal projection in the distal direction will reduce the likelihood of aberrant regeneration and neuroma formation. Within the spinal cord, white matter destruction is the primary culprit leading to paralysis. Likewise, axon growth that emulates the original rostral-caudal anatomy is preferred.
iii) *Suppress the inhibitors of regeneration or stimulate regeneration (especially in the CNS):* Biomaterials will need to either stimulate nerve regeneration or negate the growth inhibiting microenvironment following CNS injury. Pharmaceutics aimed to mitigate inflammation and secondary injury are further warranted. If significant neural tissue is lost, cellular therapies that involve harvesting cells, *in vitro* expansion and reintroduction into the lesion may be necessary. Facilitating PNS regeneration via additional presentation of trophic support may also accelerate distal target reinnervation.

Table 1. Selected peptide sequences and effects on the nervous system.

Peptide sequence	Outcomes	Reference
IKVAV	Hippocampal cell adhesion	[20]
YIGSR	Increased hippocampal neurite length Neuroblastoma cell adhesion	[20], [21]
GDPGYIGSR/GQAASIKVAV (50:50)	DRG neurite outgrowth	[22]
GGGGGGYIGSR or GGGGGGIKVAV	Increased neurite length on hippocampal cells	[20]
RGD, GRGDS	Supports neuron adhesion Encouraged axonal ingrowth at lower dosage levels. Supports Schwann and glial cell adhesion	[17], [61] [23]
CDPGYIGSR	DRG increased neurite outgrowth	[24]
CQAASIKVAV	DRG adhesion and neurite outgrowth	[25]
KHIFSDDSSE	Adhesion of astrocytes but not fibroblasts	[26]
RNIAEIIKDI	Neurite Extension	[27]
RADA16	Return of optic nerve function after injury	[28]
CDPGYIGSR or CSRARKQAASIKVAVSAD	Improved PNS regeneration in rats	[29]

3. Peptide Conjugated Biomaterials for Cell Attachment and Improving Interfacial Interactions

3.1. *The extracellular matrix as an engineering template*

The natural extracellular matrix serves multiple structural and functional roles. The ECM provides physical support, a substrate for attachment, is a repository for growth factors and participates in cell mechanostransduction. Interactions between cells and the surrounding matrix are key in maintaining appropriate phenotype [11] and are also dynamic – the ECM stimulates cells, and in turn, cells actively remodel the matrix. The ECM offers innate advantages as a restorative material because of its biocompatibility, structure and presence of cell-recognition binding domains needed for attachment, growth and differentiation [12].

Biological engineers have recognized ECM as an ideal model for manipulation. Indeed, naturally sourced biomaterials (especially collagens, fibrin and acellularized tissue) have a long track record in biomedical applications [13]. However, there is still concern regarding pathogenic transmission of naturally sourced materials, as well as restricted processing. Moreover, the ultrastructure and composition of the final product is limited to the derived source.

New methods aimed to combine the cell recognition properties of natural biomaterials with the scalability and customization of synthetic materials is becoming prevalent. Hybrid constructs reduce the risk of immunogenicity, biologic contaminants and can be engineered to release desirable pharmaceutics or biologics (including cells). The mechanical and microstructural properties can also be tailored to mimic biologic analogs. This section reviews emerging techniques in biomaterial science that have promising implications in neural engineering.

3.2. *ECM-derived peptide sequences*

Within the nervous system ECM, there are a significant number of biomolecules that have been isolated which modulate cell behavior and survival. Two well studied compounds are laminin and fibronectin. Laminin is ubiquitous in basement membrane and mediates attachment, cell spreading, growth, differentiation and neuronal survival [14]. Fibronectin has also been shown to facilitate Schwann cell adhesion and migration as well as neuron adhesion [15], [16]. Both of these proteins have been used extensively *in vitro*, especially as coatings for non-adhesive substrates. However, extraction of these glycoproteins is difficult and expensive. Secondly, high molecular weight proteins tend to adsorb randomly onto a surface and the optimum presentation of the binding domains is not always realized.

An alternative to using whole molecule proteins is the synthesis of short peptide sequences that retain the bioactivity of the native whole protein (Table 1). Multiple sites within laminin-1 have been identified and synthesized for *in vitro* and *in vivo* applications. RGD, which is also common to fibronectin and vitronectin, has generated a wealth of data in nervous system models as well other tissue types. *In vitro,* studies show RGD can promote neuron adhesion and neurite outgrowth [17] in two and three dimensions [18]. Binding affinities and peptide concentration also affect neurite growth characteristics, with higher concentrations actually impeding growth [18]. However, the binding sites for RGD are expressed by many cell types and RGD has been proven to enhance glia and fibroblast adhesion [19]. *In vivo*, competition between inflammatory cells, stromal cells, glia and neurons for the RGD oligomer may subsequently produce unforeseen consequences.

Within the α_1 chain of laminin resides YIGSR, a sequence shown to interact with a 67-kDa receptor on cell surfaces [30]. YIGSR can improve neuroblastoma cell adhesion [21], while slight modifications to YIGSR by adding an amide-terminated arginine (YIGSR-NH_3) improves bioactivity [31]. It is thought that additional amino groups flanking the active binding site can enhance cell recognition by providing a more natural presentation.

The pentapeptide IKVAV located on the α_1 chain has also been extensively researched. *In vitro*, IKVAV supports cell adhesion, neurite outgrowth, progenitor cell differentiation and angiogenesis. Unlike RGD, which is considered a universal binding site, IKVAV appears to be cell discriminatory, as glia and fibroblasts exposed to IKVAV show reduced adhesion compared to neuronal counterparts [32]. This property is especially notable since neural prosthetics for chronic stimulation/recording have problems with glial scar encapsulation. Another peptide oligomer, RNIAEIIKDI (p20), has also demonstrated cell adhesion and neurite outgrowth in rat CNS neurons [33].

3.3. *Hydrogels for CNS application*

With recent advances in nanofabrication, the realization of three-dimensional designer scaffolds with synthetic polymers or a pure peptide base is possible. Hydrogels, defined as cross-linked polymeric networks that retain water, have been a prominent field of research. Hydrogel matrices also offer several unique structural and compositional advantages. First, hydrogel architectures tend to be nanoscale, which more closely mimic fibrin or collagen networks typically found *in vivo*. These similarities may enhance scaffold integration. Secondly, the high water content of hydrogels facilitate ion and nutrient exchange and the elasticity is reminiscent of soft tissues [34]. Pure peptide scaffolds are biodegradable and the byproducts of chemical breakdown are free amino acids, which can be metabolized by adjacent cells or excreted in urine. Finally, synthetic peptides are free of biological contaminants and have reduced immunogenic responses [35].

Multiple *in vitro* studies involving hybrid peptide-hydrogels have shown potential for CNS applications. For example, photopolymerizable PEG (polyethylene glycol) hydrogels conjugated with RGDS, IKVAV and YIGSR ligands were used to evaluate cell adhesion and neurite extension with a PC-12 cell system. Neurite extension of PC12 cells was greatest on RGDS-PEG hydrogels compared to PEG-IKVAV. Cells adhered to but did not extend neurites on hydrogels with YIGSR [36]. The degree of cell adhesion changed as a parameter of peptide concentration and longer neurites were observed on more compliant hydrogels. Acrylamide based gels patterned with IKVAV also showed excellent adhesion properties, where cultured neurons remained on functionalized surfaces for over 4 weeks and formed viable synapses [37].

In other cases, pure peptide scaffolds have been designed from a "bottoms up" supramolecular chemistry approach. Silva et al. [38], synthesized

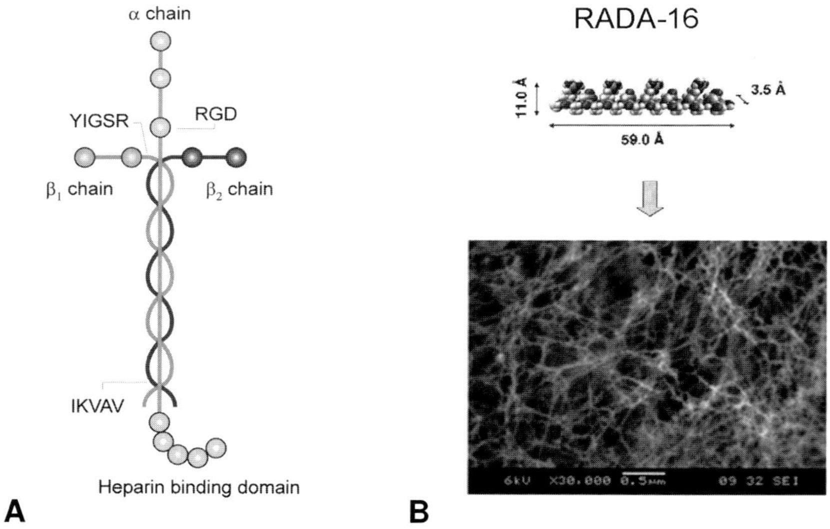

Fig. 4. (A) A schematic outline of laminin protein. Several important binding sites within laminin have been identified for application in peptide engineering. (B) Top: Molecular model of a self-assembling peptide sequence named RADA-16. Bottom: Scanning electron micrograph of the nanofibrillar hydrogel formed by RADA-16 aggregates. Reprinted with permission from [99].

nanofibrous hydrogels using self-assembly of IKVAV based peptide amphiphiles. The biomimetic scaffolds can be triggered to polymerize *in situ*, with the addition of an aqueous buffer solution. They showed IKVAV motifs could direct differentiation in neural progenitor cells while simultaneously inhibiting astrocyte differentiation. Further support for this scaffold in CNS repair was provided with a spinal cord compression model. *In vivo* treatment with IKVAV self-assembled nanofibers reduced astrogliosis, cell death and recruited oligodendrocytes at the injection site [39]. Regeneration of both ascending and descending axons as well as behavioral changes was observed. Accompanying literature with IKVAV-hyaluronic acid conjugates, also demonstrate axonal ingrowth/regeneration, glial cell invasion and neovascularization in the rat cerebellum [40].

Alternatively, Behnke et al., 2007 used a repeating peptide sequence of RADA-16 (Figure 4) to develop self-assembled nanoscaffolds [28]. Using a severed optic nerve *in vivo* model, RADA-16 was injected into the site of injury and was later shown to induce axon regeneration. Lesioned hamsters partially recovered lost vision as determined by behavioral tests. The self-assembled nanostructures were also found to be non-toxic and did not elicit an inflammatory response in brain. Follow up studies showed these same scaffolds supported neuronal migration [41].

The physiochemical properties of hydrogels also make them excellent candidates for caging cells. In traumatic brain injury (TBI) or spinal cord lesions, cavities formed from mechanical damage or tumor removal can lead to severe functional loss. Stem cell therapy has emerged as a viable avenue of research to replenish lost neurons [42]. These approaches generally involve harvesting neural progenitor cells, *in vitro* expansion/differentiation and subsequent re-implantation into the defect. Preliminary investigations with peptide hydrogels have shown promise for use in cell encapsulation techniques. Hydrogels, such as those described by Semino et al. were used to entrap neural progenitor cells [41]. In another instance, globular domains derived from laminin were coupled to keratin hydrogels. Neurosphere forming cells adhered to the hybrid keratin constructs and proliferated at a high survival rate [43].

In summary, functionalized hydrogels with optimum epitope densities provide a tunable approach to filling void defects as well as delivery of biologics. The chemical and mechanical properties of hydrogels can be modified to elicit cell-specific behavior such as attachment, neurite extension, migration and cell differentiation.

3.4. *Nerve guidance conduits for PNS*

In the PNS, the biomechanical environment places a different set of criteria on implantable devices. Therapeutic designs must cope with low level mechanical perturbations (tensile forces) within the PNS environment. While hydrogels or in-situ polymerization may be feasible, these techniques must be mated to other integration schemes. For example, a common method for PNS repair is the use of nerve guidance conduits (NGCs). NGCs are tubes or comparable structures that bridge the proximal and distal segments of a damaged nerve. NGCs are designed to eliminate the use of autologous nerve grafts, which are the clinical gold standard for gap repairs. Within the NGC is an enclosed space that permits the natural regenerative process to take effect.

Numerous biomaterials have been investigated as potential NGC candidates. NGCs have been made from natural and synthetic polymers including collagen, polyesters, silicone, alginate, chitosan and acellularized tissue (see ref [44] for review). Many of these polymers are poor substrates for cell adhesion. Peptide conjugation therefore improves interfacial interactions and reduces the likelihood of a foreign body response. Peptide conjugates have been used to coat NGC interior surfaces to facilitate cell adhesion and migration. For instance, chitosan was covalently bonded to CDPGYIGSR or CSRARKQAASIKVAVSAD sequences and molded into a nerve tube [29]. In animal tests with a 15mm gap defect in sciatic nerve, peptide modified tubes showed similar results when compared to laminin coated conduits. However, peptide and laminin grafts did not quite match the functional outcomes of autologous standards. A similar study with crab-derived chitosan and a YIGSR conjugate also demonstrated axonal sprouting and bridging of the graft [45]. New chemical techniques have also allowed peptide conjugation onto polyester based materials such as polycaprolactone (PCL) [46].

The data with peptide modified NGCs are promising. However, it is now recognized that within the PNS, simple conduits do not provide sufficient guidance cues required for adequate functional outcome. Additional growth promoting factors as well as built-in anisotropies that facilitate axon guidance are necessary to improve regeneration speeds and quality regeneration.

4. Coupling Peptide Scaffolds with Directional Information

Thus far, we have discussed peptide modified synthetics that primarily promote cell adhesion and neurite formation. Many of these studies exhibit excellent *in vitro* outcomes while others have shown some success with mammalian models.

In the PNS, however, simple conduits are inadequate for meaningful functional reconnection. In the nervous system, directed regeneration that emulates the undamaged anatomy is preferred. Misdirected fiber projection in the PNS can lead to aberrant regeneration or neuromas [5]. Within the domain of the spinal cord, directional encoding has beneficial implications, such as emulating the rostral-caudal geometry of white matter tracts. Restoration of the original tissue architecture is essential in promoting appropriate target recognition. We discuss strategies that have been used to demonstrate cell orientation and biased neurite extension. These approaches can be merged with previously discussed peptide combinations. The multitude of available chemical tools capable of synthesizing the desired peptide-polymer conjugates can be found elsewhere [47].

4.1. *Spatial gradients and micropatterning*

Target recognition of axonal projections is thought to be encoded in gradients of biomolecular origin. Axons respond to a myriad of soluble and substrate bound guidance cues and many of these mechanisms have been elucidated *in vitro* [48]. Axonal growth cones function as dynamic sensors and some studies suggest soluble chemical gradients of ~0.1% can be detected across the growth cone surface [49]. Growth cone attraction to changes in peptide concentration was highlighted by Adams et al., when immobilized IKVAV gradients were used to steer axonal projections [50]. Dorsal root ganglia neurons were able to detect a 25% difference in spatial peptide density within a 30 μm reference. The majority of neurites grew towards higher density peptide gradients and actually paused to "assess" the choice before resuming to normal growth speed. Comparable results were reported with a PPFLMLLKGSTR binding motif derived from human laminin-5. In this case, PC-12 cells extended neurites toward the higher peptide concentration gradient embedded within a collagen scaffold [51].

Early studies by Letourneau (1975) showed neurons could "select" between heterogeneous materials [52]. This concept was later refined, but similar approaches that exploit surface binding preferences are common. Adhesivity modulation of the substrate by patterning alternative stripes of pro-adhesive vs. non-adhesive proteins have been used to align glia and neurons. For example, Matsuzawa et al. used a UV-photomasking technique to create oscillating stripes of RDIAEIIKDI with alkylsilane [53]. Embryonic hippocampal neurons demonstrated substratum-controlled changes in morphology and generally extended axons along the peptide bands.

Soft photolithographic techniques such as microcontact printing (elastomeric stamping) have been used to transfer stripes of IKVAV oligopeptide onto [54] glass or silicon oxide substrates. Hippocampal neurons on biofunctionalized surfaces formed networks under serum-free conditions and remained functional for more than a week. Alternating stripes of laminin and BSA spaced 20 μm apart were used to induce Schwann cell alignment *in vitro* [55]. Data showed that 70% of the Schwann cells were oriented with respect to the micropattern after just one hour while 94% were oriented at 24 hours [55]. Further studies found that DRGs grown on top of aligned Schwann cells extended neurites along the Schwann cell monolayer [56]. This unique co-culture system may be more representative of *in vivo* interactions and may therefore be a good model for elucidating cellular dynamics.

4.2. *Synergisms with topographical cues*

Peptide gradients can be an effective way to control cell behavior. However, extending micropatterning and immobilization of ligand gradients to three-dimensions can be challenging. Alternatively, another technique often used for modulating cell orientation and neurite outgrowth is contact guidance. Contact guidance refers to a phenomenon where physical anisotropies within the substrate induce cell orientation locomotion changes [57]. In the nervous system, contact guidance exists *in vivo* and has a developmental role in growth and regeneration [58], [59]. Contact guidance has several distinct advantages over other methods for controlling cell behavior. For example, physical guidance is local, affecting cells directly interfacing with the surface. Depending on the polymeric system, topographical cues can be permanent or degradable. In tissue engineering, the following geometric schemes have been used to elicit desired outcomes in the nervous system.

4.2.1. *Thin films with micro or nanoscale patterning*

Traditional photolithographic processes borne of silicon microfabrication have been used to etch unidirectional grooves and channels onto compatible substrates (generally glass or silicon oxide). These seminal studies have provided insight into the range of topographic stimuli required to induce desired cell orientation [60],[61]. Soft lithographic methods, including casting and replica molding with PDMS and polymeric systems have changed the way patterns can be fabricated on substrates more suitable for use *in vivo* (Figure 5) For example, using a replica molding method, Li et al. manufactured grooves spaced from 1-2μm apart with depths of 150-300nm on degradable PLLA [62]. PC-12 cells and chick sympathetic neurons cultured onto these surfaces demonstrated neurite alignment (up to 70%) as well as increased extension rates of 10-30%. Miller et al., used laminin coated PLGA and PLDA with transferred microgrooves to demonstrate 95% alignment in DRG neurons [63]. Similarly, PC-12 cells grown on PPFLMLLKGSTR (laminin-derived) functionalized PLGA microgrooves showed neurite elongation parallel to the grooves. Neurites had a tendency to reside within the channels and tighter pitched grooves improved angular alignment [64].

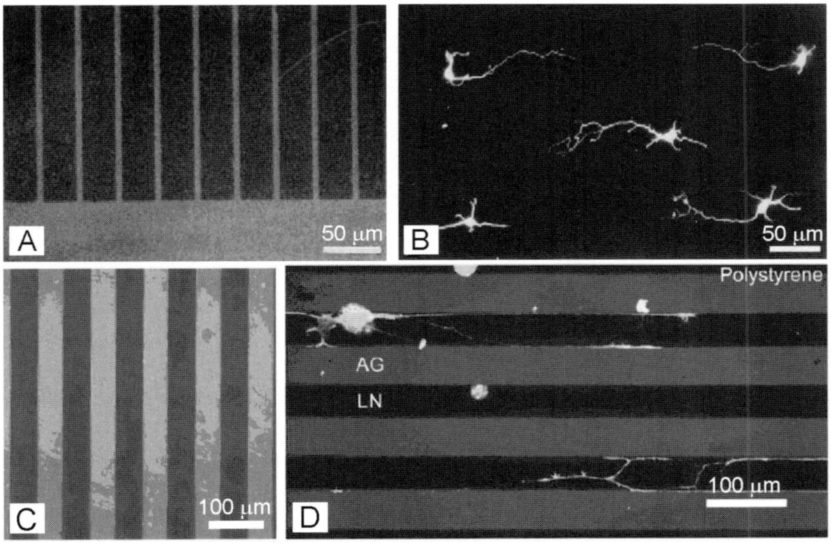

Fig. 5. (A) Striped substrate configuration prior to coupling with p20 peptide. (B) Hippocampal cells grew preferentially along the p20 coated regions. (C) Alternating stripes of laminin and aggrecan microstamped onto a glass surface. (D) DRGs cultured onto laminin and aggrecan stripes show preferred cell adhesion and orientation of laminin bands. (A), (B) Reprinted with permission from [100]. (C),(D) Reprinted with permission from [101].

4.2.2. *Microchannel and microtubular architectures*

Microtubular scaffolds for neural engineering have been an active research niche because tubular arrays mimic the native endoneurial architecture in PNS. Ma and Zhang first synthesized linear microchannels within PLLA and PLGA using a thermally induced phase separation technique. Scaffolds with porosities of 97% were achieved, but these and other properties including diameter of the microtubules, the tube morphology and orientation could be controlled. A similar freeze drying technique employed by Stokols and Tuszynski created alginate matrices with long linear pores [65]. These scaffolds were capable of releasing NGF and supported PC-12 differentiation *in vitro*. Subsequent implantation of these matrices in lesioned spinal cord showed good host integration, cell penetration into the channels and linear axon growth within the channels [66].

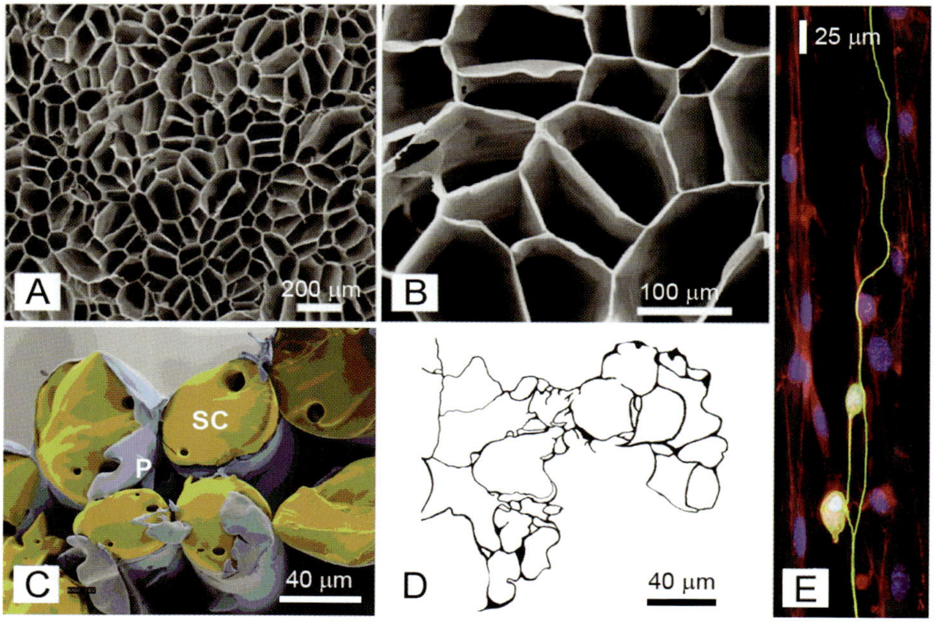

Fig. 6. (A) Cross sectional image of multi-channeled agarose scaffolds manufactured by a freeze drying technique. (B) Higher magnification of the scaffolds show thin walls separating the linear pores. (C) SEM cross section of poly-l-lactic acid (PLLA) based microtubular scaffolds manufactured with selective dissolution (yellow/SC: sucrose core, blue/P: PLLA coating). (D) Corresponding cross section of (C) reveal the membranous walls following core dissolution. (E) Immunofluorescent imaging of Schwann cells (red: actin, blue: nucleus) and chick DRG (yellow: neurofilament) co-cultures on scaffolds shown in (D). Cells and neurite aligned along the long axis of the tubular constructs. (A), (B) Reprinted with permission from [65]. (C)-(E) Reprinted with permission from [67].

Using a PLLA polymer system, Li et al. used a novel selective dissolution process with sucrose cores to create semi-permeable microtubular scaffolds with diameters between 8-100μm [67]. These 3-D scaffolds guided Schwann cell orientation along tubule surfaces as well as DRGs neurite alignment (Figure 6). For spinal cord repair, Tsai et al. devised hydrogel tubes composed of poly(2-hydroxyethyl methacrylate-co-methyl methacrylate (PHEMA-MMA) [68]. Spinal cord continuity was observed 4 and 8 weeks post transection. Serotonergic axons and bridging tissue were found to enter the PHEMA channels. Retrograde axonal tracing revealed regeneration of axons from reticular, vestibular, and raphe brainstem motor nuclei. PHEMA channels exhibited minimal scarring at the material-tissue interface and less scarring at the channel-dura interface compared to ePTFE. This pioneering present study was the first to demonstrate regeneration of brainstem motor nuclei axons into an unfilled synthetic hydrogel following complete spinal cord severance.

4.2.3. *Micro and nanofibrillar constructs*

An analog to microtubular geometry is the solid fibrillar structure. It has been well understood that curvature induced by microscale fibrils can be used to induce cell migration and morphological changes [69]. Cytoskeletal inflexibility is thought to be responsible for the alignment behavior observed in cultured cells [70].

Numerous techniques have been used to create synthetic microfibers of varying diameters. For example, PLGA microfibers were fabricated using a microfluidic spinning apparatus where PLGA strands were precipitated from a PLGA/DMSO mix exposed to a glycerol/water solution. Porous fibers with diameters on the order of 20-230μm were created. Neural progenitor cells seeded onto the PLGA scaffolds were found to extend processes along the microfibers [71]. In another study, Cai et al [72] used wet spinning to fabricate PLDLA (75:25) fibers in the range of 60-80μm to implant in a rat sciatic nerve model. Gap lesions of 18mm were bridged with implants containing these microfiber filaments (NGC). At 10 weeks post-op, improved tissue cable formation and Schwann cell migration was observed in the experimental groups. When compared to corresponding silicone conduits, tubes impregnated with micro-filaments enhanced myelinated axon regeneration. Myelin staining indicated PLDLA conduits supported axon myelination in both qualitative and quantitative measures vs empty silicone controls.

Recently, the process of electrospinning has become popular in creating nanofibrous mats and scaffolds for tissue engineering (Figure 7). Electrospinning can be used to create fiber diameters in the micron regime or even down to a few nanometers [73]. Several groups have used electrospun chitosan to create a neural scaffold. Wang et al., 2008 characterized nanofibrous chitosan and showed increased tensile strength on aligned vs. unaligned mats [74]. Schwann cells cultured onto aligned scaffolds displayed parallel orientation. Using a sciatic nerve defect, implanted chitosan mats demonstrated functional and electrophysiological recovery to levels approaching the autograft. A similar study conducted by Kim and colleagues used a much larger 17mm gap lesion in rat sciatic nerve [75]. Acrylonitrile-co-methylacrylate (PAN-MA) fibers were electrospun into aligned and unaligned configurations. Histological and

Table 2. List of common neurotrophins.

Factor	Target Cell	Neuron Function	Receptors	Reference
Nerve growth factor: NGF	Small-diameter unmyelinated axons, glial cells, various	Sympathetic, nociception, thermoception, various sensory	Trk A, p75	[80, 81]
Brain-derived neurotrophic factor: BDNF	Medium- to large-diameter axons	Motor, mechanoreception	Trk B, p75	[82, 83]
Neurotrophin 3: NT-3	Medium- to large-myelinated axons	Motor, priopriocеption, mechanoreception	Trk B,C, p75	[82, 84, 85]
Neurotrophin 4/5: NT-4/5	Small, unmyelinated axons	Motor, sympathetic, other sensory	Trk B, p75	[81, 86]
Glial-derived neurotrophic factor: GDNF	Dopaminergic neurons	Motor, sensory, various	GFRα1	[87, 88]
Ciliary neurotrophic factor: CNTF	Large myelinated axons, astrocytes, various	Motor, sensory, sympathetic	CNTFR	[89]

functional measures showed greater axonal regeneration and ingrowth on aligned substrates but not on unaligned surfaces. This study clearly showed that given the same surface area, an aligned architecture can facilitate PNS regeneration. Newer revisions to the electrospinning process has permitted the creation of pure protein or peptide block copolymer [76] that emulate the natural basement membrane morphology [77].

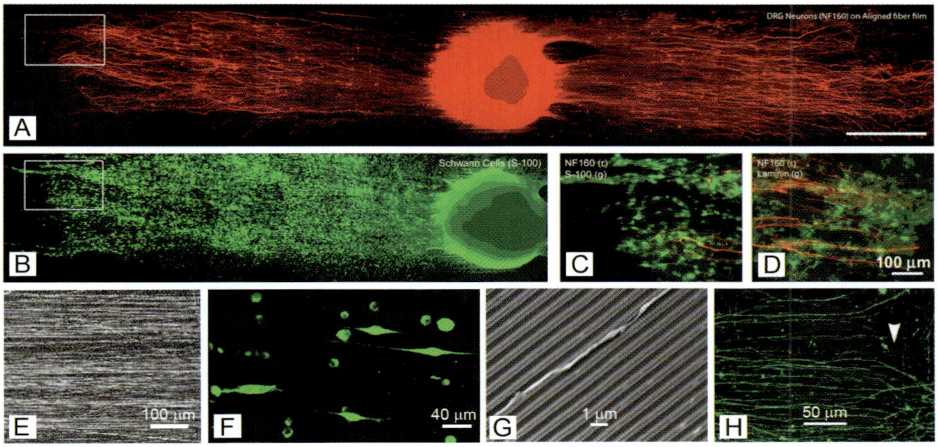

Fig. 7. (A) DRG neurons cultured onto an electrospun PAN-MA nanofiber mat. Red staining highlights neurofilament. (B) Schwann cells on the same PAN-MA scaffolds show extended morphologies. (C) Magnified neurofilament (red) and Schwann cell staining (green) of box outlined in (B). (D) A double immunostained composite of aligned axons (NF160, red) and newly deposited laminin (green). (E) Electrospun fibers of PLLA. (F) Neural stem cells cultured (2 days) onto PLLA fibers shown in (E). (G) Scanning electron micrograph of mouse DRG atop a microgrooved surface. (H) Immunostaining of DRGs on surfaces in (G) show good alignment. Arrow denotes the end of the patterned topography. (A)-(D) Reprinted with permission from [75]. (E), (F) Reprinted with permission from [102]. (G), (H) Reprinted with permission from [103].

5. Biomolecule Release from Peptide — Conjugated Scaffolds

5.1. *Growth factors and suppression of inhibitory cues*

Growth factors are potent molecules that play critical roles in development, maintenance and survival of normal tissue. Controlled delivery of growth factors has drawn special interest as a method to overcome the growth suppressing nature of the adult CNS. The function and target of common growth factors in the nervous system are shown in Table 2. While an in-depth review of neurotrophins is beyond the scope of this chapter, we will briefly discuss how emerging techniques with peptides conjugates can be refined for molecular delivery. It is believed that synergistic effects between the instructional benefits of peptide motifs with growth factors can overcome some of the obstacles to regeneration.

Secondly, within the mature CNS, there have been a number of identified physical and biological inhibitors to regeneration. For example, Nogo-A and chondroitin sulfate proteoglycans are only two of many agents that induce growth cone collapse or prevent neurite growth activity. Blocking the inhibitors with anti-NogoA antibodies [78] or chondroitinase can improve compensatory sprouting from spared axons and enhance sprouting of damaged fibers [79]. Again, inclusion of these agents within a growth permissive scaffold should mitigate problems associated in CNS regeneration.

5.2. *Release strategies*

Several schemes have been proposed for delivering neurotrophins *in vivo*. Incorporation of the target biomolecule during the polymerization step of the polymer/hydrogel is quite common. Essentially, the desired compound is trapped within the matrix of the scaffold. The release mechanism is diffusion mediated. With degradable materials, surface or bulk erosion of the polymer releases the entrapped drug, albeit in potentially sporadic pulses [90].

Using this matrix release model, Piantino et al. [91] incorporated NT-3 into a photopolymerizable hydrogel for use in spinal cord trauma. Rats treated with NT-3 loaded hydrogels exhibited greater axon regeneration in the corticospinal and raphespinal tracts when compared to controls. BBB scoring as well as a horizontal walking behavior test showed superior outcomes compared to untreated group. In another study, BDNF released from microchanneled agarose scaffolds promoted greater spinal cord axon regeneration compared to the same construct sans BDNF [66]. Loaded hydrogels may also be used as coatings for neural recording electrodes [92] whereby the growth factors would recruit and stimulate neurite growth towards the electrode and create intimate contact with the biomaterial interface.

In addition to matrix loaded delivery, impregnated microparticles have shown viability for nervous system application. Microparticles have several implementation advantages since the particles are fabricated independently and can be later embedded into hydrogels or NGCs. Secondly, the release kinetics of microspheres can be modified by changing polymer porosity, particle size and biomaterial. This property allows for potential multi-stage regulated delivery. Saltzman et al. showed controlled release of NGF from EVA and PLGA microspheres over a period of 2 months and 2 weeks, respectively [93]. In other instances, PLGA microspheres within a collagen matrix were capable of releasing NGF over a 75 day interval [94]

Growth factors can be immobilized onto substrate surfaces or within hydrogels. This strategy localizes the growth factor and reduces the risk of systemic release. Achyuta et. al. fixed both laminin and NGF and noticed PC-12 neurite outgrowth was similar to that observed on surfaces with immobilized laminin and soluble NGF. [95]. In other reports, NGF has been successfully tethered to a variety of other polymers including pHEMA [96], polypyrrole [97] and PEO-PPO [98].

6. Conclusions

Even after decades of modern research, the neurobiology governing nervous system regeneration is still being deciphered. The microenvironment within the developing nervous system is clearly different from the mature state. While the CNS and PNS place different constraints in tissue engineering, the over-arching aims following injury are quite similar: sufficient directed regeneration that leads to appreciable functional recovery. Therapies designed to treat debilitating neurologic pathologies are going to involve combined approaches that systematically address the many biochemical and cellular barriers to recovery.

Within this therapeutic framework, peptide conjugates are versatile treatment tools that serve several functions. Bioactive scaffolds can direct a host of cell-specific interactions while simultaneously act as reservoirs for exogenous compound delivery. Additionally, functionalized biomaterials can provide the necessary mechanical and physical requirements that maintain tissue integrity.

Other frontiers such as stem cell therapy have potentially promising futures, but not enough is currently known to safely wield the power. The factors that dictate cell differentiation are wide ranging and complex. However, early studies indicate certain peptide motifs can guide progenitor cell differentiation and preserve phenotypic fate. These results demonstrate the utility of bioactive materials as mainstays for stem cell rehabilitation. In the coming years, it is hoped that new insights in neuroscience will be integrated into material designs equipped to treat diseased or damaged tissue. Smart materials are expected to play a pivotal role in such medical breakthroughs.

Acknowledgments

We would like to thank Michel Schweinsberg for his contribution in artwork.

References

[1] Sherwood, C.C., et al., "Evolution of increased glia-neuron ratios in the human frontal cortex," *Proc Natl Acad Sci U S A*, Vol. 103, No. 37, 2006, pp. 13606-13611.

[2] Colon-Ramos, D.A., and K. Shen, "Cellular conductors: glial cells as guideposts during neural circuit development," *PLoS Biol*, Vol. 6, No. 4, 2008, pp. e112.

[3] Sunderland S., and K. Bradley, "The cross-sectional area of peripheral nerve trunks devoted to nerve fibres," *Brain*, Vol. 72, 1949, pp.428–449

[4] Taniuchi, M., H.B. Clark, and E.M. Johnson, Jr., "Induction of nerve growth factor receptor in Schwann cells after axotomy," *Proc Natl Acad Sci U S A*, Vol. 83, No. 11, 1986, pp. 4094-4098.

[5] Sumner, A.J., "Aberrant reinnervation," *Muscle Nerve*, Vol. 13, No. 9, 1990, pp. 801-803.

[6] Lundborg, G., "A 25-year perspective of peripheral nerve surgery: evolving neuroscientific concepts and clinical significance," *J Hand Surg [Am]*, Vol. 25, No. 3, 2000, pp. 391-414.

[7] Richardson, P.M., U.M. McGuinness, and A.J. Aguayo, "Axons from CNS neurons regenerate into PNS grafts," *Nature*, Vol. 284, No. 5753, 1980, pp. 264-265.

[8] Tello F., "La influencia del neurotropismo en la regeneracion de los centros nerviosos," *Trab Lab Invest Biol,* Vol. 9, 1911, pp. 123-159.

[9] Rossignol, S., et al., "Spinal cord injury: time to move?," *J Neurosci*, Vol. 27, No. 44, 2007, pp. 11782-11792.

[10] Liuzzi, F.J., and R.J. Lasek, "Astrocytes block axonal regeneration in mammals by activating the physiological stop pathway," *Science*, Vol. 237, No. 4815, 1987, pp. 642-645.

[11] Sellaro, T.L., et al., "Maintenance of hepatic sinusoidal endothelial cell phenotype in vitro using organ-specific extracellular matrix scaffolds," *Tissue Eng*, Vol. 13, No. 9, 2007, pp. 2301-2310.

[12] Lutolf, M.P., and J.A. Hubbell, "Synthetic biomaterials as instructive extracellular microenvironments for morphogenesis in tissue engineering," *Nat Biotechnol*, Vol. 23, No. 1, 2005, pp. 47-55.

[13] Badylak, S.F., D.O. Freytes, and T.W. Gilbert, "Extracellular matrix as a biological scaffold material: Structure and function," *Acta Biomater*, Vol. 5, No. 1, 2009, pp. 1-13.

[14] Chen, Z.L., and S. Strickland, "Laminin gamma1 is critical for Schwann cell differentiation, axon myelination, and regeneration in the peripheral nerve," *J Cell Biol*, Vol. 163, No. 4, 2003, pp. 889-899.

[15] Baron-Van Evercooren, A., et al., "Fibronectin promotes rat Schwann cell growth and motility," *J Cell Biol*, Vol. 93, No. 1, 1982, pp. 211-216.

[16] Baron-Van Evercooren, A., et al., "Nerve growth factor, laminin, and fibronectin promote neurite growth in human fetal sensory ganglia cultures," *J Neurosci Res*, Vol. 8, No. 2-3, 1982, pp. 179-193.

[17] Zhang, Z., et al., "Neurite outgrowth on well-characterized surfaces: preparation and characterization of chemically and spatially controlled fibronectin and RGD substrates with good bioactivity," *Biomaterials*, Vol. 26, No. 1, 2005, pp. 47-61.

[18] Schense, J.C., and J.A. Hubbell, "Three-dimensional migration of neurites is mediated by adhesion site density and affinity," *J Biol Chem*, Vol. 275, No. 10, 2000, pp. 6813-6818.

[19] Davis, D.H., et al., "Immobilization of RGD to < 1 1 1 > silicon surfaces for enhanced cell adhesion and proliferation," *Biomaterials*, Vol. 23, No. 19, 2002, pp. 4019-4027.

[20] Tong, Y.W., and M.S. Shoichet, "Enhancing the neuronal interaction on fluoropolymer surfaces with mixed peptides or spacer group linkers," *Biomaterials*, Vol. 22, No. 10, 2001, pp. 1029-1034.
[21] Dhoot, N.O., et al., "Peptide-modified alginate surfaces as a growth permissive substrate for neurite outgrowth," *J Biomed Mater Res A*, Vol. 71, No. 2, 2004, pp. 191-200.
[22] Yu, T.T., and M.S. Shoichet, "Guided cell adhesion and outgrowth in peptide-modified channels for neural tissue engineering," *Biomaterials*, Vol. 26, No. 13, 2005, pp. 1507-1514.
[23] Liu, W.Q., et al., "RGD-mediated adhesive interactions are important for peripheral axon outgrowth in vivo," *Neurobiol Dis*, Vol. 34, No. 1, 2009, pp. 11-22.
[24] Borkenhagen, M., et al., "Three-dimensional extracellular matrix engineering in the nervous system," *J Biomed Mater Res*, Vol. 40, No. 3, 1998, pp. 392-400.
[25] Shaw, D., and M.S. Shoichet, "Toward spinal cord injury repair strategies: peptide surface modification of expanded poly(tetrafluoroethylene) fibers for guided neurite outgrowth in vitro," *J Craniofac Surg*, Vol. 14, No. 3, 2003, pp. 308-316.
[26] Kam, L., et al., "Selective adhesion of astrocytes to surfaces modified with immobilized peptides," *Biomaterials*, Vol. 23, No. 2, 2002, pp. 511-515.
[27] Schense, J.C., et al., "Enzymatic incorporation of bioactive peptides into fibrin matrices enhances neurite extension," *Nat Biotechnol*, Vol. 18, No. 4, 2000, pp. 415-419.
[28] Ellis-Behnke, R.G., et al., "Nano neuro knitting: peptide nanofiber scaffold for brain repair and axon regeneration with functional return of vision," *Proc Natl Acad Sci U S A*, Vol. 103, No. 13, 2006, pp. 5054-5059.
[29] Suzuki, M., et al., "Tendon chitosan tubes covalently coupled with synthesized laminin peptides facilitate nerve regeneration in vivo," *J Neurosci Res*, Vol. 72, No. 5, 2003, pp. 646-659.
[30] Graf, J., et al., "A pentapeptide from the laminin B1 chain mediates cell adhesion and binds the 67,000 laminin receptor," *Biochemistry*, Vol. 26, No. 22, 1987, pp. 6896-6900.
[31] Ranieri, J.P., et al., "Spatial control of neuronal cell attachment and differentiation on covalently patterned laminin oligopeptide substrates," *Int J Dev Neurosci*, Vol. 12, No. 8, 1994, pp. 725-735.
[32] Massia, S.P., M.M. Holecko, and G.R. Ehteshami, "In vitro assessment of bioactive coatings for neural implant applications," *J Biomed Mater Res A*, Vol. 68, No. 1, 2004, pp. 177-186.
[33] Liesi, P., et al., "Identification of a neurite outgrowth-promoting domain of laminin using synthetic peptides," *FEBS Lett*, Vol. 244, No. 1, 1989, pp. 141-148.
[34] Tsang, V.L., and S.N. Bhatia, "Three-dimensional tissue fabrication," *Adv Drug Deliv Rev*, Vol. 56, No. 11, 2004, pp. 1635-1647.
[35] Lupi, O., "Prions in dermatology," *J Am Acad Dermatol*, Vol. 46, No. 5, 2002, pp. 790-793.
[36] Gunn, J.W., S.D. Turner, and B.K. Mann, "Adhesive and mechanical properties of hydrogels influence neurite extension," *J Biomed Mater Res A*, Vol. 72, No. 1, 2005, pp. 91-97.
[37] Hynd, M.R., et al., "Directed cell growth on protein-functionalized hydrogel surfaces," *J Neurosci Methods*, Vol. 162, No. 1-2, 2007, pp. 255-263.
[38] Silva, G.A., et al., "Selective differentiation of neural progenitor cells by high-epitope density nanofibers," *Science*, Vol. 303, No. 5662, 2004, pp. 1352-1355.
[39] Tysseling-Mattiace, V.M., et al., "Self-assembling nanofibers inhibit glial scar formation and promote axon elongation after spinal cord injury," *J Neurosci*, Vol. 28, No. 14, 2008, pp. 3814-3823.
[40] Wei, Y.T., et al., "Hyaluronic acid hydrogels with IKVAV peptides for tissue repair and axonal regeneration in an injured rat brain," *Biomed Mater*, Vol. 2, No. 3, 2007, pp. S142-146.
[41] Semino, C.E., et al., "Entrapment of migrating hippocampal neural cells in three-dimensional peptide nanofiber scaffold," *Tissue Eng*, Vol. 10, No. 3-4, 2004, pp. 643-655.

[42] Shear, D.A., et al., "Neural progenitor cell transplants promote long-term functional recovery after traumatic brain injury," *Brain Res*, Vol. 1026, No. 1, 2004, pp. 11-22.
[43] Nakaji-Hirabayashi, T., K. Kato, and H. Iwata, "Self-assembling chimeric protein for the construction of biodegradable hydrogels capable of interaction with integrins expressed on neural stem/progenitor cells," *Biomacromolecules*, Vol. 9, No. 5, 2008, pp. 1411-1416.
[44] Dalton, P.D., and J. Mey, "Neural interactions with materials," *Front Biosci*, Vol. 14, No., 2009, pp. 769-795.
[45] Itoh, S., et al., "Effects of a laminin peptide (YIGSR) immobilized on crab-tendon chitosan tubes on nerve regeneration," *J Biomed Mater Res B Appl Biomater*, Vol. 73, No. 2, 2005, pp. 375-382.
[46] Santiago, L.Y., et al., "Peptide-surface modification of poly(caprolactone) with laminin-derived sequences for adipose-derived stem cell applications," *Biomaterials*, Vol. 27, No. 15, 2006, pp. 2962-2969.
[47] Gauthier, M.A., and H.A. Klok, "Peptide/protein-polymer conjugates: synthetic strategies and design concepts," *Chem Commun (Camb)*, Vol. No. 23, 2008, pp. 2591-2611.
[48] Keynes, R., and G.M. Cook, "Axon guidance molecules," *Cell*, Vol. 83, No. 2, 1995, pp. 161-169.
[49] Rosoff, W.J., et al., "A new chemotaxis assay shows the extreme sensitivity of axons to molecular gradients," *Nat Neurosci*, Vol. 7, No. 6, 2004, pp. 678-682.
[50] Adams, D.N., et al., "Growth cones turn and migrate up an immobilized gradient of the laminin IKVAV peptide," *J Neurobiol*, Vol. 62, No. 1, 2005, pp. 134-147.
[51] Yao, L., et al., "The effect of laminin peptide gradient in enzymatically cross-linked collagen scaffolds on neurite growth," *J Biomed Mater Res A*, Vol. No., 2009.
[52] Letourneau, P.C., "Cell-to-substratum adhesion and guidance of axonal elongation," *Dev Biol*, Vol. 44, No. 1, 1975, pp. 92-101.
[53] Matsuzawa, M., et al., "Directional neurite outgrowth and axonal differentiation of embryonic hippocampal neurons are promoted by a neurite outgrowth domain of the B2-chain of laminin," *Int J Dev Neurosci*, Vol. 14, No. 3, 1996, pp. 283-295.
[54] Klein, C.L., M. Scholl, and A. Maelicke, "Neuronal networks in vitro: formation and organization on biofunctionalized surfaces," *J Mater Sci Mater Med*, Vol. 10, No. 12, 1999, pp. 721-727.
[55] Thompson, D.M., and H.M. Buettner, "Schwann cell response to micropatterned laminin surfaces," *Tissue Eng*, Vol. 7, No. 3, 2001, pp. 247-265.
[56] Thompson, D.M., and H.M. Buettner, "Neurite outgrowth is directed by schwann cell alignment in the absence of other guidance cues," *Ann Biomed Eng*, Vol. 34, No. 1, 2006, pp. 161-168.
[57] Weiss, L., "Cell contact phenomena," *In Vitro*, Vol. 5, No., 1970, pp. 48-78.
[58] Super, H., and E. Soriano, "The organization of the embryonic and early postnatal murine hippocampus. II. Development of entorhinal, commissural, and septal connections studied with the lipophilic tracer DiI," *J Comp Neurol*, Vol. 344, No. 1, 1994, pp. 101-120.
[59] Nordlander, R.H., J.W. Gazzerro, and H. Cook, "Growth cones and axon trajectories of a sensory pathway in the amphibian spinal cord," *J Comp Neurol*, Vol. 307, No. 4, 1991, pp. 539-548.
[60] Clark, P., et al., "Cell guidance by ultrafine topography in vitro," *J Cell Sci*, Vol. 99 (Pt 1), No., 1991, pp. 73-77.
[61] Rajnicek, A., and C. McCaig, "Guidance of CNS growth cones by substratum grooves and ridges: effects of inhibitors of the cytoskeleton, calcium channels and signal transduction pathways," *J Cell Sci*, Vol. 110 (Pt 23), No., 1997, pp. 2915-2924.
[62] Li, J., H. McNally, and R. Shi, "Enhanced neurite alignment on micro-patterned poly-L-lactic acid films," *J Biomed Mater Res A*, Vol. No., 2008.

[63] Miller, C., S. Jeftinija, and S. Mallapragada, "Synergistic effects of physical and chemical guidance cues on neurite alignment and outgrowth on biodegradable polymer substrates," *Tissue Eng*, Vol. 8, No. 3, 2002, pp. 367-378.
[64] Yao, L., et al., "Effect of functionalized micropatterned PLGA on guided neurite growth," *Acta Biomater*, Vol. 5, No. 2, 2009, pp. 580-588.
[65] Stokols, S., and M.H. Tuszynski, "The fabrication and characterization of linearly oriented nerve guidance scaffolds for spinal cord injury," *Biomaterials*, Vol. 25, No. 27, 2004, pp. 5839-5846.
[66] Stokols, S., and M.H. Tuszynski, "Freeze-dried agarose scaffolds with uniaxial channels stimulate and guide linear axonal growth following spinal cord injury," *Biomaterials*, Vol. 27, No. 3, 2006, pp. 443-451.
[67] Li, J., T.A. Rickett, and R. Shi, "Biomimetic nerve scaffolds with aligned intraluminal microchannels: a "sweet" approach to tissue engineering," *Langmuir*, Vol. 25, No. 3, 2009, pp. 1813-1817.
[68] Tsai, E.C., et al., "Synthetic hydrogel guidance channels facilitate regeneration of adult rat brainstem motor axons after complete spinal cord transection," *J Neurotrauma*, Vol. 21, No. 6, 2004, pp. 789-804.
[69] Smeal, R.M., et al., "Substrate curvature influences the direction of nerve outgrowth," *Ann Biomed Eng*, Vol. 33, No. 3, 2005, pp. 376-382.
[70] Dunn, G.A., and J.P. Heath, "A new hypothesis of contact guidance in tissue cells," *Exp Cell Res*, Vol. 101, No. 1, 1976, pp. 1-14.
[71] Hwang, C.M., et al., "Microfluidic chip-based fabrication of PLGA microfiber scaffolds for tissue engineering," *Langmuir*, Vol. 24, No. 13, 2008, pp. 6845-6851.
[72] Cai, J., et al., "Permeable guidance channels containing microfilament scaffolds enhance axon growth and maturation," *J Biomed Mater Res A*, Vol. 75, No. 2, 2005, pp. 374-386.
[73] Wang, H.S., G.D. Fu, and X.S. Li, "Functional polymeric nanofibers from electrospinning," *Recent Pat Nanotechnol*, Vol. 3, No. 1, 2009, pp. 21-31.
[74] Wang, W., et al., "Effects of Schwann cell alignment along the oriented electrospun chitosan nanofibers on nerve regeneration," *J Biomed Mater Res A*, Vol. No., 2008.
[75] Kim, Y.T., et al., "The role of aligned polymer fiber-based constructs in the bridging of long peripheral nerve gaps," *Biomaterials*, Vol. 29, No. 21, 2008, pp. 3117-3127.
[76] Grafahrend, D., et al., "Biofunctionalized poly(ethylene glycol)-block-poly(epsilon-caprolactone) nanofibers for tissue engineering," *J Mater Sci Mater Med*, Vol. 19, No. 4, 2008, pp. 1479-1484.
[77] Neal, R.A., et al., "Laminin nanofiber meshes that mimic morphological properties and bioactivity of basement membranes," *Tissue Eng Part C Methods*, Vol. 15, No. 1, 2009, pp. 11-21.
[78] Schwab, M.E., "Nogo and axon regeneration," *Curr Opin Neurobiol*, Vol. 14, No. 1, 2004, pp. 118-124.
[79] Fawcett, J.W., "Overcoming inhibition in the damaged spinal cord," *J Neurotrauma*, Vol. 23, No. 3-4, 2006, pp. 371-383.
[80] Jenq, C.B., and R.E. Coggeshall, "Long-term patterns of axon regeneration in the sciatic nerve and its tributaries," *Brain Res*, Vol. 345, No. 1, 1985, pp. 34-44.
[81] Chao, M.V., R. Rajagopal, and F.S. Lee, "Neurotrophin signalling in health and disease," *Clin Sci (Lond)*, Vol. 110, No. 2, 2006, pp. 167-173.
[82] Snider, W.D., and D.E. Wright, "Neurotrophins cause a new sensation," *Neuron*, Vol. 16, No. 2, 1996, pp. 229-232.
[83] Terris, D.J., et al., "Brain-derived neurotrophic factor-enriched collagen tubule as a substitute for autologous nerve grafts," *Arch Otolaryngol Head Neck Surg*, Vol. 127, No. 3, 2001, pp. 294-298.

[84] Soppet, D., et al., "The neurotrophic factors brain-derived neurotrophic factor and neurotrophin-3 are ligands for the trkB tyrosine kinase receptor," *Cell*, Vol. 65, No. 5, 1991, pp. 895-903.
[85] Tessarollo, L., et al., "Targeted mutation in the neurotrophin-3 gene results in loss of muscle sensory neurons," *Proc Natl Acad Sci U S A*, Vol. 91, No. 25, 1994, pp. 11844-11848.
[86] Klein, R., et al., "The trkB tyrosine protein kinase is a receptor for neurotrophin-4," *Neuron*, Vol. 8, No. 5, 1992, pp. 947-956.
[87] Munson, J.B., and S.B. McMahon, "Effects of GDNF on axotomized sensory and motor neurons in adult rats," *Eur J Neurosci*, Vol. 9, No. 6, 1997, pp. 1126-1129.
[88] Barras, F.M., et al., "Glial cell line-derived neurotrophic factor released by synthetic guidance channels promotes facial nerve regeneration in the rat," *J Neurosci Res*, Vol. 70, No. 6, 2002, pp. 746-755.
[89] Sendtner, M., et al., "Ciliary neurotrophic factor," *J Neurobiol*, Vol. 25, No. 11, 1994, pp. 1436-1453.
[90] Wang, P.P., J. Frazier, and H. Brem, "Local drug delivery to the brain," *Adv Drug Deliv Rev*, Vol. 54, No. 7, 2002, pp. 987-1013.
[91] Piantino, J., et al., "An injectable, biodegradable hydrogel for trophic factor delivery enhances axonal rewiring and improves performance after spinal cord injury," *Exp Neurol*, Vol. 201, No. 2, 2006, pp. 359-367.
[92] Jhaveri, S.J., et al., "Release of nerve growth factor from HEMA hydrogel-coated substrates and its effect on the differentiation of neural cells," *Biomacromolecules*, Vol. 10, No. 1, 2009, pp. 174-183.
[93] Saltzman, W.M., et al., "Intracranial delivery of recombinant nerve growth factor: release kinetics and protein distribution for three delivery systems," *Pharm Res*, Vol. 16, No. 2, 1999, pp. 232-240.
[94] Rosner, B.I., et al., "Rational design of contact guiding, neurotrophic matrices for peripheral nerve regeneration," *Ann Biomed Eng*, Vol. 31, No. 11, 2003, pp. 1383-1401.
[95] Achyuta, A.K., et al., "Synergistic effect of immobilized laminin and nerve growth factor on PC12 neurite outgrowth," *Biotechnol Prog*, Vol. 25, No. 1, 2009, pp. 227-234.
[96] Kapur, T.A., and M.S. Shoichet, "Chemically-bound nerve growth factor for neural tissue engineering applications," *J Biomater Sci Polym Ed*, Vol. 14, No. 4, 2003, pp. 383-394.
[97] Gomez, N., and C.E. Schmidt, "Nerve growth factor-immobilized polypyrrole: bioactive electrically conducting polymer for enhanced neurite extension," *J Biomed Mater Res A*, Vol. 81, No. 1, 2007, pp. 135-149.
[98] Yim, E.K., and K.W. Leong, "Proliferation and differentiation of human embryonic germ cell derivatives in bioactive polymeric fibrous scaffold," *J Biomater Sci Polym Ed*, Vol. 16, No. 10, 2005, pp. 1193-1217.
[99] Nagai, Y., et al., "Slow release of molecules in self-assembling peptide nanofiber scaffold," *J Control Release*, Vol. 115, No. 1, 2006, pp. 18-25.
[100] Matsuzawa, M., P. Liesi, and W. Knoll, "Chemically modifying glass surfaces to study substratum-guided neurite outgrowth in culture," *J Neurosci Methods*, Vol. 69, No. 2, 1996, pp. 189-196.
[101] Hodgkinson, G.N., P.A. Tresco, and V. Hlady, "The differential influence of colocalized and segregated dual protein signals on neurite outgrowth on surfaces," *Biomaterials*, Vol. 28, No. 16, 2007, pp. 2590-2602.
[102] Yang, F., et al., "Electrospinning of nano/micro scale poly(L-lactic acid) aligned fibers and their potential in neural tissue engineering," *Biomaterials*, Vol. 26, No. 15, 2005, pp. 2603-2610.
[103] Johansson, F., et al., "Axonal outgrowth on nano-imprinted patterns," *Biomaterials*, Vol. 27, No. 8, 2006, pp. 1251-1258.

CHAPTER 14

HYBRID BIOMATERIALS FOR ENGINEERING VASCULAR TISSUES

Thomas C. Flanagan[1], Sebastian Olszewski[2], Julia Frese[2] and Stefan Jockenhoevel[2*]

[1]*School of Medicine & Medical Science, Health Sciences Centre, University College Dublin, Belfield, Dublin 4, Ireland*

[2]*Department of Applied Medical Engineering, Helmholtz Institute for Biomedical Engineering, RWTH Aachen University, Pauwelsstrasse 20, 52074 Aachen, Germany*

[*]*E-mail: jockenhoevel@hia.rwth-aachen.de*

1. Introduction

Vascular disease is the most frequent cause of death in Western society [1]. The most common presentation is atherosclerosis, a slow, complex inflammatory disease process resulting in a thickening of the inner arterial lining. Occluded vessels resulting from coronary and peripheral atherosclerosis can lead to ischemic tissue in the heart and lower limb, respectively, which may result in myocardial infarction or lower limb loss. In such patients, the capacity for intrinsic tissue repair is severely compromised, and surgical intervention is generally required to restore blood flow to the tissues. Potential treatments of occluded coronary or peripheral vessels include anti-thrombotic therapy, angioplasty/stent deployment, arterial by-pass grafting and therapeutic angiogenesis.

In the cases of both coronary and peripheral artery occlusion, normal blood flow can be restored to the tissue using balloon angioplasty, in which a catheter is advanced to the site of obstruction using minimally-invasive percutaneous techniques, and the balloon is subsequently inflated to compress the atherosclerotic plaque against the arterial wall. In these cases, however, the arteries frequently undergo restenosis (re-narrowing) [2] – a reparative process that occurs after injury to the endothelium. The incidence of restenosis can be significantly reduced by implanting an expandable stainless steel or nitinol stent at the occlusion site during the angioplasty procedure. Despite advances in the design and development of stent materials, however, including some degree of clinical success for drug-eluting stents [3], angioplasty techniques are still hindered by late thrombosis events and in-stent restenosis, and intense research is ongoing in an effort to develop more biocompatible materials.

In cases of coronary arteries with greater than 70% occlusion, by-pass grafting is generally performed. Synthetic vascular conduits composed of polyethylene terephthalate (Dacron™), expanded polytetraflouroethylene (ePTFE, Teflon™) and polyurethane have been successfully used in the replacement of large-calibre (≥5 mm) vessels [4]. However, small-calibre vessels (<5 mm) constructed from synthetic materials for coronary artery by-pass have poor intermediate and long-term patency rates, attributed to thrombogenic occlusion of the lumen caused by the blood-contacting surface [5, 6]. Autologous grafts, including the internal thoracic artery and saphenous vein, remain the standard for by-pass or replacement of small-calibre vessels. However, many patients do not have an autologous vessel suitable for use due to pre-existing pathological conditions or prior surgical harvest.

The urgent requirement to develop alternative vascular structures and to regenerate tissue following ischemia has led to the development of 'living' grafts through the field of tissue engineering [7]. Tissue engineering design strategies are typically based on the seeding of a scaffold material (biological, synthetic, or a composite of both) with a suitable source of living cells in an appropriate three-dimensional configuration, which is subsequently conditioned using various external stimuli, including biochemical or mechanical factors. Each of the three essential components of the technique have important, specific functions: the cells, or viable component of the construct, will ultimately develop and remodel the tissue/graft, and in the case of vascular constructs, should form a thrombo-resistant coating on the luminal surface. The scaffold material is designed to deliver cells and other molecules to the implantation site, where they are maintained in a suitable anatomic configuration, while biochemical or mechanical stimulation acts to guide optimal cellular and physical properties via controlled gene expression, differentiation, tissue development and remodeling. Indeed, 'hybrid' biomaterials can be engineered with additional biological recognition motifs for interaction with cell receptors and the control of cell signaling cascades and responses, or for local and controlled delivery of cells, proteins or gene vectors.

With regard to the cellular elements in vascular tissue engineering, many of the current strategies are focused on the replacement/approximation of the archetypal blood contacting surface – the vascular endothelium. The presence of an endothelial lining in the small-calibre vascular graft is absolutely essential to graft viability, as it inhibits thrombosis and contributes to long-term graft patency. The endothelium can also control blood flow and vessel tone [8], prevent infection and inflammation of the underlying graft wall, as well as transmit mechanical and other signals to the underlying smooth muscle cells (SMCs) [9, 10]. To form a functional endothelial monolayer, numerous attempts have been made to coat the lumen of synthetic grafts with cultured endothelial cells [11-13]. Such approaches demonstrated moderate improvement of graft patency, but ultimately require implantation of a permanent foreign, non-degradable structure. To develop tissue-engineered vascular grafts, endothelial cells have been cultured together with SMCs on natural or synthetic biodegradable polymer scaffolds, or self-assembled extracellular matrix (ECM) [14-19]. The vascular grafts can subsequently undergo dynamic conditioning protocols *in vitro* to enhance their mechanical properties prior to implantation. However, there is still substantial loss of endothelial cells from the graft surfaces under dynamic flow conditions. In addition, the production of vascular grafts in this manner is a time-consuming and expensive process, while there are also concerns for phenotypic alterations of endothelial cell populations after long periods *in vitro*.

In addition to the development of small-calibre vascular grafts for restoring normal blood flow to ischemic tissues, researchers in the vascular tissue engineering field are investigating methods of generating intrinsic vasculature within larger tissue constructs or within regenerating tissue (therapeutic angiogenesis) [20-22]. The most critical hindrance to the clinical application of implantable tissue-engineered grafts is the inability to sustain large numbers of viable cells within a construct once implanted into the host. *In vivo*, most cells within implanted tissue-engineered constructs do not survive distances of a few hundred micrometers from the nearest capillary as the limits of oxygen diffusion are exceeded, and such cells are dependent on neovascularisation to survive within the construct. Equally, cells within ischemic tissues require therapeutic intervention to restore or regenerate collateral vessels for tissue survival. Novel strategies are being pursued to stimulate the body's natural mechanisms of blood vessel formation for the treatment of myocardial ischemia and lower limb ischemia by delivering angiogenic growth factors via hybrid biomaterials.

Based on the current literature, this book chapter focuses on two exciting applications of hybrid biomaterials for the restoration of blood flow to damaged tissues. The first application is the recruitment of autologous endothelial progenitor cells (EPCs) to vascular grafts or stents composed of hybrid biomaterials. The second application is the development of a tissue microvasculature subsequent to ischemia, or for the purpose of developing large volume, implantable tissue-engineered structures.

2. Endothelialisation of Vascular Prostheses

The need to produce thrombo-resistant small-calibre vascular grafts for clinical application led to the innovative use of endothelial cells to pre-coat the graft lumen prior to implantation [11-13]. The majority of research on the promotion of endothelial cell seeding on vascular structures has involved coating the luminal graft surface with individual ECM proteins or protein mixtures [23, 24]. Such surface treatments have enhanced cellular retention on synthetic structures but there still remains a need for improved materials or adhesion factors that improve cell attachment and prevent subsequent cell loss under flow conditions [25]. Further drawbacks of this approach include the fact that autologous endothelial cells are a requirement for successful application of this technique due to the immunological concerns presented by donor endothelial cells [7]. As a result, an intact vessel must be harvested from another site in the patient in a prior surgical procedure in order that healthy endothelial cells can be isolated for subsequent seeding on the replacement graft. In addition, the currently used synthetic fabric grafts composed of Dacron™ or ePTFE cannot be remodelled by the patient's cells. Poor compliance together with an inability to remodel can prevent long-term adaptation of the vessel within the implantation site, which may ultimately lead to occlusion by intimal hyperplasia [7].

These limitations have driven intense research into the development of alternative graft materials and identification of more suitable endothelial cell sources. Graft material properties can be modified through hybridisation or biofunctionalisation to more closely approximate the ECM and promote desirable protein and cellular interactions. The ECM acts not only as a structural scaffold material but also contains a myriad cell signalling motifs and growth factors that guide cell attachment and cellular responses [26]. The environment in the immediate vicinity of the cell provides defined structural cues that determine cell-specific behaviour, including attachment, proliferation, differentiation, and the protein synthesis needed for tissue organisation and remodeling. Structural features of the ECM, including bioresponsive motifs, have inspired the design of hybrid biomaterials as tissue engineering scaffolds. One strategy in vascular tissue engineering is to ligate endothelium-derived molecules or their cell interacting domains to the surface of vascular grafts to mimic features of the ECM and thereby assist specific cell adhesion [27]. Concerning alternatives to endothelial cells harvested from a patient biopsy, endothelial progenitor cells (EPCs) have emerged in the last decade as a promising cell source for an autologous, biocompatible lining of vascular prostheses via *in situ* endothelialisation techniques, whereby the cells are 'captured' from the bloodstream by recognition motifs on hybrid biomaterials [28-31].

There has been much focus on the potential utility of EPCs for therapeutic vascular regeneration since their discovery in adult peripheral blood by Asahara and colleagues [32]. A number of reports have since highlighted a number of subpopulations within the EPC community [33, 34], with the mononuclear cell fraction containing at least two distinct EPC subpopulations; 'early' EPCs present in culture within 4-7 days, exhibit characteristics of both endothelial cells and monocytes, and do not proliferate well in culture. In contrast, 'late' EPCs (or endothelial colony-forming cells) emerge in culture after 2-3 weeks, display the characteristic 'cobblestone' morphology of endothelial cells, and demonstrate excellent proliferative capacity in long-term culture.

Evidence suggests that EPCs home to sites of neovascularisation from the bone marrow and differentiate into mature endothelial cells, subsequently contributing to the endothelial repair process [32]. While there are low numbers of circulating EPCs in the vasculature at any given instance (less than 0.01% of peripheral blood mononuclear cells) [35], the numbers can be increased or 'mobilised' from the bone marrow in response to many factors [36], including local ischemia [37], oestrogen [38], statins [39], erythropoietin [40], angiopoietin-1, stroma-derived factor-1 (SDF-1) and vascular endothelial growth factor (VEGF) [41], amongst others. EPCs are characterised by the expression of stem cell (CD133, CD34) and endothelial cell markers (VEGF receptor 2, CD31, VE-cadherin, von Willebrand factor), and by uptake of labelled acetylated low-density lipoprotein (ac-LDL) [42, 43].

Recent approaches to immobilise autologous EPCs to the luminal surface of implanted vascular grafts have included modification/hybridisation of the biomaterial surface with specific ligands to capture the cells from the circulating blood.

2.1. *EPC capture using cRGD peptides*

Cell adhesion molecules or ligands impart a level of signaling that controls the regulation of gene expression and cellular organization. Bioactivity of a synthetic polymer scaffold can be modified with covalently-attached adhesion peptide sequences, such as arginine-glycine-aspartic acid (RGD) or tyrosine-isoleucine-glycine-serine-arginine (YIGSR) [44]. Such sequences are present on a number of ECM proteins, forming a physical link between the ECM and the cells via integrin cell surface receptors [45]. Incorporated sequences function to improve cell adhesion, spreading and more sophisticated functions, whilst also enabling integrin-mediated activation of a number of cell signaling pathways that are critical to tissue development and remodeling [46]. Previous published data has demonstrated the expression of integrins with binding motifs for cyclic RGD (cRGD) on EPCs [47, 48], and it is thought that homing and differentiation of EPCs are largely dependent on integrin binding and the resulting signaling cascade that is triggered [49]. Therefore, coating of biomaterials by EPC attracting peptides such as cRGD may be useful for endothelialization of synthetic surfaces by EPCs.

Blindt and colleagues recently described a novel stent coating loaded with integrin-binding cRGD peptide (GPenGRGDSPCA) [28]. The cyclic structure of the peptide is believed to more closely approximate the conformation of the natural ligand, and was established by a disulfide bond between penicillamine (Pen) and cysteine. The authors hypothesized that EPCs would be attracted and bound to the stent because they express specific integrins that have high affinity for the RGD sequence. Through *in vitro* and *in vivo* porcine studies, the authors demonstrated that the cRGD peptides embedded in the coating of the stainless steel stent promoted stimulation of cell outgrowth and shear-resistant attachment of EPCs to the stent, as well as acting as chemoattractants for EPCs. Effective re-endothelialisation was achieved comprising labelled infused porcine EPCs as well as endogenous $CD34^+$ cells. Subsequent analyses for vessel occlusion *in vivo* revealed that there was no significant beneficial effect of the cRGD stent at 4 weeks after implantation. However, after 12 weeks, the mean neointimal area in the cRGD-loaded stent was significantly lower (2.2 ± 0.3 mm^2) compared to the unloaded (3.8 ± 0.4 mm^2) or bare metal stent (3.8 ± 0.3 mm^2). Additionally, the cross-sectional area of stenosis was significantly lower with the cRGD-loaded stent (33 ± 5 %) in comparison with the controls - unloaded (54 ± 6 %) and bare metal stent (53 ± 3 %), respectively.

In this study [28], Blindt and colleagues demonstrated proof of concept for their innovative approach of a cRGD-loaded stent coating. The feasibility and biocompatibility of the novel graft has been shown in a well-established porcine model for arterial injury. In addition to performing in equal measure to state-of-the-art bare metal stents for short-term application, the cRGD stent also exhibited a significantly better long-term protection from neointimal hyperplasia. The authors concluded that a 3-month observation in their porcine model was comparable to data from 12-18 month follow-up in humans, which underscores the possibility for good long-term efficacy of the grafts.

However, further *in vivo* studies with an extended follow-up period must be undertaken to entirely survey the issue of long-term feasibility. In addition, the transfer of the presented data to a human model is limited by the fact that the animals lacked any spontaneous atherosclerosis. Thus, the observed beneficial effects of the cRGD stent might be only representative for healthy arteries, as mentioned by the authors themselves. In relation to vascular graft development using biological peptides as opposed to vascular stents, the group of Seifalian [29] has developed compliant poly(carbonate-urea)urethane (PCU) grafts containing covalently bonded RGD-containing peptides. The authors demonstrated that the addition of the RGD motif resulted in improved attachment and differentiation of $CD133^+$ cells, and may be more suitable for *in situ* endothelialisation of vascular grafts in comparison to the naked PCU graft. Although both of the aforementioned studies establish a very promising strategy, the clinical potential of this approach is currently limited due to the fact that integrins – the receptors ultimately interacting with the RGD peptide – are not confined to EPCs, and hybrid materials need to be optimised to promote the specific adhesion of EPCs only. The group of Patterson and colleagues have used phage display screening methods to identify and select novel EPC-specific peptide ligands with high specificity [30, 31]. The group identified the threonine-proline-serine (TPS) motif as an important ligand binding to cell surface receptors on human blood outgrowth endothelial cells (HBOEC). A subsequent study employing a hybrid biomaterial consisting of TPS-peptide (TPSLEQRTVYAK) immobilised to methacrylic terpolymers demonstrated attachment of HBOEC, but not human umbilical vein endothelial cells (HUVEC), appearing to show specificity for endothelial cells of progenitor origin [31].

In situ endothelialisation of vascular grafts and stents composed of hybrid biomaterials is a novel and exciting area of research that aims to eliminate the need for surgical biopsies and extended *in vitro* culture protocols for producing autologous endothelial cells that will render implanted grafts biocompatible. Various peptides and techniques have been identified to promote endothelial cell capture from the circulation and hold promise for the development of next generation vascular prostheses.

3. Tissue-Engineered Microvascular Networks

The further application of hybrid biomaterials in the field of vascular tissue engineering is the development of a tissue microvasculature subsequent to ischemia, or for the purposes of developing large volume, implantable tissue-engineered structures. To date, the engineering of less complex tissue such as skin grafts, cartilage and urinary bladder have been successfully approved for clinical use [50]. These products are either avascular tissue (cartilage) or thin enough for cell survival due to their proximity to the nearest capillary (150-200 μm). Following implantation, spontaneous vascular ingrowth is a part of the inflammatory healing process induced in the first instance by the surgical procedure. Furthermore, the seeded cells increase the transcription of angiogenic growth factors as a reaction to hypoxia to benefit the vasculogenesis process [51]. This spontaneous vascular ingrowth from the host is an extensive process which can take up to several weeks [52].

In order to achieve a sufficient vascular system within thick engineered tissue, a better understanding of the mechanisms involved through cell source, scaffold material and angiogenic factors is necessary. The importance of combining these key players requires the development of natural hybrid biomaterials with possibilities for inducing vasculogenesis.

Biodegradable and biocompatible materials can be manufactured with a uniform quality and have controllable structure comparable to the body's own proteins. The ideal hybrid material should promote cell and growth factor adhesion, as well as the induction and maintenance of appropriate cell phenotype.

3.1. *Cell sources*

The construction of blood vessels is promoted by the processes of vasculogenesis and angiogenesis. The process of angiogenesis is the formation and remodeling of vessels into more complex networks from pre-existing vessels. On the other hand, vasculogenesis is defined as the initial differentiation of precursor cells into endothelial cells and the subsequent formation of a microvascular network. The vasculogenesis process occurs during embryonic development and adult vascular growth and can be divided into five consecutive steps [53]:

1. Endothelial cells are generated from precursor cells, called angioblasts.
2. Endothelial cells form the vessel primordia and cellular aggregates, without lumen development.
3. A primitive endothelial tube is formed, composed of polarised endothelial cells.
4. A primary vascular network is formed from an array of developing endothelial tubes.
5. Pericytes and vascular SMCs are recruited.

In comparison to thick vascular walls of arteries and veins, a capillary is composed of a single layer of endothelial cells surrounded by a basal membrane and a single layer of pericytes [54]. The formation of capillaries is depended on endothelial cells which are present at the interface between blood and surrounding tissue regulate the exchange of gases, fluids, nutrients and waste products and take part in the maintenance of hemostasis and process of inflammation [21, 55].

The migration, proliferation and differentiation of endothelial cells are inhibited by the cell-cell contact and their intimate contact with the ECM. Endothelial cells are normally stable with a cell turnover rate of months up to three years for human endothelial cells [56]. Changes of this state occur by mechanical shear stress of blood flow as well as the biochemical stimulation and signaling by angiogenic growth factors.

Various sources of endothelial cells have been used for *in vitro* and *in vivo* models of angiogenesis and vasculogenesis [57-59]. Further cell source options are endothelial cells derived from hemotopoetic stem cells and the circulating EPCs.

3.2. *Growth factors*

A popular approach to induce capillary growth in tissue-engineered constructs is the use of growth factors embedded in synthetic or natural matrices as recombinant proteins, genes or factor-overexpressing genetically-engineered cell transplants. Through basic research and clinical therapeutic experience, a group of angiogenic molecules was identified and their role in the initiation of new blood vessel growth has been speculated. A number of these factors exert their activity directly on endothelial cells and initiate capillary formation, and include vascular endothelial growth factor (VEGF), fibroblast growth factor (FGF) and hepatocyte growth factor (HGF). The ‘indirect’ angiogenic factors, platelet-derived growth factor (PDGF), transforming growth factor-β (TGF-β) or angiopoietin (Ang) stabilize the newly formed capillaries by recruiting pericytes and SMCs.

The incorporation of growth factors into the scaffold material can allow continuous stimulation of vascular tissue growth. The delivery can be classified by the release process, which is either driven by passive diffusion or coupled to the degradation rate of the material [60].

Various release systems of porous degradable solid scaffolds have been formed from polyesters of lactic acid (PLA), glycolic acid (PGA) and poly lactide-co glycolide (PLG). In one study, VEGF or FGF-1 was combined with polymer particles prior to scaffold processing, and a sustained release of growth factor through the degradation process was demonstrated within a short time period [61]. To achieve a more optimized, slow release period, a further technique was developed. This approach allowed the encapsulation of growth factors in microspheres before scaffold processing. The combination of both techniques achieves a more mature angiogenesis process by delivery of two or more growth factors within one scaffold. The combination of VEGF and PDGF shows a rapid formation of vascular networks. While VEGF was released during the initial degradation phase and stimulated the growth of a primitive vascular network, PDFG was subsequently released from encapsulated microspheres and stimulated network development and support by recruiting SMCs [62].

An alternative method for angiogenic factor delivery employs the co-culture of endothelial cells with a further cell type, such as fibroblasts or SMCs seeded within a fibrin gel [63]. Fibroblasts act as the growth factor delivery vehicle and participate in the stimulation and stabilization of new capillaries by the production of TGF-β or angiopoietin.

To increase the biofunctionality of the synthetic polymers and therefore to mimic the surrounded ECM, various strategies have been developed by attaching specific peptides to the polymer surface. In normal tissue, the ECM is a network of scaffolding components including different collagen types, fibronectin, laminin, hyaluronic acid and fibrin [64]. Various ECM peptides sequences which determine the influence of cell behavior have been grafted on synthetic materials to enhance the biological properties. RGD peptide, a synthetic peptide from fibronectin, has been reported to increase endothelial cell and EPC adhesion after incorporation to polycarbonate or polyurethane [29].

Therefore, the components of ECM are obtained as naturally extracted or chemically synthesized proteins for the purpose of augmenting the biological properties of tissue engineering scaffolds. Cultured endothelial cells have been shown to form capillary-like structures with lumens on collagens, fibrin, fibronectin and laminin [65].

An alternative approach for capillary network development was shown when Chinese hamster ovary cells were transfected with VEGF cDNA. These cells were encapsulated in microspheres and co-implanted with cell-seeded matrices in mice. VEGF was secreted in a large amount over a period of several weeks and increased the vascularisation near the cell seeded matrices [66]. In addition, the use of naked plasmid DNA and viral vectors for recombinant expression of angiogenic growth factors can increase blood vessel formation in the developing tissue. Several studies investigated the sustained delivery of either plasmid DNA encoding PDGF [67], or VEGF [68] and subsequent cell transfection resulted in capillary formation.

3.3. *Neovascularization in tissue-engineered constructs*

The previously presented strategies to enhance capillary growth within a tissue-engineered construct can be used for pre-vascularization before implantation. This method requires the determination of ideal culture conditions for different endothelial cell sources. Neovascularization of tissue-engineered constructs can be performed by adding endothelial cells to tissue constructs seeded with other cell types, resulting in the formation of capillary networks. This strategy was first described and performed for a skin equivalent [69]. Dermal fibroblasts, keratinocytes and human umbilical vein endothelial cells (HUVECs) were co-cultured on a chitosan-collagen scaffold. The skin equivalent promoted spontaneous formation of capillary-like structures with typical intercellular junctions. Further studies illustrated that the pre-vascularized skin equivalent could be anastomosed to the host vascular system within 4 days after implantation. In contrast, the process of vascularization of a non-prevascularized graft took up to 14 days [70]. This time difference results from the need of the host blood vessel to grow to the deeper regions of the construct as no vascular structures are present in the skin equivalent.

In bone tissue engineering the direct contact of endothelial cells and osteoblasts seems to be essential to form capillary-structures in a three-dimensional scaffold. The formation of microvasculature could be observed when endothelial cells were seeded in co-culture with human osteoblasts or with human osteoblast cell line MG-63. These results support the assumption that osteoblasts produce signals which are essential for the survival of endothelial cells and the formation of vascular structures [71]. The pre-vascularization strategies have also been applied to the development of cardiac muscle [72], skeletal muscle [73] and bladder [74].

Vascularization of large tissue engineered constructs is to date still one of the main limitations in tissue engineering. Various strategies, including the interaction of cell sources, different growth factors and synthetic and natural polymers, are currently being investigated for pre-vascularisation of large, volume tissue-engineered structures *in vitro*, or for the recruitment of a neovasculature *in situ* using therapeutic angiogenesis for collateral vessel formation in ischemic tissue. The development of hybrid biomaterials to provide optimized growth factor delivery will provide significant advances in this field.

References

[1] Writing Group Members, et al., "Heart Disease and Stroke Statistics 2009 Update: A Report from the American Heart Association Statistics Committee and Stroke Statistics Subcommittee," *Circulation*, Vol. 119, 2009, pp. e21-e181.

[2] Cwikiel, W., "Restenosis After Balloon Angioplasty and/or Stent Insertion: Origin and Prevention," *Acta Radiologica*, Vol. 43, No. 5, 2003, pp. 442-454.

[3] Maluenda, G., G. Lemesle, and R. Waksman, "A Critical Appraisal of the Safety and Efficacy of Drug-Eluting Stents," *Clinical Pharmacology and Therapeutics*, Vol. 85, No. 5, 2009, pp. 474-480.

[4] Kannan, R.Y., et al., "Current Status of Prosthetic Bypass Grafts: A Review," *Journal of Biomedical Materials Research Part B: Applied Biomaterials*, Vol. 74, No. 1, 2005, pp. 570-581.

[5] Bergan, J.J., et al., "Randomization of Autogenous Vein and Polytetrafluoroethylene Grafts in Femoral-Distal Reconstruction," *Surgery*, Vol. 92, No. 6, 1982, pp. 921-930.

[6] Sayers, R.D., et al., "Long-Term Results of Femerotibial Bypass with Vein or Polytetrafluoroethylene," *British Journal of Surgery*, Vol. 85, No. 7, 1998, pp. 934-938.

[7] Nerem, R.M., and D. Seliktar, "Vascular Tissue Engineering", *Annual Review of Biomedical Engineering*, Vol. 3, 2001, pp. 225-243.

[8] Furchgott, R.F., and J.V. Zawadski, "The Obligatory Role of Endothelial Cells in the Relaxation of Arterial Smooth Muscle by Acetylcholine," Nature, Vol. 288, No. 5789, 1980, pp. 373-376.

[9] Cybulsky, M.I., and M.A. Gimbrone Jr., "Endothelial Expression of a Mononuclear Leukocyte Adhesion Molecule During Atherogenesis," *Science*, Vol. 251, No. 4995, 1991, pp. 788-791.

[10] Casscells, W., "Migration of Smooth Muscle and Endothelial Cells. Crtitical Events in Restenosis," *Circulation*, Vol. 86, No. 3, 1992, pp. 723-729.

[11] Herring, M., A. Gardner, and J. Glover, "A Single-Staged Technique for Seeding Vascular Grafts with Autogenous Endothelium," *Surgery*, Vol. 84, No. 4, 1978, pp. 498-504.

[12] Zilla P., et al., "Endothelial Cell Seeding of Polytetrafluoroethylene Vascular Grafts in Humans: A Preliminary Report," *Journal of Vascular Surgery*, Vol. 6, No. 6, 1987, pp. 535-541.

[13] Meinhart, J.G., et al., "Clinical Autologous In Vitro Endothelialization of 153 Infrainguinal ePTFE Grafts," *Annals of Thoracic Surgery*, Vol. 71, No. 5 Suppl., 2001, pp. S327-S331.

[14] L'Heureux, N., et al., "A Completely Biological Tissue-Engineered Human Blood Vessel," *FASEB Journal*, Vol. 12, No. 1, 1998, pp. 47-56.

[15] Niklason, L.E., et al., "Functional Arteries Grown In Vitro," *Science*, Vol. 284, No. 5413, 1999, pp. 489-493.

[16] Hoerstrup, S.P., et al., "Tissue Engineering of Small Caliber Vascular Grafts," *European Journal of Cardiothoracic Surgery*, Vol. 20, No. 1, 2001, pp. 164-169.
[17] Berglund, J.D., et al., "A Biological Hybrid Model for Collagen-Based Tissue Engineered Vascular Constructs," *Biomaterials*, Vol. 24, No. 7, 2003, pp. 1241-1254.
[18] Wu, H.C., et al., "Coculture of Endothelial and Smooth Muscle Cells on a Collagen Membrane in the Development of a Small-Diameter Vascular Graft," *Biomaterials*, Vol. 28, No. 7, 2007, pp. 1385-1392.
[19] Tschoeke, B., et al., "Tissue-Engineered Small-Caliber Vascular Graft Based on a Novel Biodegradable Composite Fibrin-Polylactide Scaffold," *Tissue Engineering Part A*, Vol. 15, No. 8, 2009, pp. 1909-1918.
[20] Lei, Y., et al., "Therapeutic Angiogenesis: Devising New Strategies Based on Past Experiences," *Basic Research in Cardiology*, Vol. 99, No. 2, 2004, pp. 121-132.
[21] Ko, H.C., B.K. Milthorpe, and C.D. McFarland, "Engineering Thick Tissues – The Vascularisation Problem," *European Cells & Materials*, Vol. 14, 2007, pp. 1-19.
[22] Kaully, T., et al., "Vascularization – The Conduit to Viable Engineered Tissue," *Tissue Engineering Part B*, Vol. 15, No. 2, 2009, pp. 159-169.
[23] Kaehler, J., et al., "Precoating Substrate and Surface Configuration Determine Adherence and Spreading of Seeded Endothelial Cells on Polytetrafluoroethylene Grafts," *Journal of Vascular Surgery*, Vol. 9, No. 4, 1989, pp. 535-541.
[24] Sugawara, Y., et al., "Rapid Post-Incubation Endothelial Retention by Dacron Grafts," *Journal of Surgical Research*, Vol. 67, No. 2, 1997, pp. 132-136.
[25] Bhat, V., et al., "Improving Endothelial Cell Adhesion to Vascular Graft Surfaces: Clinical Need and Strategies," *Journal of Biomaterials Science, Polymer Edition*, Vol. 9, No. 11, 1998, pp. 1117-1135.
[26] Haralson, M.A., and J.R. Hassell, "The Extracellular Matrix: An Overview." In *Extracellular Matrix: A Practical Approach*, pp. 1-30, Haralson, M.A., and J.R. Hassell (eds.), New York: Oxford University Press, 1995.
[27] Lutolf, M.P., and J.A. Hubbell, "Synthetic Biomateials as Instructive Extracellular Microenvironments for Morphogenesis in Tissue Engineering," *Nature Biotechnology*, Vol. 23, No. 1, 2005, pp. 47-55.
[28] Blindt, R., et al., "A Novel Drug-Eluting Stent Coated with an Integrin-Binding Cyclic Arg-Gly-Asp Peptide Inhibits Intimal Hyperplasia by Recruiting Endothelial Progenitor Cells," *Journal of the American College of Cardiology*, Vol. 47, No. 9, 2006, pp. 1786-1795.
[29] Alobaid, N., et al., "Nanocomposite Containing Bioactive Peptides Promote Endothelialisation by Circulating Progenitor Cells: An In Vitro Evaluation," *European Journal of Vascular & Endovascular Surgery*, Vol. 32, No. 1, 2006, pp. 76-83.
[30] Veleva, A.N., S.L. Cooper, and C. Patterson, "Selection and Initial Characterization of Novel Peptide Ligands that Bind Specifically to Human Blood Outgrowth Endothelial Cells," *Biotechnology and Bioengineering*, Vol. 98, No. 1, 2007, pp. 306-312.
[31] Veleva, A.N., D. E. Heath, S.L. Cooper, and C. Patterson, "Selective Endothelial Cell Attachment to Peptide-Modified Terpolymers," *Biomaterials*, Vol. 29, No. 27, 2008, pp. 3656-3661.
[32] Asahara, T., et al., "Isolation of Putative Progenitor Endothelial Cells for Angiogenesis," *Science*, Vol. 275, No. 5302, 1997, pp. 964-967.
[33] Gulati, R., et al., "Diverse Origin and Function of Cells with Endothelial Phenotype Obtained from Adult Human Blood," *Circulation Research*, Vol. 93, No. 11, 2003, pp. 1023-1025.
[34] Rehman, J., et al., "Peripheral Blood "Endothelial Progenitor Cells" are Derived from Monocyte/Macrophages and Secrete Angiogenic Growth Factors," *Circulation*, Vol. 107, No. 8, 2003, pp. 1164-1169.

[35] Smadja, D.M., et al., "Endothelial Progenitor Cells: Characterization, In Vitro Expansion, and Prospects for Autologous Cell Therapy," *Cell Biology and Toxicology*, Vol. 23, No. 4, 2007, pp. 223-239.
[36] Aicher, A., M.A. Zeiher, and S. Dimmeler, "Mobilizing Endothelial Progenitor Cells," *Hypertension*, Vol. 45, No. 3, 2005, pp. 321-325.
[37] Adams, V., et al., "Increase of Circulating Endothelial Progenitor Cells in Patients with Coronary Artery Disease after Exercise-Induced Ischemia," *Arteriosclerosis, Thrombosis and Vascular Biology*, Vol. 24, No. 4, 2004, pp. 684-690.
[38] Strehlow, K., et al., "Estrogen Increases Bone Marrow-Derived Endothelial Progenitor Cell Production and Diminishes Neointima Formation," *Circulation*, Vol. 107, No. 24, 2003, pp. 3059-3065.
[39] Vasa, M., et al., "Increase in Circulating Endothelial Progenitor Cells by Statin Therapy in Patients with Stable Coronary Artery Disease," *Circulation*, Vol. 103, No. 24, 2001, pp. 2885-2890.
[40] Bahlmann, F.H., et al., "Erythropoietin Regulates Endothelial Progenitor Cells," *Blood*, Vol. 103, No. 3, 2004, pp. 921-926.
[41] Moore, M.A., et al., Mobilization of Endothelial and Hematopoietic Stem and Progenitor Cells by Adenovector-Mediated Elevation of Serum Levels of SDF-1, VEGF, and Angiopoietin-1," *Annals of the New York Academy of Sciences*, Vol. 938, 2001, pp. 36-47.
[42] Hill, J.M., et al., "Circulating Endothelial Progenitor Cells, Vascular Function, and Cardiovascular Risk," *New England Journal of Medicine,* Vol. 348, No. 7, 2003, pp. 593-600.
[43] Hristov, M., W. Erl, and P.C. Weber, "Endothelial Progenitor Cells: Mobilization, Differentiation, and Homing," *Arteriosclerosis, Thrombosis and Vascular Biology*, Vol. 23, No. 7, 2003, pp. 1185-1189.
[44] Hubbell, J.A., "Biomaterials in Tissue Engineering," *Biotechnology (NY)*, Vol. 13, No. 6, 1995, pp. 565-576.
[45] van der Flier, A., and A. Sonnenberg, "Function and Interactions of Integrins," *Cell and Tissue Research*, Vol. 305, No. 3, 2001, pp. 285-298.
[46] Kim, B.S., and D.J. Mooney, "Development of Biocompatible Synthetic Extracellular Matrices for Tissue Engineering," *Trends in Biotechnology*, Vol. 16, No. 5, 1998, pp. 224-230.
[47] Walter, D.H., et al., "Statin Therapy Accelarates Reendothelialization: A Novel Effect Involving Mobilization and Incorporation of Bone Marrow-Derived Endothelial Progenitor Cells," *Circulation*, Vol. 105, No. 25, 2002, pp. 3017-3024.
[48] Peled, A., et al., "The Chemokine SDF-1 Activates the Integrins LFA-1, VLA-4, and VLA-5 on Immature Human CD34(+) Cells: Role in Transendothelial/Stromal Migration and Engraftment of NOD/SCID Mice," *Blood*, Vol. 95, No. 11, 2000, pp. 3289-3296.
[49] Avci-Adali, M., et al., "New Strategies for In Vivo Tissue Engineering by Mimicry of Homing Factors for Self-Endothelialisation of Blood Contacting Materials," *Biomaterials*, Vol. 29, No. 29, 2008, pp. 3936-3945.
[50] Nichols, J.E., and J. Cortiella, "Engineering of a Complex Organ: Progress Toward Development of a Tissue-Engineered Lung," *Proceedings of the American Thoracic Society*, Vol. 5, No. 3, 2008, pp. 723-730.
[51] Levy, A.P., N.S. Levy, and M.A. Goldberg, "Hypoxia-Inducible Protein Binding to Vascular Endothelial Growth Factor mRNA and its Modulation by the Von Hippel-Lindau Protein," *Journal of Biological Chemistry*, Vol. 271, No. 41, 1996, pp. 25492-25497.
[52] Jabbarzadeh, E., and C.F. Abrams, "Strategies to Enhance Capillary Formation Inside Biomaterials: A Computational Study," *Tissue Engineering*, Vol. 13, No. 8, 2007, pp. 2073-2086.

[53] Drake, C.J., J.E. Hungerford, and C.D. Little, "Morphogenesis of the First Blood Vessels," *Annals of the New York Academy of Sciences*, Vol. 857, 1998, pp. 155-179.
[54] Moon, J.J., and J.L. West, "Vascularization of Engineered Tissues: Approaches to Promote Angiogenesis in Biomaterials," *Current Topics in Medicinal Chemistry*, Vol. 8, No. 4, pp. 300-310.
[55] Lin, Y., D.J. Weisdorf, A. Solovey, and R.P. Hebbel, "Origins of Circulating Endothelial Cells and Endothelial Outgrowth from Blood," *Journal of Clinical Investigation,* Vol. 105, No. 1, 2000, pp. 71-77.
[56] Hirschi, K.K., et al., "Vascular Assembly in Natural and Engineered Tissues," *Annals of the New York Academy of Sciences*, Vol. 961, 2002, pp. 223-242.
[57] Dutt, K., et al., "Three-Dimensional Model of Angiogenesis: Co-Culture of Human Retinal Cells with Bovine Aortic Endothelial Cells in the NASA Bioreactor," *Tissue Engineering*, Vol. 9, No. 5, 2003, 893-908.
[58] Burg, K.J., et al., "Comparative Study of Seeding Methods for Three-Dimensional Polymeric Scaffolds," *Journal of Biomedical Materials Research*, Vol. 51, No. 4, 2000, pp. 642-649.
[59] Frye, C.A., and Patrick Jr., C.W., "Isolation and Culture of Rat Microvascular Endothelial Cells," *In Vitro Cellular & Developmental Biology – Animal*, Vol. 38, No. 4, 2002, 208-212.
[60] Zisch, A.H., M.P. Lutolf, and J.A. Hubbell, "Biopolymeric Delivery Matrices for Angiogenic Growth Factors," *Cardiovascular Pathology*, Vol. 12, No. 6, 2003, pp. 295-310.
[61] Kannan, R.Y., et al., "Roles of Tissue Engineering and Vascularisation in the Development of Micro-Vascular Networks: A Review," *Biomaterials*, Vol. 26, No. 14, 2005, pp. 1857-1875.
[62] Richardson, T.P., et al., "Polymeric System for Dual Growth Factor Delivery," *Nature Biotechnology*, Vol. 19, No. 11, 2001, pp. 1029-1034.
[63] Griffith, C.K., et al., "Diffusion Limits of an In Vitro Thick Prevascularised Tissue," *Tissue Engineering*, Vol. 11, No. 1-2, 2005, pp. 257-266.
[64] Badylak, S.F., "The Extracellular Matrix as a Biologic Scaffold Material," *Biomaterials,* Vol. 28, No. 25, 2007, pp. 3587-3593.
[65] Sieminski, A.L., and K.J. Gooch, "Biomaterial-Microvasculature Interactions," *Biomaterials*, Vol. 21, No. 22, 2000, pp. 2232-2241.
[66] Laschke, M.W., et al., "Angiogenesis in Tissue Engineering: Breathing Life into Constructed Tissue Substitutes," *Tissue Engineering*, Vol. 12, No. 8, 2006, pp. 2093-2104.
[67] Shea, L.D., et al., "DNA Delivery from Polymer Matrices for Tissue Engineering," *Nature Biotechnology*, Vol. 17, No. 6, 1999, pp. 551-554.
[68] De Coppi, P., et al., "Angiogenic Gene-Modified Muscle Cells for Enhancement of Tissue Formation," *Tissue Engineering*, Vol. 11, No. 7-8, 2005, pp. 1034-1044.
[69] Black, A.F., et al., "In Vitro Reconstruction of a Human Capillary-Like Network in a Tissue-Engineered Skin Equivalent," *FASEB Journal,* Vol. 12, No. 13, 1998, pp. 1331-1340.
[70] Tremblay, P.L., et al., "Inosculation of Tissue-Engineered Capillaries With the Host's Vasculature in a Reconstructed Skin Transplanted on Mice," *American Journal of Transplantation*, Vol. 5, No. 5, 2005, pp. 1002-1010.
[71] Rivron, N.C., et al., "Engineering Vascularised Tissues In Vitro," *European Cells & Materials*, Vol. 15, 2008, pp. 27-40.
[72] Kelm, J.M., et al., "Design of Custom-Shaped Vascularized Tissues Using Microtissue Spheroids as Minimal Building Units," *Tissue Engineering*, Vol. 12, No. 8, 2006, pp. 2151-2160.
[73] Levenberg, S., et al., "Engineering Vascularized Skeletal Muscle Tissue," *Nature Biotechnology*, Vol. 23, No. 7, 2005, pp. 879-884.
[74] Schultheiss, D., et al., "Biological Vascularized Matrix for Bladder Tissue Engineering: Matrix Preparation, Reseeding Techniques and Short-Term Implantation in a Porcine Model," *Journal of Urology*, Vol. 173, No. 1, 2005, pp. 276-280.

CHAPTER 15

DYNAMIC CELL CULTURE METHODS FOR FUNCTIONALIZED BIOMATERIALS

Bonnie C. Landy and Vassilios I. Sikavitsas*

School of Chemical, Biological and Materials Engineering, Bioengineering Center, University of Oklahoma, Norman, OK 73019, USA

**E-mail: vis@ou.edu*

1. Introduction

Tissue engineering is a complex and constantly adapting field, necessitating a multi-disciplinary, inclusive approach to create tissues which can most resemble those found in the human body. As the process of tissue growth *in vivo* is influenced by a multitude of factors, so tissue engineering can incorporate a variety of strategies. The field stems from the desire to replace or repair damaged tissues by the combination of cells, a carrier on which cell and tissue growth can occur, and mechano-chemical stimuli to promote tissue growth in a functional manner [1]. Once the neotissue is formed, it would be implanted, where it may integrate and be remodeled to be indistinguishable from the native tissue.

The selection of an appropriate cell type for a functional engineered tissue is critical because, under the proper culture conditions, those cells will be forming the extracellular matrix in the neotissue. The structure and properties of the matrix can depend heavily upon both the cell type and the culture conditions. In addition, *ex vivo* cell expansion may be necessary to achieve high cell density in a cultured construct, requiring cells with a high proliferative capability.

Cells used for tissue engineering applications require a surface on which to adhere for survival, proliferation, and extracellular matrix (ECM) synthesis. This surface is usually provided by a scaffold, a biocompatible material which can provide both chemical and mechanical microenvironments to mimic those of a specific tissue. The properties of the scaffold can greatly influence the function, proliferation, migration, and differentiation of the cultured cells, which then translates into the properties of the engineered tissue and the *de novo* ECM [2]. It is now possible to design materials for this purpose which could serve multiple functions: to be a bioactive support for growing cells and to be a resorbable template for the growing tissue [3]. By using a biodegradable scaffold material, the construct can degrade as it is replaced by the extracellular matrix formed by the cultured cells. In turn, the cells could respond with enhanced adhesion, proliferation, or ECM production due to the presence of a bioactive surface. One of the most effective ways to transform a biomaterial's surface into a bioresponsive microenvironment is to incorporate biomimetic moieties, motifs from biological macromolecules that elicit specific cellular responses similar to that *in vivo* [4]. Sometimes an entire protein or glycosaminoglycan is used, such as collagen, heparin, or morphogenetic growth factors, to gain increased cell growth, adhesion, and most importantly, signaling that leads to the desirable differentiated phenotype. However, specific domains, or even short sequences of these proteins have been found to be effective, regulating cell adhesion or signaling moieties in much the same way as the parent protein. Functionalizing a biomaterial surface with an oligopeptide may reduce protein denaturation which can occur from random folding of a protein on the surface [5].

However, a three-dimensional functional tissue cannot be produced using merely a biomimetic surface; a cell culture system should also provide stimuli similar to those experienced under physiological conditions. This can often be provided by using a dynamic cell culture system, a method of growing cells which may incorporate fluid flow to increase nutrient and waste transport and provide homogenous cell distribution, or alternatively to introduce electrical or mechanical stimulation by stretching or compression. The use of a bioreactor is integral to tissue engineering, as it can provide the mechanical macro- and micro-environment in which the tissue can be optimally regenerated [6,7] . A variety of bioreactor designs exist which demonstrate the ability to increase transport as well as possibly mimic physiological conditions to stimulate cell growth. Multiple designs are explored in the following sections, as well as the combined use of these cell culture systems with functionalized biomaterials in order to engineer successful tissue grafts.

2. Bioreactors for Dynamic Cell Culture

Engineered tissues cultured statically typically consist of a Petri dish with cell culture medium surrounding a scaffold onto which has been poured a suspension of cells. The attraction of this system lies primarily in its simplicity: it is inexpensive, easily kept sterile, easily maintained, and generally less challenging to use. However, the transport of nutrients into a construct and the movement of waste away from cells are limited to diffusion [8, 9, 10]. Static culture may only be a viable option for constructs of rather small dimensions, although the cells are usually found only at the periphery of the construct, predominantly on one side [11,12]. In addition, the bioreactor can create a microenvironment which provides favorable cell growth and differentiation, resulting in favorable ECM structure.

2.1. *Bioreactor functionality*

One of the primary obstacles to overcome by using a bioreactor was mass transport limitations in the interior of cell seeded porous scaffolds. Several bioreactor systems have been proposed and their majority introduced fluid flow in some way, improving transport of oxygen, nutrients, and signaling molecules when compared to the traditional static culture. The introduction of convective forces in fluid flow based bioreactor designs, in general reduced cell morbidity in the central section of porous scaffolds, supported cell migration, and even improved cell signaling by decreasing steep concentration gradients of bioactive molecules in the cell culture medium [13]. It was found that cellular spheroids larger than 1 mm in diameter showed a necrotic, hypoxic core when cultured statically, only obtaining viable cells in a layer at the outer edge [14]. Clearly, for a functional engineered tissue graft, structures greater than 1 mm in diameter are necessary, so mass transport limitations are a serious hurdle for producing viable tissues. The various bioreactor designs described in the following sections clearly demonstrate improvement over the mass transport limitations of static cultures.

Another benefit of dynamic cell culture systems is to aid in the distribution of cells throughout the scaffold. Often, the traditional dropwise cell seeding process can generate disproportionally high seeding densities at the exterior of porous scaffolds. In addition, the distribution of cells has been linked to the distribution of matrix created within the construct, leading to the conclusion that cells seeded more homogenously may result in a more uniform final tissue [15, 16, 17, 20, 42]. It has been shown that higher seeding efficiencies and uniformities can be obtaining using a dynamic method of seeding and culture [13]. Convection from seeding a dilute cell suspension in a spinner flask onto a matrix may result in improved seeding efficiencies compared to static seeding, but oscillatory perfusion of a cell suspension through a matrix can sometimes result in higher seeding efficiencies [18, 19, 20, 21, 22].

Mechanical forces, which are known to be integral in cell signaling *in vivo*, can also increase the biosynthetic activity of cells *in vitro*, possibly improving the quality or accelerating the process of regenerating tissues [23,24,25]. Stimulation can occur in several bioreactor designs in the form of shear stresses caused by fluid flow. In addition, some bioreactors seek to mimic the physiological environment of the specific tissue by introducing compressive or tensile loading. Pulsatile radial stretch can be favorable for vascular grafts, compressive loading for cartilage, tensile and torsional stress for ligaments and tendons, and shear forces for bone tissues [26, 27, 28, 29, 30, 31, 32, 33, 34, 35, 36, 74, 69] . Although it is known that these forces greatly influence the behavior of the cultured cells, it is difficult to compare specific mechanical regimes (duration, frequency, intensity, etc.) from different bioreactors. Often the hydrodynamic or mechanical conditions differ among bioreactor designs, resulting in a complex body of data from which it is difficult to draw definite conclusions about the cellular response to an exact mechanical regime. However, bioreactors can also provide a controlled environment in which to study the complex cellular processes which are driven by mechanical conditions, sometimes enhanced by mathematical modeling of the specific forces on cells [37, 38]. Therefore, bioreactors will continue to be one of the key intersections of biology and engineering, where complex 3D hydrodynamics can be characterized and their effects on biological components can be studied.

2.2. *Various designs of bioreactors*

The choice of bioreactor design can be one based on many factors: tissue type, cell type, material, or physiological conditions. Most bioreactors rely on fluid convection to improve nutrient and oxygen transport into a construct while using fluid flow or a mechanical stimulator to expose the cell seeded scaffolds to shear, compressive, or tensile forces. This section describes some of the more common bioreactors used in tissue engineering.

2.2.1. *Spinner flask*

One of the earliest and simplest bioreactor systems was the spinner flask. To improve upon the mass transfer limitations in static cultures, the spinner flask incorporates a stirring mechanism to induce convection. This hydrodynamic force may suspend tissue engineering scaffolds or microcarriers in the solution, or they may be immobilized with needles, submerged in the medium. Stirring can be caused by a magnetic stir bar, a shaft impeller, or a pendulum which is usually pulled through the fluid by magnetic attraction on a stir plate, causing continuous mixing in the culture vessel. Throughout the media volume, this stirring provides a nearly homogenous mixture for oxygen and nutrients, although the velocity of the fluid varies drastically around the vessel. This results in variable shear stresses for immobilized constructs, possibly reaching relatively high shear forces at the surface of a construct. The hydrodynamics of the system are conditions of turbulent mixing, characterized by eddies at the surface of constructs, improving nutrient transport into a porous scaffold [12]. However, it has been shown that this improved transport may not reach into the core of a construct, leaving diffusion as the main mechanism of transport beyond the outer edges [39].

2.2.2. *Rotating vessel bioreactor*

One of the more popular bioreactor designs involves inducing fluid flow by rotation of the culture vessel, as with the rotating wall vessel (RWV). The RWV bioreactor was originally developed by National Aeronautics and Space Administration (NASA) scientists in order to study the effects of microgravity upon tissues and cells while on the gravity of earth [40, 41]. They were later used to promote three-dimensional cell growth without the presence of damaging high shear forces experienced in spinner flask cultures. The violent forces involved with other seeding and culture methods such as shaker and spinner flasks do not always allow adequate attachment interactions between cell and polymer. The basic design includes one inner, static, gas-permeable cylinder which is surrounded by a larger, rotating, impermeable cylinder. The cell culture medium and the culturing constructs are located in the annular region. This design allows gas exchange through the inner cylinder while the rotating outer cylinder provides the force needed to generate the mostly laminar fluid flow [42]. This design allows for the scaffolds near the outer edge to experience a very narrow range of shear forces, though there is a very low velocity area at the inner cylinder. The RWV can be a much more consistent method of dynamic cell culture, as it has been reported that the hydrodynamic culture conditions are fairly homogenous [43].

Media exchange can also occur through a modified design, the rotating wall perfused vessel bioreactor (RWPV), which includes both a rotational inner cylinder and a disk limiting perfusion inlet to the region nearest the outer cylinder's wall. The rate of fluid perfusion seems to have little effect on the mean shear conditions experienced by the constructs [44]. An alternate design features the cell culture chamber linked to the media using Albuflow porous fiber bundles (Fresenius Medical Care), and the reactor resulted in higher glucose availability and slower lactate formation when compared to a non-perfused rotary culture of lymphoblastoma cells [45]. It also resulted in a stable culture of human hepatocytes with regard to liver function markers and cell growth when cells were cultured on microcarrier beads for a bioartificial liver (BAL) [46]. In addition, it was designed to function as a stand-alone, independently heated and controlled device for potentially mobile applications with disposable tubes and culture chambers.

In addition, the solid-state rotating bioreactor features the rotation of both cylinders at the same rate, resulting in scaffold shear due to gravitational and centrifugal forces within the volume. The volume of culture medium moves as a solid body around the horizontal axis, which results in laminar flow and minimal shear force on the constructs. These are especially useful for cell aggregation systems because the very low hydrodynamic forces allow for lengthier cell-cell interactions. In addition, their simplicity and efficacy translate well into large-scale systems [47].

2.2.3. *Flow perfusion systems*

The perfusion of media in a bioreactor can result in multiple desirable phenomena: extensive nutrient transport into regions in the core of constructs, a relatively narrow range of shear stresses, the ability to simply recycle media, and a wide range of hydrodynamic conditions can be achieved by changing flow rate. Generally the media is either perfused through a chamber in which the scaffold is located or through the scaffold itself. The first design does provide continuous recirculation of nutrients in the media, but it may not satisfy transport needs into the construct itself. This is, however, an especially applicable bioreactor for use with thin tissues, such as vascular grafts. In addition, it can then also provide some mechanical conditioning similar to the pulsatile action of blood *in vivo* [67].

An option for thicker engineered tissues utilizing a porous scaffold is to provide nutrients and oxygen to the core using fluid perfused through the scaffold itself. Usually flow is restricted to one axis of the scaffold by placing the scaffold into a cassette or holder. The scaffolds are then contained in a chamber through which media is pumped. These scaffolds can be cultured in parallel by using individual circuits of tubing connected to a multi-head peristaltic pump or multiple-syringe pump [48, 49]. This design of bioreactor has been used extensively for bone tissue engineering, as the fluid flow through the porous network also stimulates osteoblastic cells through shear stress [50, 51, 52, 53, 54, 34]. This can cause improved differentiation of the cells, resulting in increased matrix synthesis, both from mechanotransduction and transport of chemical signals. In addition, this bioreactor can be beneficial for cell seeding techniques, resulting in a more homogenous distribution of cells throughout a scaffold [19, 20, 21, 22]. The increased transport of nutrients and oxygen can help maintain cell viability in long-term cultures, as high cell density is vital to engineered tissues [55].

3. Functionalized Materials used with Bioreactors

The complexities of tissue growth *in vivo* necessitate that a multi-faceted approach be employed in order for a tissue engineered construct to be mechanically, chemically, and biologically viable. One of the most promising advances in tissue engineering is the inclusion of bioactive molecules into an otherwise inert scaffold material [4]. By incorporating peptides or whole proteins which contribute to cell attachment and signaling, the properties of the final construct can be improved. For example, one peptide sequence found to be integral in cell adhesion and signaling is Arginine-Glycine-Aspartic acid (RGD) sequence, which is found in many important adhesive proteins of the ECM including fibronectin and vitronectin [56, 57]. It has been shown that this short fragment can mediate cell interactions with biomaterial surfaces similar to its parent glycoprotein, and that its presence modulates cell adhesion to fibronectin [58, 59, 60, 61, 62, 63, 64]. Full-length proteins can also be attached, adsorbed, or entrapped on a biomaterial, resulting in cell interactions specific to the molecule. The combination of chemical signals required and the dynamic culture conditions is specific to each tissue. In this section, some of the most recent uses of bioreactors for culture of functionalized tissue engineered constructs will be highlighted, with special consideration to the non-functionalized or static controls.

3.1. *Cardiovascular tissue*

It is well known that the behavior of cells and the properties of their extracellular matrix depend upon their culture conditions. For cardiovascular tissue, this is especially important because the cells and their construct need to withstand the shear forces and pressures associated with the cardiovascular system. For vascular grafts, native tissue can withstand physiological pressure of up to 120 mmHg, has burst strength of up to 1680 mmHg, and has suture retention strength of 270 g [26]. Engineered heart valves must be able to open and close at an approximate frequency of 1 Hz and maintain structure and function under shear stresses and bending forces inherent with blood flow at a pressure of 80-120 mmHg [65]. Therefore, major areas of interest for cardiovascular tissue engineering include the mechanical strength and organization of the ECM and the differentiated function of the endothelial cell layer, which are pivotal to the success of an engineered cardiovascular tissue.

3.1.1. *Vascular grafts*

The bioreactors for vascular grafts serve multiple purposes: to seed the scaffold homogenously, to provide nutrients to cells throughout the scaffold, to organize the cells and the extracellular matrix they produce, and to mechanically condition and stimulate the cells. The need for tissue engineered vascular grafts is primarily for small diameter vessels (<5 mm), as larger ones can oftentimes be grafted with a fully synthetic material, such as expanded polytetrafluoroethylene and DACRON, with excellent patency. Other methods have included using extracellular matrix components, such as collagens, fibronectin, laminin, and vitronectin to form a meshwork scaffold. In this way, one can create a scaffold from the biological components which would normally comprise vasculature. One way to create scaffolding from these components is to decellularize an allogeneic or xenogeneic graft. Although these tissues can be remodeled *in vivo*, an advantage over synthetic fiber-woven scaffolds, patients still undergo a variety of negative post-implantation effects. A possibility for achieving long-term success of a vascular graft is to promote endothelialization and to resist acute thrombosis. It is possible that endothelialization could be optimized by the combination of a bioactive material with a dynamic culture system, which can provide biochemical and mechanical stimuli to a vascular graft construct, promoting proliferation, tissue differentiation, and upregulation of extracellular matrix components, as well as organization of the cells and their products [66, 67]. Cummings *et al.* displayed that 10% cyclic mechanical strain at a frequency of 1 Hz to a collagen-fibrin hybrid construct resulted in significantly improved mechanical properties [68]. The hybrid collagen-fibrin hydrogel matrix, molded around a silicone sleeve, contained suspended rat aortic smooth muscle cells. Some constructs were then mechanically strained by a pressure pulse in a previously developed bioreactor for 4 days after 48 hours in static culture [69]. The hybrid matrix displayed desirable mechanical characteristics over hydrogels of only collagen or fibrin, and the cyclically strained samples performed better than statically cultured samples. A similar method utilizing shear rather than strain was employed by Shirota *et al.* to determine the potential of human endothelial progenitor cells (EPCs) from circulating peripheral blood to line microporous polyurethane grafts coated with a photoreactive gelatin layer. After seeding the EPCs to the construct statically for 4 days, hydrodynamic shear stress was applied using a circulatory loop. This apparatus yielded a flow rate of 60 mL/min, which resulted in a calculated shear stress of 30 dyne/cm^2 for 12 hours. This simple system resulted in elongated EPCs which were aligned in the direction of flow. The cells were tightly adhered and appeared in a confluent monolayer, similar to native artery.

Tissue engineered vascular grafts can be made more physiologically analogous by incorporating two pivotal types of cells into a perfused vascular engineering graft, both smooth muscle and endothelial cells. Jeong *et al.* used a hybrid scaffold of jellyfish collagen with poly(lactide-co-glycolide) (PLGA) fibers to demonstrate the benefits of both a hybrid biomaterial and a dynamic culture system [70]. Tubular scaffolds were formed by molding and drying collagen gels, then electrospinning PLGA fibrous layers on the abluminal surface. First, rabbit aorta smooth muscle cells were seeded by injection and held under static conditions in a pulsatile perfusion bioreactor for 2 days. Then, the scaffolds were subjected to pressure flow of 25 mmHg with a pulse of 1 Hz for 14 days. After the SMC culture, rabbit endothelial cells were seeded into the lumen and allowed to adhere for 90 minutes before the flow rate was increased gradually up to 0.1 mL/s over 7 days. The perfusion was found to significantly influence cell alignment in the direction parallel to flow when compared to the randomly aligned static cultures. This alignment appears in arteries *in vivo* and is critical for the contractile functions of these cells [71].

The emphasis for most tissue engineered products is to culture the proper cell types *in vitro* prior to implantation of the functional tissue. Tillman *et al.* demonstrated this using conditioning of poly(ε-caprolactone) (PCL) and collagen hybrid electrospun scaffolds seeded with both endothelial and smooth muscle cells in a pulsatile perfusion bioreactor for a total of 9 days [72]. The cells adhered to the surface of the graft even under the physiological pulsatile conditions and resulted in a structure similar to native vessel. When exposed to an *in vivo* sheep blood model, the ECs lining the luminal surface of the conditioned grafts only showed minimal platelet adherence, key for *in vivo* patency of grafts. In addition, the structural integrity of 7 out of 8 (87.5%) unseeded constructs of the same materials successfully maintained pulsatile arterial flow up to 1 month after implantation *in vivo*.

In a similar way, Zhang *et al.* used silk-based vascular grafts seeded with human coronary artery smooth muscle cells and human aortic endothelial cells sequentially with a Matrigel® coating between to mimic the basement membrane [73]. The silk and Matrigel® together increased endothelium coverage and retention when in dynamic flow. In addition, the dynamic flow conditions resulted in improved cell proliferation and alignment, extracellular matrix production, and cell phenotype. Flow rate in the peristaltic pumped perfusion system was increased from 5 to 35 mL/min over 7 days, and then maintained at 35 mL/min for up to another 7 days. The expression of mRNA for SMC contractile markers was between 3.9 and 15.3 fold higher for the dynamic cultures at days 7 and 14. Maintaining the contractile phenotype of the SMCs *in vitro* is an important obstacle for vascular graft engineering [74,75]. An additional exciting prospect for this system is its ability to be further modified by the facile attachment of RGD-peptides or other peptides or proteins, a method previously determined feasible [76,77]. It is clear that by combining hybrid vascular scaffolds with co-culture in a dynamic setting, the most structurally and functionally successful tissue engineered vascular graft can be achieved on an individual basis of requirements [78]. In addition, by focusing on specific peptide sequences incorporated into a biomimetic material, it has been shown possible to reduce thrombogenicity of an ECM graft while still promoting endothelial cell attachment and culture on the biomaterial surface [79].This research is an indication of the direction for hybrid vessel grafts where bioresponsive surfaces can promote attachment and proliferation of desired cells while avoiding the responses of undesired cell types.

3.1.2. *Heart valves*

Tissue engineering of heart valves can be complex due to their precise mechanical function and forceful fluid environment [65]. In addition, the specialized cellular and ECM components need the ability to be remodeled in response to changes in mechanical forces, just as a heart valve *in vivo* adjusts [80]. The usefulness of a bioreactor becomes clear in conditioning tissues to withstand and function in the physiological environment. Previously, tissue engineered heart valve bioreactors have been shown to induce extracellular matrix formation, increase structural integrity, improve cell organization and surface [81,82,83]. This is done through the use of a pulsatile flow system which pumps the culture medium through the construct in conditions that resemble the standard systolic and diastolic pressures [84]. There are many critical parameters with such a system, including the level of pulsation [85]. It is now possible that by combining bioresponsive materials with dynamic systems, a more complete and functional heart valve could be constructed. Huang *et al.* created a decellularized porcine valve construct which was coated with fibronectin and seeded with cells transduced with the gene for hepatocyte growth factor (HGF) [86]. This system included both a hybrid xenogeneic/ECM component scaffold as well as cells programmed to express a growth factor shown to induce proliferation and motility in endothelial cells [87]. The constructs were cultured with the transduced marrow stromal cells in a pulse duplicator system, where the media flow and pressure were gradually increased for up to 8 weeks [83]. High levels of endothelial cell retention even under high flow and pressure were demonstrated on the construct, due to the presence of HGF and fibronectin. Although extensive cell growth was observed, little active matrix synthesis occurred, so longer studies are necessary to evaluate the construct further. It is clear that a bioreactor system is integral in creating a mechanically sound engineered heart valve, but also that hybrid materials may be required to maintain cell density and function so that ECM remodeling of a construct can occur both *in vitro* and *in vivo*.

3.1.3. *Cardiac tissue*

The successful growth of heart muscle *in vitro* could be used to treat cases of acute myocardial infarction by implanting the constructs to enhance the contractile function of the left ventricle. The field has been therefore focused on creating functional tissue constructs rather than the entire complex organ. This requires a suitable scaffold as well as a cell source which can demonstrate significant contractile ability as well as proliferative capabilities. Primary cardiac myocytes are non-proliferative, so adult-derived stem cells as well as human embryonic stem cells are also being investigated [88]. In addition, neonatal and/or embryonic primary cardiac cells retain their contractile ability in 3D culture. Papadaki *et al.* used rat neonatal cardiac myocytes on a variety of materials in multiple culture conditions to investigate the feasibility of engineered cardiac tissue [89]. By using a PGA mesh which had been surface-hydrolyzed in NaOH then coated with laminin, they cultured cells in both a stirred flask and a rotating vessel to compare culture conditions based on cellularity, conduction velocity, maximum signal amplitude, maximal capture rate, and excitation threshold. Compared with previous studies in their laboratory, the system parameters which resulted in the most functional tissue were using laminin-coated surface-hydrolyzed PGA scaffolds seeded with a high concentration of cardiac myocytes, rotating bioreactors, and low-serum medium [90].

Similarly, a polymer-collagen scaffold was used by Park *et al.* to develop cardiac tissue [91]. Three different polymers were combined into a gas-foamed construct: two PCL:PLA copolymers of differing ratios and PLGA in a weight ratio of 1:1:4. This combination was determined to be a bioresorbable scaffold to provide mechanical stability and elasticity. The scaffold was then immersed in collagen I solution for 3 hours, then punched to create an array of microchannels. The scaffolds were inoculated with neonatal heart cells suspended in Matrigel® and cultured in a perfusion bioreactor as previously developed [92,93]. Particularly, the combination of the perfusion system and the composite scaffold provided a high and uniform cell density over the control materials (i.e. the PLGA sponge and the collagen sponge) and the orbitally mixed dish culture system. The perfusion was believed to improve mass transport in the construct interior while the composite scaffold enabled cell attachment and infiltration due to both the elasticity of the construct (from PCL) and the hydrophilicity of the surface (from the collagen) combined with the mechanical integrity of the polymer composite. In addition, the composite scaffolds had the highest expression of cardiac markers and demonstrated the electromechanical coupling of cells and the establishment of contractile function. It was concluded that the elasticity imparted by the inclusion of PCL, the cell attachment increase caused by collagen, and the mechanical integrity inherent in PLGA combined with the superior mass transfer of a perfusion system resulted in a novel engineered cardiac tissue.

3.2. *Bone*

Bone is another tissue which demands specific mechanical properties *in vivo*. Because of this, the materials used for bone tissue engineering are often polymers, meant to biodegrade as mineralized extracellular matrix replaces it, and ceramics, which have excellent mechanical loading capabilities. However, these materials do not always display a bioactive surface for cellular adhesion, proliferation, and differentiation. There are many methods to modify materials, including chemically, using cross-linking, hydrolysis, or aminolysis, or physically, by adsorbing or entrapping a molecule [5, 94, 95, 96]. In addition, culturing osteoblastic or mesenchymal stem cells on these materials is most improved when dynamic cell culture methods are used. A bioreactor provides mechanical forces which can mimic the mechanical stimuli experienced by bone cells *in vivo*, and so can result in improved cell differentiation and therefore function [32, 97, 50]. Also, various bioreactors are often used to improve seeding homogeneity, such as in Bokhari *et al.* [98]. They used foam scaffolds made of high internal phase emulsions polymer, or PolyHIPE polymer (PHP), modified with hydroxyapatite combined with a cell adhesion-promoting peptide. The peptide RAD16-I is self-assembling at physiological pH by changing the concentration of NaCl or KCl. It contains an Arg-Ala-Asp (RAD) peptide, which has been studied in several different cell types [99]. These peptides self-assemble into nanofibers that can surround cells in a way that mimics the physiological 3-D ECM. The authors studied the culture of primary rat osteoblasts on these materials using a dynamic seeding method using flow perfusion of 25 μL/min from a syringe pump, after which the constructs were cultured for up to 35 days in a spinner flask. The dynamic seeding improved the distribution of cells within the scaffold, and they proliferated and remained viable up to 35 days, implying that both the seeding and long term dynamic methods were effective. In addition, the RAD16-I increased the depth of cell growth at 35 days. The RAD16-I also influenced mineralization, as there was elevated alkaline phosphatase, osteopontin, and bone nodule production in the PHP foams. The immobilization of the RAD16-I peptide created a favorable environment for the osteoblasts while the dynamic culture method resulted in even cell distribution and effective nutrient transport.

In Roeker *et al.*, a dynamic rotating bed bioreactor is used with a functionalized ceramic material. A commercially available porous zirconium dioxide ceramic, Sponceram®, is combined with polyvinylsaccharides (2-deoxy-*N*-methacrlamido-D-glucose) coupled to BMP-2, a bioactive protein, adsorbed onto the surface of the scaffolds [100]. In addition to 2-D tests with various combinations of these materials, 3-D samples were cultured for 7 weeks in a Z®RP platform, a rotating-bed bioreactor located in a GMP conform breeder with control unit. The scaffolds were fixed onto a vertical shaft, rotating alternately through medium and atmosphere. When cultured with an osteoblastic model cell line, some bone specific markers were upregulated in the polyvinylsaccharide-BMP-2 conjugated scaffolds compared with scaffolds only adsorbed with BMP-2. This led the authors to conclude that the polyvinylsaccharide acted as a spacer for the bioactive molecule, providing flexibility and proximity to the cells for the ligands.

A similar bioreactor was used in von Walter *et al.*, along with fibronectin bound to a TiO_2/perlite composite, termed "Ecopore" [101]. When cultured with human primary osteoblasts in a revolving bioreactor with cell culture incubation vessels clamped parallel to the revolution axis, cell proliferation appeared to primarily occur at the peripheral zone of the scaffolds. The cell seeding proved more effective on the fibronectin coated Ecopore material. In addition, the dynamic method of seeding and culturing scaffolds led to a more uniform attachment of the cells on the entire visible surface of the constructs when compared to traditional static seeding. However, the authors concluded that the pore size of Ecopore should be optimized to better accommodate cell ingrowth and nutrient transport into the interior of the material.

In Alvarez-Barreto *et al.*, a perfusion bioreactor was used to seed cells on a functionalized scaffold and to culture them long-term in a stimulatory environment [102]. The base material is poly(L-lactic acid) (PLLA), a biodegradable and widely used polymer for tissue engineering. However, it can only support cell adhesion to a certain degree because of the lack of functional groups for cell interaction [8]. Through a method previously described, poly (L-lysine) (polyK) is entrapped on the surface of the PLLA foams [103]. A peptide, RGDS, was then linked to the polyK by creating a disulfide bond using N-succinimidyl 3-(2-pyridyldithio) propionate (SPDP). These functionalized scaffolds were seeded with rat mesenchymal stem cells (MSCs) using an oscillatory flow perfusion process previously found to result in favorable cell distribution throughout the scaffold as well as increased cell adhesion strength [20]. This was carried out in a parallel six-chamber flow perfusion bioreactor featuring recirculating media, and fluid flow confined by a cassette holding the scaffold in place. This flow perfusion design was used in multiple studies of MSC cultures in three-dimensional scaffolds, as seen in Figure 1 [48, 50, 52, 104,105, 106, 107, 108, 109, 110, 111, 112]. The markers of osteogenesis were measured as alkaline phosphatase activity (ALP) and mineral deposition. The levels of ALP and calcium were significantly higher under the dynamically cultured methods when compared to statically cultured samples. Furthermore, the addition of polyK and RGDC resulted in higher cell density, ALP and calcium levels. The effect of RGD on osteoblastic differentiation of MSCs appeared to occur in a dose dependent manner, similar to other studies [113, 114, 115]. Also, the combination of shear forces with the peptide RGD increased MSC osteogenesis synergistically when compared with their individual effects, which also agrees with previous studies [116]. However, the authors did find that there was a critical level of RGD which produced the most promising cellular responses at varying flow rates. Clearly the link between cell adhesion peptides and stimulatory shear forces can be better elucidated by optimizing the conditions for cell adhesion, cell detachment, and cell differentiation.

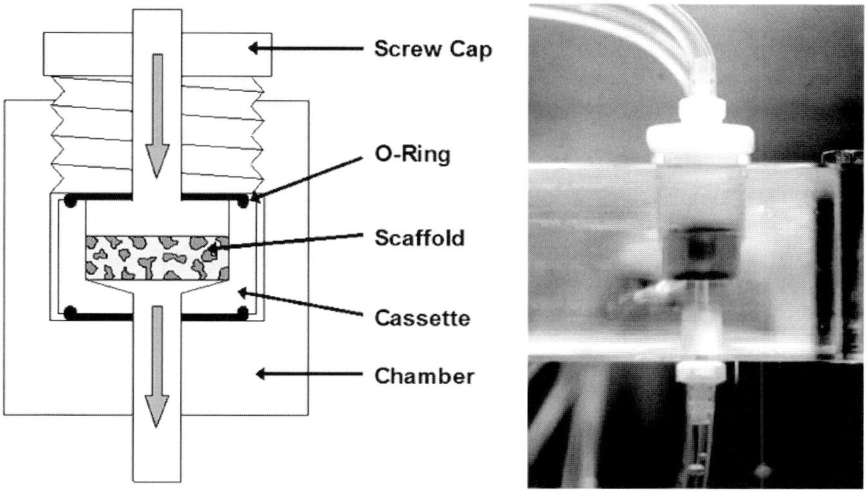

Fig. 1. The flow perfusion chamber used for both seeding and culture of PLLA functionalized porous scaffolds for bone tissue engineering in Alvarez-Baretto *et al.* [102]. Adapted from [48].

3.3. *Cartilage*

Cartilage is a complex tissue characterized by its high water content, its resistance to pressure, and its ability to withstand repetitive compressive and shear loading. These qualities are attributed to its unique extracellular matrix (ECM), composed of primarily collagen and proteoglycans, allowing the material to remain saturated with water and dissolved ions. It has limited capabilities for regeneration *in vivo*, so this tissue requires special considerations when attempting to regenerate it *in vitro*. Mechanical stimulation of cartilage tissue engineered constructs is known to effect the metabolic activity of the chondrocytes as well as result in an improved biochemical composition of the constructs when compared to nonloaded, static constructs [117, 118]. This occurs through the physical deformation of the matrix transferring to the encapsulated cells, which respond due to a process called mechanotransduction. With appropriate strain or shear load and frequency, this response can be elicited to improve chodrocytic or progenitor cell differentiation and phenotype expression, resulting in improved matrix components and structural integrity. Angele *et al.*

explored this using a composite hyaluronan-gelatin composite sponge to culture human mesenchymal progenitor cells under cyclic mechanical compression [119]. The scaffold material had been developed to include derivatized hyaluronan, which could provide matrix stability as well as encourage chondrogenic differentiation, with gelatin, shown to improve cell attachment, differentiation, and proliferation *in vitro* [120]. These scaffolds were shown to induce chondrogenic differentiation of mesenchymal progenitor cells with TGF-β1 included in the culture medium, evidenced by the composites showing extensive extracellular matrix with cartilage-like morphology which stained positive for type II collagen. This material was later cultured under uniaxial, unconfined sinusoidal compressive loading at 0.33 Hz and a peak stress of 7994 Pa for a period of 4 hours/day for the first 7 days of culture for samples harvested at 1, 7, 14, or 21 days. The chondrogenic markers for type II collagen, aggrecan, and type I collagen were all upregulated for all time points when compared to non-loaded controls, and DNA content and type X collagen expression was consistent between the loaded and non-loaded groups. The expression for the loaded samples versus the non-loaded samples was the highest at 14 days of culture, at +386% for aggrecan, +221% for type I collagen, and +687% for type II collagen. The loaded samples showed a significant increase in proteoglycan content after 21 days of culture, but not at the earlier time points. The authors concluded that an appropriate load enhanced the chondrogenic differentiation of mesenchymal progenitor cells, which may in turn increase the formation of an appropriate matrix, resulting in a construct with both biochemical and mechanical stability.

Compressive strain was also investigated by Appelman *et al.* using scaffolds which incorporated both poly(ethylene glycol) (PEG) and bioactive molecules to combine a hydrated hydrogel structure with direct cell-attachment sites for enhanced chondrogenic differentiation and exploration of the effects of combined mechanical and chemical stimuli [121]. Four groups of scaffold material were used: PEG-Fibrinogen, PEG-Albumin, PEG-Proteoglycan, and PEG only control. Fibrinogen and albumin conjugated materials had been previously characterized [122,123], but the PEG-Proteoglycan material prepared using Michael-type addition is novel for cartilage tissue engineering. Since proteoglycans make up 25-35% of the dry weight of articular cartilage, and contribute strongly to chondrocyte-matrix interactions *in vivo*, they were chosen to explore the effects of both biochemical signaling with mechanical stimulation. The authors encapsulated cells in the different gels then used a pneumatic bioreactor system with pistons which directly applied a maximum 15%

compressive strain to the samples. The constructs were stimulated 3 times each day for 1 hour on and 2 hours off at 1 Hz with constant media perfusion. The authors found that although the compressive modulus of all materials decreased with time, the stimulated constructs showed up to 45.4% higher moduli (occurred in the PEG-Fibronectin material) than the unstimulated controls. The authors concluded that both the molecular composition and architecture of a scaffold influences the mechanotransduction of chondrocytes under compressive strain, and that, as determined by the compressive modulus of the different groups, the mechanical stimulation improved the chondrocyte ECM production. Also, as the different bioactive molecules performed differently in mechanical testing, they also believe there to be a correlation between cell adhesion points on a scaffold and enhanced mechanotransduction.

A simpler, and therefore less susceptible to contamination, option for dynamic cell culture remains the spinner flask. It is especially useful to help distribute cells throughout a novel material to gauge cell attachment and viability. Chang *et al.* employed this dynamic cell culture method on a new tri-copolymer designed to incorporate biomimetic signals for cell attachment while being a degradable substrate [124]. The components gelatin, chondroitin-6-sulfate, and hyaluronan were combined in ratios similar to that seen in hyaline cartilage. Adult porcine chondrocytes were injected into the constructs, and then cultured in a spinner flask or Petri dishes for 2, 3, 4, and 5 weeks. An initial higher shear rate was used in order to more evenly distribute the cells within the construct, and the distribution of chondrocytes was found to be more homogenous in constructs cultured in the spinner flask than in the Petri dishes. In addition, the authors found the tri-copolymer supported chondrocyte ECM production, as evidenced by staining of the new matrix, and by polarized imaging collagen fibers with an organized structure, distinct from the amorphous gelatin of the scaffold. Also, immunohistochemical staining supported the presence of S-100 protein and type II collagen, which implies the retention of the chondrogenic phenotype.

The spinner flask can also be used to accommodate dynamic cell culture in a microsphere aggregation system. This system has been especially utilized with functionalized materials designed for cartilage by Hunt *et al.*, investigating both moieties to improve cell attachment as well as time release of growth factors [125,126]. These systems incorporate microspheres, a growth system which affords large surface area, which can lead to more rapid cell expansion and higher overall cell numbers than traditional culture. In addition, the use of flow intermittency allows cultured microspheres to aggregate, creating constructs which have cell density throughout. Furthermore, microcarrier expansion of chondrocytes promotes redifferentiation of cells to the functional phenotype [127]. The RGD motif (in the peptide GRGDSPK) can be cross-linked to the surface of PLLA microspheres [126], and TGF-β1 can be incorporated by a water/oil/water (W/O/W) double-emulsion, solvent extraction method. When cultured in a commercially available pendulum stirred-type spinner flask at 50 rpm for 5 minutes in flow and 15 minutes in stasis, human chondrosarcoma cell line OUMS-27 cells proliferated and aggregated on the microspheres. The size of the aggregates grew progressively over 14 days for all microcarrier types, polystyrene control, PLLA + RGD, PLLA + TGF-β1, and PLLA plain. The incorporation of the RGD motif increased aggregate size after 7 days, most likely due to increased cell attachment to the surface of the microcarriers. The release of TGF-β1 also increased aggregate size after 7 days of culture, and it also increased sulfated GAG production the most between 7 and 14 days of culture. Both bioactive molecule incorporations resulted in increased cell attachment, with the added benefit that the PLLA scaffold would degrade with time, leaving only new tissue. Cartilage is a multi-faceted, highly-functional tissue featuring a very specialized architecture, especially for articular cartilage, which can best be engineered using both materials which have been functionalized to increase cell attachment and differentiation as well as a dynamic system in which to provide mechanical stimulation and nutrient resources.

3.4. *Ligaments and tendons*

Bioreactors for the use of mechanical stimulation have long been utilized for ligament tissue engineering due to the beneficial effect strain can have on the cellular phenotype [128]. In addition, growth factors can have a profound effect upon the function of cells, notably basic fibroblast growth factor (bFGF) and growth and differentiation factor 5 (GDF-5) along with others for ligament and tendon tissue applications [129, 130, 131]. The McAllister *et al.* group has created a 95% porous polycaprolactone (PCL) scaffold which provides an initial burst release of growth factor followed by lower dose release. This scaffold is coated with a combination solution of collagen and the growth factor of interest and allowed to dry between multiple applications. In Petrigliano *et al.*, bFGF coating was used on the PCL scaffolds for cultures of rat bone marrow stromal cells (BMSC). Scaffolds were subjected to loading of 6% uniaxial cyclical strain at a frequency of 0.125 Hz for 23 hours/day, conditions found to be previously favorable [132,133]. A lower dose (100 ng) of bFGF or uniaxial cyclic strain alone both proved positive mRNA expression over the control (no bFGF, no strain) scaffolds, as measured by collagen types I and III and tenascin-C. The scaffolds which underwent both uniaxial strain culture and initially contained 500 ng of bFGF resulted in the highest expression of collagen types I and III and tenascin-C mRNA. In addition, histology also showed that either the inclusion of bFGF or strain caused BMSCs to elongate, but there was no additive or synergistic effect on cell morphology with the two combined. In Farng *et al.*, GDF-5 was used to determine whether the growth factor and mechanical stimulation would influence cellular differentiation and proliferation on the PCL scaffolds using a mouse bone marrow stromal cell line [134]. Neither mechanical strain nor GDF-5 alone increased cell proliferation, but when combined, cell activity was 1.7 times greater than the untreated (no strain, no GDF-5) controls. However, the combination of GDF-5 and strain only produced an increase in the expression of collagen III mRNA, while the stimuli alone caused collagen I and scleraxis mRNA to also be upregulated. It is clear that chemical signals or mechanical strain alone could aid in the creation of a tissue engineered ligament construct, but there is still potential for optimization of the combination of both stimuli.

To enhance initial cell-matrix interactions with a ligament scaffold, Chen *et al.* modified a silk fibroin material with the RGD peptide [135]. The silk protein material, when prepared as a wire-rope matrix, had been characterized as a suitable scaffold for ligament tissue engineering due to its physiologically applicable mechanical properties that can be maintained *in vitro*, and the fact that, after it is implanted, it will degrade slowly [136]. It can be modified by covalent coupling of RGD peptides by activation with 1-ethyl-3-(dimethylaminopropyl) carbodiimide hydrochloride (EDC) and N-hydroxysuccinimide (NHS), followed by incubation with the peptide solution. These scaffolds were cultured in a bioreactor system which provides a suitable environment for construct growth as well as applying mechanical stimulation with both linear and rotational displacement [137]. When cultured with human bone marrow stromal cells (BMSC), the silk matrices exhibited a higher cell density and enhanced cell spreading when modified with the peptide, both 1 hour and 1 day after seeding, but the peptide did not appear to influence cell growth rates from 7 to 14 days of culture. Collagen type I was produced significantly more in RGD-modified matrices after 14 days of culture, and collagen transcription levels at day 7 were elevated on the modified matrices. However, these are not entirely conclusive evidence of the differentiation lineage of the BMSCs, as these are also typical of the fibroblastic phenotype. Overall, the incorporation of a peptide known to enhance cell adhesion and migration seemed to augment the already promising silk fibroin matrix as an option for ligament tissue engineering.

Engineered tendons, similar to ligaments, can display significantly enhanced mechanical and morphological properties when subjected to mechanical loading. The cyclic loading of tendon cells or mesenchymal stem cells, tenocyte progenitors, can cause the cells to align with the strain axis on a construct and result in higher construct stiffness. Tensile strain has been studied on a variety of materials, ranging from collagen gels to decellularized biological scaffolds, such as small intestine submucosa (SIS) and human umbilical vein (HUV) constructs, as well as silk and synthetic materials [138, 139, 140, 141,142]. However, it is clear that multiple variables relating to the mechanical stimulation, frequency, strain amplitude, duration, and daily cycle number, can all influence the characteristics of the final construct [143,144]. Functionalization of a scaffold material has been shown to be possible by Kardestuncer *et al.* by tethering the popular RGD motif to silk in order to augment the tendon-bone interface to promote both adhesion of tenocytes and mineralization [145]. It is possible that future endeavors with tendon tissue engineering will involve both mechanical stimulation and also hybrid scaffolding materials to promote mechanical integrity and cell adhesion, proliferation, and matrix synthesis.

3.5. *Hepatic tissue*

Dynamic cell culture is especially relevant to hepatocyte culture, as they are a cell type characterized by high metabolism and so need a constant nutrient and oxygen source to maintain viability and phenotype stability [146, 147]. Tsang *et al.* explored the use of fluid perfusion through a photopatterned hydrogel with encapsulated hepatocytes [148]. The adhesive RGDS peptide was incorportated into a PEG hydrogel after the screening of multiple adhesive peptides. Hepatocytes, RGDS, and the PEGDA crosslinking oligomer were photopatterened in a triple layered construct which allowed media perfusion through its fluidic channels. When placed in a previously designed perfusion circuit at a flow rate of 0.5 mL/min, viable cells were visible through all three layers at days 1 and 3 [149]. Longer cultures were allowed, up to 12 days, to investigate albumin and urea synthesis, markers of metabolic function in the liver. The dynamically cultured constructs produced higher levels of albumin and urea than flat, unpatterned constructs with the same cell density. In addition, the hydrogels containing 20 μmol/mL RGDS demonstrated 5 fold higher urea and albumin levels than PEG-only controls in a 3 day, static study. This suggests future studies to enable progress toward "organ printing," where combining multilayer photopatterning with optimized cell adhesion and function could result in a viable tissue.

Huang *et al.* also used a rapid-prototyping technique to create a 3-D scaffold with the ability to be cultured in a perfusion bioreactor [150]. Using a fully-automated selective laser sintering (SLS) process, porous, salt-leached polycaprolactone (PCL) tetrahedral scaffolds were created with and without macro-sized flow channels. Then, two different forms of seeding were investigated: avidin-biotin binding and collagen treatment. For the AB method, the Hep G2 cells were treated with the biotin compound and the avidin was allowed to adsorb into the scaffolds for 2 hours, followed by injection of the cell suspension and a centrifugation seeding process [151]. The media perfusion began at a flow rate of 2 mL/min for 2 hours, followed by 5 mL/min for the remainder of the culture period. The initial seeding efficiency was slightly higher using the AB seeding on the 3-D construct, but the remarkable differences occurred at day 9 of culture, when the construct with fluid channels and AB binding showed significantly higher cell numbers. In addition, the constructs with channels and AB binding showed clear advantages in cell function, through glucose consumption and albumin production, over the constructs with no channels and over those treated with collagen adhesion. The monolayer control culture nearly lost the ability to remove ammonium, one of the most important functions for bioartificial liver function. The cells adhered using the AB binding in the perfusion showed a higher detoxification capacity than the other perfusion cultures, but lower than that of a shaking 3-D PCL disk culture. The perfusion culture and the enhanced cell adhesion through avidin-biotin binding both enable the cells to grow and function, showing promise for the development of *in vitro* liver tissues [150].

4. Future Perspectives

It can be concluded that in most cases presented, the combination of a biomimetic material as a scaffold with a physiologically relevant mechanical microenvironment, results in a more functional, homogenous engineered tissue. There are obviously still obstacles for the development of tissue engineered grafts displaying the properties of native tissue, but the field continues to advance to overcome the many complexities inherent in designing a biologically relevant product.

The concentration, distance, and method of functionalization are all important factors when incorporating a biomolecule on a scaffold's surface. Furthermore, these characteristics multiply when more than one biomolecule are introduced. However, just as the native ECM contains many components, it is possible that a variety of biomolecules or bioactive motifs should be immobilized to the material. Moreover, it is concentration gradients which instruct developing organs, and they can also be used to create complex engineered tissues and tissue interfaces [152].

It is possible that in the future bioreactors could also be adapted to combine stimuli to culture hybrid grafts of tissue interfaces. In this way, the organization of the neotissue may more closely resemble the anatomical interface. For example, to create an osteochondral graft consisting of both bony and cartilaginous portions, one cell type could be used: mesenchymal stem cells. Then, the tissue-specific stimulation could cause regions of the construct to grow in apposition to one another. Tissue-specific growth factors would also need to be incorporated, necessitating a complex bioreactor with capabilities for multiple stimuli [153, 154].

Finally, for tissue engineering to become clinically applicable, manufacturing techniques need to be scaled up to accommodate a sterile, rapidly accessible product. This will also involve close communication between bioengineers and the surgeons who perform implantations of the engineered grafts. It should be noted that in many instances, the grafts will be patient specific, whether with cells, composition, size, or shape making the development of industrial-scale processes a challenge that is currently in progress.

The continuation of research incorporating synergistically both chemical and mechanical stimuli by combining functionalized materials with dynamic cell culture systems can only bring us closer to the realization of fully functional engineered grafts. As our understanding of the consequences of each stimulus grows, so can our understanding of how stimuli act in concert to shorten the time of generating an engineered tissue graft.

References

[1] Langer, R. and Vacanti J. P., "Tissue Engineering," *Science*, Vol. 260, No. 5110, 1993, pp. 920-6.

[2] Bonassar, L. J. and Vacanti C. A., "Tissue Engineering: The First Decade and Beyond," *J Cell Biochem Suppl*, Vol. 30-31, No. 1998, pp. 297-303.

[3] Hench, L. L. and Polak J. M., "Third-Generation Biomedical Materials," *Science*, Vol. 295, No. 5557, 2002, pp. 1014-7.

[4] Lutolf, M. P. and Hubbell J. A., "Synthetic Biomaterials as Instructive Extracellular Microenvironments for Morphogenesis in Tissue Engineering," *Nat Biotechnol*, Vol. 23, No. 1, 2005, pp. 47-55.

[5] Shin, H., Jo S. and Mikos A. G., "Biomimetic Materials for Tissue Engineering," *Biomaterials*, Vol. 24, No. 24, 2003, pp. 4353-64.

[6] Martin, I., Wendt D. and Heberer M., "The Role of Bioreactors in Tissue Engineering," *Trends Biotechnol*, Vol. 22, No. 2, 2004, pp. 80-6.

[7] Nerem, R. M., "Cell-Based Therapies: From Basic Biology to Replacement, Repair, and Regeneration," *Biomaterials*, Vol. 28, No. 34, 2007, pp. 5074-7.

[8] Ishaug, S. L., *et al.*, "Bone Formation by Three-Dimensional Stromal Osteoblast Culture in Biodegradable Polymer Scaffolds," *J Biomed Mater Res*, Vol. 36, No. 1, 1997, pp. 17-28.

[9] Sikavitsas, V. I., Bancroft G. N. and Mikos A. G., "Formation of Three-Dimensional Cell/Polymer Constructs for Bone Tissue Engineering in a Spinner Flask and a Rotating Wall Vessel Bioreactor," *J Biomed Mater Res*, Vol. 62, No. 1, 2002, pp. 136-148.

[10] Botchwey, E. A., *et al.*, "Tissue Engineered Bone: Measurement of Nutrient Transport in Three-Dimensional Matrices," *J Biomed Mater Res A*, Vol. 67A, No. 1, 2003, pp. 357-367.

[11] Goldstein, A. S., *et al.*, "Effect of Convection on Osteoblastic Cell Growth and Function in Biodegradable Polymer Foam Scaffolds," *Biomaterials*, Vol. 22, No. 11, 2001, pp. 1279-88.

[12] Gooch, K. J., *et al.*, "Effects of Mixing Intensity on Tissue-Engineered Cartilage," *Biotechnol Bioeng*, Vol. 72, No. 4, 2001, pp. 402-7.

[13] Gordana Vunjak-Novakovic, L. E. F., Robert J. Biron, Robert Langer,, "Effects of Mixing on the Composition and Morphology of Tissue-Engineered Cartilage," *AIChE J*, Vol. 42, No. 3, 1996, pp. 850-860.

[14] Sutherland, R. M., *et al.*, "Oxygenation and Differentiation in Multicellular Spheroids of Human Colon Carcinoma," *Cancer Res*, Vol. 46, No. 10, 1986, pp. 5320-9.

[15] Holy, C. E., Shoichet M. S. and Davies J. E., "Engineering Three-Dimensional Bone Tissue in Vitro Using Biodegradable Scaffolds: Investigating Initial Cell-Seeding Density and Culture Period," *J Biomed Mater Res*, Vol. 51, No. 3, 2000, pp. 376-82.

[16] Kim, B. S., *et al.*, "Optimizing Seeding and Culture Methods to Engineer Smooth Muscle Tissue on Biodegradable Polymer Matrices," *Biotechnol Bioeng*, Vol. 57, No. 1, 1998, pp. 46-54.

[17] Weinand, C., *et al.*, "Conditions Affecting Cell Seeding onto Three-Dimensional Scaffolds for Cellular-Based Biodegradable Implants," *J Biomed Mater Res B: App Biomat*, Epub Apr 2009.

[18] Li, Y., *et al.*, "Effects of Filtration Seeding on Cell Density, Spatial Distribution, and Proliferation in Nonwoven Fibrous Matrices," *Biotechnol Prog*, Vol. 17, No. 5, 2001, pp. 935-44.

[19] Wendt, D., *et al.*, "Oscillating Perfusion of Cell Suspensions through Three-Dimensional Scaffolds Enhances Cell Seeding Efficiency and Uniformity," *Biotechnol Bioeng*, Vol. 84, No. 2, 2003, pp. 205-14.

[20] Alvarez-Barreto, J. F., *et al.*, "Flow Perfusion Improves Seeding of Tissue Engineering Scaffolds with Different Architectures," *Ann Biomed Eng*, Vol. 35, No. 3, 2007, pp. 429-42.

[21] Du, D., Furukawa K. and Ushida T., "Oscillatory Perfusion Seeding and Culturing of Osteoblast-Like Cells on Porous Beta-Tricalcium Phosphate Scaffolds," *J Biomed Mater Res A*, Vol. 86A, No. 3, 2008, pp. 796-803.

[22] Alvarez-Barreto, J. F. and Sikavitsas V. I., "Improved Mesenchymal Stem Cell Seeding on Rgd-Modified Poly(L-Lactic Acid) Scaffolds Using Flow Perfusion," *Macromol Biosci*, Vol. 7, No. 5, 2007, pp. 579-88.

[23] Butler, D. L., Goldstein S. A. and Guilak F., "Functional Tissue Engineering: The Role of Biomechanics," *J Biomech Eng*, Vol. 122, No. 6, 2000, pp. 570-5.

[24] Bonassar, L. J. and Vacanti C. A., "Tissue Engineering: The First Decade and Beyond," *J Cell Biochem Suppl*, Vol. 30-31, No. 1998, pp. 297-303.

[25] Martin, I., Wendt D. and Heberer M., "The Role of Bioreactors in Tissue Engineering," *Trends Biotechnol*, Vol. 22, No. 2, 2004, pp. 80-6.

[26] Niklason, L. E., *et al.*, "Functional Arteries Grown in Vitro," *Science*, Vol. 284, No. 5413, 1999, pp. 489-93.

[27] Davisson, T., *et al.*, "Static and Dynamic Compression Modulate Matrix Metabolism in Tissue Engineered Cartilage," *J Orthop Res*, Vol. 20, No. 4, 2002, pp. 842-8.

[28] Waldman, S. D., *et al.*, "Effect of Biomechanical Conditioning on Cartilaginous Tissue Formation in Vitro," *J Bone Joint Surg Am*, Vol. 85-A Suppl 2, No. 2003, pp. 101-5.

[29] Mauck, R. L., *et al.*, "Functional Tissue Engineering of Articular Cartilage through Dynamic Loading of Chondrocyte-Seeded Agarose Gels," *J Biomech Eng*, Vol. 122, No. 3, 2000, pp. 252-60.

[30] Garvin, J., *et al.*, "Novel System for Engineering Bioartificial Tendons and Application of Mechanical Load," *Tissue Eng*, Vol. 9, No. 5, 2003, pp. 967-79.

[31] Stehle, J., *et al.*, "Effects of Cyclic Stretching on Anterior Cruciate Ligament-Constructs Fabricated from Human Mscs and Collagen Type I Gels," *J Biomech*, Vol. 39, No. Supplement 1, 2006, pp. S60-S60.

[32] Hillsley, M. V. and Frangos J. A., "Review: Bone Tissue Engineering: The Role of Interstitial Fluid Flow," *Biotech Bioeng*, Vol. 43, No. 7, 1994, pp. 573-581.

[33] Meinel, L., *et al.*, "Bone Tissue Engineering Using Human Mesenchymal Stem Cells: Effects of Scaffold Material and Medium Flow," *Ann Biomed Eng*, Vol. 32, No. 1, 2004, pp. 112-122.

[34] Sikavitsas, V. I., Temenoff J. S. and Mikos A. G., "Biomaterials and Bone Mechanotransduction," *Biomaterials*, Vol. 22, No. 19, 2001, pp. 2581-93.

[35] Elder, B. D. and Athanasiou K. A., "Hydrostatic Pressure in Articular Cartilage Tissue Engineering: From Chondrocytes to Tissue Regeneration," *Tissue Eng Part B Rev*, Vol. 15, No. 1, 2009, pp. 43-53.

[36] Moreau, J. E., *et al.*, "Sequential Biochemical and Mechanical Stimulation in the Development of Tissue-Engineered Ligaments," *Tissue Eng Part A*, Vol. 14, No. 7, 2008, pp. 1161-72.

[37] Singh, H. and Hutmacher D. W., "Bioreactor Studies and Computational Fluid Dynamics," *Adv Biochem Eng Biotechnol*, Vol. 112, No. 2009, pp. 231-49.

[38] Wendt, D., *et al.*, "Bioreactors in Tissue Engineering: Scientific Challenges and Clinical Perspectives," *Adv Biochem Eng Biotechnol*, Vol. 112, No. 2009, pp. 1-27.

[39] Philippe Sucosky, D. F. O., Jason B. Brown, G. Paul Neitzel,, "Fluid Mechanics of a Spinner-Flask Bioreactor," *Biotech Bioeng*, Vol. 85, No. 1, 2004, pp. 34-46.

[40] Wolf DA Schwarz RP, Analysis of gravity-induced particle motion and fluid perfusion flow in the NASA-designed rotating zero-head-space tissue culture vessel. NASA Technical Paper. 3143, 1-12 (1991)

[41] Unsworth, B. R. and Lelkes P. I., "Growing Tissues in Microgravity," *Nat Med*, Vol. 4, No. 8, 1998, pp. 901-7.

[42] Freed, L. E., *et al.*, "Chondrogenesis in a Cell-Polymer-Bioreactor System," *Exp Cell Res*, Vol. 240, No. 1, 1998, pp. 58-65.

[43] Williams, K. A., Saini S. and Wick T. M., "Computational Fluid Dynamics Modeling of Steady-State Momentum and Mass Transport in a Bioreactor for Cartilage Tissue Engineering," *Biotech Prog*, Vol. 18, No. 5, 2002, pp. 951-963.

[44] Begley, C. M. and Kleis S. J., "The Fluid Dynamic and Shear Environment in the Nasa/Jsc Rotating-Wall Perfused-Vessel Bioreactor," *Biotech Bioeng*, Vol. 70, No. 1, 2000, pp. 32-40.

[45] Wurm, M., *et al.*, "Development of a Novel Perfused Rotary Cell Culture System," *Tissue Eng*, Vol. 13, No. 11, 2007, pp. 2761-2768.

[46] Wurm, M., *et al.*, "Introduction of a Novel Prototype Bioartificial Liver Support System Utilizing Small Human Hepatocytes in Rotary Culture," *Tissue Eng Part A*, Vol. 15, No. 5, 2009, pp. 1063-1073.

[47] Cormier, J. T., *et al.*, "Expansion of Undifferentiated Murine Embryonic Stem Cells as Aggregates in Suspension Culture Bioreactors," *Tissue Eng*, Vol. 12, No. 11, 2006, pp. 3233-45.

[48] Bancroft, G. N., Sikavitsas V. I. and Mikos A. G., "Design of a Flow Perfusion Bioreactor System for Bone Tissue-Engineering Applications," *Tissue Eng*, Vol. 9, No. 3, 2003, pp. 549-54.

[49] Xie, Y., *et al.*, "Three-Dimensional Flow Perfusion Culture System for Stem Cell Proliferation inside the Critical-Size Beta-Tricalcium Phosphate Scaffold," *Tissue Eng*, Vol. 12, No. 12, 2006, pp. 3535-43.

[50] Bancroft, G. N., *et al.*, "Fluid Flow Increases Mineralized Matrix Deposition in 3d Perfusion Culture of Marrow Stromal Osteoblasts in a Dose-Dependent Manner," *Proc Natl Acad Sci U S A*, Vol. 99, No. 20, 2002, pp. 12600-5.

[51] Cartmell, S. H., *et al.*, "Effects of Medium Perfusion Rate on Cell-Seeded Three-Dimensional Bone Constructs in Vitro," *Tissue Eng*, Vol. 9, No. 6, 2003, pp. 1197-203.

[52] Sikavitsas, V. I., *et al.*, "Mineralized Matrix Deposition by Marrow Stromal Osteoblasts in 3d Perfusion Culture Increases with Increasing Fluid Shear Forces," *Proc Natl Acad Sci U S A*, Vol. 100, No. 25, 2003, pp. 14683-8.

[53] Riddle, R. C. and Donahue H. J., "From Streaming-Potentials to Shear Stress: 25 Years of Bone Cell Mechanotransduction," *J Orthop Res*, Vol. 27, No. 2, 2009, pp. 143-9.

[54] Schwartz, Z., *et al.*, "Osteoblast Response to Fluid Induced Shear Depends on Substrate Microarchitecture and Varies with Time," *J Biomed Mater Res A*, Vol. 83, No. 1, 2007, pp. 20-32.

[55] Dvir, T., *et al.*, "A Novel Perfusion Bioreactor Providing a Homogenous Milieu for Tissue Regeneration," *Tissue Eng*, Vol. 12, No. 10, 2006, pp. 2843-52.

[56] Pierschbacher, M. D. and Ruoslahti E., "Cell Attachment Activity of Fibronectin Can Be Duplicated by Small Synthetic Fragments of the Molecule," *Nature*, Vol. 309, No. 5963, 1984, pp. 30-3.

[57] Pierschbacher, M. D. and Ruoslahti E., "Variants of the Cell Recognition Site of Fibronectin That Retain Attachment-Promoting Activity," *Proc Natl Acad Sci U S A*, Vol. 81, No. 19, 1984, pp. 5985-8.

[58] Cook, A. D., *et al.*, "Characterization and Development of Rgd-Peptide-Modified Poly(Lactic Acid-Co-Lysine) as an Interactive, Resorbable Biomaterial," *J Biomed Mater Res*, Vol. 35, No. 4, 1997, pp. 513-23.

[59] Garcia, A. J., Ducheyne P. and Boettiger D., "Effect of Surface Reaction Stage on Fibronectin-Mediated Adhesion of Osteoblast-Like Cells to Bioactive Glass," *J Biomed Mater Res*, Vol. 40, No. 1, 1998, pp. 48-56.

[60] Rezania, A. and Healy K. E., "The Effect of Peptide Surface Density on Mineralization of a Matrix Deposited by Osteogenic Cells," *J Biomed Mater Res*, Vol. 52, No. 4, 2000, pp. 595-600.

[61] Kurihara, H. and Nagamune T., "Cell Adhesion Ability of Artificial Extracellular Matrix Proteins Containing a Long Repetitive Arg-Gly-Asp Sequence," *J Biosci Bioeng*, Vol. 100, No. 1, 2005, pp. 82-7.
[62] Jung, H. J., *et al.*, "Effect of Rgd-Immobilized Dual-Pore Poly(L-Lactic Acid) Scaffolds on Chondrocyte Proliferation and Extracellular Matrix Production," *Artif Organs*, Vol. 32, No. 12, 2008, pp. 981-9.
[63] Sawyer, A. A., Hennessy K. M. and Bellis S. L., "Regulation of Mesenchymal Stem Cell Attachment and Spreading on Hydroxyapatite by Rgd Peptides and Adsorbed Serum Proteins," *Biomaterials*, Vol. 26, No. 13, 2005, pp. 1467-75.
[64] Zhu, J., *et al.*, "Design and Synthesis of Biomimetic Hydrogel Scaffolds with Controlled Organization of Cyclic Rgd Peptides," *Bioconjug Chem*, Vol. 20, No. 2, 2009, pp. 333-9.
[65] Barron, V., *et al.*, "Bioreactors for Cardiovascular Cell and Tissue Growth: A Review," *Ann Biomed Eng*, Vol. 31, No. 9, 2003, pp. 1017-30.
[66] Ratcliffe, A. and Niklason L. E., "Bioreactors and Bioprocessing for Tissue Engineering," *Ann N Y Acad Sci*, Vol. 961, No. 2002, pp. 210-5.
[67] Williams, C. and Wick T. M., "Perfusion Bioreactor for Small Diameter Tissue-Engineered Arteries," *Tissue Eng*, Vol. 10, No. 5-6, 2004, pp. 930-41.
[68] Cummings, C. L., *et al.*, "Properties of Engineered Vascular Constructs Made from Collagen, Fibrin, and Collagen-Fibrin Mixtures," *Biomaterials*, Vol. 25, No. 17, 2004, pp. 3699-706.
[69] Seliktar, D., *et al.*, "Dynamic Mechanical Conditioning of Collagen-Gel Blood Vessel Constructs Induces Remodeling in Vitro," *Ann Biomed Eng*, Vol. 28, No. 4, 2000, pp. 351-62.
[70] Jeong, S. I., *et al.*, "Tissue-Engineered Vascular Grafts Composed of Marine Collagen and Plga Fibers Using Pulsatile Perfusion Bioreactors," *Biomaterials*, Vol. 28, No. 6, 2007, pp. 1115-22.
[71] Dartsch, P. C. and Hammerle H., "Orientation Response of Arterial Smooth Muscle Cells to Mechanical Stimulation," *Eur J Cell Biol*, Vol. 41, No. 2, 1986, pp. 339-46.
[72] Tillman, B. W., *et al.*, "The in Vivo Stability of Electrospun Polycaprolactone-Collagen Scaffolds in Vascular Reconstruction," *Biomaterials*, Vol. 30, No. 4, 2009, pp. 583-8.
[73] Zhang, X., *et al.*, "Dynamic Culture Conditions to Generate Silk-Based Tissue-Engineered Vascular Grafts," *Biomaterials*, Vol. 30, No. 19, 2009, pp. 3213-23.
[74] Stegemann, J. P. and Nerem R. M., "Phenotype Modulation in Vascular Tissue Engineering Using Biochemical and Mechanical Stimulation," *Ann Biomed Eng*, Vol. 31, No. 4, 2003, pp. 391-402.
[75] Haga, J. H., Li Y. S. and Chien S., "Molecular Basis of the Effects of Mechanical Stretch on Vascular Smooth Muscle Cells," *J Biomech*, Vol. 40, No. 5, 2007, pp. 947-60.
[76] Lovett, M., *et al.*, "Silk Fibroin Microtubes for Blood Vessel Engineering," *Biomaterials*, Vol. 28, No. 35, 2007, pp. 5271-9.
[77] Sofia, S., *et al.*, "Functionalized Silk-Based Biomaterials for Bone Formation," *J Biomed Mater Res*, Vol. 54, No. 1, 2001, pp. 139-48.
[78] Sarkar, S., *et al.*, "Achieving the Ideal Properties for Vascular Bypass Grafts Using a Tissue Engineered Approach: A Review," *Med Biol Eng Comput*, Vol. 45, No. 4, 2007, pp. 327-36.
[79] Rodenberg, E. J. and Pavalko F. M., "Peptides Derived from Fibronectin Type Iii Connecting Segments Promote Endothelial Cell Adhesion but Not Platelet Adhesion: Implications in Tissue-Engineered Vascular Grafts," *Tissue Eng*, Vol. 13, No. 11, 2007, pp. 2653-66.
[80] Mendelson, K. and Schoen F., "Heart Valve Tissue Engineering: Concepts, Approaches, Progress, and Challenges," *Ann Biomed Eng*, Vol. 34, No. 12, 2006, pp. 1799-1819.

[81] Sodian, R., *et al.*, "Tissue Engineering of Heart Valves: In Vitro Experiences," *Ann Thorac Surg*, Vol. 70, No. 1, 2000, pp. 140-4.
[82] Hoerstrup, S. P., *et al.*, "Functional Living Trileaflet Heart Valves Grown in Vitro," *Circulation*, Vol. 102, No. 19 Suppl 3, 2000, pp. III44-9.
[83] Hoerstrup, S. P., *et al.*, "Tissue Engineering of Functional Trileaflet Heart Valves from Human Marrow Stromal Cells," *Circulation*, Vol. 106, No. 12 Suppl 1, 2002, pp. I143-50.
[84] Dumont, K., *et al.*, "Design of a New Pulsatile Bioreactor for Tissue Engineered Aortic Heart Valve Formation," *Artif Organs*, Vol. 26, No. 8, 2002, pp. 710-4.
[85] Mol, A., *et al.*, "The Relevance of Large Strains in Functional Tissue Engineering of Heart Valves," *Thorac Cardiovasc Surg*, Vol. 51, No. 2, 2003, pp. 78-83.
[86] Huang, S. D., *et al.*, "Synergistic Effect of Fibronectin and Hepatocyte Growth Factor on Stable Cell-Matrix Adhesion, Re-Endothelialization, and Reconstitution in Developing Tissue-Engineered Heart Valves," *Heart Vessels*, Vol. 22, No. 2, 2007, pp. 116-22.
[87] Rahman, S., *et al.*, "Novel Hepatocyte Growth Factor (Hgf) Binding Domains on Fibronectin and Vitronectin Coordinate a Distinct and Amplified Met-Integrin Induced Signalling Pathway in Endothelial Cells," *BMC Cell Biol*, Vol. 6, No. 1, 2005, pp. 8.
[88] Khait, L., *et al.*, "Getting to the Heart of Tissue Engineering," *J Cardiovasc Trans Res*, Vol. 1, No. 1, 2008, pp. 71-84.
[89] Papadaki, M., *et al.*, "Tissue Engineering of Functional Cardiac Muscle: Molecular, Structural, and Electrophysiological Studies," *Am J Physiol Heart Circ Physiol*, Vol. 280, No. 1, 2001, pp. H168-78.
[90] Bursac, N., *et al.*, "Cardiac Muscle Tissue Engineering: Toward an in Vitro Model for Electrophysiological Studies," *Am J Physiol*, Vol. 277, No. 2 Pt 2, 1999, pp. H433-44.
[91] Park, H., *et al.*, "A Novel Composite Scaffold for Cardiac Tissue Engineering," *In Vitro Cell Dev Biol Anim*, Vol. 41, No. 7, 2005, pp. 188-96.
[92] Radisic, M., *et al.*, "High-Density Seeding of Myocyte Cells for Cardiac Tissue Engineering," *Biotechnol Bioeng*, Vol. 82, No. 4, 2003, pp. 403-14.
[93] Radisic, M., *et al.*, "Medium Perfusion Enables Engineering of Compact and Contractile Cardiac Tissue," *Am J Physiol Heart Circ Physiol*, Vol. 286, No. 2, 2004, pp. H507-16.
[94] Jabbari, E., *et al.*, "Material Properties and Bone Marrow Stromal Cells Response to in Situ Crosslinkable Rgd-Functionlized Lactide-Co-Glycolide Scaffolds," *J Biomed Mater Res A*, Vol. 89, No. 1, 2009, pp. 124-37.
[95] Liu, X. and Ma P. X., "Polymeric Scaffolds for Bone Tissue Engineering," *Ann Biomed Eng*, Vol. 32, No. 3, 2004, pp. 477-86.
[96] Jagur-Grodzinski, J., "Polymers for Tissue Engineering, Medical Devices, and Regenerative Medicine. Concise General Review of Recent Studies," *Polymers for Advanced Technologies*, Vol. 17, No. 6, 2006, pp. 395-418.
[97] Abousleiman, R. I. and Sikavitsas V. I., "Bioreactors for Tissues of the Musculoskeletal System," *Adv Exp Med Biol*, Vol. 585, No. 2006, pp. 243-59.
[98] Bokhari, M. A., *et al.*, "The Enhancement of Osteoblast Growth and Differentiation in Vitro on a Peptide Hydrogel-Polyhipe Polymer Hybrid Material," *Biomaterials*, Vol. 26, No. 25, 2005, pp. 5198-208.
[99] Zhang, S., *et al.*, "Self-Complementary Oligopeptide Matrices Support Mammalian Cell Attachment," *Biomaterials*, Vol. 16, No. 18, 1995, pp. 1385-93.
[100] Roeker, S., *et al.*, "A Study on the Influence of Biocompatible Composites with Bioactive Ligands toward Their Effect on Cell Adhesion and Growth for the Application in Bone Tissue Engineering," *J Biomed Mater Res B: App Biomater*, Epub April 2009, ahead of print.

[101] von Walter, M., *et al.*, "In Vitro Behavior of a Porous Tio2/Perlite Composite and Its Surface Modification with Fibronectin," *Biomaterials*, Vol. 26, No. 16, 2005, pp. 2813-2826.

[102] Alvarez-Barreto, J. F., *et al.*, "Enhanced Osteoblastic Differentiation of Mesenchymal Stem Cells Seeded in RGD Functionalized PLLA Scaffolds and Cultured in a Flow Perfusion Bioreactor," submitted for publication 2009.

[103] Alvarez-Barreto, J. F., *et al.*, "Preparation of a Functionally Flexible, Three-Dimensional, Biomimetic Poly(L-Lactic Acid) Scaffold with Improved Cell Adhesion," *Tissue Eng*, Vol. 13, No. 6, 2007, pp. 1205-17.

[104] Gomes, M. E., *et al.*, "Influence of the Porosity of Starch-Based Fiber Mesh Scaffolds on the Proliferation and Osteogenic Differentiation of Bone Marrow Stromal Cells Cultured in a Flow Perfusion Bioreactor," *Tissue Eng*, Vol. 12, No. 4, 2006, pp. 801-9.

[105] Datta, N., *et al.*, "In Vitro Generated Extracellular Matrix and Fluid Shear Stress Synergistically Enhance 3d Osteoblastic Differentiation," *Proc Natl Acad Sci U S A*, Vol. 103, No. 8, 2006, pp. 2488-93.

[106] Holtorf, H. L., Jansen J. A. and Mikos A. G., "Flow Perfusion Culture Induces the Osteoblastic Differentiation of Marrow Stromal Cell-Scaffold Constructs in the Absence of Dexamethasone," *J Biomed Mater Res A*, Vol. 72A, No. 3, 2005, pp. 326-334.

[107] Gomes, M. E., *et al.*, "Effect of Flow Perfusion on the Osteogenic Differentiation of Bone Marrow Stromal Cells Cultured on Starch-Based Three-Dimensional Scaffolds," *J Biomed Mater Res A*, Vol. 67A, No. 1, 2003, pp. 87-95.

[108] Gomes, M. E., *et al.*, "In Vitro Localization of Bone Growth Factors in Constructs of Biodegradable Scaffolds Seeded with Marrow Stromal Cells and Cultured in a Flow Perfusion Bioreactor," *Tissue Eng*, Vol. 12, No. 1, 2006, pp. 177-88.

[109] Pham, Q. P., *et al.*, "Analysis of the Osteoinductive Capacity and Angiogenicity of an *in vitro* Generated Extracellular Matrix," *J Biomed Mater Res A*, Vol. 88A, No. 2, 2009, pp. 295-303.

[110] Sikavitsas, V. I., *et al.*, "Influence of the *in Vitro* Culture Period on the *in Vivo* Performance of Cell/Titanium Bone Tissue-Engineered Constructs Using a Rat Cranial Critical Size Defect Model," *J Biomed Mater Res A*, Vol. 67A, No. 3, 2003, pp. 944-951.

[111] van den Dolder, J., *et al.*, "Flow Perfusion Culture of Marrow Stromal Osteoblasts in Titanium Fiber Mesh," *J Biomed Mater Res Part A*, Vol. 64A, No. 2, 2003, pp. 235-241.

[112] Sikavitsas, V. I., *et al.*, "Flow Perfusion Enhances the Calcified Matrix Deposition of Marrow Stromal Cells in Biodegradable Nonwoven Fiber Mesh Scaffolds," *Ann Biomed Eng*, Vol. 33, No. 1, 2005, pp. 63-70.

[113] Comisar, W. A., *et al.*, "Engineering Rgd Nanopatterned Hydrogels to Control Preosteoblast Behavior: A Combined Computational and Experimental Approach," *Biomaterials*, Vol. 28, No. 30, 2007, pp. 4409-17.

[114] Hosseinkhani, H., *et al.*, "Osteogenic Differentiation of Mesenchymal Stem Cells in Self-Assembled Peptide-Amphiphile Nanofibers," *Biomaterials*, Vol. 27, No. 22, 2006, pp. 4079-86.

[115] Yang, F., *et al.*, "The Effect of Incorporating Rgd Adhesive Peptide in Polyethylene Glycol Diacrylate Hydrogel on Osteogenesis of Bone Marrow Stromal Cells," *Biomaterials*, Vol. 26, No. 30, 2005, pp. 5991-8.

[116] Holtorf, H. L., Jansen J. A. and Mikos A. G., "Ectopic Bone Formation in Rat Marrow Stromal Cell/Titanium Fiber Mesh Scaffold Constructs: Effect of Initial Cell Phenotype," *Biomaterials*, Vol. 26, No. 31, 2005, pp. 6208-16.

[117] Gemmiti, C. V. and Guldberg R. E., "Fluid Flow Increases Type Ii Collagen Deposition and Tensile Mechanical Properties in Bioreactor-Grown Tissue-Engineered Cartilage," *Tissue Eng*, Vol. 12, No. 3, 2006, pp. 469-79.

[118] Mauck, R. L., *et al.*, "Influence of Seeding Density and Dynamic Deformational Loading on the Developing Structure/Function Relationships of Chondrocyte-Seeded Agarose Hydrogels," *Ann Biomed Eng*, Vol. 30, No. 8, 2002, pp. 1046-56.

[119] Angele, P., *et al.*, "Cyclic, Mechanical Compression Enhances Chondrogenesis of Mesenchymal Progenitor Cells in Tissue Engineering Scaffolds," *Biorheology*, Vol. 41, No. 3-4, 2004, pp. 335-46.

[120] Angele, P., *et al.*, "Engineering of Osteochondral Tissue with Bone Marrow Mesenchymal Progenitor Cells in a Derivatized Hyaluronan-Gelatin Composite Sponge," *Tissue Eng*, Vol. 5, No. 6, 1999, pp. 545-54.

[121] Appelman, T. P., *et al.*, "The Differential Effect of Scaffold Composition and Architecture on Chondrocyte Response to Mechanical Stimulation," *Biomaterials*, Vol. 30, No. 4, 2009, pp. 518-25.

[122] Gonen-Wadmany, M., Oss-Ronen L. and Seliktar D., "Protein-Polymer Conjugates for Forming Photopolymerizable Biomimetic Hydrogels for Tissue Engineering," *Biomaterials*, Vol. 28, No. 26, 2007, pp. 3876-86.

[123] Dikovsky, D., Bianco-Peled H. and Seliktar D., "The Effect of Structural Alterations of Peg-Fibrinogen Hydrogel Scaffolds on 3-D Cellular Morphology and Cellular Migration," *Biomaterials*, Vol. 27, No. 8, 2006, pp. 1496-506.

[124] Chang, C. H., *et al.*, "Gelatin-Chondroitin-Hyaluronan Tri-Copolymer Scaffold for Cartilage Tissue Engineering," *Biomaterials*, Vol. 24, No. 26, 2003, pp. 4853-8.

[125] Curran, S. J., *et al.*, "Expansion of Human Chondrocytes in an Intermittent Stirred Flow Bioreactor, Using Modified Biodegradable Microspheres," *Tissue Eng*, Vol. 11, No. 9-10, 2005, pp. 1312-22.

[126] Chen, R., *et al.*, "The Use of Poly(L-Lactide) and Rgd Modified Microspheres as Cell Carriers in a Flow Intermittency Bioreactor for Tissue Engineering Cartilage," *Biomaterials*, Vol. 27, No. 25, 2006, pp. 4453-60.

[127] Malda, J., *et al.*, "Expansion of Bovine Chondrocytes on Microcarriers Enhances Redifferentiation," *Tissue Eng*, Vol. 9, No. 5, 2003, pp. 939-48.

[128] Skutek, M., *et al.*, "Cyclic Mechanical Stretching Modulates Secretion Pattern of Growth Factors in Human Tendon Fibroblasts," *Eur J Appl Physiol*, Vol. 86, No. 1, 2001, pp. 48-52.

[129] Hankemeier, S., *et al.*, "Modulation of Proliferation and Differentiation of Human Bone Marrow Stromal Cells by Fibroblast Growth Factor 2: Potential Implications for Tissue Engineering of Tendons and Ligaments," *Tissue Eng*, Vol. 11, No. 1-2, 2005, pp. 41-9.

[130] Moreau, J. E., *et al.*, "Growth Factor Induced Fibroblast Differentiation from Human Bone Marrow Stromal Cells in Vitro," *J Orthop Res*, Vol. 23, No. 1, 2005, pp. 164-74.

[131] Wolfman, N. M., *et al.*, "Ectopic Induction of Tendon and Ligament in Rats by Growth and Differentiation Factors 5, 6, and 7, Members of the Tgf-Beta Gene Family," *J Clin Invest*, Vol. 100, No. 2, 1997, pp. 321-30.

[132] Petrigliano, F. A., *et al.*, "The Effects of Local Bfgf Release and Uniaxial Strain on Cellular Adaptation and Gene Expression in a 3d Environment: Implications for Ligament Tissue Engineering," *Tissue Eng*, Vol. 13, No. 11, 2007, pp. 2721-31.

[133] Puk, C. K., *et al.*, "The Effects of Short-Term Stimulation on Fibroblast Spreading in an in Vitro 3d System," *J Biomed Mater Res A*, Vol. 76, No. 4, 2006, pp. 665-73.

[134] Farng, E., *et al.*, "The Effects of Gdf-5 and Uniaxial Strain on Mesenchymal Stem Cells in 3-D Culture," *Clin Orthop Relat Res*, Vol. 466, No. 8, 2008, pp. 1930-7.

[135] Chen, J., *et al.*, "Human Bone Marrow Stromal Cell and Ligament Fibroblast Responses on Rgd-Modified Silk Fibers," *J Biomed Mater Res A*, Vol. 67, No. 2, 2003, pp. 559-70.

[136] Altman, G. H., *et al.*, "Silk Matrix for Tissue Engineered Anterior Cruciate Ligaments," *Biomaterials*, Vol. 23, No. 20, 2002, pp. 4131-41.

[137] Altman, G. H., *et al.*, "Cell Differentiation by Mechanical Stress," *FASEB J*, Vol. 16, No. 2, 2002, pp. 270-2.

[138] Cao, Y., *et al.*, "Generation of Neo-Tendon Using Synthetic Polymers Seeded with Tenocytes," *Transplant Proc*, Vol. 26, No. 6, 1994, pp. 3390-2.

[139] Webb, K., *et al.*, "Cyclic Strain Increases Fibroblast Proliferation, Matrix Accumulation, and Elastic Modulus of Fibroblast-Seeded Polyurethane Constructs," *J Biomech*, Vol. 39, No. 6, 2006, pp. 1136-44.

[140] Androjna, C., Spragg R. K. and Derwin K. A., "Mechanical Conditioning of Cell-Seeded Small Intestine Submucosa: A Potential Tissue-Engineering Strategy for Tendon Repair," *Tissue Eng*, Vol. 13, No. 2, 2007, pp. 233-43.

[141] Butler, D. L., *et al.*, "Functional Tissue Engineering for Tendon Repair: A Multidisciplinary Strategy Using Mesenchymal Stem Cells, Bioscaffolds, and Mechanical Stimulation," *J Orthop Res*, Vol. 26, No. 1, 2008, pp. 1-9.

[142] Abousleiman, R. I., *et al.*, "Tendon Tissue Engineering Using Cell-Seeded Umbilical Veins Cultured in a Mechanical Stimulator," *Tissue Eng Part A*, Vol. 15, No. 4, 2009, pp. 787-95.

[143] Feng, Z., *et al.*, "Construction of Fibroblast-Collagen Gels with Orientated Fibrils Induced by Static or Dynamic Stress: Toward the Fabrication of Small Tendon Grafts," *J Artif Organs*, Vol. 9, No. 4, 2006, pp. 220-5.

[144] Joshi, S. D. and Webb K., "Variation of Cyclic Strain Parameters Regulates Development of Elastic Modulus in Fibroblast/Substrate Constructs," *J Orthop Res*, Vol. 26, No. 8, 2008, pp. 1105-13.

[145] Kardestuncer, T., *et al.*, "Rgd-Tethered Silk Substrate Stimulates the Differentiation of Human Tendon Cells," *Clin Orthop Relat Res*, Vol. 448, No. 2006, pp. 234-9.

[146] Balis, U. J., *et al.*, "Oxygen Consumption Characteristics of Porcine Hepatocytes," *Metab Eng*, Vol. 1, No. 1, 1999, pp. 49-62.

[147] Catapano, G., *et al.*, "The Effect of Oxygen Transport Resistances on the Viability and Functions of Isolated Rat Hepatocytes," *Int J Artif Organs*, Vol. 19, No. 1, 1996, pp. 61-71.

[148] Tsang, V. L., *et al.*, "Fabrication of 3d Hepatic Tissues by Additive Photopatterning of Cellular Hydrogels," *FASEB J.*, Vol. 21, No. 3, 2007, pp. 790-801.

[149] Allen, J. W. and Bhatia S. N., "Formation of Steady-State Oxygen Gradients in Vitro: Application to Liver Zonation," *Biotechnol Bioeng*, Vol. 82, No. 3, 2003, pp. 253-62.

[150] Huang, H., *et al.*, "Avidin-Biotin Binding-Based Cell Seeding and Perfusion Culture of Liver-Derived Cells in a Porous Scaffold with a Three-Dimensional Interconnected Flow-Channel Network," *Biomaterials*, Vol. 28, No. 26, 2007, pp. 3815-23.

[151] Kojima, N., Matsuo T. and Sakai Y., "Rapid Hepatic Cell Attachment onto Biodegradable Polymer Surfaces without Toxicity Using an Avidin-Biotin Binding System," *Biomaterials*, Vol. 27, No. 28, 2006, pp. 4904-10.

[152] Singh, M., Berkland C. and Detamore M. S., "Strategies and Applications for Incorporating Physical and Chemical Signal Gradients in Tissue Engineering," *Tissue Eng Part B Rev*, Vol. 14, No. 4, 2008, pp. 341-66.

[153] Grayson, W. L., *et al.*, "Engineering Custom-Designed Osteochondral Tissue Grafts," *Trends Biotechnol*, Vol. 26, No. 4, 2008, pp. 181-9.

[154] Burdick, J. A. and Vunjak-Novakovic G., "Engineered Microenvironments for Controlled Stem Cell Differentiation," *Tissue Eng Part A*, Vol. 15, No. 2, 2009, pp. 205-219.

SUBJECT INDEX